John O'Donel Alexander

Arthropods and Human Skin

Foreword by Arthur Rook

With 256 Figures and 115 Tables

Springer-Verlag
Berlin Heidelberg New York Tokyo 1984

John O'Donel Alexander, MB, ChB, FRCP (Glasgow)
Emeritus Consultant Dermatologist, Glasgow Royal Infirmary and Lately Honorary Clinical Lecturer in Dermatology, University of Glasgow

ISBN-13: 978-1-4471-1358-4 Springer-Verlag Berlin Heidelberg New York Tokyo

Library of Congress Cataloging in Publication Data
Alexander, John O'Donel
Arthropods and human skin.
Bibliography: p. Includes index.
1. Skin—Inflammation. 2. Bites and stings. 3. Arthropoda, Poisonous. I. Title. [DNLM: 1. Arthropods. 2. Ectoparasitic Infestations. 3. Bites and Stings. 4. Skin Diseases—diagnosis. WR 360 A434a] RL231.A44 1984 616.9'68 84-5571
ISBN-13: 978-1-4471-1358-4 e-ISBN-13: 978-1-4471-1356-0
DOI: 10.1007/978-1-4471-1356-0

Softcover reprint of the hardcover 1st edition 1984

Filmset by Polyglot Pte Ltd
Printed by William Clowes Limited, Beccles, Suffolk

2128/3916 543210

Foreword

To the entomologist all insects have six legs; the layman tends to use the term "insect" to include the eight-legged spiders and mites. All these creatures are correctly classified as arthropods. Many thousands of the hundreds of thousands of recognised species of arthropods are found in the human environment—domestic, occupational and recreational. Those species which are obligate parasites of man, the human scabies mite and the head and body lice, produce familiar clinical syndromes. They remain important in medical practice and have been the subject of a great deal of recent research. This is beginning to throw much light on the immunological mechanisms which largely determine the reactions of the host. Dr. Alexander has provided a detailed survey of this work.

The wasps, bees, ants and other Hymenoptera which may sting man in self-defence can cause painful, even fatal reactions. The recent work on this important subject has also been thoroughly reviewed.

Every dermatologist of experience will admit that he sees many patients in whom he makes a diagnosis of "insect bites", if he has the confidence to do so, or of "papular urticaria" or "prurigo" when he lacks such confidence, mainly because he is at a loss to know which arthropod is likely to be implicated. In his survey of the enormous literature in the entomological, public health and dermatology journals Dr. Alexander has provided an invaluable guide in which the solutions to these clinical mysteries can be sought.

This book will be indispensable for the dermatologist in practice and for those concerned with environmental health.

Addenbrookes Hospital, Cambridge, 1984 Arthur Rook

Preface

Ever since I began practising Dermatology, some 40 years ago, I have felt the need for good reference books. Clinical experience is an excellent teacher, especially with the competitive stimulus of working alongside others of equal experience with differing interpretation of findings, but reference sources of quality are still very necessary when trying to elucidate the problems of the common as well the lesser known dermatoses.

Ebeling, in his book *Urban Entomology*, has remarked that millions of individuals are stung by venomous arthropods each year and many thousands are seriously upset. Such large numbers cannot be ignored, yet many of those disorders associated with arthropods are often no more than a name in an index, and even the scantiest of details are lacking in all but the biggest dermatological textbooks. This is not really surprising because Dermatology is such a vast subject, and even in the largest tomes only a limited space can be devoted to the effects of arthropods.

From the clinical point of view many arthropods cause only minor lesions in some patients. Diseases which do not endanger a patient's life are frequently ignored, but there is no doubt that even trivial lesions can assume a serious aspect if they are very numerous. Even the humble flea can make life intolerable for long periods of time. Many a fisherman has had his day's sport or even his whole holiday ruined by the attentions of the black fly, *Simulium*. On the other hand, whilst the clinical features of the disorders of the skin caused by arthropods form the basic theme of this book, it must not be forgotten that many arthropods, apart from being the vectors of disease-producing bacteria, viruses, rickettsiae or protozoa, can cause serious, even fatal reactions in their own right (e.g. bees, wasps, some spiders, scorpions). It is important that those dealing with skin disorders should be fully aware of the nature of such severe reactions, especially if they are dealing with an unexpected infestation such as, for example, lepidopterism.

Some arthropod-induced disorders are normally important only in certain areas. For example, necrotic arachnidism does not occur in Europe and has only been recognised as occurring in North America relatively recently; yet it has been a well-known hazard in several South American countries for a long time. Similarly myiasis in one form or another is well known in some regions and not at all in others. Such disorders, however, are now beginning to assume greater importance for dermatologists in areas where they do not usually occur because of the enormous increase in worldwide air travel. Persons returning from holidays or business trips in tropical countries may present with skin disorders of arthropod origin unknown in their home locality but common enough in the area they have been visiting. The lesions may seem quite bizarre to their regular medical attendant or his specialist colleague.

Knowledge of the clinical appearance, history and mode of onset of these arthropod-induced skin lesions in obviously of primary importance, but a sound general acquaintance with the appearance, biology and habits of the creatures themselves is equally valuable. It makes for a much better understanding of the skin eruptions, improves the likelihood of the correct diagnosis being reached and at the same time allows the physician to explain matters to his patient with some real authority. No one would question the value of knowledge of the development and life cycle of the malaria parasite in the management and control of malaria. The same principle is just as relevant in the understanding and management of those skin disorders caused directly or indirectly by arthropods. It is especially applicable to management and was succinctly expressed by Rook when he said, "The efficiency of any measures of disinfestation cannot, except by chance, be greater than the operator's knowledge of the life history and habits of the parasite concerned." A simple example will illustrate this. Head lice live, feed and breed on the scalp, whereas body lice, whilst feeding on the host, live and breed on the host's clothing. The management of infestation by these two parasites is dependent on this knowledge.

This book is intended to answer the problems raised above and to fill the hiatus in textbooks by supplying the necessary clinical, histopathological, immunological, epidemiological and entomological details necessary for a sound understanding of the quite numerous eruptions caused by arthropods on the human skin. For convenience it has been arranged systematically in accordance with the zoological classification of the species concerned. It is felt that having all this information encompassed in one volume, together with an extensive bibliography, will be useful not only to dermatologists and general physicians but also to hospital pathologists and immunologists and to public health authorities. It will be evident from a perusal of the references for each chapter that a great deal of painstaking research has been carried out in the past in the laboratories of parasitologists, entomologists and veterinary workers. It is a pleasure to acknowledge the vital role they have played in elucidating many of the problems in this field and it is hoped that this book may also be of some use to them.

Glasgow, Scotland, 1984 John O'Donel Alexander

Acknowledgements

This book would have been impossible for me to write without help and advice, the acknowledgement of which is indeed a pleasure. The generosity with which my friends and correspondents have responded to requests for assistance has been heart-warming. My special thanks are due to two colleagues. Arthur Rook, in spite of his own heavy writing commitments, most generously read every chapter as it was completed and gave me invaluable advice, particularly as to what had been left out and, perhaps more important, what should have been omitted. He most tactfully curbed my natural tendency to ungrammatical verbosity. Alan Lyell, with whom I have worked for many years as a close clinical colleague, was equally prodigal with his time. He, too, read the entire book, giving much practical advice and criticism and often suggesting lines of thought which I had overlooked. He was responsible for taking a great many pictures of my own and his patients. Both of these colleagues have sustained my efforts right up to the moment of completion of the manuscript and I am most grateful.

My thanks are due to many others for specific assistance including the following:

Dr. B. Heilesen (Copenhagen), Dr. A. M. Hughes (Infestation Control Laboratories, M.A.F.F.), Prof. M. T. James (Washington State University), Prof. M. M. J. Lavoipierre (University of California, Davis), Dr. J. W. Maunder (London School of Hygiene and Tropical Medicine), Dr. R. L. Smiley (Systematic Entomology Laboratory, U.S. Department of Agriculture, Beltsville, Maryland) and Dr. R. V. Southcott (Adelaide, Australia) all gave me unrestricted access to their publications and illustrations.

Prof. A. R. Ahmed (University of California, Los Angeles), Dr. Suzanne Alexander (Consultant Dermatologist, Barking, Essex), Prof. J. T. Baxter [Royal (Dick) School of Veterinary Studies, University of Edinburgh], Dr. T. O. Browning (University of Adelaide, Australia), Dr. Mary Bunney (Consultant Dermatologist, Edinburgh), Dr. J. R. Condy (Harare, Zimbabwe), Dr. D. C. Crosti (Milan), Dr. Vincent Derbes (Tulane University, New Orleans), Dr. W. S. Douglas (Consultant Dermatologist, Monklands General Hospital, Lanarkshire), Prof. A. J. Duggan (Director, Wellcome Museum of Medical Sciences, London), Prof. W. Ebeling (University of California, Los Angeles), Prof. A. Fain (Institute of Tropical Medicine, Antwerp), Dr. A. S. Field (Prince Henry Hospital, Little Bay, New South Wales), Dr. R. A. Fulton (Consultant Dermatologist, Limavady, Northern Ireland), Dr. J. H. Frenken (Amsterdam, now in Andorra), Dr. M. D. Gallagher (Oman Natural History Museum, Sultanate of Oman), Prof. E. M. Grosshans (Strasbourg), Dr. Patrick Hall-Smith (Consultant Dermatologist, Brighton), Prof. F. F. Hellier (University of Leeds), Dr. Harry Hoogstraal (U.S. Naval Medical Research Unit, Cairo), Dr. I. T. Jackson (Mayo Clinic, Rochester, Minnesota), Dr. D. J. Lewis [Hon. Associate of the British Museum (Natural History)], Dr. T. Lewis (Rothamstead Experimental Station, Harpenden), Dr. J. C. P.Logan (Consultant Dermatologist, Stobhill Hospital, Glasgow), Prof. R. N. MacKie (University of Glasgow), Prof. Z. Maretic (Pula, Jugoslavia), Prof. M. J. Marples (Woodstock), Dr. N. Morley (Consultant Dermatologist, Glasgow), Prof. W. B. Nutting (University of Massachusetts), Prof. A. Radford (Flinders University, South Australia), Dr. T. Reunala (Helsinki), Prof. Ney Romiti (Santos, Brazil), Dr. Brian Russell

(Consultant Dermatologist, Saffron Walden, Essex), Dr. A. L. Schroeter (Mayo-Clinic, Rochester, Minnesota), Mr. J. A. Green (Sales Manager, Stafford-Miller Ltd, Hatfield), Dr. H. V. Smith (University of Glasgow), Prof. J. H. Theis (University of California, Davis), Dr. R. N. Titchener (West of Scotland Agricultural College, Auchincruive, Ayrshire), Dr. D. van Neste (Catholic University of Louvain, Belgium), Mr. P. J. Waldie (Dept. of Medical Illustration, Stobhill Hospital, Glasgow), Dr. M. Walkey (Queen Mary College, University of London) and Dr. M. Young (Consultant Dermatologist, Greenock) all supplied or were instrumental in supplying original prints of illustrations from their publications or of hitherto unpublished pictures.

Information on local arthropods, on special subjects, on nomenclature, drugs and historical data were provided by Dr. Harry Arnold (Honolulu), Prof. J. L. Cloudsley-Thomson (Birkbeck College, University of London), Dr. R. M. Dobson Dept. of Zoology, University of Glasgow), Dr. M. S. K. Ghauri (Commonwealth Institute of Entomology), Dr. Elmo Hardy (Hawaii), Prof. Carl Holubar (University of Vienna and Hadasseh University Jerusalem), Prof. K. Mellanby (Monkwood Experimental Station, Huntingdon), Dr. D. MacFarlane (Commonwealth Institute of Entomology, London), Mrs. J. McCabe (Drug Information Centre, Glasgow Royal Infirmary) Prof. M. K. Polano (Zoeller, Netherlands), Mr. Mark Shaw (Dept of Natural History, Royal Scottish Museum, Edinburgh), Dr. F. R. Wanless [British Museum (Natural History)], Ciba-Geigy Pharmaceuticals Division (Horsham, Sussex), Jantzen Pharmaceuticals (Marlow, Bucks), Napp Laboratories (Watford) and Rentokil Ltd (Giffnock, Glasgow). Translations were kindly made by Dr. E. Desselberger (German), Dr. I. Lominska (Polish), Dr. M. Ratzer (Csech) and Mr. M. Goh (Chinese) and I am grateful to all four.

Dr. John Thomson has allowed me freedom of access to the Dermatological slide collection at Glasgow Royal Infirmary, which has been most useful. Mr W. Towler, lately of the Medical Illustration Unit of the University Department of Surgery at Glasgow Royal Infirmary, and latterly Mr. W. Paterson and his staff (Messrs. F. Speirs, W. Burns, T. Ross and Mrs Kelly) have between them produced many black and white prints from negatives, colour prints and colour transparencies, loaned or supplied by many of the persons mentioned above. Their work, which was invaluable, was carried out with meticulous care to ensure the best possible results. Without their cooperation the illustrations could not have been produced and I am very grateful. I have to thank many individuals, Journal editors and publishers for granting me permission to reproduce illustrations from their copyright publications. The sources of these illustrations have been acknowledged in the relevant legends.

The large number of references cited in the bibliography at the end of each chapter has entailed much work for library staff in collecting, tracing and photocopying them. I must thank especially the librarians of the Royal College of Physicians and Surgeons of Glasgow; of Glasgow University; of the British Medical Association; of the Institute of Dertmatology of St. John's Hospital for Diseases of the Skin, London and of the British Library at Boston Spa for their help. Many obscure references were obtained only by continued persistence on their part. The libraries and institutions abroad which furnished material for them are also to be thanked.

The manuscript was typed by Mrs. Anne Dunlop, whose care and accuracy has saved a lot of time and she too is to be thanked.

Michael Jackson of Springer-Verlag came into the picture at a late stage but has been most helpful and encouraging and has smoothed matters of publishing detail in a most knowledgeable and efficient manner. I owe a special debt of gratitude to his sub-editor Mrs. J. Watt of Bristol whose meticulous attention to detail has immeasurably improved the manuscript, correcting accidental contradictions between the script and the references, in many instances ensuring that the latter were absolutely accurate and at the same time contriving to improve phraseology where there was doubt as to the exact meaning. I have also to thank Roger Dobbing for his expertise and advice on the technicalities of publication, the results of which are here for all to see.

Contents

1 Introduction

Much has been made, and rightly so, of the role played by arthropods as vectors of infectious diseases. The physical effects of the arthropods themselves on the human skin receive much less attention. When a person is attacked by an arthropod, regardless of whether an infection is transferred or not, there is of necessity a wound, however trivial, on the skin of the victim. Doctors, especially general practitioners and dermatologists, are frequently confronted by patients whose skin lesions appear to be due to the bite, sting or other activity of some arthropod. The identity of the arthropod responsible may or may not be obvious, but once a diagnosis of "insect bite" has been conveyed to the patient, questions will follow. What sort of creature is responsible? What does it look like? How or why did it attack the patient? What can be done about it? Will it happen again and how can it be avoided? Will it get better? This book is designed to answer these questions.

The diagnosis of an arthropod-induced lesion is often made only in a negative manner by the process of exclusion. This is surprising considering the large number of species which can damage man's skin. It is hoped that the information gathered together here will encourage a more positive attitude.

Several interrelated factors must be taken into account. The clinical lesions can be variable in character. They may be single or multiple, local or generalised. There may sometimes be a diagnostic distribution, but on the other hand the same eruption can be induced by quite different species. The onset may be abrupt or gradual. The attack may be made in the night when the victim is asleep or in the daytime when he or she is at work, at home, caring for pets or even going for a walk.

Histological changes may be diagnostic. Portions of arthropods may be seen in biopsy specimens, whilst others show characteristic cellular infiltration. Immunological reactions play an important role. The changing nature of these reactions with the development of antibodies alters the clinical presentation. In other patients the dominant symptoms may be the result of the pharmacological action of chemicals in the arthropod saliva or venom.

Arthropods may become an occupational hazard in some instances. At other times an epidemic of skin lesions in man may be due to a sudden proliferation of a particular species or perhaps to an epizootic infestation in pet animals which has transferred to their owners.

In Chapter 2 there is a brief general description and discussion of these clinical, histopathological, immunological and epidemiological factors, each of which is later discussed in more detail in the chapters dealing with individual orders of arthropods.

As mentioned in the Preface, little is said in most textbooks about skin disorders caused by arthropods. This applies especially to entomological detail. The present volume seeks to remedy this. Quite apart from the zoological identity of a particular species it is most helpful for the clinician to have some knowledge of the appearance, life cycle, breeding and general habits of the creatures which cause these skin reactions. He can then answer many of his patients' questions satisfactorily. He will be aware, for example, that forcible removal of ticks is the way to cause future trouble and that blistering beetles should not be crushed on the skin. He will know the most suitable treatment for toxic reactions, which vary considerably and do not all respond to the same treatment. He will be able to advise on what action should be taken if offending arthropods are encountered again. He can suggest the most suitable first aid kit to carry around for emergencies for those persons with hypersensitivity.

Treatment of the skin lesions themselves is generally a straightforward dermatological problem but may be ineffective unless the insects or arachnids are appropriately dealt with at the same time. Systemic effects may require emergency treatment and in very serious cases the patient may even need intensive care. The help of specialist physicians will then be necessary.

Chapter 3 supplies some basic entomological details about insect and arachnid structure and identification. Nomenclature and other terms are explained. In subsequent chapters the specific morphology, biology and "life-style" of the various orders are given. Each chapter also contains classified lists of harmful species for ease of reference.

In spite of all this information, help and advice about identification is likely to be required; it is wise to know where to contact entomologists, veterinarians and public health laboratories. A very important point in this respect is to acquire good specimens of the supposed causal arthropod whenever possible. Patients should be encouraged to collect and preserve specimens for expert examination, since their own descriptions are notoriously vague and inaccurate. Historical detail about the individual case is also valuable and patients should be questioned fully about this aspect.

Important references, especially those concerning unusual arthropod pests and their toxins, are denoted by an asterisk in the reference lists at the end of each chapter.

2 General Considerations

The skin is one of man's first lines of defence against invasion or external stimuli. It can react in a variety of ways against all kinds of stimuli, whether physical or chemical, including arthropods and their products. From the patient's point of view these result in one or more lesions on the skin accompanied by local or general symptoms. The effects may be relatively trivial, or may cause great inconvenience or even be fatal. In severe, non-fatal reactions the victim's subsequent way of life may be greatly altered.

For the clinician the diagnostic problem may be difficult. If the reaction is severe he will be presented with an acute emergency requiring prompt treatment. The management frequently depends on the correct diagnosis of the cause. When arthropods are concerned, suspicion of this is often the physician's most valuable aid. In areas where arthropods are known to cause trouble, diagnosis is fairly straightforward, but in other regions the physician must learn not to overlook them. This is a matter of education of both the medical profession and the general public.

Gordon (1950) grouped the reactions which could occur as a result of the attentions of arthropods under four headings:

1. Mechanical trauma
2. Secondary infection
3. Sensitisation phenomenona
4. Toxic effects

This is a convenient arrangement for discussion, but there are a limited number of clinical appearances that can present and similar morphological reactions can have several different arthropod causes. The distinguishing features depend on various other factors, such as number and distribution of lesions; their mode of onset and spread; what symptoms there are, such as itching, burning sensations, pain etc.; and whether or not there are any general symptoms. All these are part of general history taking and clinical examination, which rightly remain the basis on which a diagnosis is made. In taking a history the evidence of relatives or other witnesses to the occurrence should not be neglected. Many other factors have also to be considered and they have been enumerated in Tables 2.1–2.4.

In general terms the clinical (and histological) reaction is influenced by any or all of the factors outlined in Table 2.1. Children usually react more severely than adults to toxins or superficial irritants, are more liable to secondary infection and are immunologically immature. The habits of children in relation to arthropods differ from those of adults. They handle and play with them and are thus more likely to have lesions on the hands and arms than adults and are also more easily bitten by aggressive arthropods. They also have much closer contact with their pets and acquire the latter's parasites more frequently than adults. The elderly

Table 2.1. Factors directly involving the victim which may affect the reaction to arthropods

1. Age
2. Sex
3. Ethnic group
4. Familial involvement
5. Presence of other disease in the patient, e.g. skin disease or discharging lesions
6. Immunological status
7. Is the patient atopic?
8. Medicaments which may be taken

Table 2.2. Factors influencing the clinical and histopathological appearances of skin lesions caused by arthropods

1. Immune status of the patient in relation to
a) Arthropods in general
b) Specific arthropods
2. The species of arthropod
3. The interrelationship of 1 and 2
4. The pharmacological action of venom injected
5. The toxic action of venom injected
6. Contact reactions to toxic arthropod secretions
7. Scratching
8. Secondary infection

may react more severely to very toxic arthropod venoms but, on the other hand, are less liable to develop immunological reactions, especially if they have lived for a long time in an infested region.

The sex of the victim plays little part in the development of reactions to arthropods except in so far as men are more liable to exposure to certain species encountered mainly out of doors because they are more likely to have outdoor occupations. This applies particularly to tick bites and exposure to certain caterpillars. On the other hand, women and children may suffer bee and wasp stings more often because of the attraction of the latter to highly coloured clothing.

It is very doubtful if the ethnic origin of a victim has any aetiological role in attack by arthropods or in the severity of the reaction. It had been thought that perhaps some ethnic groups were more attractive to arthropods than others (or conversely that some were more repellent than others). Maibach et al. (1966) showed that substances on human skin attractive to arthropods were dissolved in sweat, whilst any repellent properties were concentrated in the surface lipids (derived from epidermal cells rather than from sebum). They found that the skin of an older person was rather less attractive than that of a younger subject and they attributed this to the increased lipid content. An anonymous Editorial writer (1940) had pointed out that there was no ethnic difference in sweat or body odour and attributed the liability to reaction in Europeans and apparent immunity of indigenous Africans to the attentions of local arthropods to acquired immunity by the latter and lack of it by the former. This opinion was confirmed by Gordon and Crewe (1948). It was not an ethnic difference but a residential one.

Familial involvement is usually a matter of similar opportunities for exposure to the same arthropod, e.g. pet parasites. If there is regular familial reaction to a variety of arthropods this may mean that the family is atopic. Atopics are alleged to be more liable to reaction to many arthropods, especially Hymenoptera. This may partly be accounted for by the use of the word "allergy", which has now become almost synonymous with the asthma, eczema, hay fever syndrome (Shulman 1967). However, the Insect Allergy Committee of the American Academy of Allergy (1965) has pointed out that severe reactions to arthropods occur in both atopics and non-atopics and only about one in three of those who are sensitive to insects are atopic. It is almost certain that the arthropods themselves cannot distinguish between those who are and those who are not atopic; persons are bitten and stung without fear or favour. Atopics may be more liable to severe reactions.

The presence of other skin disease may have an influence on the reaction to or liability to attacks of arthropods. Persons with scaly or encrusted or discharging skin lesions are certainly more attractive to dipterous flies and this increases the likelihood of myiasis in certain areas. Those who have a severe skin disorder requiring immunosuppressive therapy may react unfavourably to arthropods or may be difficult to rid of invaders because the treatment necessary is deleterious to the more serious complaint. For example, an epidemic of scabies proved exceedingly difficult to control in a hospital devoted to the treatment and management of Brazilian pemphigus (fogo selvagem) (Martins-Castro et al. 1974). Other patients with leprosy, where sensitisation may be diminished, may suffer severely from conditions such as tungiasis (W. S. Douglas 1979, personal communication).

The immune status of the patient is probably the most important single factor determining the reaction to a particular arthropod. The same general principle applies to all arthropods. The possibility that some alteration in a patient's reactions to arthropods might be dependent on his physical condition first occurred to Hebra (1868) when considering Norwegian scabies. He regarded this condition as ordinary scabies developing in a person with a different constitution. In other words "the soil" was altered. Subsequent realisation that a large number of patients with this disease were immunosuppressed in one way or another has vindicated his perspicacity. Other observations on the different effects of fleas on long-established residents and on newcomers in California (Lunsford 1949), and of *Cordylobia anthropophaga* in similar circumstances in Sierra Leone (Blacklock and Thomson 1923) led to the researches of Benson and Semenov (1930), which showed that water-soluble extracts of the proteins of bee body and bee venom gave positive skin reactions in patients with severe reactions to bee stings. Theodor (1935) and Mellanby (1946) both recognised that sensitivity acquired to *Phlebotomus* and *Aedes*, respectively, began with a delayed papular reaction. Mellanby described the five stages of immunity inherent in reactions to arthropods. Firstly there was no reaction in persons never before exposed to arthropods (or a particular species of arthropod). Then with repeated bites they began to develop sensitivity, which was initially manifested by a delayed reaction some 24 h after receiving a bite. (Theodor emphasised that this delay could be up to 3 weeks or longer.) This subsided in about 1 week. At a later stage, which might be weeks, months or even years later, a bite was followed by an immediate reaction (a weal), which subsided in a few hours to be succeeded by the delayed itching papule. After a further period of exposure the delayed reaction no longer occurred but only the immediate weal and finally no reaction appeared at all. The patient was then said to be immune.

This was confirmed exactly by Heilesen (1949). Moreover, it was suggested that the antigens responsible were, in the case of bites, contained in the arthropod saliva. Gordon (1950), and later Hudson et al. (1960) showed that there was no reaction to mosquito bites if the insects' salivary glands were extirpated or the ducts cut. Gordon also pointed out that sensitisation did not develop if mosquito bites were regular and continuous but only if repeated irregularly. Furthermore, he stressed that any immunity could be highly specific and involve only one species. These immunological changes evident clinically are due to differing histological reactions. The small itchy, erythematous papules of the delayed response are characterised histologically by minimal dermal oedema, possible focal necrosis and a dense cellular infiltrate of lymphocytes, histiocytes and numerous eosinophils. During the process of involution lymphocytes are predominant.

These exact features both clinically and histologically are seen in the persistent itching papule of papular urticaria (strophulus; lichen urticatus) and in the delayed reaction to skin tests with injected arthropod antigen (Schaffer et al. 1954). The immediate reaction clinically is a large urticarial weal which microscopically shows intense dermal oedema and a scanty infiltrate mostly of eosinophils. De Panfilis et al. (1983) observed a few Ig-bearing cells in the cellular infiltrate of the insect bite reaction. IgG-bearing cells were commoner than those bearing IgM. No IgA-carrying cells were seen. De Panfilis suggested that in situ IgG and IgM from these cells could react with insect allergens in the same manner as the local reaction to experimental arthropod bite is stimulated by circulating IgG and IgM. Rook (1961) convincingly argued that the clinical appearances and general behaviour of the eruption of papular urticaria showed all the stages of the development of these immunological reactions right up to the stage of complete immunity to the offending arthropod (nearly always fleas).

Important as the immunological reactions are, there are other types of reaction and other factors to be considered (see also Table 2.2). The antigens in saliva (in sting fluid in the case of stinging insects) have other properties, and there may be other substances present which have pharmacological or irritant properties in their own right, and can thus alter the reaction (Mann and Bates 1960). Such venoms, for that is what salivary and sting secretions often are, contain various enzymes, such as hyaluronidase, proteases, peptidases or phospholipase A; peptides, such as kinins, histamine- or heparin-releasing agents; and biogenic amines like histamine, 5-hydroxytryptamine, or acetylcholine. The general effects vary according to the concentration or total amount injected into the victim. Some of the non-protein constituents can also act as haptens and function as sensitisers, as was indeed shown with the sensitising agent in flea saliva (Benjamini and Feingold 1970). The effects of physiological substances in excess may produce severe toxic reactions. For example, multiple bee stings may cause acute histamine poisoning with acute vasodilatation, increased capillary permeability and smooth muscle stimulation, which cause oedema, diarrhoea and pain, amongst other symptoms (Murray 1964). Scorpion stings contain considerable amounts of adrenaline-like material and acetylcholine and induce the general effect of powerful autonomic nervous system stimulation with excessive salivation, sweating, bradycardia, hypertension and glycosuria (Barsoum et al. 1954). Many venoms contain spreading factors like hyaluronidase. This has the effect not only of extending the area of oedema induced by histamine, but also of spreading the inflammatory cellular infiltrate beyond the confines of the papules seen with the delayed reaction described above (Goldman et al. 1952). Other venoms contain toxic principles which induce serious pathological changes. For example, spider venom intended to paralyse or kill the spider's prey can cause not only neurological effects in man, as in latrodectism, but also acute haemolysis and intravascular coagulation, as in acute loxoscelism in South America (Macchiavello 1947). This represents the toxic reaction described by Gordon (1950). On the other hand, other toxic reactions cause severe pain, as seen in wasp and bee stings, which belong to the group Gordon included as deterrent toxins. Hägermark (1974) described the effects of bradykinin and kallikrein, both of which have been found in arthropod venoms. Bradykinin stimulates histamine release and itching, which is relieved by antihistamines, whilst kallikrein causes itch on its own, which is unrelated to histamine and not relieved by antihistamines.

Similar chemicals of the amine and peptide group are encountered in ant venoms, especially in the venom of *Solenopsis* species (fire ant). This particular venom induces focal necrosis and also has insecticidal, bactericidal and haemolytic properties. Its effects are therefore seen clinically as sterile, necrotic pustules, sometimes with a haemorrhagic element. The histological appearance of local necrosis in the upper collagen, with at first a dense cellular infiltrate of histiocytes and lymphocytes, giving place later to neutrophils and lymphocytes, is fully described in Chapter 10 (Caro et al. 1957).

Before considering Gordon's mechanical group, the contact reactions seen with some arthropods, which are the result of the deposition of noxious venom on the skin by some species, should be mentioned. These usually result in an eczematous reaction both clinically and histologically, but if the irritant is composed of a very powerful chemical, such as the quinones secreted by the giant millipedes, gangrenous burns with subsequent scarring will develop. Some ants and cockroaches secrete less irritating substances, whilst other harmful chemicals are found in the spines and urticating hairs of lepidopterous larvae (caterpillars) and in the crushed bodies of blistering beetles, any of which can cause eczematous reaction or deeper damage if the poison penetrates the epidermis. It is interesting in this context to remember that J. H. Fabré (1916), the celebrated French naturalist, invented the patch test in the 1890s when conducting experiments to discover what it was that caused a rash on his skin when he handled caterpillars. He was also the first to suggest, with experimental evidence to support his contention, that sexual attraction between arthropods was communicated by olfactory means through what are now known as pheromones. These latter substances are also indirectly responsible for multiple Hymenoptera stings, as some species leave pheromone deposits on the skin after stinging a person so as to attract others of the same species to come to their aid to defend the nest.

Gordon's first group of mechanical trauma depends on the mechanisms of attack by the individual arthropods. He divided this group into (1) reactions which were dependent on the physical size of the mouthparts of the attacking species; (2) reactions due to the continued presence on man of true parasites such as *Sarcoptes scabiei*; (3) the presence of parasitic larvae such as *Dermatobia hominis*; and (4) the effects of "accidental" parasitic larvae, under which heading he included wound myiasis caused by larvae normally parasitic on other animals, e.g. American and Old World screwworm fly larvae, blowfly larvae etc. The last group contains some species which are better included with *D. hominis* (see Chap. 8, pp. 94–99). Table 2.3 shows the general grouping of arthropods according to their manner of feeding or attacking man. Some of these are quite extraordinary. For example, Eisner and Meinwald (1966), discussing defensive secretions of arthropods, noted that whip scorpions

Table 2.3. Types of arthropods which may damage human skin

Type of arthropod	Examples
1. *Parasitic*	
a) Human	*Pediculus*; *Sarcoptes*
b) From developing forms	Myiasis-producing Diptera
c) Animal parasites	*Cheyletiella*; *Sarcoptes*; gamasids
2. *Blood-sucking arthropods*	
a) Obligatory feeders, rapid and multiple feeders	Some Diptera; fleas; some Hemiptera
b) Obligatory slow feeders. Mouthparts fixed to skin	Ticks; trombiculids
c) Casual bites from predatory species	Some Hemiptera
3. *Phytophagous arthropods which may bite man*	Thrips; some Hemiptera
4. *Arthropods which bite in self-defence*	Spiders
5. *Stinging arthropods*	
a) Social insects defending nest, or in self-defence	Hymenoptera
b) Solitary arthropods in self-defence	Scorpions
6. *Arthropods which spray contact irritants*	Some ants; cockroaches; millipedes
7. *Arthropods whose body contains irritants if crushed*	Coleoptera
8. *Arthropods which leave poison spines or hairs on the skin*	Lepidoptera; some bird-eating spiders

have venom glands with ducts which open and revolve to release their toxin in the manner of artillery gun turrets, whilst the bombardier beetle releases its venom by the explosive force of a chemical reaction. These authors pointed out that it is not uncommon for a similar toxin to be present in the venom of different species. For example, formic acid is secreted by some ants, by carabid beetles and notodontid caterpillars. On the other hand, related species may secrete quite different toxins: In millipedes, for example *p*-benzoquinone is produced by *Julida*, *Spirobolida* and *Spirostreptida* species, a cyanogen by *Polydesmida* and a phenol by *Chlorodesmida*.

Gordon noted that the fine proboscis of mosquitoes could penetrate capillaries without causing much damage, whereas tsetse flies caused considerable laceration and bleeding. Some arthropods cause much damage when the mouthparts are inserted, although a great deal of this may be due to saliva injected. However, tick mouthparts get broken off in situ, the retained portion causing pseudo-epitheliomatous hyperplasia of the epidermis and a dense underlying cellular reaction composed of neutrophils, eosinophils, plasma cells and histiocytes, and sometimes large numbers of lymphocytes arranged in a follicular pattern (Allen 1947). In this foreign body granulomatous reaction parts of the chitinous fragments of the mouthparts of the ticks are usually discernible and giant cells will be seen in their vicinity. The clinical appearance is of a raised, tender inflamed nodule, the end result being a small hard fibrous nodule. Goldman et al. (1952) have noted that when lesions caused by an arthropod of any type persist for long periods the indication is of retained fragments of body chitin. Two well-known examples are the granulomata caused by persistent scabies nodules and by *Demodex folliculorum* escaping into the dermal tissues from a ruptured hair follicle.

Parasitic larvae produce reactions which are both immunological and, latterly, furuncular. They affect different regions in succession during their migration. When larvae live in ulcerated or diseased tissue their action is to destroy the tissue with which they are in contact. Scabies and pediculi, which are true obligatory parasites of man, have more or less fixed reaction patterns, with minimal reactions superimposed in scabies. Blood-sucking and stinging arthropods produce immunological and toxic reactions generally because of repeated exposure. Phytophagous arthropods are more of a nuisance than a danger, but sheer numbers may make the nuisance almost intolerable. The toxic reactions to predators and those with toxic defensive secretions have already been discussed. In addition, the last three groups in Table 2.3 produce contact reactions which, if repeated, may also induce immunological changes.

There are epidemiological factors in arthropod bites and stings which have to be considered in general management. Some of the factors are set out in Table 2.4. The amount and type of clothing worn is often a determining factor in the distribution of multiple lesions or the site of solitary lesions. In general, people living in tropical climates wear much less clothing than do those in temperate regions and are thus more exposed to bites and stings, especially with regard to mosquitoes and the dipterous flies whose larvae cause the various form of myiasis. The effect of clothing is to confine the attacks of some arthropods, e.g. midges, black flies and mosquitoes, to exposed skin, whilst others, such as fleas, prefer to feed on covered areas. Still others actually live in the clothing and feed on the person's skin (body lice). Moreover, areas of constriction of clothing often limit the extent of arthropod attack (fleas and certain mites). Bright colours of some clothes and the scent of cosmetics, soap and hair cream may attract some arthropods and instigate attack (e.g. wasps). Some chemicals, of course, have a repellent effect, and a knowledge of these is useful in advising what to use for preventive purposes.

Table 2.4. Epidemiological factors which may influence the development of reactions to arthropods

1. *Directly related to the victim*
   a) Clothing worn or not
   b) Brightness of clothing
   c) Perfumes worn
   d) Repellents used
2. *Housing*
   a) Western type
   b) Local type
   c) Arthropod proofed
   d) Rodent proofed
3. Pets
4. Overcrowding
5. Sanitary arrangements
6. Garbage disposal
7. Housekeeping and husbandry
8. Political state of the region
   (e.g. war, famine etc.)
9. Occupation (see also Table 2.5)

Housing construction is an important item in the prevention of arthropod attack in those areas where they are prevalent. Local types of housing such as native huts, however elaborate, are as a rule dark and full of crevices, which form ideal hiding and breeding places for such creatures as cockroaches, bugs, some mosquitoes and spiders. Western-style dwellings, on the other hand, whilst still able to afford shelter for all these creatures, are much more easily protected. Fine mesh netting coverings for doors and windows will keep out most flying insects. Active crawling and walking species such as cockroaches, certain bugs and especially scorpions can easily walk into unprotected premises. Building the house about 15–30 cm off the ground helps to keep many out. Scorpions are adept climbers but can easily be excluded by the insertion of a row of glazed tiles set vertically into the outside wall right round the house. No opening should be left for other species. The hosts of some arthropods, such as mice or rats, can carry their parasites indoors and should also therefore be kept out.

Pets can also transport parasites which may attack man, and measures must be taken to keep them in abeyance. Regular grooming and regular disinfestation treatment of the animal and its bedding will prevent these parasites appearing at all.

Overcrowding, bad sanitation and poor garbage disposal provide favourable conditions for breeding many harmful arthropods. This particularly applies to Diptera, wasps, fleas, bugs and, in certain areas, scorpions. Certain species of scorpion thrive in badly constructed wood piles, untidy outhouses and litter generally. Careful regular attention by health authorities to all these factors would go a long way to eradicating many species. For individual families this means good housekeeping and good husbandry. The former includes regular cleaning of the house and furniture, the avoidance of collections of rubbish and dust behind cupboards, stoves, pictures, furniture etc., maintenance of doors, windows and skirting boards and keeping attics and cellars in good repair. Good husbandry means the avoidance of creating rubbish tips by proper garbage disposal, tidy and off-the-ground storage of wood and other materials, good land drainage and the avoidance of minor surgical procedures on livestock in arthropod-breeding seasons in myiasis areas.

Krinsky (1983) has drawn attention to the role of occupation in determining reactions to the bites of various mites and ticks; his findings form the basis for Table 2.5.

The political status of a region may influence large-scale epidemics. Where there are wars, refugee camps, poverty, starvation or drought, harmful arthropods will flourish.

It follows from what has been said that a knowledge of the appearance, habits and noxious properties of arthropods in general is most useful in the diagnosis and management of their effects on the human skin. However, entomology is a vast subject, and it is essential when there is *any* difficulty to get the expert assistance of a professional entomologist. He can identify a particular species with certainty and will know the general steps to be taken in its control. A veterinarian may also be of great help where animal parasites are concerned. The treatment of local reactions is usually straightforward; however, where systemic effects are prominent, help from a general physician may be needed. Immunotherapy is fully discussed in Chapter 10.

Table 2.5. Association of occupation with various arthropods

Occupation	Arthropods encountered
Farm worker	Biting Diptera; myiasis-producing Diptera; bird and rodent mites; *Pyemotes tritici*; *Cheyletiella* spp.; plant mites; chiggers; ticks
Forestry worker	Caterpillars; some *Pyemotes* spp.; trombiculids
Flax worker, Vineyard worker	Spiders in South America, especially *Loxosceles* spp.
Food processing worker	Rat mites; Carpoglyphidae, especially with dried fruit
Grain processing worker	*Pyemotes* species; Acaridae; Glycyphagidae; rat mites
Floriculture worker	Mite predators of phytophagous insects, e.g. *Pyemotes* spp.
Factory worker	Mites associated with any of the above processes; bird and rodent mites, especially in office workers
Dock worker	Spiders; ants; rodent mites; *Pyemotes*; Acaridae; Glycyphagidae; Carpoglyphidae (all on imported food and other products)
Restaurant worker	Acaridae; Glycyphidae; Carpoglyphidae
Bee keeper	Bees
Entomologist	Lepidoptera; some beetles; various mites; millipedes

References

Allen AC (1947) Persistent "insect bites" (dermal eosinophilic granuloma) simulating lymphoblastoma, histiocytosis and squamous cell carcinoma. Am J Pathol 24: 367–375

Barsoum GS, Nawaby M, Salama S (1954) Scorpion poisoning. Its signs, symptoms and treatment. J Egypt Med Assoc 37: 857–894

Benjamini E, Feingold BF (1970) Immunity to arthropods. In: Jackson GJ, Herman R and Onger I (eds) Immunity to parasitic animals. Appleton-Century-Crofts, New York, pp 1061–1134

Benson RL, Semenov H (1930) Allergy in its relation to bee sting. Allergy 1: 105–116

Blacklock B, Thompson MG (1923) A study of the Tumbu fly *Cordylobia anthropophaga* Grinberg in Sierra Leone. Ann Trop Med Parasitol 17: 444–510

Caro MR, Derbes VJ, Jung R (1957) Skin response to the sting of the imported fire ant (*Solenopsis saevissima*). Arch Dermatol 75: 475–488

De Panfilis G, Reali D, Manfredi G and Allegra F (1983) Dimostrazione di cellule portaturi di immunoglobuline nel contesti dell' infiltrato delle reazioni locali al artropodi. G Ital Dermatol Venereol 118: 13–15

Editorial (1940) Sweat and body odour. JAMA 114: 2238

Eisner T, Meinwald J (1966) Defensive secretions of arthropods. Science 153: 1341–1350

Fabre JH (1916) The life of the caterpillar. Translated by Teixeria de Mattos O. Dodd, Mead and Co., New York

Goldman L, Rockwell E, Richfield DF (1952) III. Histopathological studies on cutaneous reactions to the bites of various arthropods. Am J Trop Med Hyg 3: 514–525

Gordon RM (1950) Reactions produced by arthropods directly injurious to the skin of man. Br Med J II: 316–318

Gordon RM, Crewe W (1948) The mechanisms by which mosquitoes and tse-tse flies obtain their blood meal, the histology of the lesions produced and the subsequent reaction of the mammalian host, together with some observations on the feeding of *Chrysops* and *Cimex*. Ann Trop Med Parasitol 42: 334–356

Hägermark O (1974) Studies on experimental itch induced by Kallikrein and bradykinin. Acta Derm Venereol (Stockh) 54: 397–400

Hebra F von (1868) On diseases of the skin including the exanthemata. Translated by Fagge CH and Pye-Smith PH. The New Sydenham Society, London. II: 213–216

Heilesen B (1949) Studies on mosquito bites. Acta Derm Venereol (Stockh) II: 245–267

Hudson A, Bowman L, Orr CWM (1960) Effects of absence of saliva on blood feeding by mosquitoes. Science 131: 1730–1731

Insect Allergy Committee of the American Academy of Allergy (1965) Insect-sting allergy. Questionnaire study of 2606 cases. JAMA 193: 115–120

Krinsky W (1983) Dermatoses associated with the bites of mites and ticks (Arthropodi: Acari). Int J Dermatol 22: 75–91

Lunsford CJ (1949) Flea problem in California. Arch Dermatol Syphilol 60: 1184–1202

Macchiavello A (1947) Cutaneous arachnidism or gangrenous spot of Chile. Puerto Rico J Public Health Trop Med 22: 421–466

Maibach HI, Skinner WA, Strauss WG, Khan AA (1966) Factors that attract and repel mosquitoes in human skin. JAMA 196: 263–266

Mann GJ, Bates HR (1960) The pathology of insect bites; a brief review and report of eleven fatal cases. South Med J 53: 1399–1406

Martins-Castro R, Proenca N, de Salles-Gomez LF (1974) On the association of some dermatoses with South American pemphigus foliaceus. Int J Dermatol 13: 271–275

Mellanby K (1946) Man's reactions to mosquito bites. Nature 158: 554

Murray JA (1964) A case of multiple bee stings. Cent Afr J Med 10: 249–251

Rook A (1961) Papular urticaria. Pediatr Clin North Am 8: 817–833

Shaffer B Jacobson C, Beerman H (1954) Histopathological correlation of lesions of papular urticaria and positive skin test reactions to insect antigens. Arch Dermatol Syphilol 70: 437–442

Shulman J (1967) Allergic responses to insects. Annu Rev Entomol 12: 323–346

Theodor O (1935) A study of the reactions to *Phlebotomus* bites with some remarks on "Harara". Trans R Soc Trop Med Hyg 29: 273–284

3 The Structure and Classification of Mites

Mites are members of the order Acarina of the class Arachnida and are in general less well known to the medical profession than are insects such as mosquitoes, fleas, bedbugs and bees, with the notable exception of *Sarcoptes scabiei.* Some details of their structure and classification are therefore not out of place. Apart from being important vectors of several infectious diseases, they can cause a great deal of cutaneous problems in man through their own efforts.

Structure

Morphologically mites show marked differences from insects, the principal one being the almost complete absence of segmentation. Figure 3.1 illustrates this is diagrammatic form. A different nomenclature is necessary because of this difference. Basically a mite has mouthparts (the gnathosome) and a body (the idiosome). The latter, for descriptive purposes and for classification, is divided into three parts: the propodosome, from which arise the two anterior pairs of legs; the metapodosome, bearing the two posterior pairs of legs; and the opisthosome, posterior to the metapodosome. The idiosome contains the alimentary and reproductive systems and the condensed nervous system. The metapodosome and episthosome are together known as the hysterosome.

The integument or outer covering of the mite is composed of chitin, which in certain areas becomes hardened or sclerotised to form rigid plates and supports for the legs. Distributed over all parts of

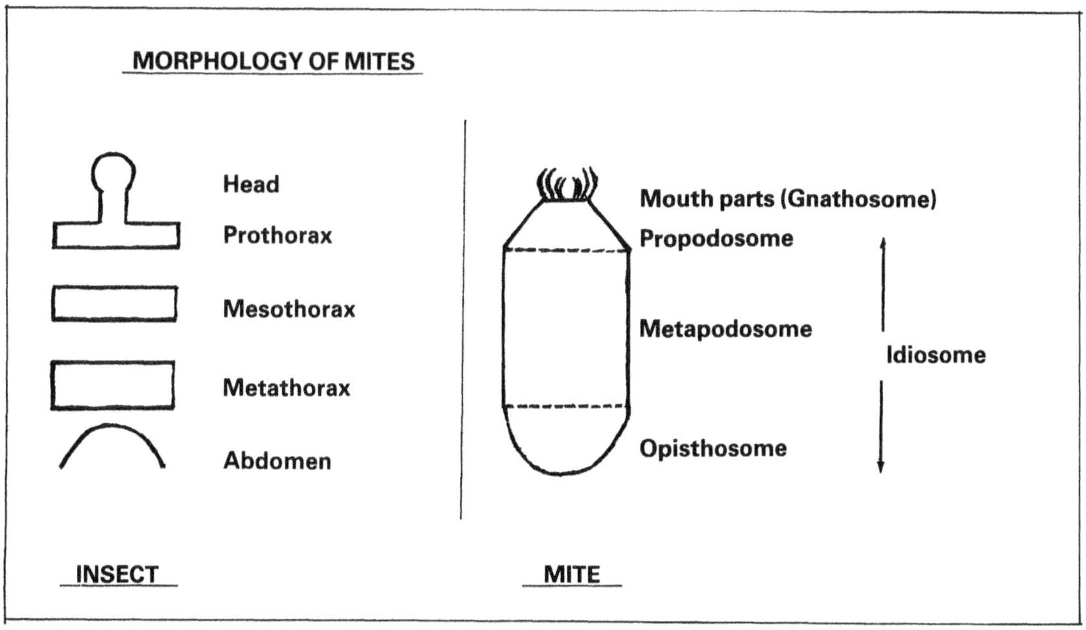

Fig. 3.1. Difference in general structure between insects and mites. The arbitrary morphological divisions of the mite body for the purposes of description are also shown. (After Gordon and Lavoipierre 1962, by kind permission of Prof. M.M.J. Lavoipierre)

the mite are numerous hairs or setae and a number of spines. The principal ones have regular positions on the various parts of the gnathosome, idiosome and legs, and their shape, size and presence or absence are important identification characteristics in the various species. In particular, the setae and spines on the tarsi of the legs have important sensory functions, which are augmented by the few special sensory organs which may be present. Their position and nomenclature are illustrated in Fig. 3.2.

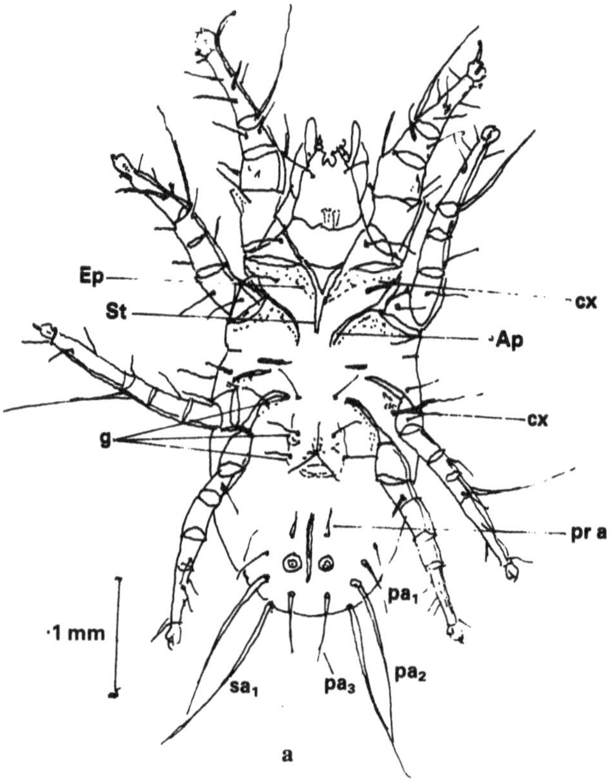

a

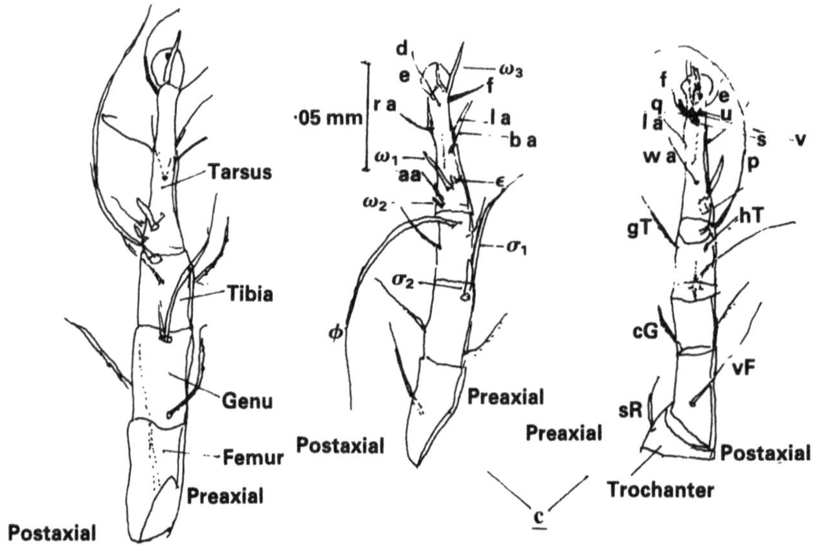

b

Fig. 3.2a–c. Setal nomenclature of mites. **a** ventral view of female *Acarus siro L*; **b** dorsal view of left leg I of female *A. Siro L*; **c** dorsal and ventral views of leg I of *A. gracilis*. *pr a*, preanal; pa_1-pa_3, postanal; *Sa i*, sacral internal; *cx*, coxal; *g*, genital; *Ap*, apodeme; *Ep*, epimeron; *St*, sternum; ω, omega 1–3 (solenidion of tarsus); ϕ, phi (solenidion of tibia); σ, sigma 1–2 (solenidion of genu); ϵ, epsilon (famulus of tarsus); *aa*, *ba*, *d*, *e*, *f*, *la*, *wa*, *p*, *q*, *s*, *u*, *v*, setae and spines of tarsus; *gT*, *hT*, setae of tibia; *cG*, *mG*, setae of genu; *vF*, seta of femur; *sR*, seta of trochanter. (After Hughes 1961, by kind permission of the author and the Ministry of Agriculture, Fisheries and Food)

The gnathosome is a complicated structure which has a base composed of the fused, sclerotised remnants of dorsal and ventral structures called tergites and sternites. In some species the tergites form dorsal plates projecting anteriorly to shield the gnathosome. The latter has two paired appendages, the chelicerae and the pedipalps. The basal segments of the pedipalps, the coxae, are fused with both tergites and sternites to complete the sclerotised base of the gnathosome (Fig. 3.3). The pedipalps have from two to five mobile portions, which vary greatly in appearance and function in the different genera and species. In some species they have a sensory function analagous to the antennae of insects, whilst in others (e.g. *Cheyletus*) they are large and adapted for grasping either prey, such as the body of another mite, or (e.g. *Cheyletiella*) the hair of the host on which the mite is parasitic. Like the legs, to which their segmentation gives them a resemblance, the pedipalps have important and often complicated arrangements of setae and spines, particularly on the terminal segment or tarsus. Examples of pedipalps are given in Fig. 3.4.

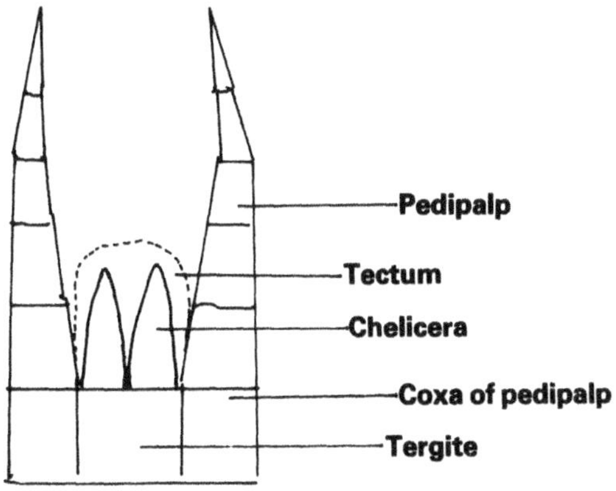

◁ **Fig. 3.3.** Structure of the gnathosome of mites in general, dorsal view. The pedipalps have a variable number of segments, depending on the species. The tectum may conceal the underlying chelicerae, partly or completely.

Fig. 3.4a–d. Examples of the gnathosome in four different types of mite. **a** *Cheyletiella* sp. (note the incurved claws of the pedipalps adapted for grasping hair); **b** *Cheyletus* sp. with pedipalps for grasping prey (note also the piercing chelicerae and the strong pedipalps); **c** the gnathosome of *Dermatophagoides* sp. with chelicerae for chewing; **d** the narrow gnathosome with long pedipalps and piercing chelicerae of *Ornithonyssus bacoti*. (The drawings of **a**, **b** and **c** are tracings from actual photographs of the respective mites obtained **a** from a dog and **b** and **c** from house dust. **d** is taken from a drawing by Hirst but considerably enlarged)

▽

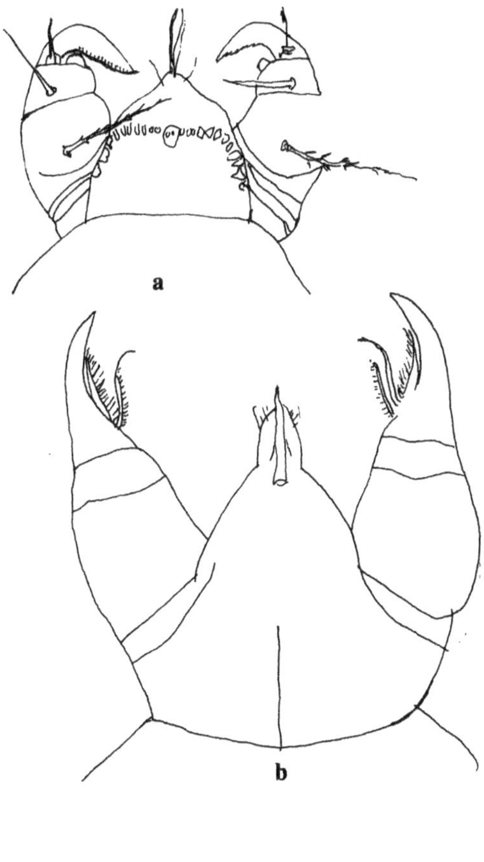

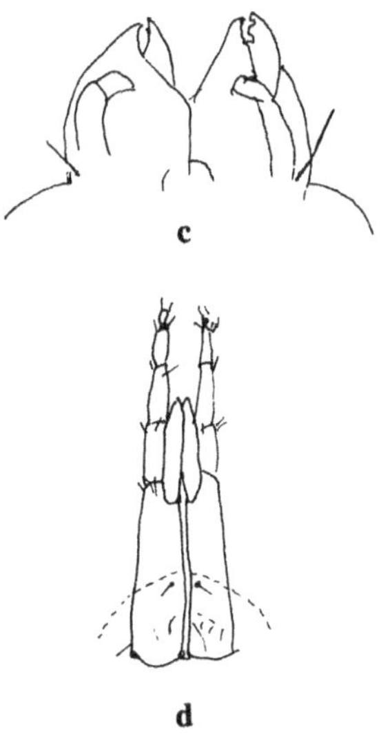

The chelicerae are three-segmented structures lying dorsally which are concerned with feeding, and their structure is modified accordingly. In some species the modification is towards chewing and grinding (as in the Acaridae), in others for piercing to suck blood or other fluids (as in the Cheyletidae or the Parasitoidae). In some species the chelicerae are concealed on the dorsal view by an enlarged sclerotised plate developed from the tergite. Apart from the chelicerae and pedipalps there are other structures, such as the labrum and the mala, which form a sort of mouth cavity continued posteriorly as a hypopharynx, the size of which is controlled by various muscles.

The idiosome is oval or rounded and may be soft, as in the Acaridae, or hardened in some areas into plates, the majority of which are situated dorsally but some may be ventral. The different species in some genera have characteristically shaped plates. They are most prominent in the suborder Parasitiformes, in the Ixodides (ticks) and Parasitoidiae (gamasid mites). They have an array of setae, the position and nomenclature of which are shown in Fig. 3.5. On the ventral surface there are also sclerotised segments formed by the fusion of the coxae of the legs with the idiosome. These structures are known as epimerons. Their shape is often of some diagnostic importance in identification. On the ventral surface are the external genitalia of the male (lying posteriorly) and the genital opening in the female (lying centrally or anteriorly). The anus is usually at the posterior end, just ventrally. The shape of the genital structures may also have diagnostic features in certain species.

The four pairs of legs (three pairs in the larvae) are numbered I, II, III and IV, from the front backwards. They have six segments—the coxa, trochanter, femur, genu, tibia and tarsus. When the coxa is fused to the idiosome to form an epimeron there are only five moveable segments, whilst if the femur is divided into two portions there may appear to be seven segments. The tarsus may terminate in a soft expansion or pulvillus, which is tipped with one or possibly more claws, which may be rigid or mobile. They have an array of setae, of which many, especially in I and II, have a sensory function (See Fig. 3.2).

The sexes are distinct, and, in addition to primary morphological sex differences, males and females may differ in size, in the shape or extent of sclerotised plates, or sometimes in the structure of the legs. Reproduction is usually ovigerous, but sometimes young may emerge from the egg or even mature before birth. (In the case of *Pyemotes* the young are born sexually mature.) Parthenogenetic reproduction is not uncommon.

Classification

Hughes (1961) has described how mites are divided into five suborders and the following brief details have been condensed from her book.

1. Notostigmata With, 1903: A single genus. Segmented hysterosome with eight dorsal stigmata
2. Holothyroidea Reuter, 1909: Single genus. Large species. Two stigmata opening above coxae III and IV
3. Parasitiformes Reuter, 1909 (Mesostigmata s. lat): Two stigmata laterally above the legs, five-segmented palps, two secretory canals opening into the hind gut
   Two divisions:
   a) Ixodides Leach, 1815 (Metastigmata) Ticks
   b) Mesostigmata G. Canestrini 1891 s. str.
4. Trombidiformes Reuter, 1909 (Prostigmata s. lat.): Two stigmata opening at base of gnathosome
   Four divisions:
   a) Tarsonemini G. Canestrini and Fanzago, 1877: Mostly insect parasites. Club-shaped pseudostigmatic organ on dorsal aspect of propodosome (e.g. *Pyemotes*)
   b) Endeostigmata Grandjean, 1937: Free-living soil mites
   c) Prostigmata Kramer, 1877: Aquatic and terrestrial forms. The latter include the Trombidiidae and the Trombiculidae ("harvest mites")
   d) Tetrapodili Bremi, 1872: Plant mites
5. Sarcoptiformes Reuter, 1909: Segmentation scarcely apparent
   Two divisions:
   a) Oribatei Duges, 1934 (Cryptostigmata): Dark, well-sclerotised with well-developed tracheae opening by stigmata or perforations
   b) Acaridiae Latreille, 1806 (Astigmata): No stigmata. Respiration by diffusion through soft cuticle.

Identification

The identification of a particular mite by placing it in its correct genus is achieved by finding the answers to a series of questions set out in the form of keys, which can be found in standard textbooks, specialist papers dealing with revisions of groups and other works involving classification. There are so many insects and mites—over a million known species—that it is obviously impossible to find all

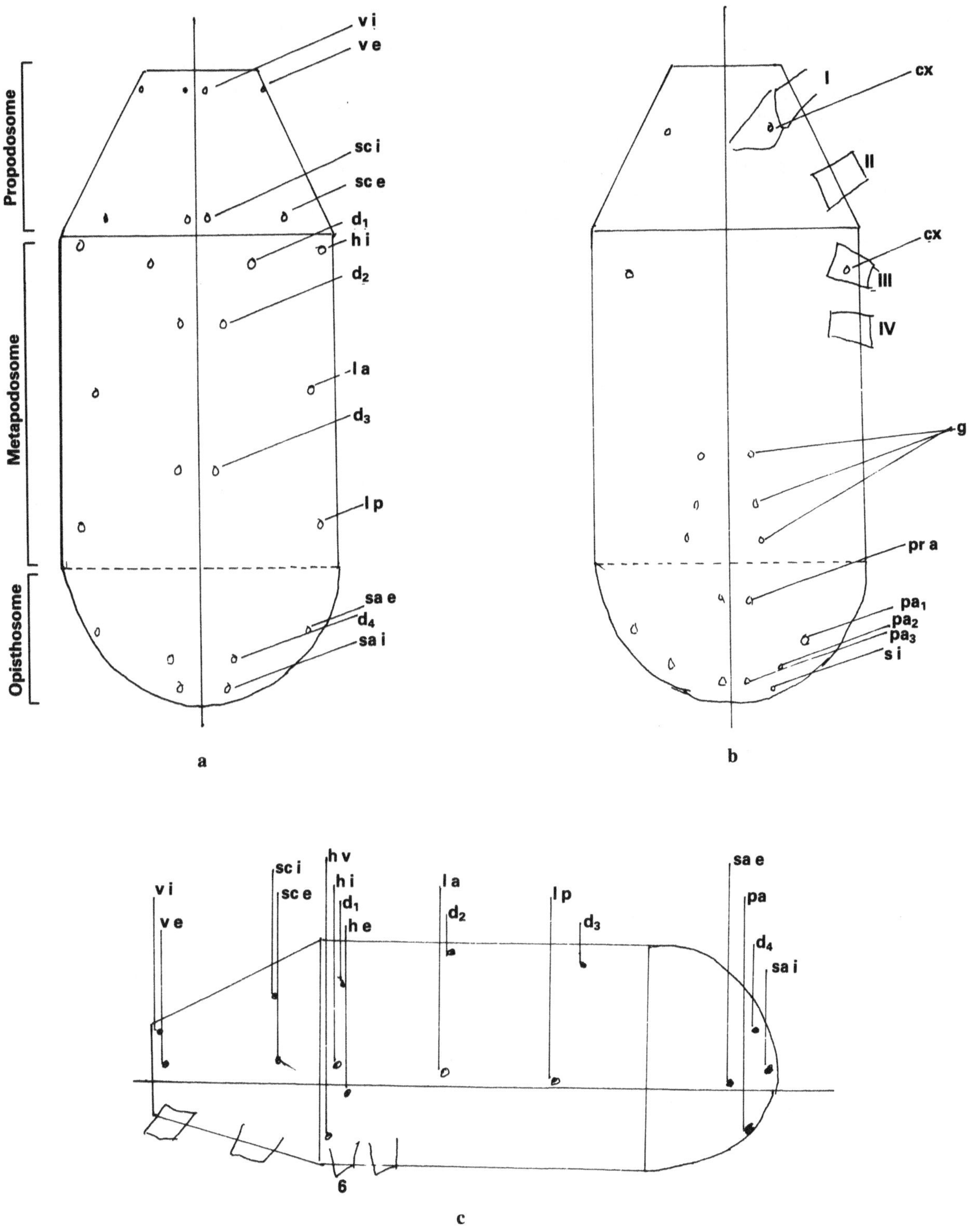

Fig. 3.5a–c. Standard arrangement of setae on the idiosome of a mite. Their numbers may vary somewhat, e.g. there may be from one to five postanal setae. The diagram does not indicate the length of the setae as these vary from species to species. **a** dorsal aspect; **b** ventral aspect; **c** lateral aspect. *v i*, *v e*, internal and external vertical; *sc i*, *sc e*, internal and external scapular; *h i*, *h e* and *h v*, internal, external and ventral humeral; *l a*, *l p*, anterior and posterior lateral; d_1–d_4, dorsal; *sa i*, *sa e*, internal and external sacral; *pra*, preanal; pa_1–pa_3, postanal; *cx*, coxal; *g*, genital.

the information in one book. However, a knowledge of the principles of identification and practice of the procedure are all that is required, except when difficulty arises, in which case an expert's assistance is essential.

The first step after having ascertained that the creature in question is an arachnid belonging to the order Acarina is to put it into the correct suborder. A key for this purpose will be found in a book such as *An Introduction to Acarology* by Baker and Wharton (1958). For those mites found in stored products Hughes (1961) gives the following key to the suborder, which will serve as an example:

1. Mites with a long whip-like solenidion (an elongated hollow chitinous tube) arising on the dorsal extremity of tibiae I and II—usually extending beyond the tarsus—Suborder Sarcoptiformes
   a) Well-sclerotised mites with a pair of prominent sensillae or pseudostigmatic organs arising from the dorsal side of the propodosome near to its posterior margin—Suborder Oribatei
   b) Feebly sclerotised mites without prominent pseudostigmatic organ—Suborder Acaridiae

—Mites without such a whip-like solenidion: 2

—Stigmata on the sides of the idiosome and usually associated with a tubular peritreme—Suborder Parasitiformes, Mesostigmata s. str.
   a) Coxae I usually cylindrical and widely removed from one another, so that the tritosternum is clearly visible—*Parasitoidea* or *Uroseius acuminatus* Koch
   b) Coxae I usually flattened and trapezoid in shape, touching or nearly touching each other, so that the tritosternum is largely concealed—*Uropodoidea*

— Stigmata opening on or at the base of the gnathosome usually difficult to see, and sometimes associated with a peritreme—Suborder Trombidiformes or Prostigmata s. lat.

Having determined the correct suborder for the specimen a similar exercise is carried out to ascertain to which superfamily, family or subfamily it belongs, repeating this procedure again when the genus is reached. A key is required for each stage. As an example of the final stage of ascertaining the correct species, here is the key elaborated by Smiley (1965) for male specimens in the genus *Cheyletiella*:

1. — Sensory organ on genu I not heart shaped and depressed at the apex; not on dogs
   — 2

   — Sensory organ on genu I heart shaped and depressed at the apex
   — *yasguri* Smiley
2. — Aedeagus originating below the level of coxa IV; on rabbits
   — 3

   — Aedeagus originating on or above the level of coxa IV; on cats
   — *blakei* sp. n
3. — Sensory organ on genu I global; aedeagus curved; on rabbits
   — *parasitovorax* (Megnin)

   — Sensory organ on genu I oblong; aedeagus straight; on rabbits
   — *furmani* sp. n.

This key was later shown by Van Bronswijk and de Kreek (1976) to require the examination of several specimens, as the shape of the sensory organ is not always clear cut.

It can readily be observed from this brief outline of the procedure necessary to identify unknown mites that a number of keys are required. Except for fairly well-defined specimens, and where the source may reduce the number of steps required for identification, only a specialist department would have all the keys available. Fortunately, the number of species which attack man is relatively small, numbered in dozens rather than tens of thousands. In cases of real difficulty only very large organisations such as the British Museum or government acarology or entomology services can carry out the identification.

Nomenclature

There is a standard code of rules governing nomenclature which has been laid down by the International Committee of Zoological Nomenclature. The following brief summary is based on a most informative chapter on this subject in *Entomology for Students of Medicine* by Gordon and Lavoipierre (1962). I am greatly indebted to Prof. M.M.J. Lavoipierre for his permission to use this material. This classification applies to all animals.

1. Each species is designated by two names, the generic and the specific, written in italics. A subspecies bears a third name, also written in italics, e.g. *Ornithonyssus bacoti*; *Pediculus humanus capitis*. Divisions above and including genera are given an initial capital letter. When a species is repeatedly indicated, only the capital letter is used, e.g. *O. bacoti*.

2. All the scientific names are in Latin form.
3. Family and subfamily names are formed by adding "idae" and "inae" respectively to the stem of the generic names, e.g. genus *Acarus*, family Acaridae.
4. Generic names are single worded and can be used alone. Subgenera are mentioned in parentheses after the generic name but never alone. If a generic name is changed the old name can be inserted in parenthesis, e.g. *Ornithonyssus* (= *Liponyssus*) *bacoti*. The equal sign must be used to avoid the name in parenthesis being mistaken for a subgenus.
5. Specific names derived from persons are written with a small initial letter, e.g. *Ornithonyssus bacoti*.
6. The author of a scientific name is the first person to publish that name. If this author's name is to be cited it comes after the scientific name but not in italics, followed by a comma and the date, thus: *Suidasia nesbitti* Hughes, 1948. If subsequently the species is transferred to another genus the author's name and date are retained but placed in parenthesis, thus: *Ornithonyssus bacoti* (Hirst 1915).[1] New species are indicated in the original description by sp. n. (or sp. nov.) e.g. *Suidasia nesbitti* sp. n. in Hughes original paper, in 1948.

References

Baker EW, Wharton GW (1958) An introduction to acarology. MacMillan Company, New York

*Gordon RM, Lavoipierre MMJ (1962) Entomology for students of medicine. Blackwell, Oxford

*Hughes AM (1961) The mites of stored food. Ministry of Agriculture, Fisheries and Food. Technical Bulletin No 9, HMSO, London

Smiley RL (1965) Two new species of the genus *Cheyletiella* (Acarina: Cheyletidae). Proc. Entomol. Soc. Washington 67: 75–79

Van Bronswijk JEMH, de Kreek EJ (1976) *Cheyletiella* (Acarina: Cheyletiellidae) of dog, cat and domestic rabbit; a review. J Med Entomol 13: 315–327

1. The reader will note that there is some inconsistency in the citing of the original authority for a scientific name. In some cases the names of the original authors were impossible to trace, and in some of the longer lists they have been deliberately omitted because of their cumbersomeness. It is evidently not always necessary to cite such authorities.

4 Thysanoptera and Dictyoptera, Suborder Blattaria

Thysanoptera

The order Thysanoptera (meaning fringe-winged), known as thrips, comprise about 5000 species with a worldwide distribution. Although mainly phytophagous, some species are predatory on other arthropods and others can occasionally cause lesions on man's skin. They are the smallest winged insects, their size in temperate climates being 1–2 mm long, although they have a range from 0.5 to 14 mm in the tropics. The principal suborders and classification are shown in Table 4.1, whilst Table 4.2 indicates those species said to have caused human reactions. Interested readers who want a comprehensive account of thrips should consult Lewis (1973), from whose work the following details have been compiled.

Morphology

Thrips have a typical insect structure of head, thorax and segmented abdomen with three pairs of legs. Apart from their narrow fringed wings they have peculiar retractable bladders on the feet, and the mouthparts are asymmetrical and arranged in a vertically directed cone appearing to arise between the first pair of legs. Figures 4.1, 4.2 and 4.3 show these general details. Feeding is achieved by the puncturing of plant cell walls by the sharp pointed mandibular stylet and the sucking up of the contents. This process is assisted by the digestive properties of saliva secreted through the mouth. Predatory species feed on their prey or on vegetable matter in this manner, but some species suck up only exuded cell contents from the surface after the cells have been rasped by the mouthparts.

Life Cycle

Eggs are laid in plant stems and leaves through incisions cut by the ovipositor. The various stages consist of egg, two larval instars, prepupa, two pupal instars and adult. The process occupies from 11 to 36 days depending on species and environ-

Table 4.1. Classification of thrips. (Compiled from Lewis 1973)

Classification	Distribution	Remarks
Terebrantia		Wings parallel at rest
1. Aeolothripidae		Many are facultative predators
a) Erotidothripinae b) Melanothripinae c) Mymaothripinae d) Aeolothripinae	Temperate zones of north and south hemispheres	
2. Merothripidae	Tropics and subtropics	Minute, usually found on windows
3. Heterothripidae	America	Flower dwellers
4. Thripidae		
a) Thripinae b) Heliothripinae	Worldwide	These contain the species of economic importance
Tubulifera		Wings crossed at rest
1. Phlaeothripidae a) Phlaeothripinae b) Megathripinae c) Urothripinae	Worldwide	Meadow and woodland dwellers

Table 4.2. Species of thrips which have been reported as having caused reactions in man. (Compiled from various sources, notably Bailey 1936 and Lewis 1973

Species	Location	Remarks	Reference
Melanthrips fusca	France	Attacked tubercular patient during febrile episodes	Artault de Vevy (1902)
Karnyothrips flavipes	Trinidad	A blood-sucking thrips	Williams (1921)
Gynaikothrips uzeli	Algiers	Always near fig trees. Conjunctival and skin irritation	Sevenet (1922)
G. ficorum	Algiers		James and Harwood (1969)
Caliothrips indicus (= *Heliothrips*)	Sudan	Sharp, painful inflammation. Non-blood sucker	Johnston (1925)
"Grain infesting" sp.	Northern	Severe itch. Thought to be seeking moisture.	Korting (1930)
Limothrips cerealium	Germany	Also affected bathers in sea	Ludwig (1912)
Thrips imaginis	Australia	Rash on face. Dry weather	Evans (1932)
Thrips tabaci (larvae and adults)	California	Workers in onion plots. Prickling on arms, face and neck. Second larval instar of *T. tabaci* sucked blood. Small dots which cleared in 1–2 days. Any exposed skin affected	Bailey (1936)
Frankiniella moultoni	California		
Taeniothrips inconsequens	California		
Scoliothrips sexmaculatus	California	Experimental tests with these predator species caused little inflammation. They showed little inclination to bite	Bailey (1936)
Leptothrips mali	California		
Aeolothrips fasciatus	California		
A. kuwanii	California		

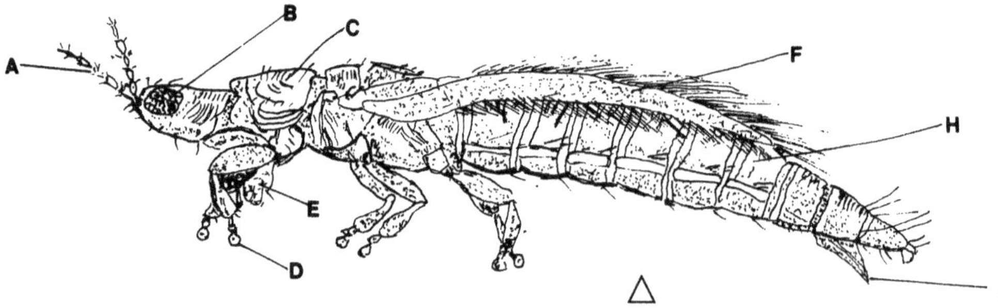

Fig. 4.1. Side view of *Anaphathrips sandersoni* to show the main morphological features. *A*, antenna; *B*, compound eye; *C*, prothorax; *D*, protrusable bladder on tip of tarsus; *E*, mouth cone; *F*, fringed wing; *G*, ovipositor; *H*, abdomen. [After Lewis 1973, by kind permission of the author and the publisher, Academic Press Inc. (London) Ltd.]

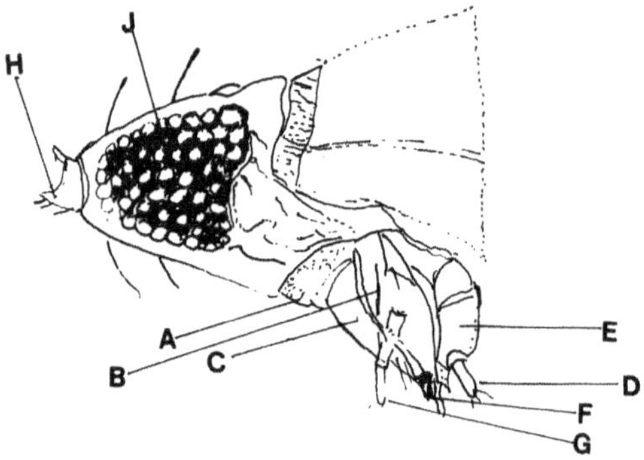

Fig. 4.2. Side view of head and mouthparts of *Chirothrips hamatus*. *A*, clypeus; *B*, maxilla; *C*, labrum; *D*, labial palp; *E*, labium; *F*, stylet; *G*, maxillary palp; *H*, base of antenna; *J*, compound eye. [After Lewis 1973, by kind permission of the author and the publisher, Academic Press Inc. (London) Ltd.]

mental temperature, the period being shorter in tropical zones. Some species have a diapause of up to a year at the second larval stage. Males are generally very much fewer than females, especially in warm climates. Parthogenesis is quite common.

Thrips are of considerable economic importance because of the damage which they inflict on crops. Some species have worldwide significance in this respect, e.g. *Thrips tabaci* or onion thrips. Other crops, including bananas, citrus fruit, cotton grass,

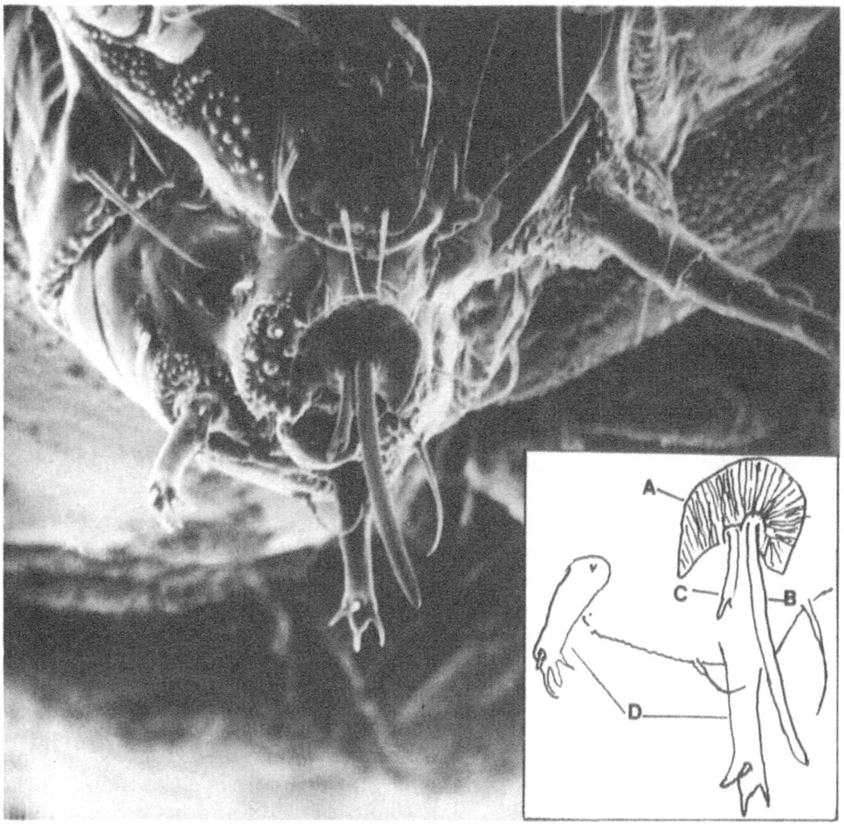

Fig. 4.3. A scanning electron microscope oblique-frontal view of the mouth-cone of *Limathrips cerealium*. The fully expanded crescent-shaped labral pad (*A* in inset) is in the middle of the micrograph and through it project the single stout left mandible (*B*) and the slimmer paired maxilla (*C*) (seen here less extended than the mandible and split at the end). Behind these mouth-parts are the downward projecting labial palps (*D*) with apparently "fingered tips", probably used for orientating the piercing organ. [From Chisholm IF (1983) Feeding mechanism, behaviour and effects of *Limothrips* sp. on cereals. (PhD thesis.) Courtesy of Dr. I.F. Chisholm and Dr. Trevor Lewis (Rothamsted Experimental Station)] Originally × 1700

wheat or fruit, can be damaged by different species in different regions. The damage may take the form of leaf roll, gall formation, scars on fruit, flower distortion etc.

Clinical Features of "Thrips Bites"

Man may be annoyed merely by the vast numbers of thrips, especially if they get into his nostrils, auditory canals or conjunctival sacs. Such events can occur in warm sultry climates during thrips migrations. If the climate at the time becomes dry, the insects are attracted to any liquid, including sweat on man's skin. They will feed on this liquid and may as a result cause itching and prickling sensations. Bailey (1936) reviewed the instances recorded up to that time (Table 4.2). The points to be noted were that the insects in general seemed to be looking for fluid. Some species, notably *Karnyothrips flavipes*, *Thrips tabaci*, *Frankiniella moultoni* and *Taeniothrips inconsequens*, all appeared able to suck blood. There was little or no clinical evidence of any lesions being produced except evanescent pinkish dots. Some itching and prickling sensations were experienced and occasionally some inflammation ensued.

A more recent report (Goldstein and Skipworth 1968) described the occurrence of some hundreds of instances of papular eruptions due to an unidentified species of thrips over a 7-year period amongst American soldiers in Hawaii. The lesions affected principally the face, neck and upper extremities but were occasionally also found on the upper anterior chest wall and thighs. They consisted of erythematous macules and papules varying in size from pinpoint to 3 mm in diameter and were surrounded by an "anaemic halo" suggesting vasoconstriction. They lasted from 6 to 10 days leaving no residual mark. Slight itch was noted in some patients but only a few required antihistamines for this. There was no fever, but in at least one instance there was a mild generalised lymphadenopathy. The patients were in otherwise excellent general health and no abnormal laboratory findings were found.

Doubt was cast on the suggestion that these lesions were due to thrip bites by Aeling (1974), who recorded 20 patients with a similar condition, which he termed "Hypoanesthetic halos in Hawaii" (HHH disease) because of the diminished sensation in the halo part of the lesion. He said that they had been seen by dermatologists in the island for at least 6 or 7 years prior to the introduction of Cuban laurel thrips. They were thought to be due to the bites of nocturnal mosquitoes. Similar lesions were also recorded in Vietnam. The exact arthropod responsible has yet to be determined.

Histopathology

In six of the patients described by Goldstein and Skipworth (1968) no abnormal epidermal changes were seen but some dermal oedema and a mild perivascular infiltrate of lymphocytes was present. There was no tissue eosinophilia, although a few extravasated erythrocytes were seen.

The patients were affected when they were "in the field", the majority in a mountain camp but some in a camp on the seashore. Most cases occurred in January (the cool season) and a few in April and May (the start of the hot season). The condition was evidently not uncommon and well known to the local dermatologists, although not all of them regarded thrips as the cause. Experimental reproduction of the lesions by exposure to these thrips was unsuccessful, in contrast to the production of a small white lump about 6 mm in diameter with a surrounding blanched area 18 mm by 12 mm reported by Williams (1921). Goldstein and his colleague pointed out that Williams' report and their own were the only ones to mention the pale halo in the lesions, which they attributed to vasoconstriction.

No treatment appeared to be required.

Control of Thrips

The thrips populations and the damage they cause are best controlled by sound agricultural and horticultural methods, the most important being an adequate water supply for crops. Contact systemic insecticides can be used, if required, and many are effective. For long-term effectiveness chlorinated hydrocarbons are tending to be replaced by more persistent organophosphorus compounds and carbamates, whilst for short-term use pyrethrum or nicotine dust are adequate. Sprays are most suitable out of doors, and dusts or aerosols in greenhouses. Lewis (1973) gives comprehensive details.

Cockroaches

Cockroaches (the word is probably derived from the Spanish *cucaracha* and the superfamily name Blattoidea from the Latin *blatta*) have one of the longest histories of continuous existence of any living creature (Patton 1931). They extend back geologically for 400 million years (Ebeling 1975) and during the carboniferous period were the dominant species of insect (Patton 1931). There are some 4000 species, of which less than 1% affect man or his environment (James and Harwood 1969). Their principal effect on man is to consume or contaminate his food supply, to render his dwellings unsavoury and theoretically to act as a vector for infectious diseases. Up to four polioviruses, 40 species of bacteria and 12 of helminths have been isolated from cockroaches but none have been proven to be conveyed to man (Guthrie and Tindall 1968). Guthrie and his colleague have pointed out that, nuisance as they are, the injury cockroaches cause to men is insignificant compared to that of the locust (in crop destruction) or the anopheline mosquito (as a vector of disease). As regards actual injury to man and the production of skin lesions cockroaches come low on the scale of injurious arthropods.

Cockroaches belong to the order Dictyoptera, suborder Blattaria, the general subdivisions of which are shown in Table 4.3. Morphologically they are typical insects with two pairs of wings, the front pair being hard and leathery, many veined and forming a dorsal canopy for the hind pair, which fold underneath like a fan (Chinery 1976). In some species (e.g. *Blatta orientalis*) the wings are well developed in the male but smaller in the female, and in others they are vestigial (James and Harwood 1969). The mouthparts are of the chewing type, cerci are usually present and the legs are not modified for any special purpose (Chinery 1976). The insects as a whole are flattened dorsoventrally, usually with a smooth surface, and are black or brown in colour, but some species are brighter orange in the tropics. There are prominent, multisegmental filiform antennae (see Fig. 4.4) (James and Harwood 1969). Cockroaches vary in size from 10 mm to over 60 mm (see Fig. 4.5).

Table 4.3. Classification of cockroaches. (Adapted from Roth and Alsop 1978)

Suborder and superfamily	Family and subfamily	Genus
Blattaria		
Blattoidea	Cryptocercidae	
	Cryptocercinae	
	Blattidae	
	Lamproblattinae	
	Tyrominiinae	
	Blattinae	*Periplaneta*; *Blatta*: *Neostylopyga*; *Deropellis*; *Pseudoderopellis*
	Polyzosterinae	*Pelmatosulpha*; *Eurycotis*; *Cutilia*; *Platyzosteria*; *Polyzosteria*; *Zonoploca*; *Megazosteria*; *Desmozosteria*; *Drymaplaneta*; *Euzosteria*
Blaberoidea	Polyphagidae	
	Polyphaginae	
	Holocompinae	
	Blattellidae	
	Anaplectinae	
	Plectopterinae	*Supella*
	Blattellinae	*Blattella*; *Parcoblatta*; *Lobopleis*
	Nictoborinae	*Megaloblatta*; *Nictobora*
	Ectobiinae	*Ectobius*
	Blaberidae	
	Panesthiinae	
	Blaberinae	*Byrsotria*; *Blacerus*
	Zeliborinae	
	Perisphaerinae	
	Epilamperinae	
	Oxyhaloinae	*Leucophaea*; *Nauphoeta*; *Gromphadorhina*
	Panchlorinae	*Panchlora*
	Diplopterinae	*Diploptera*
	Pycnoscelinae	*Pycnoscelus*

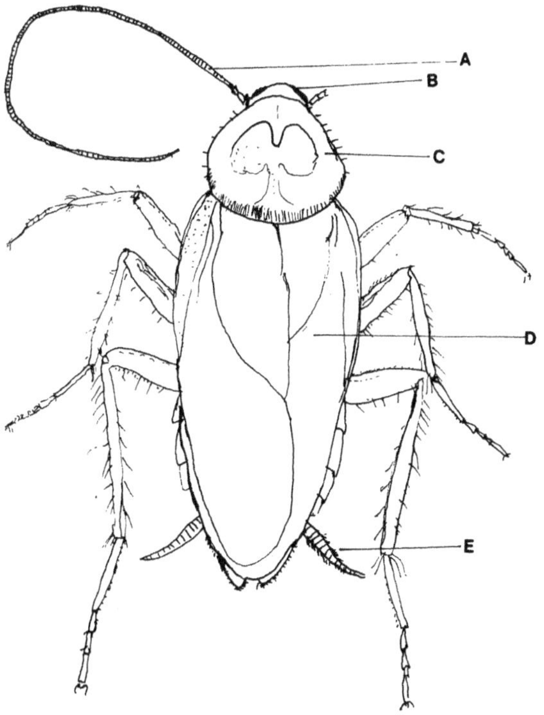

Fig. 4.4. *Periplaneta americana*, the American cockroach. *A*, filamentous antenna; *B*, compound eye; *C*, pronotum overlying the deflexed head which is almost invisible; *D*, folded wings; *E*, segmented cerci. (After Patton 1931)

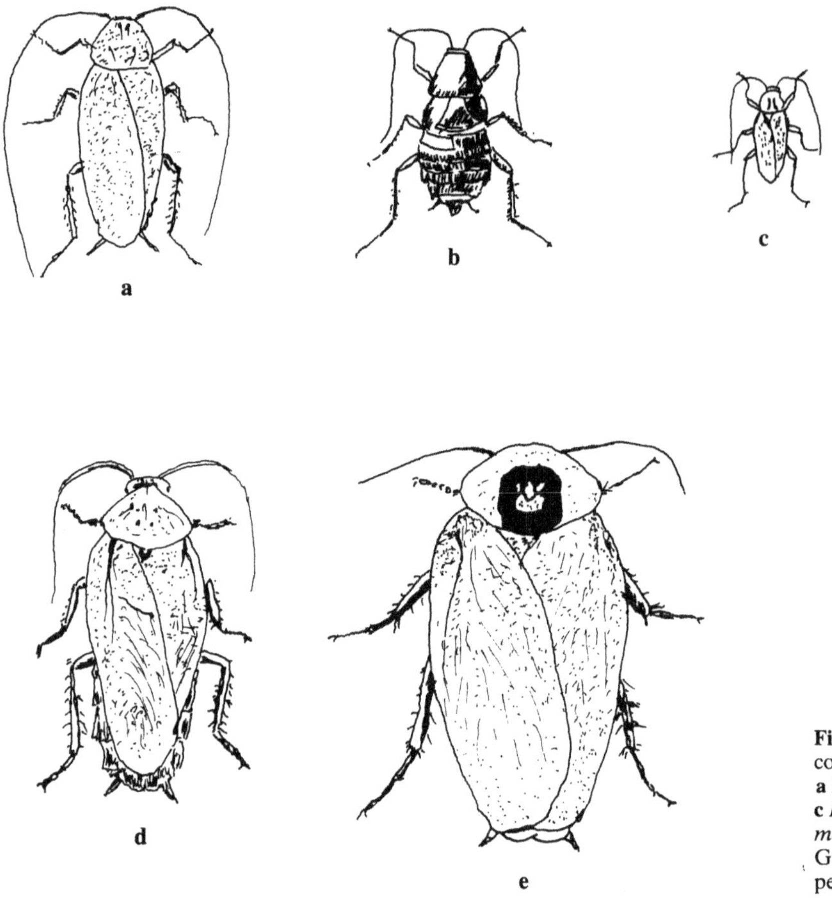

Fig. 4.5a–e. Some common cockroaches, all natural size. **a** *Periplaneta americana;* **b** *Blatta orientalis;* **c** *Blattella germanica*; **d** *Leucophaea maderae*; **e** *Blaberus craniifer*. (After Guthrie and Tindall 1968, by kind permission of the authors)

Life Cycle

The life cycle goes from egg to nymph to adult with several nymphal instars. The eggs are laid in a leathery bean-shaped sack known as an ootheca and arranged vertically in two rows inside. *Periplaneta americana*, *Blatta orientalis* and *Supella supellectilium* have about 16 eggs to the ootheca, but there are some 48 in the ootheca of *Blattella germanica.* The female carries the ootheca about for a day or two before depositing it in a sheltered spot, except in the case of *Blattella germanica* where the female carries it for several weeks. The incubation period at 30°C and 70% relative humidity is about 32 days, but at ordinary room temperature it varies with species—*P. americana*, 53 days; *B. orientalis*, 42–81 days; and *Blattella germanica*, $28\frac{1}{2}$ days (James and Harwood 1969). About 7% of eggs of *Blattella germanica* hatch whilst the female is still carrying the ootheca, but almost all the remainder hatch within 24 h of its being deposited on the ground. The nymphs of this latter species moult every 2 weeks or so, there being six or seven instars and the whole life cycle taking about 3 months. This means that at least two generations per year are produced. There are about 13 instars for *P. americana* and the life cycle takes a year. The life span of this species varies from 102 to 588 days, but individual specimens have been noted to survive for 783, 793 and 913 days, respectively (James and Harwood 1969).

Biology

Cockroaches are gregarious, the immature instars tending to congregate in one area and foraging for food from this centre. Their return is facilitated by the secretion of a clustering pheromone in the faeces (Ebeling 1975). They progress by walking, or more usually by running, and although some species are capable of flight, most only fly in emergencies (Roth and Willis 1957). They prefer to live in heated buildings in temperate climates and infest the kitchen, living room and bathroom in human dwellings. They also invade hospitals and similar institutions, food and grain stores, supermarkets and ships. Insanitary conditions encourage infestation and promote rapid breeding. In warm temperature zone summers and all the year round in the tropics they live and breed outdoors quite freely. They are often found in vast numbers in sewers and the inside of sewage manhole covers. (Roth and Willis 1957; Guthrie and Tindall 1968).

Cockroaches are nocturnal, all their feeding forays (over 100 each night) and migrations being made between 7.00 and 10.30 p.m. and for a brief period around 6 a.m. (Guthrie and Tindall 1968). Although they are more or less omnivorous, they prefer starchy and sugary material and will also consume any human food, as well as excreta, secretions (pus, sputum etc.), blood, toenails and fungi. They vomit and defaecate indiscriminately during feeding and are thus potential vectors of organisms from contaminated sources. Cockroaches also emit nauseating odours which arise from secretions by various defence glands and contaminate food and the environment. The secretions are of two types (Roth and Alsop 1978). One is a liquid secretion containing aldehydes, quinones and other chemicals discharged in response to predatory attack and acting as a contact irritant. This type is possibly irritant to man's skin. The other is a viscid, sticky substance which gums up the mouthparts of smaller intending arthropod predators. Roth et al. (1956) isolated the first of the liquid secretions, trans-2-hexenal, which is very irritant to human skin. It can be ejected by the cockroach as a spray under pressure to a distance of up to 1 m. All polyzosterine species of Blattidae (see Table 4.3) can spray such noxious fluids, which are effected, it is believed, by a build-up of haemolymph pressure which is released from the reservoir only when the closure muscles (acting as a sphincter) are deliberately relaxed. Full details of cockroach toxins can be found in Roth and Alsop (1978) (see also Chap. 24, Millipede Burns).

Table 4.4 indicates those species which are said to affect man. According to Roth and Willis (1957), these species have been shown naturally or experimentally to be vectors of organisms or to bite man.

Table 4.4. Species of cockroach which have been said to affect man or are alleged vectors. (Compiled mainly from Roth and Willis 1957; Ebeling 1975; Roth and Alsop 1978)

Species	Remarks
Periplaneta americana (L)[a]	American cockroach; flies readily; widespread
P. fuliginosus (Serville)	Smoky brown cockroach; Southern and Central USA only
P. australasiae (Fabr.)[a]	Australian cockroach; tropics and neotropics
P. brunnea Burmeister	Brown cockroach; tropical
P. ignota Shaw	Australia
Blatta orientalis L.[a]	Oriental cockroach; widespread; abundant odour
Neostylopyga rhombifolia (Stoll)	Habits resemble those of *P. americana*; Far East; USA; can spray defence secretions
Eurycotis floridana (Walker)	Woods cockroach; Southern Florida and Caribbean; sprays repellent defence secretion.
E. decipiens	Also sprays secretions; causes vertigo, nausea and lacrimation in man
Polyphaga saussurei (Dohan)	Southeast Asia
Supella supellectilium (Serville) (= *S. longipalpa* (Fabr.))	Flies readily; brown-banded cockroach; African origin; common in USA
Blattella germanica (L)[a]	German cockroach; cosmopolitan
Byrostria fumigata[a]	
Blaberus atropos (Stoll)	South America; non-domestic species
B. craniifer Burmeister	Cuba, Mexico, Florida and Central America
B. discoidalis Serville[a]	Ecuador and Puerto Rico; attacks sleepers
B. fusca Brunner	Non-domestic species
Leucophaea maderae (Fabr.)[a]	Madeira cockroach; widespread; African origin
Nauphoeta cinerea (Olivier)[a]	Lobster cockroach; African origin, now Florida, Australia and Hawaii
Gromphadorinha brunneri (Butler)[a]	
Pycnoscelus surinamensis (L)	Surinam cockroach; tropics and neotropics
Shelfordiella tartara (Saussure)	Central Asia, especially in houses with mud floors

[a] These species have been recorded as causing skin reactions and there are probably many others on this list which have done so (Roth and Willis 1957).

Clinical Features

Cockroaches cause three types of reaction in human skin: (1) bites, (2) contact reactions and (3) hypersensitivity reactions.

Bites nearly always occur in circumstances where cockroaches are, at best, inadequately controlled. They gnaw the toe- and fingernails and calloused skin of sleeping persons, devouring these insensitive structures until a tender area is reached, when the limb is sharply withdrawn (Durie 1870; Kingsley 1870; Nicols 1870; Heiser 1936; and various authors from the seventeenth to the twentieth centuries cited by Roth and Willis 1957). Many of the reported incidents occurred on board ships. Drury 1837, (cited by Roth and Willis 1957) noted that *Blaberus discoidalis* had often stripped the flesh off fingers and toes of sick and dying persons in the West Indies. Nicols experienced the nocturnal removal by cockroaches of a traumatic blister on his foot leaving a painful ulcer. Small children have been bitten on the face when asleep, the insects attracted by food particles on their lips (Patton 1931; Frings 1948, cited by Roth and Willis 1957). Popselow averred that the bites were triangular (Pawlowsky and Stein 1930). The latter two authors proved experimentally that cockroaches would gnaw the skin surface.

Contact reactions may be of two types. Firstly there is a dermatitis reaction after the cockroaches have crawled over the sleeper's exposed skin, for example on the legs (Vinson 1865) or on the face in a linear pattern (Simon 1952; both cited by Roth and Willis 1957). These were probably primary irritant reactions to the insect defence secretions (see above). Secondly there is an immediate type of urticarial reaction at the site of contact, also sometimes occurring in sleeping patients (Simon 1952), but more commonly appearing in laboratory workers and others handling cockroaches constantly (Bernton and Brown 1967; Zschunke 1978). Roth and Willis cited a colleague (M. F. Lerner) who developed such a contact urticaria on his feet from shoes contaminated when stamping on a swarming mass of cockroaches. The eruption only ceased when he stopped wearing the shoes. These reactions were probably due to hypersensitivity to a protein constituent in cockroach saliva. Pawlowsky and Stein (1930) reproduced such a reaction by a cutaneous scratch test using an extract of the insect's saliva. The reaction in Lerner's case was more likely to have been a primary irritant one.

Generalised hypersensitivity reactions are manifested by symptoms of hayfever, asthma, conjunctival irritation and sometimes by widespread urticaria. They usually result from the effects of contact or inhalant cockroach antigens in persons, such as zoologists, who have worked with these insects for a long time. The mere opening of a drawer containing cockroaches may be enough to induce symptoms (Bernton and Brown 1969; Bernton et al. 1972). Similar reactions, commonly of a respiratory type, may occur with ingestant allergens amongst the general public from food contaminated by cockroaches. Bernton and Brown (1969) indicated that these allergens are an important aetiological factor in inducing symptoms in allergic patients since it may be difficult to avoid them when there is a heavy infestation. They showed, by skin tests, that there is a positive relationship between the degree of cockroach infestation and the occurrence and severity of symptoms in such patients.

Histopathology

Pawlowsky and Stein (1930) examined skin attacked by cockroaches and skin into which the insect's saliva had been injected. The histological appearances were identical: There was epidermal cell degeneration and necrosis with underlying dermal inflammation, showing dilated capillaries filled with lymphocytes and "leucocytes" and the same cells plus immature neutrophils in the perivascular tissues.

Epidemiology

Cockroaches flourish especially well in primitive conditions. Bernton and Brown (1967) demonstrated a direct relationship between overcrowding of humans and density of cockroach population. This was shown in ethnic groups, the penurious Puerto Rican communities having a much greater infestation rate than the better-off Italian and Jewish groups. Confined populations, such as on board infested ships, are particularly at risk, whereas in communities with good hygienic standards cockroach infestation is rare.

Treatment

Bites require only simple sterile dressings. It is interesting to note that some Blattidae species secrete phenolic compounds which are antibacterial and antifungal (Roth and Alsop 1978), and one could speculate that this might account for the apparent absence of secondary infection after the majority of cockroach bites. For contact reactions simple antipruritic lotions should be sufficient, although some hypersensitivity responses may require subcutaneous adrenalin (Roth and Willis 1957).

Prevention

Prevention depends on control of the cockroach population. This is best achieved by good general housekeeping. Food should be stored in insect-proof containers, preferably in cupboards. Scraps of food should never be left lying about. Cleaning activities should be thorough and meticulous. Possible hiding places such as cracks in walls and plaster, holes in woodwork etc. should be kept in good repair. These measures apply to all types of building likely to be infested.

Established cockroach colonies may be encouraged to leave by the above measures. Their destruction may necessitate the use of insecticides. Strips of varnish incorporating pyrethrins or dichlorvos, poisoned bait for stray cockroaches, pressure sprays of pyrethrins for the hiding places and the use of persistent insecticides such as carbamates for more permanent effect are all effective (Guthrie and Tindall 1968).

References

Aeling JL (1974) Hypoanesthetic halos in Hawaii. Cutis 14: 541–544

Artault de Vevy S (1902) Pseudo-parasitisme des thrips. Bull Soc Zool Fr 27: 207–209

Bailey SF (1936) Thrips attacking man. Can Entomologist 68: 95–98

Bernton HS, Brown H (1967) Cockroach allergy II: The relation of infestation to sensitisation. South Med J 60: 852–855

Bernton HS, Brown H (1969) Insect allergy: The allergenic potential of the cockroach. South Med J 62: 1207–1210

Bernton HS, McMahon TP, Brown H (1972) Cockroach asthma. Br J Dis Chest 66: 61–66

Chinery M (1976) A field guide to the insects of Britain and Northern Europe, 2nd edn. Collins, London, pp 93–95

Durie J (1870) The cockroach. Nature 3: 27

Ebeling W (1975) Urban entomology. University of California, Division of Agricultural Science, Los Angeles, Cal, pp 217–244

Evans JW (1932) The bionomics and economic importance of *Thrips imaginis* Bagnall and special reference to the effects on apple production in Australia. Pamphlet No 30 of the Council of Scientific Industrial Research of Melbourne. Cited by Bailey (1936)

Goldstein N, Skipworth GB (1968) Papular eruption secondary to thrips bites. JAMA 203: 53–55

*Guthrie DM, Tindall AR (1968) The biology of the cockroach. Edward Arnold, London, pp 1–408

Heiser V (1936) A doctor's odyssey. Cape, London

James MT, Harwood RF (1969) In: Herms's medical entomology, 6th edn. Macmillan, London pp 115–122, 400

Johnston HB (1925) *Heliothrips indicus* (Bagnall) injurious to man in the Sudan. Entomologists Monthly Mag 61: 132-133

Kingsley C (1870) Cockroaches. Nature 3: 148

Korting A (1930) Beitrag zur Kenntnis der Lebensgewohnheiten und der phytophagen Bedeutung einiger an Gelierde lebenden Thysanopteren. Z Angew Entomol 16: 451–512. Cited by Bailey (1936)

*Lewis T (1973) Thrips: their biology, ecology and economic importance. Academic, London

Ludwig (1912) Die "Eintagsfliegen" von Loboe. Z Wiss Insekten-Biol 8: 71–72. Cited by Bailey (1936)

Nicols A (1870) The cockroach. Nature 3: 108

Patton WS (1931) Insects, ticks, mites and venomous animals of medical and veterinary importance. Part II Public health. HR Grubb, Croydon, 373–385

Pawlowsky EN, Stein AK (1930) Experimentelle Untersuchung über die Wirkung des Bisses von *Periplaneta orientalis* auf die Menschenhaut. Arch Dermatol Syphilis 162: 611–620

*Roth LH, Alsop DW (1978) Toxins of Blattaria. In: Bettini S (ed) Arthropod venoms. Springer, Berlin Heidelberg New York, pp 465–487 (Handbook of experimental pharmacology, vol 48)

*Roth LM, Willis ER (1957) The medical and veterinary importance of cockroaches. Smithsonian Miscellaneous Collections 134 (No 10), 1–147

Roth LM, Niegish WD, Stahl WH (1956) Occurrence of 2-Hexenal in the cockroach *Eurycotis floridana*. Science 123: 670–671

Senevet G (1922) Présence à Alger d'un insecte fort gênand pour l'homme. Bull Soc Hist Nat Afr Nord 13: 97–98

Williams CB (1921) A blood sucking thrips. Entomologist 54: 163–164

Zschunke E (1978) Contact urticaria, contact dermatitis and asthma from cockroaches. Arch Dermatol 114: 1715–1716

5 Infestation with Anoplura—Lice

The two genera of Anoplura or sucking lice, *Pediculus* and *Pthirus*, are obligatory parasites of man. [*Pthirus* is the correct zoological name for the pubic louse, because a misprint was inadvertently accepted by the International Committee of Zoological Nomenclature (Maunder 1983b). Nevertheless, infestation with pubic lice is correctly spelled *phthiriasis* according to the *Oxford English Dictionary*.]

Lice have a cosmopolitan distribution and are important primarily because the pediculi are vectors of typhus, trench and relapsing fevers (caused respectively by *Rickettsia prowazekii*, *R. quintana* and *Borrelia recurrentis*) and possibly of the dog tapeworm *Dipylidium carinum*, if the louse is accidentally swallowed (Maegraith 1971). They also cause much bodily discomfort to those infested and may involve enormous numbers of people. The colossal mortality from typhus in the past lead to intensive study of the louse and its biology and habits in an endeavour to control its activities. The literature is enormous. Nuttall (1917a) listed 639 publications up to 1917, and there have been at least as many since.

There is still a social stigma attached to "lousiness" and, although not directly caused by poor hygiene, pediculosis corporis is commonest in circumstances of bad hygiene. Head lice are still regarded by the public and a considerable proportion of the medical and nursing profession as a sign of dirtiness, whereas, as Maunder (1974) has rightly said, dirt does not cause lice to appear on a child's scalp. In fact they prosper more readily on a clean scalp rather than a neglected one (Maunder 1983b) and they come from another person. Pubic lice, which are still principally spread by promiscuous sexual intercourse, are discussed in more detail after *pediculi*.

Pediculus humanus

There are two forms of *Pediculus humanus*. One lives in the clothing of the infested person (*P. humanus corporis* or *P. humanus vestimentorum*) and the other on the human scalp (*P. humanus capitis*). For convenience, they will be referred to as *P. corporis* and *P. capitis* respectively. Morphologically they are so alike that even an expert of the calibre of Nuttall declared that he could not distinguish convincingly between them (Bacot 1917a). Neumann (1911) concluded that there were two distinct species and he was supported by Hase (1915), on the basis of minute morphological differences, and later by Busvine (1978) with further anatomical evidence. On the other hand, Howlett (1917) reared body lice on the scalp and head lice on the body and found that each took on the habits and characteristics of the other after three generations. Busvine (1977) also emphasised the long recognised fact that the two "species" could interbreed in captivity, although not, it seems, in nature. He considered that the head louse was probably the ancestral form deriving from the time when man was a generally hairy individual.

Morphology

Lice belonging to the genus *Pediculus* are wingless and flattened dorsoventrally. They are in general greyish (but see below) and their integument is tough and translucent (Busvine 1966). Figures 5.1 and 5.2 show the salient anatomical features. The antennae are short and three- to five-jointed, the nymphs having three joints and the adults five joints (Hase 1915). The eyes, placed laterally, are simple ocelli. The mouthparts are modified for piercing and sucking and are invaginated into the head. Anteriorly there is a small tube-like structure, the haustellum, armed with teeth, which are everted when the haustellum is extended. The

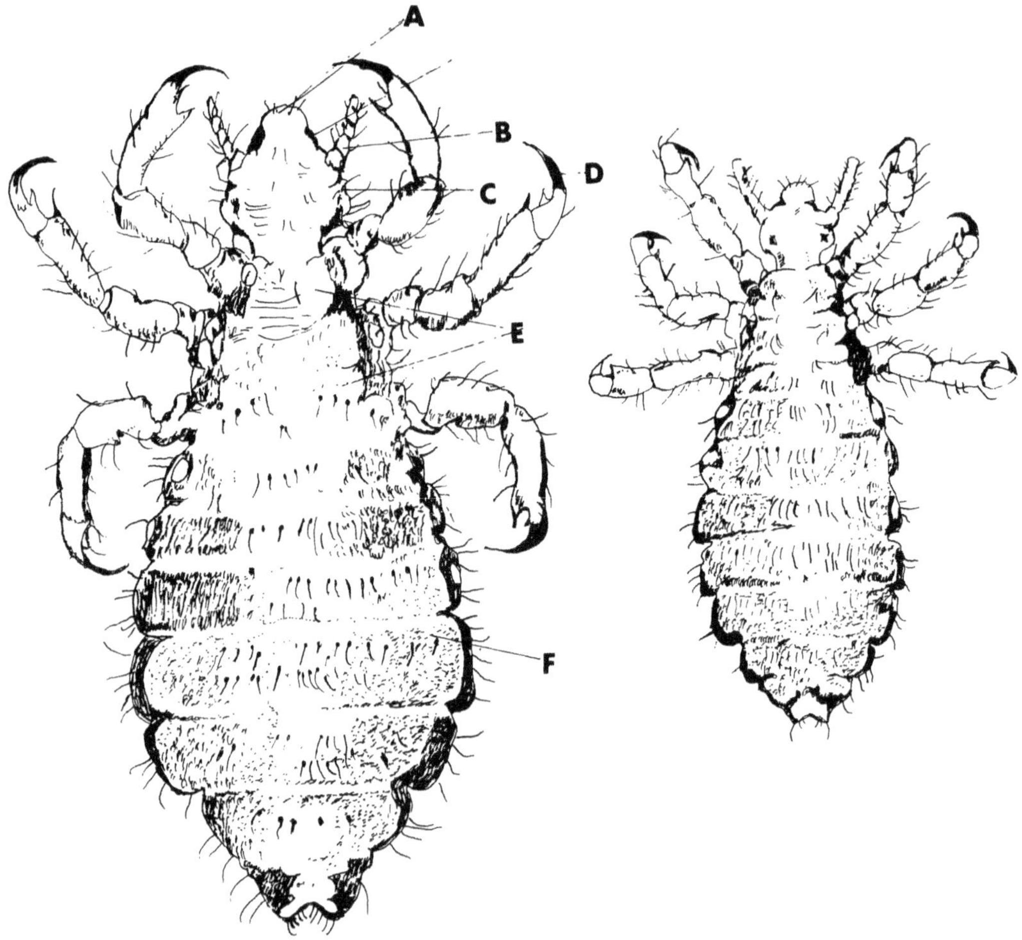

Fig. 5.1. Showing on the left a body louse and on the right a head louse drawn to the same scale. *A*, head; *B*, antenna; *C*, ocellar eye; *D*, claw on tarsus II; *E*, thorax; *F*, abdomen. (Courtesy of Stafford Miller Ltd, Hatfield)

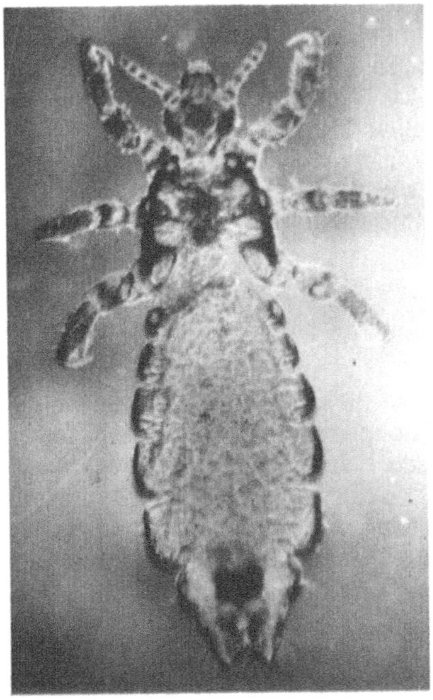

Fig. 5.2. Body louse as seen under light microscope. For comparison with Fig. 5.1.

mouth cavity consists of a buccal funnel and a cibarial pump. The cibarium is that part of the preoral cavity enclosed by the proximal part of the hypopharynx below and the clypeus in front. This cibarial cavity can be dilated by means of a dilator muscle, which pulls the roof upwards and forwards thus exerting suction and drawing food into the cavity. When the muscle relaxes, the cavity contracts and propels the contents backwards into the mouth and pharynx (Chapman 1971; Fig. 5.3). In the floor of the buccal cavity is the stylet sac housing the two stylets, which represent the mandible and maxilla, and an intermedial stylet functioning as a salivary duct. These structures act as the piercing mouthparts. There are no palps. The thoracic segments are fused and support three pairs of short legs, the tarsi of which each terminate in a claw adapted for clinging to hair. The abdomen has nine segments but the first two are rudimentary. It is twice as long as broad (compare with *Pthirus*). There are six abdominal spiracles (Buxton 1947).

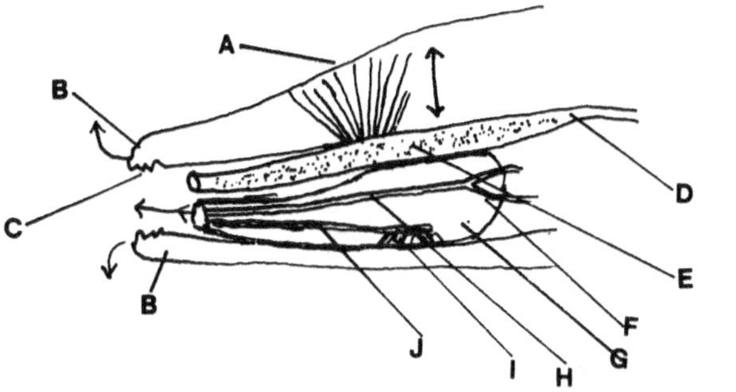

Fig. 5.3. Mouthparts of lice. *A*, cibarial dilator muscle; *B*, haustellum; *C*, teeth on haustellum (which fasten onto the skin of the host when the lips of the haustellum are everted in the direction of the *arrows*); *D*, pharynx; *E*, cavity of cibarial pump; *F*, salivary ducts; *G*, stylet sac. The *arrow* at the mouth of the stylet gutter shows the direction of its extension. The *arrow* by the cibarial dilator muscle shows how its contraction and relaxation will dilate and contract the cibarial pump. (Modified from Gordon and Lavoipierre 1962)

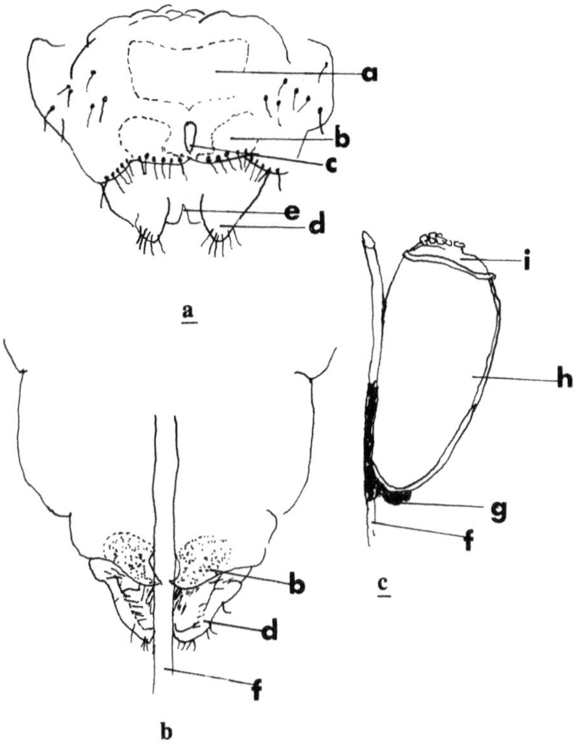

Fig. 5.4. a The posterior end of the abdomen of female *Pediculus*. **b** The method of grasping the hair by the posterior end of the abdomen for egg laying by *Pediculus*. **c** Egg cemented to hair. *a*, central shield; *b*, gonopod; *c*, genital aperture; *d*, grasping tubercles; *f*, hair; *g*, cement; *h*, egg; *i*, operculum. (Courtesy of Stafford Miller Ltd, Hatfield)

The males are rather smaller than the females in both variants in the rough proportion of five to six. The female body louse averages from 2.4 to 3.6 mm (maximum about 4 mm), whilst the corresponding head louse averages 2.4–3.3 mm. The female abdomen is rather larger than the male and terminates in two large lobes with gonopods and a central shield (Fig. 5.4). The male abdomen curves upwards at the tip so that the anal and sexual orifices are on the upper surface. This arrangement accounts for the copulatory position with the male crawling beneath the female.

Lice take on the colour of their background, greyish white if parasitic on Europeans (Fig. 5.5) and blackish on Africans and other dark-skinned races (Nuttall 1919). Moreover, the offspring from pairing black and white specimens are equally adaptable (Hase 1915; Sikora 1917). No matter to what ethnic race the host belongs, the parasite louse is the same species (Buxton 1947; see also p. 44).

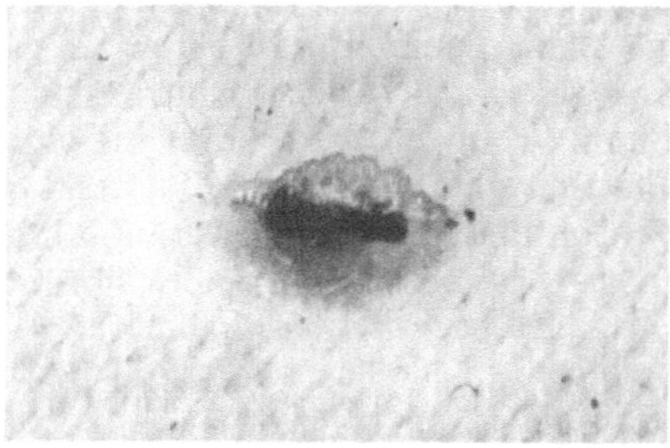

Fig. 5.5. Solitary body louse on cloth. Most of the insect seen here is abdomen. The head, thorax and legs can only be seen faintly.

Biology

Body lice live on the host's clothing and feed off his body, whilst head lice live and feed on the scalp. The method of feeding is the same in both instances, and probably the same for *Pthirus*: The haustellum is thrust forwards; the teeth penetrate the skin and are then everted and fix the mouthparts firmly to the skin. The stylets are pushed forwards by protractor muscles through the wound. Saliva is injected through one of the stylets and the latter probe for a blood vessel. When one is eventually found and pierced, blood flows; it is prevented from clotting by salivary anticoagulant and is sucked up by the action of the cibarial pump into the pharynx. The pump's action prevents reverse flow and the result is a rhythmic filling and emptying of the pump into the insect's gut (Nuttall 1917c).

Feeding under natural conditions is frequent and intermittent, four or five times daily (Maunder 1983b). According to Nuttall it starts from the moment the first nymph emerges from the egg. He also noted that lice are seldom engorged under these circumstances. This implies that they are never really hungry, that is to say they are adequately fed. They only feed to excess when they are ravenous and this often causes their death from rupture of the gut. Moreover, more blood can be extracted by frequent satisfying meals than by infrequent engorgement. Hungry lice are attracted by warmth but not if the temperature is too high. Lloyd (1919) has pointed out that lice, in addition to being slow feeders, defaecate during feeding, an action which could result in inoculation by scratching of organisms such as *Borrelia recurrentis* in the faeces.

Why are some persons attractive to lice and others not? Buxton (1947) thought it might be due to the odour or chemical composition of sweat. Features attractive to lice are body surface temperatures of 29°–30°C and relative humidity (RH) of 75%, the human body and possibly faecal odour and the darkness beneath clothing. Repellent influences are temperatures below 27°C or above 32°C, a wet sweaty surface, neutral smelling fabrics and light (Marples 1965). Some individuals are quite insusceptible to bites (MacLeod and Craufurd-Benson 1941). For oviposition, the female louse clasps either a hair or cloth fibre with the gonopods, the space between which is of the approximate diameter of a hair but is adjustable. It is assisted in holding on by claspers (Fig. 5.4b). The louse slides down the hair to the skin surface and then moves upwards again. Whilst going upwards the egg is extruded through the genital opening and at once firmly fixed to the hair by cement (Fig. 5.4c), which is secreted into the uterus by special glands and flows in front of the broader part of the egg, coating it as it is expelled. The eggs are orientated so that the cap (the operculum) points distally along the hair (Fig. 5.6). The whole process takes about 17 s; as the cement sets almost at once the louse occasionally gets fatally entangled in it. This cement cannot be dissolved without at the same time destroying the hair (Nutull 1917c).

The operculum is provided with perforations which enable the developing embryo to obtain air. Hatching is achieved by accumulation of swallowed air and amniotic fluid behind the embryo, pushing it against the operculum. The latter is pierced by tiny cutting hooks on the embryonic head and the nymph is forcibly expelled head first. This is a speedy process so as to avoid entrapping the nymph in the rapidly solidifying amniotic fluid, as may occasionally occur (Nuttall 1917c; Buxton 1947).

Body lice are gregarious and eggs tend to be laid in the same place, the female returning again and again to oviposit. For this reason the eggs (nits) are concentrated in the regions of preference of the female louse, such as the bands of trousers and skirts (especially the kilt, according to Nuttall 1917c) and the underarm and side seams of garments which are worn next to the skin (e.g. vest or shirt) (Fig. 5.7). Less common areas are jacket underarm seams, the central fork seam of the trousers and the jacket collar. On one occasion the present writer observed a solid halo of eggs, 2 cm in diameter, around each of the trouser buttons used for attaching braces, as if the button had been sewn onto a background of minute beadwork. Gratz (1973) cited the finding of Shawaby and his colleagues that in Egyptian villages it was only necessary to inspect neck bands for eggs to confirm a diagnosis of lousiness. Nuttall (1917c) also noted that in certain African tribes who wore no clothes, infestation was manifested by their necklaces being covered with eggs (nits). Most observers agree that when body lice deposit eggs on clothing they choose the inner surface nearest the skin for preference. It has been the experience of most workers that body lice occasionally deposit eggs on body hair, especially the perineal and pubic and axillary areas, and even the scalp has been involved (Nuttall 1917c). Head lice, except in very heavy infestation, seldom lay more than one egg per hair, being less liable to return to the same place to oviposit and less gregarious than body lice (Bacot 1916b). Pubic lice, on the other hand, often lay several eggs on the same hair.

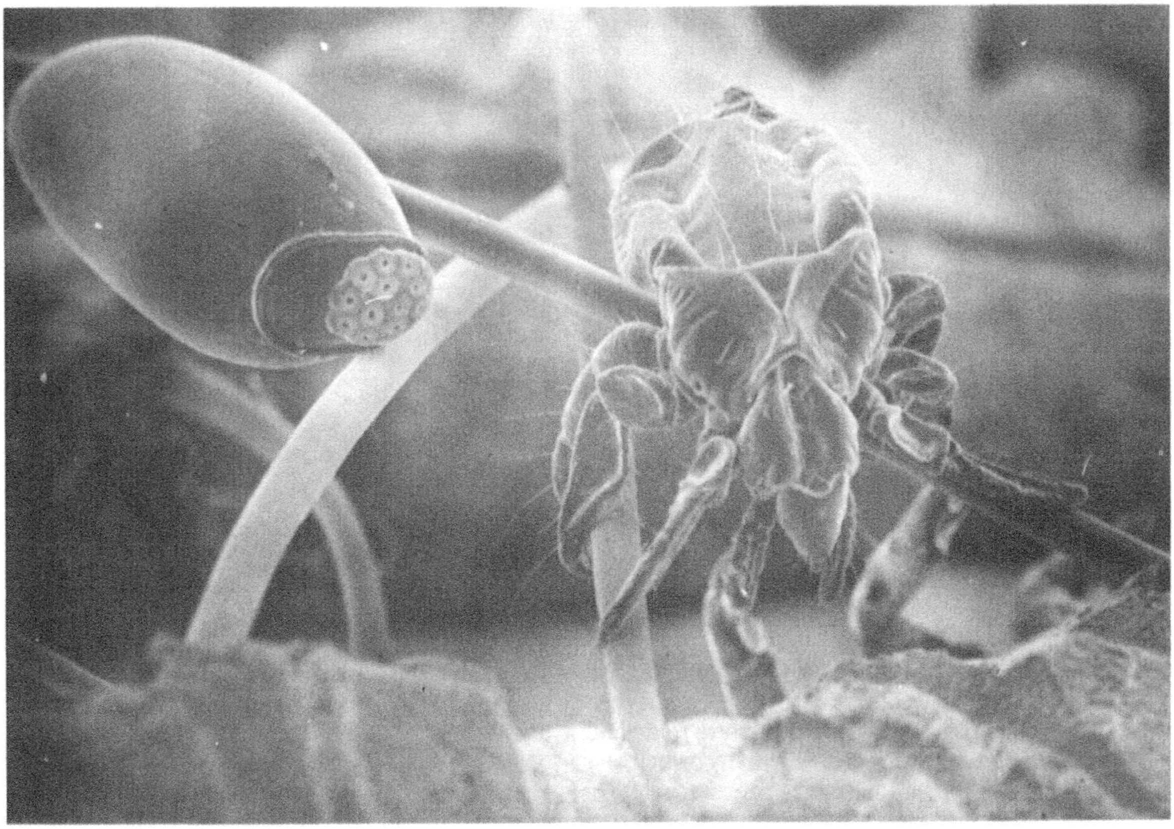

Fig. 5.6. A young head louse and an unhatched egg. This young louse has just completed its first moult. Shortly it will feed and swell to a larger size before its new skin becomes fully hardened. An unhatched egg is attached to the same hair which is supporting the louse. The exit-lid is clearly shown. This bears a group of about 16 thick-rimmed openings associated with respiration. (From Maunder 1983b, by kind permission of the author and the Editor of the *Proceedings of the Royal Institution of Great Britain*. Scanning electron micrograph taken by Mr. M.D. Smith, Department of Electron Microscopy, London School of Hygiene and Tropical Medicine)

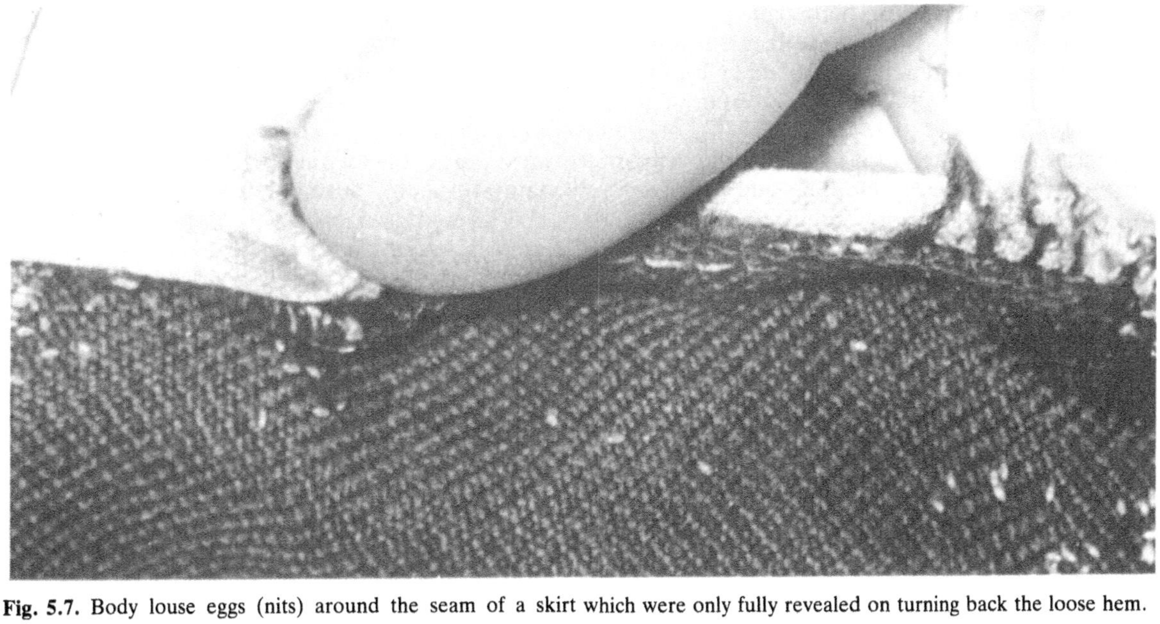

Fig. 5.7. Body louse eggs (nits) around the seam of a skirt which were only fully revealed on turning back the loose hem.

Table 5.1. Life cycle periods for the three species of Anoplura parasitic on man

Stage	*Pediculus corporis* a	b	*Pediculus capitis* a	b	*Pthirus pubis* c
Incubation period	7–9	7–10[e]	7		6–8
First nymphal	3	3–5 }			5–6 }
Second nymphal	3	4 }	$8\frac{1}{2}$		4–6 } 13–17
Third nymphal	3	3–5 }			4–5 }
Adult female to gravid female	$1–1\frac{1}{2}$	2–4			1–2
Egg to adult	17–19	17–25	15–16		22–27
Longevity	20[d]	32 male 34 female	9–10	30 male 23 female	17–22
Egg output	275–3000	295	110	141	25

[a] According to Buxton (1947) and Busvine (1977)
[b] According to Bacot (1917b)
[c] According to Nuttall (1917c)
[d] 20 days for lice in captivity. Nuttall (1917c) gave 28–29 days for similar conditions and between 30 and 46 days for different conditions of temperature and feeding. Maunder (1983b) gave 60 days as the absolute limit.
[e] Hase (1915) gave this period as 5 days at 37°C.

The approximate number of eggs laid by the females of each species under optimal conditions, together with details of the life cycle, are indicated in Table 5.1. This output can be varied principally by regularity of feeding and ambient temperature. Regular frequent feeding of captive lice produced a better egg output than infrequent feeding (Gooding 1963). Increased feeding would increase output but not fertility (Bacot 1917b), although there is a limit to this since overfeeding is injurious to the louse (see below). A rather disturbing feature noted by Fleming and Ludwig (1964) was the tendency for increased egg output to occur in insecticide-resistant lice. The hatching of eggs was greatly reduced by lowering the ambient temperature and it ceased altogether between 15.4°C and 18.6°C (59.7°–65.5°F) (Bacot 1917b). On the other hand, whilst heating to 53.6°C (128.5°F) for 5 min was fatal to lice (Buxton 1947), a similar temperature used for sterilising clothing and bedding was not always certain to kill eggs, especially if the use of the steriliser was inadequate. Dore (1916) observed that larvae had hatched from eggs which had gone through this process 7 days earlier. Such an event was immortalised by "Ian Hay" (1915), the pseudonym of Maj. Gen. Ian Hay Beith, in his book about Kitchener's volunteer army in World War I. Two Scottish soldiers were inspecting their blankets after disinfestation: First soldier, "I see they're a' there yet." Second soldier, "Aye but they must've got an awfu' fricht."

The number of lice and eggs on an individual varies greatly. Persons possibly or recently infested who take appropriate steps to deal with the matter promptly will seldom have more than one or two lice and perhaps no nits. But what about an established infestation? How many lice could one expect to find? James and Harwood (1969) and Duffy (1971) have both noted that up to 30 000 have been found in clothing of a single individual. Thomas à Becket was said to have been bathed in a wriggling mass of lice at his death (Busvine 1966). Busvine quoted Buxton as stating that under optimal conditions some four to five thousand lice could be expected on an individual within 3 months but only 10% of this figure if conditions were unfavourable. Bacot (1917a) had calculated that up to 4160 offspring could develop from a single female in its lifetime; Dore (1916) put the figure at 8000. Nuttall (1917a) estimated 1918 offspring in the lifetime of a single female and 112 778 in her daughter's lifetime of 48 days altogether. These calculations were based on average egg production and took natural wastage during development into account. The present writer has seen only two massive infestations of this order; both were on the scalp and in each there were several thousand lice, apart from nits. In the vast majority of cases there are several factors which mitigate against such large populations, whichever species is involved. Apart from mortality during development, there is a diminishing egg output both below and above the optimum temperature of 28°–32°C. No eggs hatch below 22°C and all are killed eventually between 10°C and 45°C. Egg laying is inhibited above 39°C (Nuttall 1917c). Within the inhibitory extremes but outside the optimal temperatures there is also a reduced percentage hatch and a lengthened incubation period. Relative humidity also plays a part; lice prefer an RH of 75% or less. Louse activity, including egg laying, is discouraged on moist skin surfaces (Marples 1965). These factors may all considerably reduce the total louse population. Moreover, there is a tendency for the offspring of a particular pair of lice to be all of the same sex, which will of course inhibit population growth of both head and body lice (Buxton 1947). Population excess seems to result in hostility to the females until the numbers fall to an optimal level. Maunder (1983b) has noted that there are in general four females to every male on an infested scalp, but that the proportion can be varied for other reasons, the chief being that two types of male seem to occur. One type produces offspring which are of either sex in equal numbers or even all males, whilst the other gives rise to the four to one proportion favouring females. Buxton (1941) showed that the head louse population tended to be proportional to the hair mass of the host. Other limiting factors to population growth are the destructive effects of scratching, deliberate removal of lice by the host and secondary infection. With body lice the removal of clothing at night reduces both egg laying and pairing because of the reduced ambient temperature. Marples (1965) has pointed out that removal of clothing may have a lethal effect on developing eggs, the survival of which is greatly dependent on the continuous wearing of the clothing (Hase 1915). Storage of clothing for one month totally removes all possibility of viable eggs surviving.

Movements of lice are haphazard. They meander in all directions but tend to prefer horizontal walking. Their speed increases with slight rises of temperature. According to Nuttall (1917c), under optimal conditions a louse can cover 1 m in 2 min 43 s. Long distances can be covered. Marples (1965) cites 15 ft (5 m) as the distance travelled in a meandering fashion. Hase (1915) said that migration tended to begin as the temperature approached 35°C.

Clinical Appearances of Infestation

Pediculosis Corporis

In the great majority of cases of pediculosis corporris there is only one symptom—itch. It is intermittent and is commonest at night, but not exclusively so. It can be very severe and causes indiscriminate scratching, which may be quite frantic at times (Fig. 5.8). Some persons deny itching, but, as Dubreuilh and Beille (1895) remarked, the presence of scratch marks is irrefutable proof of the incorrectness of their assertion. Massive infestation may sometimes give rise to systemic symptoms, which are discussed below (see p. 38).

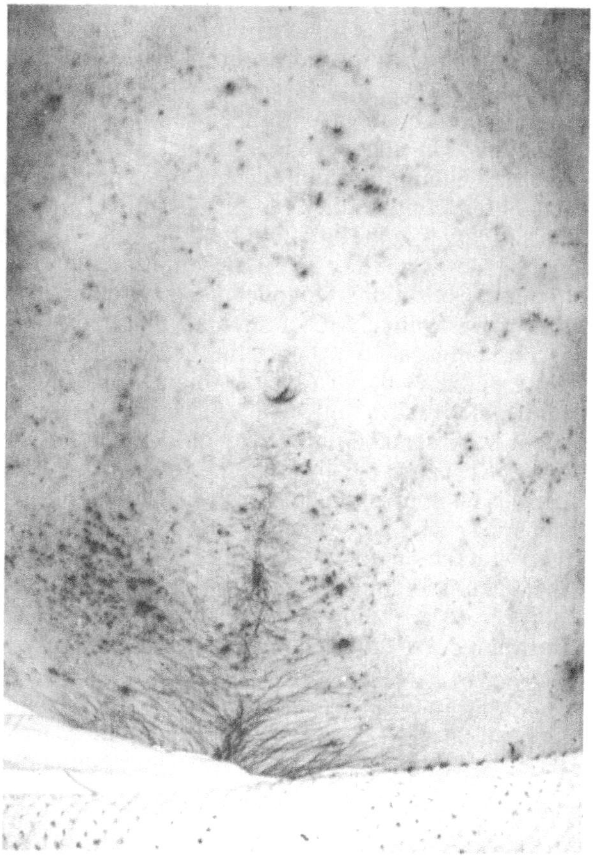

Fig. 5.8. Pediculosis corporis showing numerous excoriated bite marks and small blood crusts on the trunk in a man with a heavy infestation.

The lesion caused by the louse bite has been described by several workers (Greenough 1867; Dubreuilh and Beille 1895; Lloyd 1919; Touraine 1947; Duffy 1971) as a small red papule some 3–4 mm or less in diameter, often with a tiny central red punctum. Sometimes in debilitated persons there may be a purpuric halo (Touraine 1947). Greenough indicated that if these lesions were not scratched they would disappear in 24 h. Lloyd reported that they disappeared within an hour but often reappeared and then itched. When scratched a tiny red crust appears on the surface. Rook (1979) stated that "investigations on volunteers show that in previously unexposed subjects the bites provoke only pin-point, red macules. After 7 days or more small weals or more persistent papules develop and pruritus first becomes troublesome." This suggests much the same range of immunological reactions as that associated with other arthropod bites. In support of this are Hase's four groups of patients, arranged according to their reactions: (1) unattacked, (2) attacked and sensitive, (3) immunity acquired, and (4) symptomless but bitten continuously (cited by Nuttall 1917b). This is very like the situation described by Gordon (1950; see Chap. 2). There are differing opinions about sensitisation. Maunder (1983a) maintained that it was unlikely to occur until the victim had received at least 10 000 bites (at the rate of five per louse per day) because of the minute amounts of (antigenic) saliva injected. Sensitisation could occur with regular biting and only 20 or 30 lice present because persons may be infested for long periods without complaint. However, mild infestations may also cause itching within a few weeks. The vital factor would seem to be time rather than the amount of antigen injected, since the innoculation period for scabies is only about 1 month and the amount of antigen concerned with *Sarcoptes* is very much less than with pediculosis.

All the lesions seen are the result of scratching and chronicity. The scratch marks are quite characteristic of lousiness. They are indiscriminate, linear, often consisting of three or four parallel lines caused by the fingernails of one hand. They are all within reach of the fingers, orientated in the direction of scratching and are most pronounced on the scapular areas and the flanks; however, no region is spared except the face, forearms, hands and feet (Dubreuilh and Beille 1895).

Pigmentation is a feature of pediculosis corporis and takes two forms. In the average infestation, which is not too heavy and usually of long standing, there is a scattered pigmentation mainly on the lower trunk and most marked in the region of old lesions (see Fig. 5.9). This appearance is frequent in unsuspected cases admitted to hospital for other reasons and discovered during routine examination. The other type of pigmentation is less common but characteristic of heavy infestation. It consists of a brownish-bronze type of diffuse pigmentation, which is most marked over the genitalia, groins, upper inner thighs and pubic areas; axillae are particularly heavily pigmented and can be almost black (Greenough 1867; Greenhow 1876; Dubreuilh and Beille 1895; Touraine 1947; see Fig. 5.10). Such cases have been mistaken for Addison's disease, and the writer's case was sent to him as a possible example of mycosis fungoides.

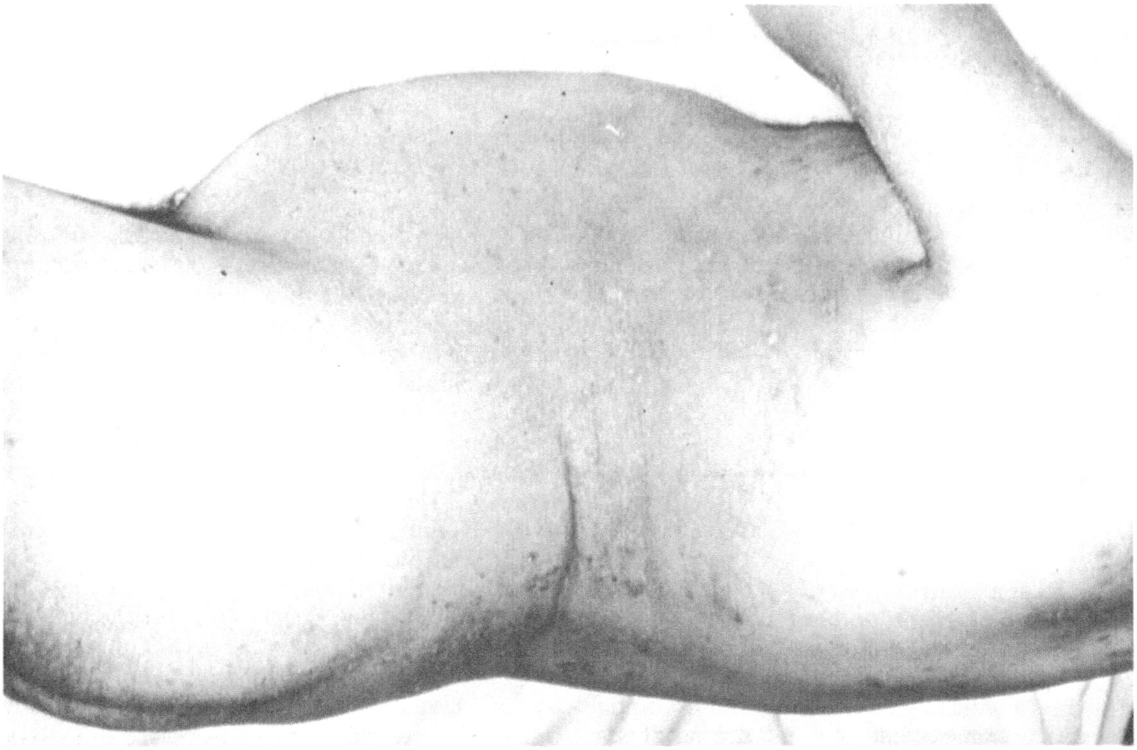

Fig. 5.9. Chronic scattered pigmentation of long-standing moderate pediculosis corporis. This appearance is not infrequently seen in patients unsuspected of being lousy who are admitted to hospital for some other reason.

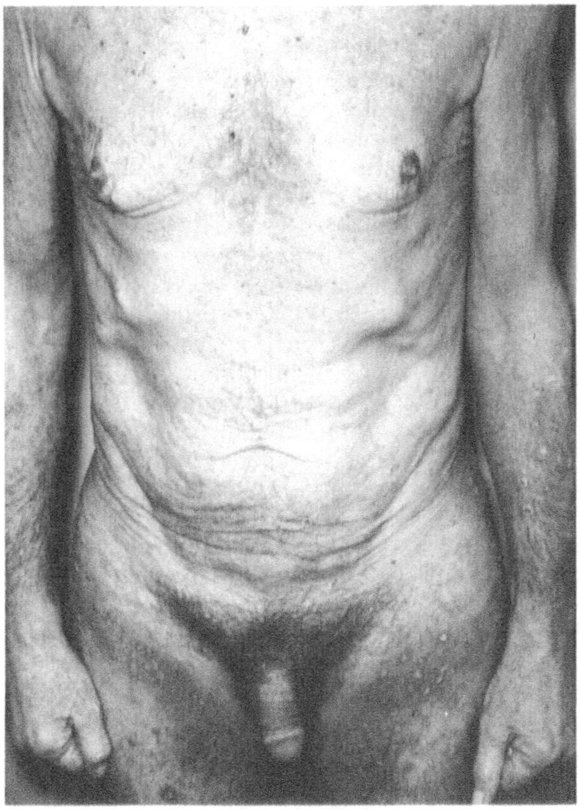

Fig. 5.10. Heavy pigmentation, especially in the pubic area, in a man with severe long-standing pediculosis corporis.

There is seldom any difficulty in recognising the true cause. It may be made more confusing by the occasional occurrence of patchy brown pigmentation of the oral mucosa (Greenhow 1876; Dubreuilh and Beille 1895). It should be remembered that in certain areas mucosal pigmentation may be racial, as in the patients reported by Brault and Montpelier (1914a,b) with mixed *Pediculus corporis* and *Pthirus pubis* infestations.

In long-standing infestation the skin takes on a rough thickened appearance with some fine furfuraceous scaling, possibly due to lack of washing as much as anything. There may be secondary infection with pustulation or impetigo. This is most marked in those areas where the skin can be damaged by the fingernails, e.g. the front of the shins (Fig. 5.11), and is due to organisms from the patient's own fingernails and not to any on the louse. In occasional cases, uncommon in mild infestation, there may be secondary eczematisation with lichenification and encrustation. In heavy or long-standing infestation there may be moderate lymphadenopathy. Nits or lice can occasionally be found on the body, usually in the axillary and pubic areas, but only with heavy infestation (Fig. 5.12). Very occasionally they may be found in the perineal area only, with no other involvement. In such cases the only complaint is pruritus ani.

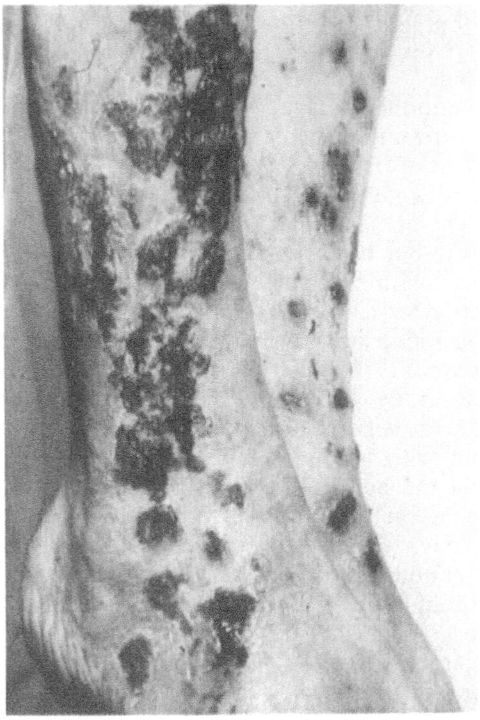

Fig. 5.11. Severe ecthymatous lesions with ulceration and encrustation in a man with pediculosis. These lesions resulted from scratching the louse bites and introducing infection with the fingernails.

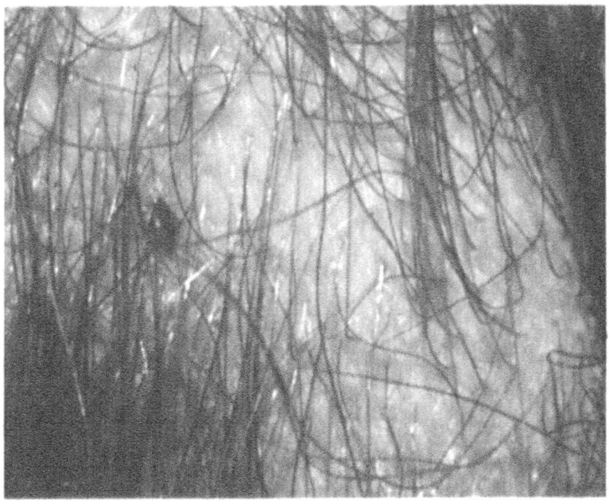

Fig. 5.12. Body louse in the pubic region in a man heavily infested with pediculosis corporis. One dark-coloured louse can be seen amongst the pubic hair at the base of the penis.

Whether these are head or body lice is difficult to say. Lydston (1892) reported such an instance as being due to *P. capitis* but produced no proof. The present writer has seen a case of long-standing pruritus ani associated with nits in the trouser seam covering the affected areas and has assumed they were those of *P. corporis*. There were no lice anywhere on the body or elsewhere in the clothing at the time.

As mentioned above, with very heavy or prolonged infestation there may be systemic effects, consisting of malaise, weakness, headache and fever and a generalised macular eruption (Duffy 1971). The present writer has not encountered this personally but has seen cases of marked anaemia associated with excessively lousy patients. A good description of similar systemic effects in persons feeding captive lice for long periods has been given by Moore (1918), by Hirschfelder and Moore (1919) and by Maunder (1983b). The reaction started with general tiredness, irritability and depression, with a continuous, dull and sometimes severe headache. Chills and fever; which was most pronounced in the afternoon, then occurred, lasting about 3 days. The fever seemed to occur sometimes within an hour of feeding lice but more often some 6 or 7 hours later. Adenopathy was evident after 1–4 days. A macular eruption rather like rubella, consisting of macules 2–3 mm in diameter, then appeared on the neck, shoulders, upper anterior chest and back. In one case this was accompanied by blisters on the forearms where the lice had fed. The symptoms in all the patients appeared to be associated with the actual feeding of the lice. Moore suggested that the syndrome resembled trench fever, which prompted him to add that some of the symptoms of the latter might be due to louse toxin. No serological studies were done or have been done to ascertain whether the reaction is due to rickettsial organisms or other infective agents, and not to this toxin. When feeding the lice was stopped, the condition cleared after 10 days or so, but recurred when feeding restarted.

Once lice have been effectively destroyed and the clothing disinfested there are no sequelae. Laurent (1901) recorded what was purported to be death due to louse bites in a child, but it is evident from the description that the cause of death was the staphylococcal scalded skin syndrome associated with secondary infection.

Pediculosis Capitis

It is generally accepted that the only complaint in the early stages of all cases and for any stage of moderate cases of pediculosis capitis is itch, which is usually localised. To this symptom in children Maunder (1977) has added restlessness, irritability, inattention and dullness at school, resulting from continuous scratching. This scratching quickly gives rise to secondary infection with tenderness or actual pain in the affected areas together with painful swelling of cervical lymph glands.

Examination of the head may show no abnormality at a superficial glance but careful inspection will reveal one or more eggs (nits) firmly attached to the hair. These are characteristically all the same size, about 1 mm long, lying at a similar angle to the hair and shiny grey in colour (Fig. 5.13; but see below, p. 39). In heavy infestations there may be huge numbers of nits (Fig. 5.14), but often only one or two can be found and these only after careful inspection of the whole scalp in detail. The areas where they are most likely to be found are just above the ears and over the suboccipital region. In older infestations they can be found on the shaft of the hair 15 cm or more from its emergence from the follicle. Their position will enable the examiner to assess how long the infestation has been present, bearing in mind that the position is

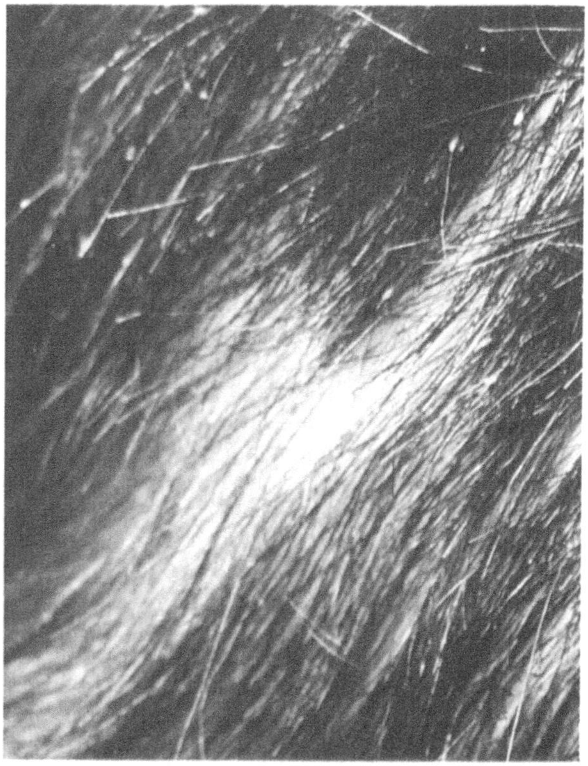

Fig. 5.13. Pediculosis capitis. Note the few scattered empty white eggs (nits) on the scalp hairs. They are all oval, lying at a slight angle to the hair to which they are attached, and are all the same size.

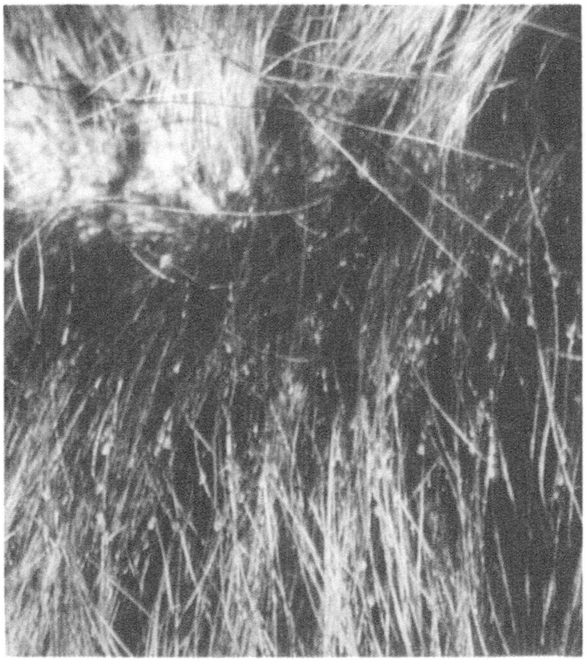

Fig. 5.14. Pediculosis capitis showing large numbers of eggs (nits) on the scalp hairs. One or two hairs are evenly coated with fragmented hair lacquer. There is also some crusting and scaling amongst the hairs. It is in areas at the roots of such hairs where active lice may be found.

fixed by an insoluble cement, that the egg was originally deposited in the angle between the hair and the scalp and that hair grows about 0.5 mm daily. Thus nits found 15 cm from the follicular orifice have been present approximately 9 months, the length of time taken for the hair to grow 15 cm. On the other hand, nits found very close to the skin surface indicate a recent infestation or continued activity of a long-standing complaint. These latter nits may contain viable embryos. Maunder (1981) has pointed out several characteristics of different sorts of head lice which have valuable diagnostic or prognostic significance. New viable eggs are laid close to the scalp and are a creamy yellow colour (see Fig. 5.8). Empty eggshells are white. Eggs which are red or black contain a dead embryo, but if the latter has not developed before death the egg assumes a flattened collapsed appearance. Very small or deformed eggs laid by dying lice may appear after treatment with anticholinesterases. Eggshells which have been present for a very long time may be worn down to only a fragment attached to the hair.

Lice may also be seen on the scalp; however, because they are mobile and because the immature forms, which are more active than the adults, greatly outnumber the adults, they may be difficult to see unless specifically sought. First-stage nymphs, which start to feed almost as soon as they are hatched are usually red because of contained blood. They resemble a pinpoint blood crust but they move—hence the name "mechanised dandruff" given to lice by soldiers. It may be necessary to watch such a blood crust for movment before reaching a decision about its nature. Older nymphs and adults are greyish or blackish according to the hair colour of the patients. They may be seen on the hair surface occasionally, but it is usually necessary to search for them amongst the hair to observe them feeding or walking about. Eggs may be found without any lice present. These have been laid by lice on a scalp inadequately treated with anticholinesterases; the mobile forms are ultimately destroyed but the eggs remain; the embryos develop but are unable to escape because they too are paralysed. Conversely lice may sometimes be seen without eggs on scalps inadequately treated with these insecticides; the residual effect kills off these lice before they can lay any eggs (Maunder 1981).

Secondary infection is almost always manifested as discrete or confluent lesions of impetigo contagiosa and may extend beyond the confines of the scalp. It is true to say that all cases of impetigo of the face and neck should raise the question of pediculosis of the scalp as being the underlying instigator. Very often the secondary infection overshadows the basic pediculosis (Fig. 5.15) and the latter can easily be overlooked by a busy, harrassed physician. Encrustation and purulent discharge together with cervical adenopathy are the salient features.

In gross infestations which have been neglected the number of lice may be very great and secondary infection may involve the whole scalp. The result is a confluent, purulent mass of matted hair, lice, nits, crusts and purulent discharge. The whole has a most unpleasant odour and looks more like a decaying bird's nest than a head of hair (Fig. 5.16). Careful inspection will reveal a gently undulating mass of lice beneath what has come to be known as plica polonica, from its prevalence in northeastern Europe at the beginning of this century. This condition is associated with poverty and neglect. The present writer has seen about half a dozen such cases in Glasgow over the past 30 years. In one particular case, of a "down and out" alcoholic man with hair about 30 cm long, secondary infection was not so pronounced, but the louse population on his scalp was astronomical. He shed lice and nits indiscriminately like largesse as he walked along. He was incidentally ill and anaemic, but recovered completely after removal of the parasites.

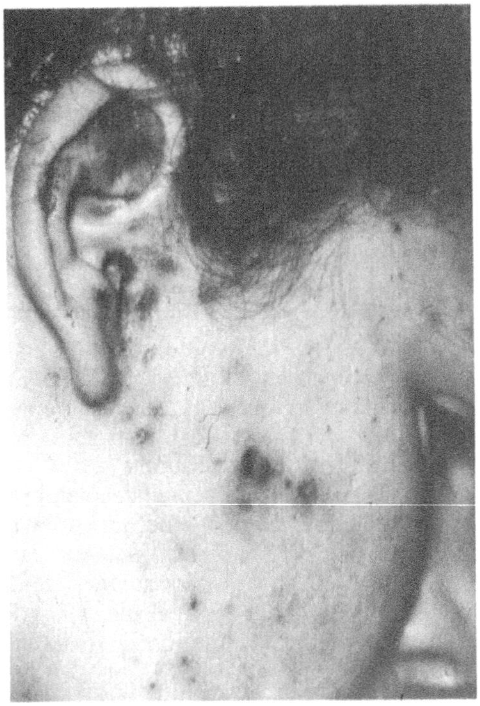

Fig. 5.15. Impetigo contagiosa of face, neck and ear extending into the scalp. This was associated with an underlying pediculosis capitis. A few nits can just be discerned amongst the tangled hair.

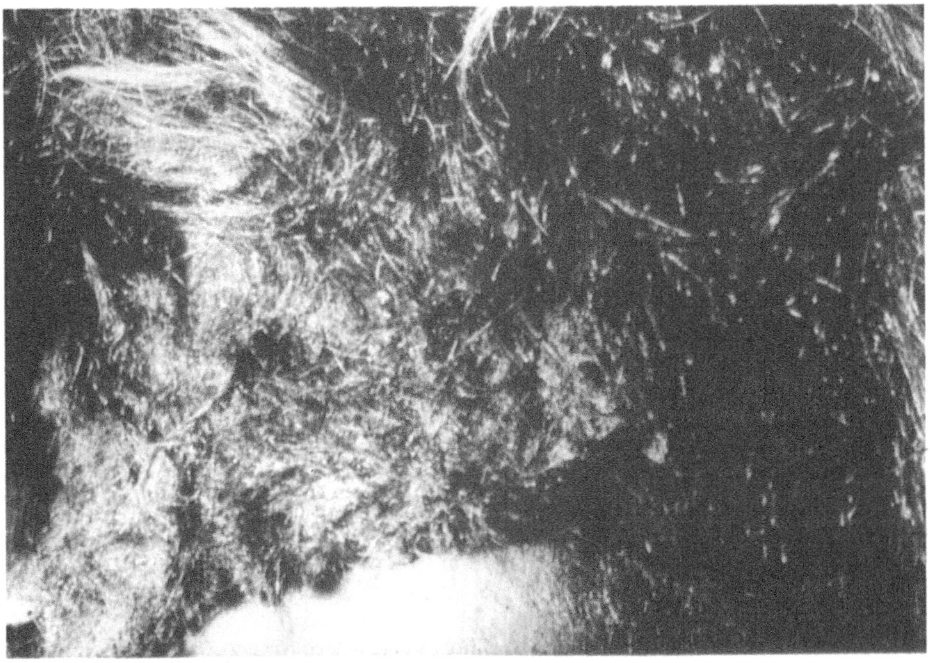

Fig. 5.16. Gross pediculosis capitis resulting in the so-called plica polonica. The entire scalp is involved and all the hair is inextricably matted together. Beneath this tangled mass will be found a smelly, purulent discharge and hundreds of lice in all stages of development.

Diagnosis

Pediculosis Corporis

Pediculosis corporis is diagnosed on two main points: (1) an excoriated, pigmented appearance of the body of the patient, as already described (see Fig. 5.9), and (2) the finding of nits and lice in the clothing. These must be deliberately sought by examining each garment separately. The most likely places to find nits are along the seams of the inner surface of the underclothes, especially vest and shirt, in trouser and skirt seams around the waist and inside the collar of shirts and jackets. It may be necessary to fold back the loose hem to see the nits (see Fig. 5.7). Active lice are most commonly seen walking or standing still on the inner surface of the innermost garment. They can appear on all garments but the number rapidly diminishes in the outer garments. They sometimes feign death (Nuttall 1917f). Very occasionally they can be encountered walking on the skin (see Fig. 5.12). A large number of red (and often dead) lice found in clothing is said to be a strong indication of typhus. Such lice have a ruptured gut as the result of presence of huge numbers of *Rickettsia prowazekii*. An occasional red louse may be seen as the result of overfeeding without typhus being present (Maunder 1981). The most remarkable situation in which to find lice is inside a plaster of Paris splint. The present writer has seen this on two occasions. In each instance the plaster had been applied for a fracture of the wrist; viable nits or lice had either been covered unsuspectingly or else the lice had crawled inside to oviposit. Whatever the explanation, they proliferated remarkably and when the casts were removed the appearance was as shown in Fig. 5.17. There were literally hundreds, possibly thousands of lice, which had appeared within 28 days and were in all stages of development. The remarkable fact was that the skin showed no clinical evidence of being lousy and there was no itch.

The differential diagnosis for pediculosis corporis includes those skin disorders in which generalised itch is prominent, such as scabies, eczema, lichen planus, dermatitis herpetiformis and symptomatic pruritus of such conditions as primary biliary cirrhosis, carcinoma of various internal organs, thyroid disease etc. If lice are found on exmination there is little difficulty, whilst the various skin conditions mentioned have their own particular features. Idiopathic itch may cause some trouble until full investigation reveals the likely cause. Scabies is said to occur along with pediculosis corporis but this is contrary to the experience of the majority of physicians.

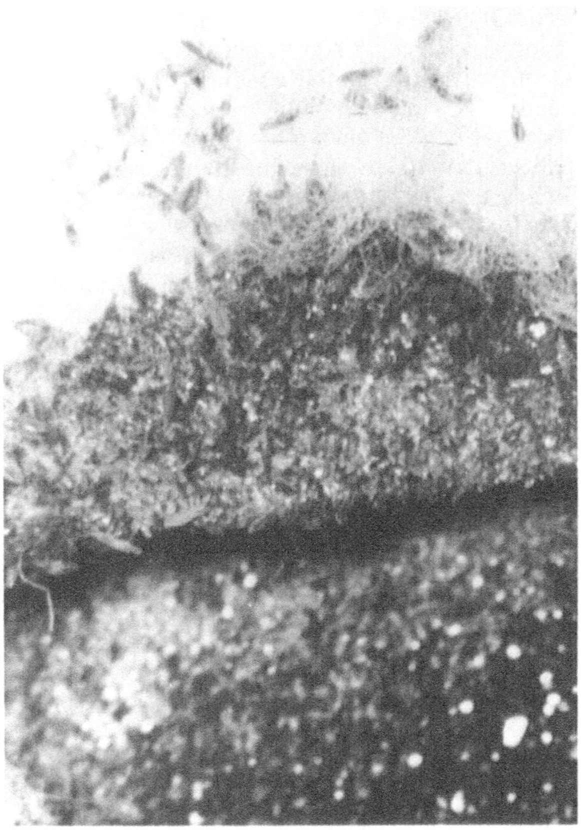

Fig. 5.17. Body lice in large numbers inside a plaster of Paris splint. The black mass in the lower half of the picture is cotton wool impregnated with altered blood and louse faeces. Many free lice can be seen on the uncontaminated cotton wool at the *top* of the picture.

Pediculosis Capitis

Pediculosis capitis is also very easy to diagnose providing it is considered in the causation of itching scalp or of impetigo of scalp, neck or face. The essential factors in making a diagnosis of pediculosis capitis are not only to consider these points but also to make a meticulous search for evidence of lice or nits. Failure to do so will inevitably result in many cases being missed. Care should be taken to avoid mistaking hair lacquer for nits. The application of lacquer is common nowadays in women's hairdressing techniques. If overdone, the lacquer will later break up into small fragments attached to the hairs, and these can be erroneously regarded as nits, as can dandruff. A hand lens may be necessary to convince oneself which is which. Dandruff (epidermal scales) is not attached to the hair, the particles are of variable size and can easily be brushed aside. Nits and lacquer are firmly fixed to the hair. Nits are of uniform size, attached to one side of the hair, ovoid in shape and about 1 mm long (see also p. 39). Lacquer encircles the hair uniformly, is of variable length from 1 to 3 or 4 mm and affects a large number of hairs (Fig. 5.18). Nothing is more embarrassing for both patient and doctor than to have a diagnosis of pediculosis made when the "nits" are, in fact, fragments of lacquer on the hair. Apart from impetigo and secondary infection, the absence of any other skin lesions such as diffuse scaling of psoriasis is noticeable. The exudation of acute eczema could be mistaken for pediculosis, except for the absence of nits or lice. Another factor of importance in this respect is the presence of other patients with pediculosis capitis within the family.

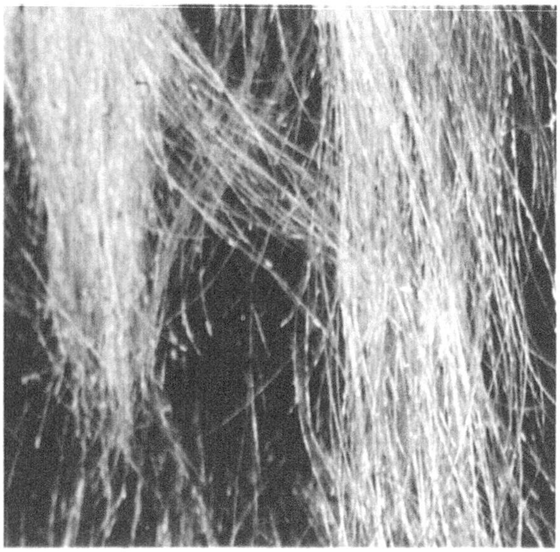

Fig. 5.18. Broken-up fragments of hair lacquer on scalp hairs. These can easily be mistaken for nits by the inexperienced or cursory examiner (see text).

Epidemiology

There are differences between the epidemiology of head and body lice which make it convenient to discuss them separately. The factors concerned play a considerable part in the persistence and spread of the two conditions so that a clear understanding is valuable in treatment and control. Treating an individual is relatively easy, but eradicating the disorder from a community is much more difficult. In order to put the importance of the two conditions into proper perspective, remembering in addition that the epidemiology of body lice is the same as that of typhus where the latter exists, it is necessary to point out that a conservative estimate of a 10% incidence of one or other or both forms of pediculosis on average throughout the world means about 400 million cases.

Pediculosis Capitis

The incidence of pediculosis capitis is cosmopolitan. One of the earliest and best surveys was that of Mellanby (1941). Noting that it was primarily a disease of children, especially preschool children, he pointed out that adults, mostly women, could also be affected at any age. Those who, like the present writer, felt that elderly women were particularly prone to the disease were probably the victims of their own unconscious bias. They were often asked to treat elderly women with head lice, but younger women preferred to treat themselves and to conceal from others the fact that they were infested. Maunder (1974) remarked that whilst the crab louse festers under the skirts of propriety the head louse shelters beneath the cloak of secrecy. Mellanby's original observation of very high incidence in preschool children has been confirmed by Coates (1971), Maunder (1974) and Donaldson (1976) (Tables 5.2 and 5.3). These reports, together with Donaldson's (1974) opinion that there was also a high incidence in adolescents, have resulted in at least 50% underestimate of the real incidence (the figures usually given for incidence being based on school returns). Maunder in fact put the probable incidence in the United Kingdom in 1974 as about one million cases (four or five times the official estimate). Other countries have equal or even-higher infestation rates (see Tables 5.4 and 5.5). Such rates would seem to justify the overall estimate given below. The incidence was found by Mellanby to be much higher in cities than in the country and greater in the city centres than in the suburbs. This finding too was confirmed by Coates (1971), but Johnson (1974) found an even distribution throughout the city of Birmingham. There is not much difference between the sexes in the very young but the incidence in older girls is proportionately higher than in boys. Pediculosis capitis in girls persists into adult life but seems to cease abruptly at puberty in boys, except perhaps in grossly neglected boys. McGuire and McNally (1972) found that for every two boys affected there were five girls (of school age only), the peak incidence being between 8 and 9 years for boys and 6 and 7 years for girls. Why men should be relatively unaffected is not known but it may be due to hormonal or other secretions on the skin surface or in the blood, which is the food of the lice.

Table 5.2. Head louse infestation rates (percentage) in primary and secondary schools in different types of area in the United Kingdom[a]

Area		Primary	Secondary	Total
Northern non-metropolitan county.	A	2.32	2.19	2.27
county	B	1.45	2.18	1.76
Southern non-metropolitan county	C	1.60	1.32	1.49
county	D	0.61	0.00	0.35
Metropolitan district	E	5.76	6.82	6.30
district	F	4.70	4.04	4.43
Outer London borough	G	0.74	1.35	1.00

[a] From Donaldson (1976), by kind permission of the author and the Editor of the *Royal Society for Health Journal.*

Table 5.3. Percentage infestation rates according to social zones in the schools in the areas listed in Table 5.2[a]

Area	Poor	Median	Good
A	2.08	2.46	0.58
B	3.12	1.43	0.26
C	2.25	1.60	0.53
D	0.57	0.64	0.00
E	10.74	4.58	3.35
F	13.41	3.11	1.06
G	1.43	1.06	0.00

[a] From Donaldson (1976), by kind permission of the author and the Editor of the *Royal Society of Health Journal.*

Table 5.4. Some survey infestation rates and other figures estimated to be the number of persons infested with pediculosis capitis

Country	Infestation rates	References
UK		
Teesside schools	Downtown 21.1% Intermediate 13.4% Suburban 0.4%	Coates (1971)
60 000 children in city fever hospitals in England	Under 5 years and girls } 50% Rural areas 5%	Mellanby (1941)
UK as a whole	Estimated 1 000 000 cases	Maunder (1974)
British Columbia		
School Area A	5–15%	Hopper (1971)
School Area B	11.5% average	
Czechoslovakia		
Schools in one area	4.7%	Palicka et al. (1971)
Chile		
53 556 persons	25.9%	Schenone et al. (1973)
Whole country	Estimated 20%	
USA		
1973	1.5 million	Taplin et al. (1982). Estimated on evidence of school incidence and sale of insecticides
1974	3.0 million	
1976	6.0 million	

Table 5.5. Incidence of body louse infestation in various countries. (Based on Gratz 1973)

Country	Remarks
Burundi (1970–1971) Lesotho (1972)	Most persons infested
Tunisia	High percentage infested
Egypt, 6 villages	13.40% of inhabitants infested
Jordan, refugee camps	1.7% infested
Yugoslavia	
Seaside village	16 of 24 families infested (1+ members)
Bosnian village	3–8% infestation
Hungary (1969–1970)	Very common, especially in gypsies
Roumania	Incidence down after eradication campaign
USSR	No data
France, vagrants	5% in 5- to 20-year-old group 15% in 15- to 60-year-old group Rare in soldiers, schools and prisons
Afghanistan	75–80% infestation rate in general population
Korea	No information about lice, but in 1951 there were 32 211 cases of typhus and in 1973 there were none
South America	Incidence increasing in mountainous areas
Mexico	100% in some villages
Guatemala	Typhus reappearing. ? result of appearance of DDT-resistant strains of lice
USA	Uncommon except in single homeless men, when incidence is about 50%

There does not appear to be any particular ethnic liability to or insusceptibility to pediculosis capitis. It is true that amongst blacks in the United States and the United Kingdom it is rare (Litt 1978), a parallel for which is the use of buffalo fat and olive oil as a deterrent against body lice by African tribes (Lloyd 1919). Maunder (1974) has indicated that the head louse in the United Kingdom and the United States has a claw structure adapted to grip hair with a round cross section (Fig. 5.19). African hair has an oval cross section, making it much more difficult for the western variety of the louse to grip. The indigenous head louse in Africa, however, is adapted to grip oval hairs.

Young children appear persistently to acquire head lice for several reasons. Firstly they are in very close contact with their mothers who may be infested. Secondly their heads are often close to those of their friends of the same age when playing, and lice can easily transfer from one to the other under such circumstances. Maunder (1983b) stressed that the vast majority of infestations occur by direct contact and pointed out that in appropriate circumstances one single louse could easily visit several heads in one day. Dispersal to other heads frequently follows copulation, but Maunder indicated that immature lice seldom migrated. Spread of lice is enhanced by conditions of overcrowding, poor housing, poverty, ignorance and lack of

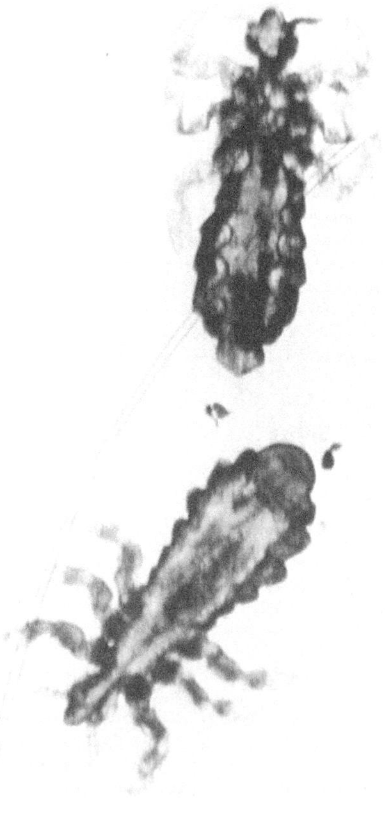

Fig. 5.19. Head lice gripping a scalp hair by specially adapted tarsal claws.

hygiene facilities—conditions which are most frequent in underdeveloped countries and refugee camps. At the same time it should be emphasised that none of these factors by themselves cause pediculosis. This applies especially to bad hygiene, which is often cited as the cause (Maunder 1977; Nitzkin 1979).

Mellanby and others have noted an increased incidence at the end of school holidays when pupils are inspected on return to school, due no doubt to the lack of supervision in the holidays by the school health authorities. At school, hat exchanging is said to be one factor encouraging spread of lice (Harding 1898) together with lack of personal clothes hooks in cloakrooms (Editorial 1979), although Maunder (1974) said that it was very unusual for pediculosis to be spread from loose hairs (with attached nits) or headgear. Mellanby felt that modern hairdressing styles which discouraged frequent combing of the hair encouraged the proliferation of head lice. Schenone et al. (1973) in Chile noted that the degree of infestation was approximately proportional to the length of the hair, although Maunder (1974) insisted that the lice seldom visited the distal parts of the hair voluntarily and that large masses of hair could actually impede transmission from scalp to scalp. The incidence of pediculosis capitis is increased by the upheaval of national crisis, as was seen amongst evacuee children in the United Kingdom between 1940 and 1943 (Blackstock 1944). The increase in tourism and migrant labour and the emergence of insecticide-resistant strains of lice have also had an influence in producing higher infestation rates.

Insecticide resistance is encouraged by too frequent use of insecticide for prophylactic purposes and by inadequate treatment. This was shown by two consecutive surveys by Wright and Brown (1957) and by Wright and Pal (1965).

Mellanby (1942) showed that in a group of 93 children boys had 12.7 active lice per scalp and girls 16.8 on average. The highest count was 142, but 65% of the children had less than 10. These figures were apparently very similar to figures obtained by Buxton in children in Asia and Africa. Mellanby made the important observation that children with very few lice were potent sources of spread of infestation, presumably because they escaped notice at first. Maunder (1977), on the other hand, defined a heavy infestation as the presence on the scalp of 200 or more active forms of lice, 10% of which would be adult females. At the time of writing he estimated that there were probably about 20 000 cases of such heavy infestation amongst children in the United Kingdom and another 200 000 milder cases.

Pediculosis Corporis

Gratz (1973) remarked that whilst a great deal of work had been done on studying the epidemiology of typhus, little attention had been paid to lousiness as a subject in itself. He studied the incidence of pediculosis corporis world wide, paying special attention to typhus areas. The results of his studies have been tabulated in Table 5.5. It can be seen from this that body louse infestation is still very common in certain areas. May (1973) considered that there was a symbiosis between the body louse and man, which was greatly helped by the wearing of warm heavy clothing. Hence the incidence of pediculosis corporis was particularly high in circumstances where heavy clothing was necessary, such as cold climates and high altitudes. Of particular significance were the mountainous regions of Ethiopia and Burundi, where the inhabitants wear large heavy cloaks of wool and cotton cloth (two in winter) reinforced at night by other coverings. Similar heavy woollen ponchos are worn by the villagers of the high Andes, and wool and camel hair garments by the Touaregs of North Africa, who seldom if ever change them and never wash. All these populations have other common characteristics. They are all poverty stricken, live in grossly overcrowded, very primitive huts or tents and in isolation. Such conditions greatly favour louse proliferation. The actual season is of little importance except in so far as severe cold encourages more clothing to be worn, thus maintaining the temperature and relative humidity of the body surface (Buxton 1947). Guterriez (1973) noted that in Bolivia 43% of the population, who were impoverished Indians, lived at about 2500 m altitude and were 100% infested. A similar state of affairs existed in a Peking poor house in the winter (Pang 1945). Individual or national poverty seems to predispose to lousiness (Meheus et al. 1974). Overcrowding by itself also seems to encourage the spread of body lice. MacLeod and Craufurd-Benson (1941) emphasised that it is almost impossible to escape infestation in a verminous environment. In countries where the overall incidence of pediculosis corporis is low, the infestation is usually acquired by sleeping in an infested bed or wearing infested garments (Lloyd 1919; Buxton 1947). Even the outer garments of a heavily infested person contain active lice and viable eggs. Many authorities have emphasised that the wearing of clothing for long periods without ever changing, as is the case with vagrants or those living in primitive conditions (see above), is conducive to the wellbeing of the louse population. Maunder (1983b) noted as a corollary that those who have the means for regular changes of clothing seldom ever become lousy, because weekly changes of clothing inhibit the development of lice. Buxton noted that lousiness was also common in the feeble minded, in persons of low intellect, ill health and vitamin deficiency. A poor nutritional state reduces the protective effects of self grooming. In those areas where infestation with body lice is prevalent, persons with less than 10 lice outnumber those with between 11 and 100 and they in turn are more numerous than those with between 101 and 1000 (Buxton 1941).

Treatment and Prevention

Proper and effective treatment is a community problem since individuals can be cleared fairly easily of infestation. As in antiscabies campaigns a set of ground rules has gradually evolved, based on experience, knowledge of the biology and habits of the louse, the epidemiology of infestation, the function and use of insecticides and resistance to them. Treatment of a confirmed case of pediculosis capitis requires first of all the choice of a suitable medicament. The innumerable possibilities are shown in Tables 5.6 and 5.7, but at present in the United Kingdom two substances are regarded as better than the others—malathion and carbaryl. They are both best used as alcoholic lotions at a concentration of 0.5%. They are applied a few drops at a time, massaged into the scalp and roots of the hair. The whole scalp should be systematically covered, particular attention being paid to the areas above and behind the ears and the suboccipital region. About 10–20 ml is sufficient for one patient. The lotion should be allowed to dry naturally and *left undisturbed for 12 h*, and then washed out. Using heat to dry hair inactivates the anticholinesterase insecticides, as does the chlorine in the water of swimming baths. Some of the insecticide will have been adsorbed onto the hair and, in the case of malathion at least, persist sufficiently to act as 100% deterrent for 2 weeks (Cole et al. 1977). Both of these substances are 100% effective and safe, although carabyl has not yet been approved for general release in the United States. Combing out the hair after treatment is cosmetically desirable but not absolutely essential. The best implement is a Sackers comb, which is metal with fine tines and a sharp blade at the base of the tines, so designed to cut any hair with a nit cemented to it and therefore likely to catch on the blade during combing. Since the epidemiological evidence indicates that at least half of the patients affected are of preschool age, the simplest plan is to treat the whole family, as for scabies (Editorial 1976). However, this may not always be acceptable, in which case only persons positively identified as infested must be treated. This, of course, necessitates home inspection, either by the patient's doctor or preferably by a nursing visitor, who should have more time. A follow-up inspection is essential and this is best done 10 days after treatment because it allows time for any egg which escapes death to hatch but is too short to allow it to mature and reach the reproductive stage. It also enables re-infestation to be recognised. Shampoos containing malathion or carbaryl are almost useless because they are washed off after a few minutes. This is too short a period for them to exert an insecticidal effect and prevents any residual effect at all (Maunder 1981).

Table 5.6. Some older and traditional measures against pediculosis and phthiriasis

Treatment	Remarks	References
Kerosene with olive oil	Very good	Dubreuilh and Beille (1895)
Kerosene	Good, but said to be ineffective ovicide	Nuttall (1917f)
Petrolatum	Smeared all over for pediculosis of scalp; good deterrent for body lice	Jamieson (1895)
1 in 40 carbolic acid solution	Soak hair for 1 h, wash off; 100% effective; used for 20 years	Whitfield (1912)
Cresol powder	Said to be effective	Schoppler (1915)
Naphthalene, Sulphur, Cresylic acid, Iodoform	All used as powders; ineffective against lice except when in close contact	Bacot (1916a)
Creosote in soap base	Ovicidal	Bacot (1917a)
Mercury powder	Not 100% effective; absorbable; dangerous	Dore (1916); Mantegna et al. (1982)

Table 5.7. Modern insecticides which have been used in the treatment of pediculosis and phthiriasis. Classification according to Busvine (1980)

Insecticide and group	Remarks	References
Stomach poisons:		
Butazolidine	Given to host orally or injection; poisons mobile feeding stages	Shawarby et al. (1964); Cole and Van Natta (1964)
Tanderil		Cole and Van Natta (1964)
Cotrimoxazole		Shashindran et al. (1978)
Contact poisons (insects):		
1. *Vegetable origin*		
Rotenone (derris)		Busvine and Buxton (1942)
Pyrethrum		
2. *Miscellaneous synthetics*:		
Lethane	Used in 1940s and 1950s	Busvine and Buxton (1942)
Lauryl thiocyanate	Effective if left undisturbed on scalp for 10 days	
3. *Pyrethroids*[a]	Enhanced by synergists; from pyrethrum; not much used; expensive	
4. *Organochlorines*:		
DDT and analogues[a]	Originally very effective; ecological objections now	Numerous; Hurlbutt et al. (1952)
HCH:[c]	Very effective but now much resistance; toxic (see Chap. 15)	Lamizana and Mouchet (1976); Davies et al. (1983); Polano (1983); Taplin (1983)
Lindane[a]		
Chlordane[a]		
Dieldrin[a]		
5. *Anticholinesterases*:		
Organophosphorous compounds:	Enzyme inhibitors by combination with enzyme; reversible but only slowly	Maunder (1971a,b); Busvine (1980)
Malathion[a]		
Dichlorvos[a]		
Carbamates:	Enzyme inhibitors by competition with acetylcholine; reversible	Clark and Cole (1967); Maunder (1971a); Busvine (1980)
Carbaryl[a]		
Propoxur[a]		
Synergists:	Mostly used with pyrethroids and carbaryl; act by detoxifying enzymes.	Cole (1973); Clark and Cole (1967)
Sulphoxide		
Piperonyl butoxide		
Contact poisons (mites and ticks):	Said to be effective	Touraine (1947); Blackstock (1944) Karacic and Yawalkar (1982)
Benzyl benzoate		
Crotamiton		
Fumigants:		
Methyl bromide	Very effective and safe	Grothaus and Cole (1973)
Ethyl formate	Reasonably safe	
Dichlorvos[b]	Very effective but not ovicidal	
Insect-development inhibitors:		
Juvenile hormones and analogues[a]	Inhibit development of eggs and maturity of stages	Takahashi et al. (1973); Vinson (1973)
Dehydrants:		Tarshish and Blinstrub (1963)
Sorptive dusts	Adsorb lipids from the insect surface causing fatal loss of water	

[a] Resistance to these compounds has developed to a greater or lesser degree.
[b] An organophosphorous compound but used for its vapour and too slow here.
[c] HCH, hexachlorocyclohexane, commonly known as benzene hexachloride, although it is not a benzene derivative.

Should the hair be cut or shaved off? At one time this measure was almost regarded as mandatory, but is not practised nowadays because of the unnecessary adverse psychological effect. However, under exceptional circumstances, e.g. plica formation, it may still be the only remedy because it becomes impossible to comb the hair. Such patients are probably better treated as hospital inpatients.

Hopper (1971), in British Columbia, advised excluding infested children from school and only readmitting them after inspection has shown them to be cured. Although apparently sensible, a quarantine policy may raise difficulties such as family embarrassment and is in fact pointless, since the average duration of pediculosis capitis in children is 4 months (Maunder 1983b). It implies parental responsibility for treatment, a good idea in itself but necessitating proper instruction or supervision. The alternative is mass treatment at school clinics, but this would omit preschool children. Better education of the general public should overcome this difficulty. Whether it should be necessary to have legal enforcement of identification and treatment of all contacts, as suggested by Coates (1971), is still debatable. Failure of an antilouse campaign might make the taking of such powers more favourable.

The management of a head louse eradication campaign is an exercise in logistics. The basic requirements are set out in Table 5.8. Regarding pediculosis capitis as an infectious disease for practical purposes is likely to procure cooperation from the public and instil a sense of urgency into a campaign. Public education is a prime factor and the best way to overcome social prejudice. It also helps children and encourages them to take part in the treatment of their younger siblings. Teachers need to be well informed to instruct pupils and encourage their cooperation as well as to identify infested children. Chemists should be made aware of the problem and requested to keep supplies of the favoured medicaments available and to encourage those seeking self-medication to ask for medical advice first of all. Family doctors and nurses, especially the latter, are the key persons around whom a campaign may collapse if they are inadequately managed and the ones who can ensure its success if sufficiently well informed. The detailed information available in medical and nursing textbooks and curricula is nearly always sadly deficient. Further basic education on the subject is essential. The importance of public cooperation should be impressed on both these professional groups and also on community authorities. A diagnosis of infestation, however, should not be made unless proof is available, and a proper explanation should be given to the patients and their parents. Good public relations are very important. Propaganda through the media and by posters should help to reinforce an educational programme. It should also point out, amongst other things, that pediculosis capitis and dirty habits are not synonymous, and also that the practice of exchanging headgear and combs amongst children is inadvisable. An eradication campaign should be timed to start actual treatment in the second term of the academic year, so as to allow time for the preliminary publicity and education, and should be supplemented by home visiting and inspection of preschool children, in case there should turn out to be difficulties about family treatment. Considerable preparation is necessary and the detailed plan of campaign must be familiar to all those taking part. It goes without saying that proper records should be kept of all those treated, together with details of family incidence, districts and schools most heavily involved etc. This information will give a good picture of the pretreatment state of infestation. A 10-day follow-up should be carried out as mentioned above for sporadic cases, with a survey about 3 months later to assess the results. Table 5.9 shows the details of the organisation of a campaign carried out in Birmingham in 1974 as an example.

Subsequent prevention of further outbreaks involves routine inspections of all schools; intermittent home visiting, say once every 3 months;

Table 5.8. Principles to be followed in conducting a campaign against head lice infestation. (Based on Donaldson 1976)

1. Regard pediculosis capitis as an infectious disease
2. Conduct education programme about louse infestation for parents; teachers, doctors, nurses, chemists and older children
3. Conduct propaganda campaign using posters, press, television and radio
4. Ensure regular systematic inspection of school children
5. Ensure regular systematic home visiting and inspection of preschool children and mothers

Table 5.9. Basis of campaign carried out in Birmingham in 1974. (Johnson 1974)

Team of 20 specially trained nursing assistants	
Preliminary work	
Family doctors and chemists notified	
Training sessions for school health staff	
Letter to all head teachers	
Explanatory leaflet to all children	one week before the inspection date for each school area
Explanatory letter to all parents	
Publicity campaign	
Campaign	
Region covered systematically from north to south	
All schools in each clinic area inspected on the same day	
All inspections in classrooms	
Infested pupils given individual instructions and medicament for the whole family by school nurse	
Infested pupils inspected next day, by smelling, to detect medicament on scalp. If not treated, sent home until treated. (In Birmingham 90% treated on first day)	
Absentees excluded on return until passed as free of infestation by the school nurse	

continued propaganda about the need for constant vigilance by parents, teachers and the children themselves; the provision of personal pegs for clothing in cloakrooms in schools; and emphasising the necessity to report any suspected case at once so as to obtain treatment and avoid spread. Nuttall's advice in 1917 still holds good—unremitting attention by medical and nursing personnel, especially the latter, is essential to maintain control. Maunder (1977) has laid great emphasis on the importance of correcting biased attitudes to pediculosis capitis amongst teachers, doctors, nurses and local authorities, which often greatly interfere witth the management of outbreaks. The whole subject is emotively beset with fear of either insects or social embarrassment. This is compounded by the changing trend to higher incidence amongst the professional middle classes and the fallacy of equating lice with dirt. Overcoming such entrenched attitudes is essential to successful eradication. This is sometimes particularly applicable to health authorities, who do not care to admit that lice are a problem in areas under their jurisdiction.

The management of outbreaks of pediculosis corporis involves much the same general principles, but in this instance the lice are in the clothing and bedding. Hot air and steam disinfestation have been in use since World War I and, when necessary, are still available in the United Kingdom in areas controlled by large municipal authorities. However, since steam disinfestation is rather damaging to some items of clothing, hot air is probably the cheapest, safest and best method for large-scale treatment. At a temperature of only 65°C for 15 min all lice and eggs can be killed (Nuttall 1917c). It is essential, however, that the temperature be monitored by thermometer during the whole process. Heat can be applied on a individual basis by using a hair dryer inside a container but must also be monitored by thermometer. Maunder (1983a) advocated the use of tumble driers as a most efficient way of destroying lice and eggs in clothing. The temperature at which they operate is high enough to be lethal to lice. Dry cleaning is apparently equally effective, the solvents used all being efficient insecticides. Fumigation with methyl bromide or ethyl formate can also be used. It is simple to do and relatively safe, although there is a slight fire risk with ethyl formate (Grothaus and Cole 1973). Full details are given in Chapter 26. Dichlorvos is unsatisfactory for treating louse-infested clothing because of its slow action and very poor ovicidal properties in the circumstances required. Whatever method is used, *all* clothing and bedding of infested persons should be treated.

Apart from the actual disinfestation of clothing, the general principles of treatment, in respect of refugee camps, military camps, prisons and other institutions where pediculosis corporis is likely to flourish, include regular inspection, regular bathing with adequate facilities provided, segregation of newcomers until pronounced free of infestation and the provision of trained, reliable and permanent personnel to carry out disinfestation. These operators should themselves be subject to routine inspection (based on Nuttall 1917c).

Control of pediculosis corporis depends more on prevention than anything else. This additionally involves the use of insecticides either impregnated into clothing or dusted onto the clothing and individuals. The best insecticides are those which leave some on the material to give a residual effect. Cole et al. (1971), using sleeve tests, listed the most effective as Montecatini L561, Abate, Mobam and malathion in that order, with residual effects lasting 5–6, 3 and 2 weeks respectively. None of the materials impregnated caused irritation to those wearing them. Carbamates are less persistent and have less residual effect, but Sussman et al. (1969) showed that carbicide, a 5% carbamate powder in a synergistic base, was more effective than malathion.

Other interesting potential means of controlling lice include juvenile hormones and their analogues, which interfere with embryogenesis or inhibit the development of mature lice (Vinson 1973), and dehydrant chemicals, which adsorb the lipid from the surface epicuticle of the arthropod integument and render it incapable of retaining water. All these methods and insecticides are discussed in detail in Chapter 26. One method, beautifully effective in its simplicity but impractical on a large scale, remains to be described. Debreuil (1917) recorded coming across an unkempt vagrant in a clearing in a wood. He was lying stark naked on the ground. All his clothes were draped carefully over an ant mound and he himself was stretched out over another. He claimed that the ants had consumed every vestige of parasite from his person and clothing, all of which he inspected carefully before dressing again. Debreuil also cited a similar case of a missionary in the Sudan who said that army ants performed the same service on any sleeping individual in their path, but additionally they bit the host as well!

Pthirus pubis

Morphology and Biology

The pubic louse *Pthirus pubis* has been known for centuries (Rosenmayer 1886). It is quite distinct in appearance and habits from the two pediculi species. Figure 5.20 illustrates its principal morphological features. It has a narrow head with six-segmented antennae and lateral eyes. The thorax

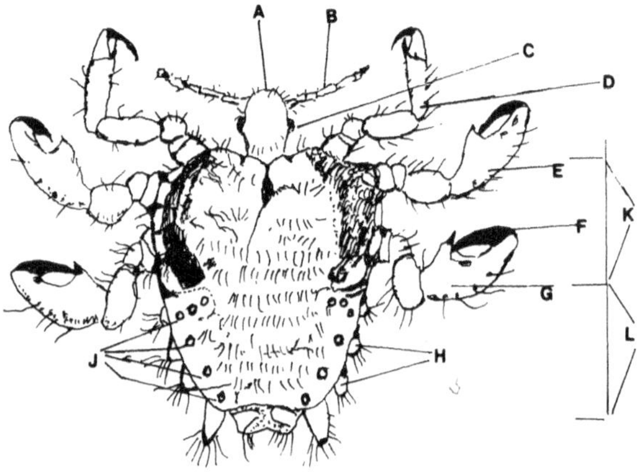

X 50

Fig. 5.20. *Pthirus pubis*—morphological features. *A*, head; *B*, antenna; *C*, eye; *D*, *E*, *G*, fixed part of tarsal claws; *F*, mobile finger of tarsal claw; *H*, abdominal protuberances; *J*, spiracular openings; *K*, thorax; *L*, abdomen. (Courtesy of Stafford Miller Ltd, Hatfield) × 50

and abdomen appear almost fused, each separately being broader than long, but the body as a whole is slightly longer than broad. Of the three pairs of legs the first pair is relatively slender. Each leg ends in a powerful claw, hinged on the tarsus and opposed to a spur on the opposite side of the latter. This is an adaptation for gripping hair (Fig. 5.21). The arrangement of spiracles is shown in Fig. 5.20. On many of the abdominal segments there are lateral protrusions, each ending in a cluster of setae. The louse as a whole is flattened dorsoventrally. The life cycle from egg to adult is from 22 to 27 days. The incubation period of the egg is 7–8 days, whilst the rest of the cycle is taken up with larval and nymphal development. The average adult life is 17 days for females and 22 days for males (Nuttall 1917e). It lives exclusively on man and prefers a humid atmosphere.

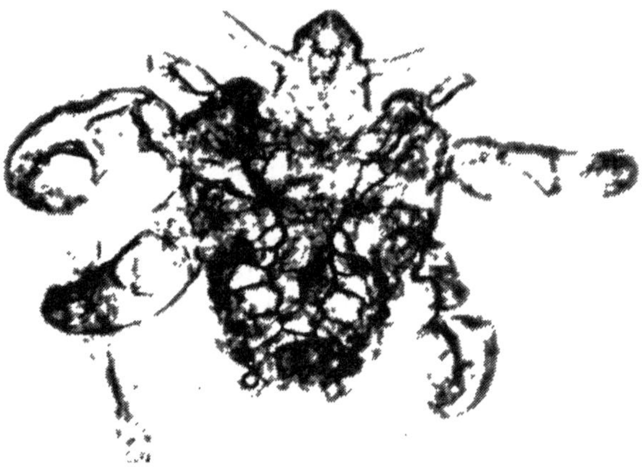

Fig. 5.21. Pubic louse gripping hair with its stout claws on legs II and III.

According to Marples (1965), *P. pubis* tolerates a higher relative humidity than do pediculi and is untroubled by sweat. On the other hand, Nuttall (1917e) reported that it became restless on exposure to light and that it quickly died in a dry atmosphere. It fixes itself to pubic hairs, inserts its mouthparts into a capillary and remains like this feeding intermittently (Marples 1965). Nuttall reported that young larvae cling to only a single hair but that all other stages grasp a hair on either side with the second and third pair of legs. The pubic and axillary hair are far enough apart to suit the span of the louse (2 mm), whereas it avoids the scalp because the hairs are too close together (1 mm). It tends to remain attached to one place for hours or days at a time but when it moves it is sluggish and prefers to move from one hair to another without letting go on both sides at the same time. This can be demonstrated if one attempts to remove a pubic louse with the point of a needle. According to Busvine (1977), its maximum daily movement is about 10 cm. Whilst it feeds it also defaecates continuously around its point of attachment (James and Harwood 1969). It does not transmit any other disease (Maegraith 1971).

Clinical Appearances of Phthiriasis Pubis

The only complaint as a rule is itching, which may be intense and occurs only in infested areas of the body. To some extent its intensity increases with heavier infestation. Some patients apparently do not itch. A possible explanation for this may be that the infestation has been discovered by observation or routine medical inspection during the incubation period, which, according to Fisher and Morton (1970), is about 30 days. These authors discovered some 36 unsuspected cases by routine examination at a clinic for sexually transmitted diseases. Orkin (1974) suggested the itch might be due to sensitisation but gave no evidence for this assertion; if it were the case one would expect the itch to be generalised more frequently. It may commence from the moment that the lice are first seen by the patient and may persist after successful treatment (Dubreuilh and Beille 1895).

The pubic and axillary areas are those commonly affected; however, the lice may spread to the perineum, thighs, very occasionally the lower legs, to the trunk, especially around the umbilicus and, in men, the nipple areas, to the upper arms, but rarely to the wrists. In very heavy infestations in adult men the beard and moustache area may rarely be involved. The eyelashes and eyebrows may also be affected in heavily infested adults but more often in children without pubic or axillary hair. Kirschner (1982) has suggested that eyelash involvement may be on the increase with greater sexual promiscuity, but it was not reported by Fisher and Morton (1970) from their clinic. Involvement of the scalp is very rare for the reasons already given, but Witkowski and Parish (1979) and Maunder (1983b) considered it was probably common. Goldman (1948) stated that it only occurred in children with eyelash involvement; indeed, this was the case in the only instance seen by the present writer. In most instances where the scalp has been involved only the marginal areas are affected (Elgart and Higdon 1973), but in three patients described by Brault and Montpellier (1914a, b) in Morocco, the involved areas were inside the scalp margins and consisted of circumscribed, slightly pigmented plaques. Patton (1931), citing Delanoe, observed that amongst the poor Jewish community in Mazagan in Morocco, all members of families infested with *P. pubis* showed more or less permanent symptomless involvement of the eyelashes.

The individual lesions produced by pubic lice are usually not discernible, the only indication being the actual lice themselves and the eggs (see Fig. 5.22). Kern (1952) recorded a severe bullous reaction in the pubic and genital region, with pubic lice also present in the axillae and cubital fossae. Bullae reappeared during a relapse. The lice are very difficult to see unless specifically sought, preferably with a lens. They look like small 1 to 2-mm brownish-grey specks in the hairy areas involved. They are seldom seen moving. According to James and Harwood (1969), they may remain stationary for days, the mouthparts embedded in the skin and the claws firmly grasping a hair on either side. The eggs are fastened to the hair in a similar way to that of the head louse, often several eggs to the same hair.

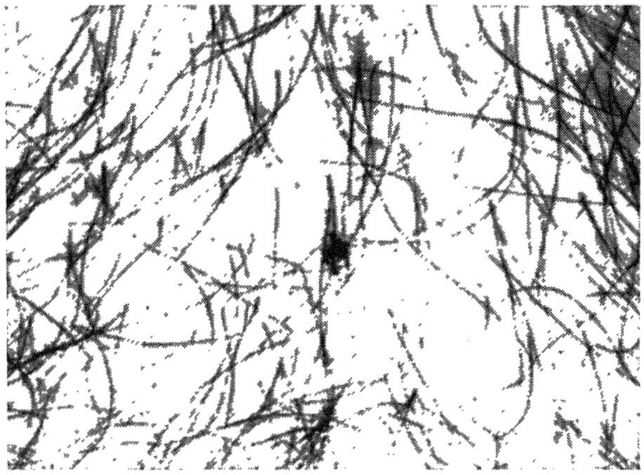

Fig. 5.22. Pubic louse fastened to the skin amongst axillary hair. One or two eggs (nits) may be seen attached to the hairs in the *top right-hand corner* of the picture.

There may be evidence of scratching but it is not nearly so noticeable as with body lice. It is also very localised, confined to the areas of infestation. Secondary infection or eczematisation when present have a similar distribution. The eyelid infestation is often heavy and gives the impression of marked yellowish encrustation (Fig. 5.23), which,

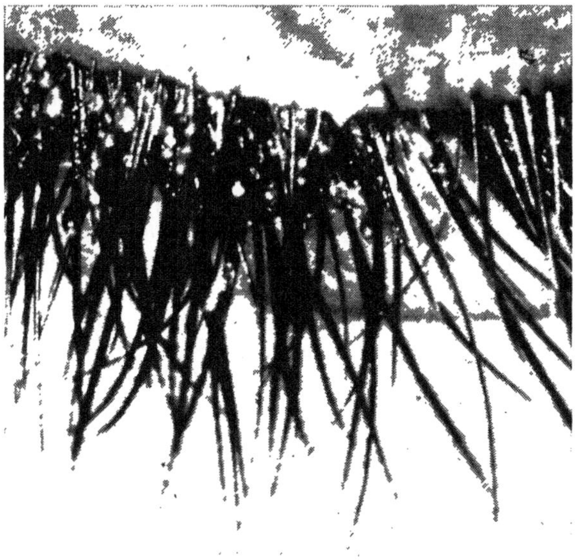

Fig. 5.23. Eggs (nits) of pubic lice attached to eyelashes. They can be made out as shining, greyish, oval globules. There are also some serous crusts mixed with them. (From Morley 1982, by kind permission of the author and the Edition of *Practitioner*)

when severe, may be accompanied by oedema of the lids, rendering the eyes invisible (Blair 1863). Careful examination will show that the crusts are in fact lice attached to the lashes and skin, together with nits, some serous exudation and minute reddish-brown faecal deposits (Stelwagon 1881). On the scalp, unless one can find the actual louse, it will be difficult to distinguish between the eggs of head and pubic lice. In fact only an entomologist familiar with both species would be able to do so. Both types of louse have been found on the same scalp (Brault and Montpellier 1914a). Conversely, Payot (1918) has remarked that not all eggs on pubic hairs are those of pubic lice.

A unique lesion, which only occurs in association with phthiriasis pubis, is the slate-grey or bluish-grey macule (known as maculae caeruleae, *tâches bleues*, *tâches bleuâtres* or *tâches ombrées*). These lesions were first recorded in association with pubic lice by Professor Falot and his pupils at the Naval School of Medicine in Toulon in 1868 (Besnier 1880). They are 0.5–1 cm in diameter, somewhat irregular in shape, always macular, and can occur anywhere on the body except the forearms, hands, feet, ankles and head (Payne 1890). They are best seen by standing back a little from the patient in a good light. They do not blanch on pressure. Dubreuilh and Beille (1895) regarded their presence as evidence of a long-standing infestation, and Nuttall (1917d) agreed that they would not appear until the infestation was 2–3 weeks old. Jamieson (1899) thought they were common in persons with blonde colouring and a "transparent" skin. Dubreuilh and Beille had seen a louse in the centre of one of these spots on more than one occasion. This supports the contention of Maunder (1983b) that they are caused by the louse feeding in the same area for long periods. Duguet (1880, cited by Besnier 1880) thought that the macules arose from the effect of something in the insect's body, as he had reproduced them earlier by the injection of louse extract into the skin. Tièche (1908) was able to reproduce these spots by confining a louse to a limited area of skin by means of an entomological cage. He reported that they appeared more readily in nervous persons with moist sweaty skins. He also noted that if the skin became irritated (did he mean inflamed?) they disappeared. The consensus of opinion is that the pigmentation is caused by a human blood pigment produced by the action of some substance in louse saliva acting on haemoglobin (Nuttall 1917d).

When phthiriasis pubis is very severe the patient may be febrile (Safdi and Farrington 1947); on the other hand, Touraine (1947) asserted that pubic lice tended to disappear during a febrile episode of some other illness, reappearing when the fever subsides. Perhaps he was referring to itch.

Epidemiology

Pubic louse infestation is not so common as pediculosis capitis but is nevertheless widespread. It appears to fluctuate in incidence over long periods. Fisher and Morton (1970) analysed 215 cases encountered at a clinic for sexually transmitted diseases in Sheffield over an interrupted period of 6 years. During that time the incidence amongst the patients attending the clinic rose from 0.8% in 1954 to 3.2% in 1968. It was most frequent in females between the ages of 15 and 19 years and in males over 20 years. It was confined to Caucasoid types, being very uncommon in Africans and Mohammedans because of their custom of shaving the body hair. Epstein (1975) considered it to be relatively rare amongst his private patients, the incidence being 0.15%. This compared with 2.46% for scabies and 2.99% for psoriasis of the pubic area. Minogue (1935) suggested that most men and many women, however respectable, had "more than a passing acquaintance with *Pthirus pubis*", but in view of the figures given this must be regarded as a gross (and cynical) exaggeration.

Phthiriasis pubis is spread by close physical contact, usually sexual intercourse, but also, much less commonly, by bed sharing by mother and child or by brothers or sisters. The children in such cases are infested on the eyelashes. Trouessart (1891) records an instance of a 5-month-old infant being infested from a wet nurse, the lice affecting the eyelashes and the scalp behind the ears. Spread may also possibly occur, very occasionally, through contact on a lavatory seat with egg-infested pubic hairs which have been loosened by scratching (Nuttall 1917d).

An increase in promiscuity is usually blamed nowadays for the increasing incidence of pubic lice infestation (e.g. "hippie love-in", quoted by Gratz 1973). This connection is suggested, according to Fisher and Morton (1970), by the fact that the sex ratio and marital status of those affected run parallel to those of persons with gonorrhoea. However, promiscuity cannot always be blamed. Minogue (1935) recorded an epidemic of cases occurring amongst patients in a mental ward, which was only cleared after weeks of intensive therapy when it was realised that the source of re-infestation was located in the scalps of two patients. Once they were treated the epidemic ceased.

Histopathology

The only report available is that for the bullous eruption described by Kern (1952). The bullae were subepidermal with some destruction of the basement membrane and contained albumen, globulin and fibrin and a few inflammatory cells. There was some oedema below the bullae. The appearances were reported by Dr. Fred Weidman, the skin histopathologist, to be like those of bullous urticaria. A biopsy of a *tâche bleue* (Safdi and Farrington 1947) showed a normal epidermis and corium, but an occasional chromatophore cell laden with brown pigment was seen in the papillae.

Treatment

The aim of treatment is essentially to kill the lice and eggs. The oldest method of treatment was to shave the affected parts, thus removing the support for the lice. It has fallen into disrepute because of inconvenience and discomfort. Other old-fashioned but effective treatments have included mercury oilment, paraffin oil, xylol and benzene (see also Table 5.6). All of these remedies can cause an irritant dermatitis, and mercury has the added serious disadvantage of causing renal damage by percutaneous absorption if overused (Mantegna et al. 1982). Since it is possible to obtain such preparations without a doctor's prescription the dangers are obvious. The modern treatment consists of one or other of several insecticides. Dichloro-diphenyl-trichloroethane (DDT) was very effective but has now been generally abandoned. 1,2,3,4,5,6-Hexachlorocyclohexane (HCH) is very effective but must be repeated as it is not ovicidal; if the infestation is severe there may be some risk in this (see Chap. 15, pp. 272–273). A preparation containing 1% malathion or 1% carbaryl as a lotion to be washed off after 12 h is effective. It is persistent and also kills ova, and is much less toxic than HCH. It can be used anywhere except on the eyelids. For use on the eyelids golden eye ointment (yellow oxide of mercury ointment) is quite acceptable but probably considerably less effective than 0.75% physostigmine ophthalmic ointment, as recommended by Ackermann (1968) and Orkin (1974). It is an anticholinesterase preparation which is toxic to lice. It is advisable to consult with an ophthalmologist before prescribing it.

References

Ackerman AB (1968) Crabs: the resurgence of *Phthirus pubis*. N Engl J Med 278: 950–951

Bacot AW (1916a) The use of insecticides against lice. Br. Med J II: 447–450

Bacot AW (1916b) Notes on *Pediculus humanus* (vestimenti) and *Pediculus capitis*. Br Med J I: 788–789

Bacot AW (1917a) The louse problem. Br Med J I: 296–297

Bacot AW (1917b) A contribution to the bionomics of *Pediculus humanus* (vestimenti) and *Pediculus capitis*. Parasitology 9: 228–258

Besnier E (1880) Review of "Sur les tâches bleus: leur production artificielle et Par Duguet, Gazette des hôpitaux 1880 Avril 20" leur valeur semeilogique. Ann Dermatol Syphiligr (Paris) 10: 542–543

Blackstock E (1944) Treatment of pediculosis capitis. Br Med J I: 114–115

Blair J (1863) An unusual case of phthiriasis. Aust Med Gazette 8: 174–175

Brault JJ, Montpellier J (1914a) Infestation du cuir chevelu de l'adulte par le *Phthirus pubis*. Bull Soc Fr Dermatol Syphiligr 25: 78–80

Brault JJ, Montpellier J (1914b) Nouveau cas d'infestation du cuir chevelu de l'adulte par le *Phthirus pubis*. Bull Soc Fr Dermatol Syphiligr 25: 206–207

Busvine JR (1966) Insects and hygiene, 2nd edn. Methuen, London, pp 240–252

Busvine JR (1977) Pediculosis: biology of the parasites. In: Orkin M, Maibach HI, Parrish LC and Schwartzman RM (eds) Scabies and pediculosis. Lippincott, Philadelphia, pp 143–152

Busvine JR (1978) Evidence from double infestation for the specific status of human head lice and body lice (Anoplura). Systematic Entomol 3: 1–8

*Busvine JR (1980) Insects and hygiene, 3rd edn. Chapman and Hall, London

Busvine JR, Buxton PA (1942) A new method of controlling the head louse. Br Med J I: 464–466

Buxton PA (1941) In: Discussion of prevention and treatment of parasitic disease. Some recent work on the louse. Br J Dermatol 53: 145–148

Buxton PA (1947) The louse: an account of the lice which infest man and their medical importance and control, 2nd edn. Edward Arnold, London

Chapman RF (1971) The insects; structure and function, 2nd edn. English Universities Press, London

Clark PH, Cole MM (1967) Resistance of body lice to carbaryl. J Econ Entomol 60: 398–400

Coates KG (1971) Control of head infestation in school children. Community Med 126: 148–149

Cole MM (1973) Synergistic compounds. In: Proceedings of an international symposium on the control of lice and louse-borne diseases. PAHO/WHO scientific publ No 263. Pan-American Health Organisation, Washington DC, p 195

Cole MM, Van Natta DL (1964) Tests with systemic insecticides in rabbits as toxicants for body lice. J Econ Entomol 57: 67–70

Cole MM, Hirst JM, Gilbert IH, Adams CT (1971) Sleeve tests of insecticides for control of body lice in 1969–70. J Econ Entomol 64: 761–762

Davies JE, Dedhia HV, Morgade C, Barquet A, Maibach H (1983) Lindane poisonings. Arch Dermatol 119: 142–144

Debreuil C (1917) Les poux et le chemineau. Bull Nationale Acclimatisation 44: 318–322

Donaldson RJ (1974) Discussion. In: Head infestation—a community problem. Proceedings of a symposium held at the

Royal Society of Medicine, London, 13 Mar 1974. Sponsored by Napp Laboratories
Donaldson RJ (1976) The head louse in England. Prevalence amongst school children. R Soc Health J 96: 55–57
Dore NA (1916) "Lice". Br Med J 1: 630
Dubreuilh W, Beille L (1895) Parasites animaux de la peau humaine. Masson et Cie, Paris
Duffy DM (1971) Ectoparasitic infestations. Cutis 7: 161–168
Editorial (1976) Lice—Yes lice again a problem. Infect Dis 6: 1, 7, 10
Editorial (1979) Head lice in the seventies. Lancet II: 130–131
Elgart ML, Higdon RS (1973) Pediculosis pubis of the scalp. Arch Dermatol 107: 916–917
Epstein E (1975) Pediculosis pubis. Med Aspects Hum Sexual 9: 12–37
Fisher RI, Morton RS (1970) *Phthirus pubis* infestation. Br J Vener Dis 46: 326–329
Fleming MB, Ludwig D (1964) Effects of temperature and parental age on the life cycle of the body louse, *Pediculus humanus humanus*. Ann Entomol Soc Am 57: 560–653
Goldman L (1948) *Phthirus pubis* infestation of the scalp and cilia in young children. Arch Dermatol Syphilol 57: 274
Gooding RH (1963) Studies on the effect of frequency of feeding upon the biology of a rabbit adapted strain of *Pediculus humanus*. J. Parasitol 49: 516–521
Gordon RM, Lavoipierre MMJ (1962) Entomology for students of medicine. Blackwell, Oxford
Gratz NG (1973) The current status of louse infestations throughout the world. In: Proceedings of an international symposium on the control of lice and louse-borne diseases. PAHO/WHO Scientific publ No 263. Pan-American Health Organisation, Washington DC, pp 23–31
Greenhow H (1876) A case of vagabond's discolouration simulating the bronzed skin of Addison's disease. Trans Clin Soc Lond 9: 44–47
Greenough FR (1867) Pediculosis vestimentorum. Boston Med Surg J 77: 241–246
Grothaus RH, Cole MM (1973) Use of fumigants for control of body lice. In: Proceedings of an international symposium on control of lice and louse-borne diseases. PAHO/WHO Scientific publ No 263, Pan-American Health Organisation, Washington DC, pp 192–195
Guterriez LG (1973) Discussion on louse-borne diseases world wide: epidemic typhus. In: Proceedings of an international symposium on control of lice and louse-borne diseases. PAHO/WHO scientific publ No 263. Pan-American Health Organisation, Washington DC, pp 60–73
Harding GF (1898) Pediculosis. Boston Med Surg J 138: 95
*Hase A (1915) Beitrage zu einer Biologie der Klederlaus (*Pediculus corporis* de Geer—*vestimenti* Nitzch). Z Angew Entomol 2: 265–359
Hay I (1915) The first hundred thousand, being the unofficial chronicle of a unit of "K(1)". Blackwood, Edinburgh
Hirshfelder AD, Moore W (1919) Clinical studies on the effects of louse bites—*Pediculus corporis*. Arch Intern Med 23: 419–430
Hopper JMH (1971) An epidemic of nits. Can J Public Health 62: 159–160
Howlett FH (1917) Notes on head and body lice and upon temperature reactions of lice and mosquitoes. Parasitology 10: 186–188
Hurlbutt HS, Altman RM and Nibley C (1952) D.D.T. resistance in Korean body lice. Science 115: 11–12
James MT, Harwood RF (1969) Herms's medical entomology, 6th edn. Macmillan, London, pp 136–143
Jamieson WA (1895) The treatment of pediculosis vestimentorum. Br J Dermatol 7: 248–249
Jamieson WA (1899) The cause of the reappearance of pediculi vestimentorum after apparently thorough treatment. Br J Dermatol 11: 193–194
Johnson NM (1974) Planning a campaign against head infestation. In: Head infestation—a community problem. Proceedings of a symposium held at the Royal Society of Medicine, London, 13 Mar 1974, pp 16–19. Sponsored by Napp Laboratories
Karacic I, Yawalkar SJ (1982) A single application of crotamiton lotion in the treatment of patients with pediculosis capitis. Int J Dermatol 21: 611–613
Kern AB (1952) Bullous eruption due to pediculosis pubis. Arch Dermatol Syphilol 65: 334–339
Kirschner MH (1982) *Phthirus pubis* infestation of the eyelids. JAMA 248: 428
Lamizana MT, Mouchet J (1976) La pediculose en milieu scolaire dans la region Parisienne. Med Maladies Infect 6: 48–52
Laurent (1901) A child killed by lice. Lancet II: 819
Litt JZ (1978) The quiddity of the head louse. Arch Dermatol 114: 1099
Lloyd L (1919) Lice and their menace to man. Henry Frowde Oxford University Press, London
Lydston FG (1892) Pediculi capitis as a cause of pruritus vulvae. J Cutan and Genito-Urinary Dis 10: 339–400
McGuire J, McNally AJ (1972) Head infestation in school children: extent of the problem and treatment. Commun Med 128: 374–375
MacLeod J, Craufurd-Benson HJ (1941) Observations on natural populations of the body louse, *Pediculus humanus corporis* DeG. Parasitology 33: 278–299
Maegraith BG (1971) In: Adams and Maegraith: Clinical tropical diseases, 5th edn. Blackwell, Oxford, pp 384–385
Mantegna M, Marasa L, Amato G (1982) Dalla Ptiriasi all'eritrodermia. Ann Ital Dermatol Clin Speriment 36: 279–286
Marples MJ (1965) The ecology of the human skin. Thomas, Springfield, Ill, pp 247–333
*Maunder JW (1971a) Resistance to organochlorine insecticides in head lice and trials using alternative compounds. Med Officer 125: 27–29
Maunder JW (1971b) Use of malathion in the treatment of lousy children. Community Med 126: 145–147
*Maunder JW (1974) The louse. In: Head infestation—a community problem. Proceedings of a symposium held at the Royal Society of Medicine, London, 13 Mar 1974, pp 9–16. Sponsored by Napp Laboratories
Maunder JW (1977) Social influences affecting the control of infestation of the person. In: Proceedings of the fifth British pest control conference, Stratford-upon-Avon
*Maunder JW (1981) Novel phenomena arising from the use of acetyl-cholinesterase inhibiting insecticides against human lice. Community Med 3: 31–37
Maunder JW (1983a) Pediculosis corporis: an updating of attitudes. Environ Health May: 130–131
*Maunder JW (1983b) The appreciation of lice. Proc R Inst Great Britain 55: 1–31
May JM (1973) Some cultural traits in the ecology of louse borne-typhus. In: Proceedings of an international symposium on the control of lice and louse-borne diseases. PAHO/WHO scientific Publ No 263. Pan-American Health Organisation, Washington DC, pp 89–94
Mehous AZ, Mubiligi V, Rugamba E (1974) A louse borne typhus epidemic in the prefecture of Butan, Rwanda. East Afr Med J 51: 675–681
Mellanby K (1941) The incidence of head lice in England. Med Officer 65: 39–43
Mellanby K (1942) Natural population of the head louse (*Pediculus humanus capitis*: Anoplura) on infected children in England. Parasitology 34: 180–184

Minogue S (1935) Pediculi pubis. Med J Aust 1: 23
Moore W (1918) An interesting reaction to louse bites. JAMA 71: 1481–1482
Morley WN (1982) Skin infestation. Practitioner 226: 1241–1246
Neumann LG (1911) Notes sur les pediculides. Arch Parasitol 14: 401–414
Nitzkin JL (1979) Head lice and hygiene. Lancet II: 910
*Nuttall GHF (1917a) Bibliography of *Pediculus* and *Phthirus*. Parasitology 10: 1–42
Nuttall GHF (1917b) The part played by *Pediculus humanus* in the causation of disease. Parasitology 10: 43–79
*Nuttall GHF (1917c) The biology of *Pediculus humanus*. Parasitology 10: 80–185
Nuttall GHF (1917d) The pathological effects of *Phthirus pubis*. Parasitology 10: 375–382
*Nuttall GHF (1917e) The biology of *Phthirus pubis*. Parasitology 10: 383–405
Nuttall GHF (1917f) Combating lousiness among soldiers and civilians. Parasitology 10: 411–588
Nuttall GHF (1919) The biology of *Pediculus humanus*. Supplementary notes. Parasitology 11: 210–220
Orkin M (1974) Pediculosis to-day. Minn Med 53: 848–852
Palicka P, Malis L, Zwyrtek K (1971) To the problem of scabies and pediculosis incidence in Karvina region (in Czech). Cesk Epidemiol Mikrobiol Immunol 20: 116–120
Pang KH (1945) Studies on typhus fever epidemic occurring in a poor house. Chin Med J 62: 334–346
Patton WS (1931) Insects, ticks, mites and venomous animals of medical and veterinary importance. Part II Public health. HR Grubb, Croydon
Payne JF (1890) Maculae caeruleae and other symptoms produced by *Pediculi pubis*. Br J Dermatol 2: 209–212
Payot F (1918) Contribution a l'étude du *Phthirus pubis* (Linne. Leach) (Morpion, Schamlasu, Fitzlares, Piattola, Crab louse.) Bull Soc Vaud Sci Nat 53: 127–161
Polano MK (1983) Pediculosis therapy. J Am Acad Dermatol 8: 120–121
Rook A (1979) Skin diseases caused by arthropods and other venomous or noxious animals. In: Rook A, Wilkinson DS and Ebeling FJG (eds) Textbook of dermatology, 3rd edn. Blackwell, Oxford
Rosenmayer L (1886) Ueber Pediculosis palpebrarum. Munch Med Wochensch 33: 145–146
Safdi SA, Farrington J (1947) Constitutional reactions and maculae caeruleae attending phthiriasis pubis. Am J Med Sci 214: 308–311
Schenone H, Falaha F, Villarroel F, Rojas A, Szekely R, Rojo M, Palomino H (1973) La infestacion por *Pediculus humanus capitis* en Santiago de Chile. Bol Chil Parasitol 28: 31–33
Schoppler H (1915) Der Kresolpuder, ein Schutz- und Vertelgungspuder des Ungeziefers im Felde. Munch Med Wochensch 62: 1137–1138
Shashindran CH, Ghandihi IS, Krishnasamy S, Ghosh NN (1978) Oral therapy of pediculosis capitis with cotrimoxazole. Br J Dermatol 98: 699–700
Shawarby AA, Mahdi AH, Sader S, Mahmoud W (1964) Laboratory and field trials of phenylbutazone as a systemic lousicide in man. J Egypt Public Health Assoc 39: 97–106
Sikora H (1917) Über Anpassung der Lause an ihre Umgebung. Arch Schiffs Tropenhyg 21: 172–173
Stelwagon HW (1881) A case of phthiriasis palpebrarum Arch Dermatol 7: 301–302
Sussman HF, Cooke SR, Bloem V (1969) Human louse infestation. Treatment with carbaryl. Arch Dermatol 100: 82–83
Takahashi M, Mihari M, Ohtaki T, Mori K (1973) Lethal effect of synthetic analogues of juvenile hormone on the body lice, *Pediculus humanus corporis*. Jpn J San Zool 23: 243–246
Taplin D (1983) Pediculosis therapy. J Am Acad Dermatol 8: 120–121
Taplin D, Castillero RM, Soiegel J, Mercer S, Rivera AA, Schachner L (1982) Malathion treatment of *Pediculus humanus var capitis* infestation. JAMA 247: 3103–3105
Tarshis B, Blinstrub R (1963) Preliminary studies in the use of sorptive dusts for the control of the human lice, *Phthirus pubis* (L) and *Pediculus humanus capitis* DeGeer. Am J Trop Med Hyg 12: 91–95
Tièche (1908) Zur Kenntnis der Maculae caeruleae. Arch Dermatol Syphilis 91: 327-336
Touraine A (1947) Les traitements actuels des parasitoses animales de la peau. Baillière, Paris
Trouessart M (1891) Sur une phthiriase du cuir chevelu, causée chez un enfant de cinq mois, par le *Phthirus inguinalis*. CR Acad Sci (Paris) 113: 1067–1069
Vinson JN (1973) IID Experimental louse control methods. In: Proceedings of an international symposium on the control of lice and louse-borne diseases. PAHO/WHO scientific publ No 263. Pan-American Health Organisation, Washington DC, pp 208–241
Whitfield A (1912) A method of rapidly exterminating *Pediculi capitis*. Lancet II: 1648–1649
Witkowski JA, Parish LC (1979) Pthiriasis capitis. Int J Dermatol 18: 559–560
Wright JW, Brown AWA (1957) Survey of possible insecticide resistance in body lice. Bull WHO 16: 9–31
Wright JW, Pal R (1965) Second survey of the insecticide resistance in body lice 1958063. Bull WHO 33: 485–501

6 Infestation by Hemiptera

Those who have been forced to sleep in a bed alive with hungry bed bugs know how interesting these parasites can make it and how active they become as soon as the light is extinguished.
(Lugger 1896)

Bugs (order Hemiptera) have been associated with man and his habitation since time immemorial. To the European this means the bedbug, *Cimex lectularius*, which has a cosmopolitan distribution, giving place in the tropics to a related species *C. hemipterus* (Patton and Cragg 1913). In the world as a whole, important as bedbugs are, this is a narrow view of bug infestation. Many other species, especially in the Americas, infest human dwellings or may attack man in other places. They cause great annoyance and some act as vectors of disease. A search of the literature, greatly helped by Ryckman and Bentley (1979), has revealed that over 100 species of bug have been recorded as having attacked man in various parts of the world. Many of these records, whilst authentic, have not been followed up adequately. They have appeared in systematic surveys of geographic regions (Banks 1919; de Bergevin 1925; Bequaert 1925; Lewis 1958), in systematic entomological studies (Readio 1927; Usinger 1934; Wood 1941, 1942a, 1953) or as listed species in books on medical entomology (Patton and Cragg 1913; Matheson 1950; Chandler 1955). Tables 6.1 and 6.2 list the less important ones, namely phytophagous bugs or occasionally waterbugs, with appropriate references. Tables 6.3 and 6.4 indicate reduviid bugs which have similarly attacked man.

Most of the phytophagous species have bitten in self-defence and their "bites" are often painful. The term "bite" is used in relation to bugs in the same way as it is used for mosquitoes. The insect actually pierces the skin with its proboscis (i.e. the injury inflicted is a stab wound and not a true bite), usually injecting some saliva in the process, and may or may not suck blood subsequently. However, the term "bite" has become accepted by common usage and will be used here. In the majority of instances bites by phytophagous bugs are single; however, occasionally with some species, e.g. *Erythronema comes* (Cicadellidae), *Ceresa bubalis* (Membracidae), *Anthocoris musculus* (Coreidae), the irritating effects are the result of large numbers of insects attacking simultaneously, like, for example, midge bites. Reference to Tables 6.1 and 6.2 indicates that whilst all those species listed have been recorded as biting, a few suck blood (*Nephotettix apicalis*, four species of Miridae, two *Clerada* species and one nabid bug). Many species have caused a noticeable local reaction. In most persons any pain caused is trivial and may be accompanied or replaced by itching or burning or tingling. In the case of the few belostomatid bites recorded the pain was very severe. Some bites show a tiny red central punctum. Others develop tenderness and some swelling and may even become secondarily infected. The bites of some Miridae species are very evanescent, as fleeting as gnat or midge bites. One species of Cicadellidae bugs has caused an urticarial eruption. None of this group of bugs leaves any permanent evidence of bites, with the exception of the Belostomatidae, which may cause tissue destruction and scarring. This is doubtless due to the potency of the proteolytic enzymes contained in the saliva (see below).

Turning to the bugs listed in Tables 6.3 and 6.4, there are three groups to be considered: the bedbugs of the Cimicidae family, the haematophagous reduviid bugs and the predaceous reduviid bugs. Before considering any individual bugs in detail there are some general aspects of considerable importance which can best be discussed as a whole.

Morphology of Bugs

The two species of bedbugs depicted in Fig. 6.1a and b closely resemble each other. They are brown, usually dark brown, flattened from above and measure approximately 4.5 mm by 2.5 mm. The head is squat, with the eyes placed laterally and

Table 6.1. Homopterous (phytophagous) bugs recorded as having bitten man. Additional features apart from the actual bite are shown in the second column

Species	Clinical remarks	Geographical areas	References
Coreidae			
Leptocoris irritans	Research worker bitten		Usinger (1934)
Anthocoridae			
Anthocorus sylvestria		Europe; Brazil	Matheson (1950); Bequaert (1925)
A. kingi	Painful; irritation; swelling	Brazil; Sudan	Bequaert (1925); Lewis (1958)
A. congolense		Brazil	Bequaert (1925)
A. musculus	Hop pickers attacked	New York	Torre-Bueno (1931)
Triphleps insidiosus		Brazil; North America	Bequaert (1925); Matheson (1950)
T. tantalus	Severe bite	India	Misra (1924)
Cardiasthesus elegans		Panama	Matheson (1950)
Lycoris campestris	Like bedbug bites	Brazil; North America; Czechoslovakia	Bequaert (1925); Matheson (1950); Stys and Daniel (1957)
Miridae			
Brachynotocoris puncticornis		Brazil	Bequaert (1925)
Trigonotylus brevipes		Brazil	Bequaert (1925)
Plagiognathus obscurus		Brazil; North America	Bequaert (1925); Matheson (1950)
Hyaloides vitropennis	Small lump at site	New York	Torre-Bueno (1931)
Lygus pratensis	Blood-sucker; itch; sharp; weal; swelling; tender	Europe; North America	Matheson (1950), Myers (1929); Readio (1927)
Camptotylus yersini		Sudan	Lewis (1958)
Psallus sp.		Sudan	Lewis (1958)
Creontiades pallidifer		Sudan	Lewis (1958)
Diaphnidia pellucida	On hickory trees	California	Usinger (1934)
Chlamydalis associatus	Sucks blood	California	Usinger (1934)
Orthotylus flavospissus	Sucks blood	California	Usinger (1934)
Haematocapsus bipunctata	Sucks blood	California	Usinger (1934)
Phylus melanocephalus	Like a gnat bite	California	Usinger (1934)
Lopidea marginalis	Marked evanescent irritation	California	Usinger (1934)
Irbisia setans	Brief red spot	California	Usinger (1934)
Cicadellidae			
Nephotettix apicalis	Noctural blood-sucker	Philippines	Banks (1919)
N. bipunctata		Philippines	Banks (1919)
Empoasca mali	Sharp; local swelling tender; red; punctum		Becker (1918) Readio (1927)
Athysaurus sp.	Urticaria	North Africa	de Bergevin (1925)
Eutettix tenellus	Research worker bitten	California	Usinger (1934)
Erythronema comes	Back and hands; mild itch; red; punctum	California	Usinger (1934)
Euscelis exitiosus	Mild itch; persistent redness	USA	Crosby (1926)
Membracidae			
Ceresa bubalis	Back and hands of apple pickers	Eastern USA	Usinger (1934)
Cercopidae			
Phrynomorphus indicus	Irritation	Madras	Donovan (1920)

the proboscis arising centrally and folded ventrally beneath the head and prothorax. The four-jointed antennae arise midway between the eyes and the proboscis. The head articulates directly with the thorax, which has three divisions as shown. The prothorax has lateral flanges reaching forwards partially to envelop the head. The meso- and metathorax are partly concealed by the elytra—the rudimentary remnants of the wings. The three pairs of legs arise ventrally, one from each thoracic segment. The lemon-shaped abdomen has eight segments. On the ventral surface of the right side of the abdomen in the female there is an indentation, which is the opening of the copulatory pouch, or organ of Berlese (see Fig. 6.1c, *k*).

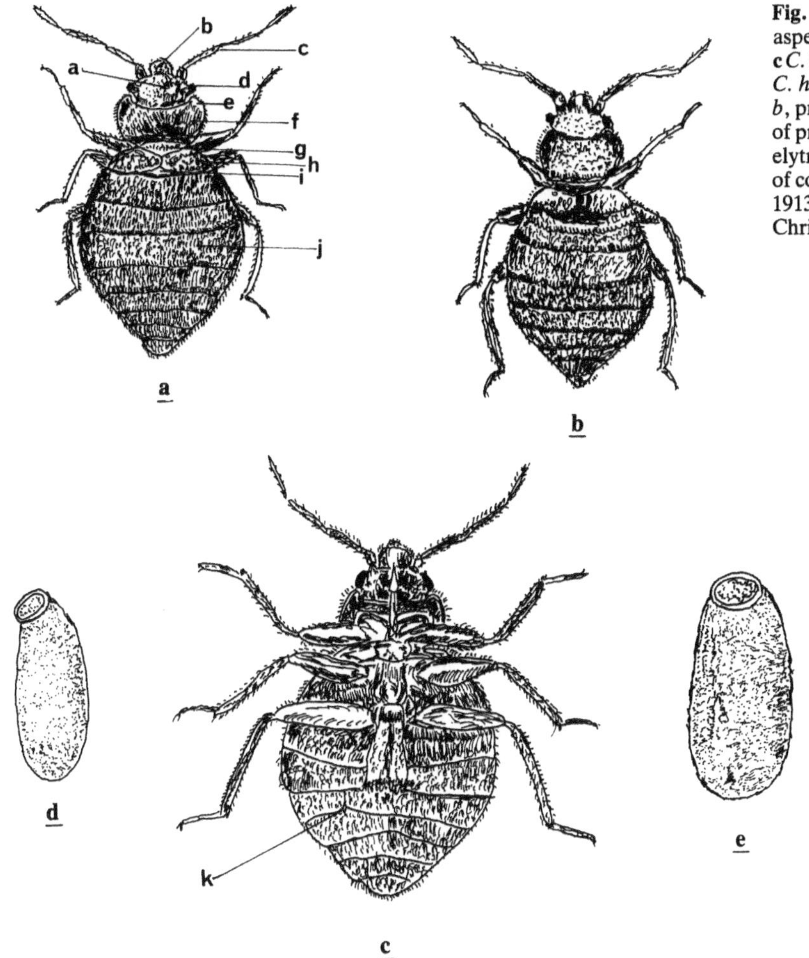

Fig. 6.1. a *Cimex lectularius*, male, dorsal aspect. **b** *C. hemipterus*, male, dorsal aspect. **c** *C. hemipterus*, female, ventral aspect. **d** Egg of *C. hemipterus*. **e** Egg of *C. lectularius*. *a*, head; *b*, proboscis; *c*, antenna; *d*, eye; *e*, lateral wing of prothorax; *f*, prothorax; *g*, mesothorax; *h*, elytron; *i*, metathorax; *j*, abdomen; *k*, opening of copulatory pouch. (After Paton and Cragg 1913, by kind permission of the publisher, The Christian Literature Society for India)

Table 6.2. Heteropterous (phytophagous) bugs recorded as having bitten man. Additional features apart from the actual bite are shown in the second column

Species	Clinical remarks	Geographical areas	References
Lygeidae			
Clerada apicicornis	Blood-suckers; like flea bites; in houses	Brazil; Hawaii; many other tropical areas	Bequaert (1925); Matheson (1950); Ferreira and Dean (1938); Illingworth (1916)
C. nidicola	Blood-suckers; like flea bites; in houses	Brazil; Hawaii; many other tropical areas	Bequaert (1925); Matheson (1950); Ferreira and Dean (1938); Illingworth (1916)
Leptodemus minutus		Brazil; North Africa	Bequaert (1925); Lewis (1958); de Bergevin (1925); Foley (1929)
L. bicolor	Like sandfly bite; irritation and fever	Sudan	Lewis (1958)
Artheneis alutacea		North Africa	Foley (1929)
Geocoris lenoni		Brazil; North Africa	Bequaert (1925); de Bergevin (1925); Matheson (1950)

Table 6.2. *(continued)*

Species	Clinical remarks	Geographical areas	References
G. scutellaris		Brazil; North Africa	Bequaert (1925); de Bergevin (1925); Matheson (1950)
Pyrrhocoridae			
Dysdercus superstitiosis		Brazil; North Africa	Bequaert (1925); Matheson (1950); Blacklock (1923)
Enicocephalidae			
Hemicephalus basalis	Very irritating severe bite	India	Misra (1924)
Nabidae			
Nabis capsiformis	Blood-sucker	Cosmopolitan in tropics	Bequaert (1925); Matheson (1950); Kinnear (1909)
N. roscipennis	Weal 1 cm	USA	Ewing (1928)
Notonectidae			
"Species"	Severe bites if handled roughly		Matheson (1950); Imms (1938)
Belostomatidae			
Benacus grisens	Painful; burning; oedema; erythema	USA	Ewing (1928)
Benacus "sp".	Very painful; local tissue destruction	USA	Brues (1972)
Lethocerus americana		USA	Matheson (1950)
L. del-ponte		Tropical America	Readio (1927)

Table 6.3. Haematophagous reduviid bugs of the family Triatominae recorded as having bitten man. The most important ones are discussed in the text, but for the others any necessary remarks about clinical details are given in the second column. Unless marked otherwise, all are infected with *Trypanosoma cruzi*

Species	Clinical remarks	Geographical area	References
Triatominae			
Triatoma rubrofasciata		Cosmopolitan	Numerous
T. sanguisuga		North America; Philippines	Numerous
T. infestans[a]		Argentina; Brazil	Numerous
T. protracta		Western and southwestern USA	Numerous
T. gerstaeckeri		Western USA, esp. Texas	Chandler (1955); Howard (1900); Lathrop and Ominsky (1965); Wood (1941)
T. brasiliensis		South America	Chandler (1955); Pick and Roubaud (1954); Lehane and Schofield (1976)
T. dimidiata[a]		Mexico; Ecuador; Central America	Chandler (1955); Howard (1900)
T. sordida		South America	Chandler (1955)
T. geniculata		Panama	Chandler (1955)
T. flavida	Inflammation at bite site	Cuba	Hoffman (1923)
T. maculipennis		Mexico	Howard (1900)
T. variegata[b]		Southern USA	Howard (1900)
T. rubida	Reaction variable	Mexico; western USA	Chandler (1955); Keh (1956); Wood (1942b)
T. rubida uhleri	Morbilliform or PU-like; itch; urticaria to blisters with anaphylactoid symptoms	Arizona and western USA	Kofoid and Whittaker (1936); Patton and Cragg (1913); Wehrle (1939)
T. phyllosoma		Mexico	Gordon and Lavoipierre (1972); Lehane and Schofield (1976)
T. maculata[a]		Venezuela	Lehane and Schofield (1976)
T. lenti			Lehane and Schofield (1976)
T. villiceps			Lehane and Schofield (1976)

Table 6.3. (*continued*)

Species	Clinical remarks	Geographical area	References
T. heidemanni[b]		Central and southern USA; Texas	Patton and Cragg (1913); Wood (1942b)
T. longipes		Texas; Arizona	Wood (1942b)
T. indictum[b]			Wood (1941)
T. protracta woodi		Southwestern USA	Wood (1941, 1942b)
T. barberi[a]		Mexico	Ghauri (1973)
Paratriatoma hirsuta		California	Wood (1942a); Keh (1956)
Panstrongylus megistus[a]		Brazil; Guyana (British Guiana)	Numerous
P. geniculatus		Brazil; Panama	Ghauri (1973)
P. herreri		Peru	Ghauri (1973)
P. rufotuberculatus		Venezuela	Ghauri (1973)
Dipetalogaster maxima		Mexico	Ghauri (1973); Costa et al. (1981)

[a] Known vector of Chagas' disease.
[b] Not infected with *Trypanosoma cruzi*.

Table 6.4. Other haematophagous reduviid bugs and also Cimicidae recorded as having bitten man. Where items are included in the second column these species are not discussed in the text.

Species	Clinical remarks	Geographical areas	References
Reduviinae			
Reduvius personatus		Widespread	Numerous
R. mayeli		Brazil	Bequaert (1925)
Rhodnius prolixus[a]		Northern South America	Numerous
R. pallescens[a]	Allergic reactions not uncommon	Brazil; Panama	Gorgas Mem. Inst. (1976)
R. neglectus			Lehane and Schofield (1976)
Platymeris rhadamanthus	Painful; sprays foul-smelling fluid, very painful for eyes	Zanzibar	Edwards (1960); Vanderplank (1958)
Mietes profana		Australia	McKeown (1942)
Aphelonotus simplex		Brazil	Bequaert (1925)
Sinea diadema	Evanescent pain and bleeding	USA	Judd (1959)
Eremorescia lewisi	Painful bite	Sudan	Lewis (1958)
Piezzolettus afer	Pain; irritation; swelling	Sudan	Lewis (1958)
Zelus exsanguis	Intense pain 30 min; swelling; persistent blister	USA	Wray (1959)
Harpactorinae			
Arilus cristatus		USA	Numerous
Acholla multispinosa	Bites in self-defence but for food in special circumstances		Readio (1927)
Piratinae			
Rasahus biguttatus		Brazil; USA	Numerous
R. thoracicus		Brazil; western USA	Numerous
Melanolestes picipes		Eastern USA	Numerous
M. abdominalis			Howard and Schwarz (1901); Matheson (1950)
Pirates affinis		India	Misra (1924)
Ectomocoris ululans	Bite persistent, needle-like; infection	Philippines	Banks (1919)
E. atrox	Very painful bite if handled	Brazil; North Africa	Bequaert (1925); de Bergevin (1925)
Apiomerinae			
Apiomeris spissipes	Very painful; self-defence; 1 h to 2 weeks	North America	Readio

Table 6.4. (*continued*)

Species	Clinical remarks	Geographical areas	References
Stenopodinae			
Stenopoda cinerea	Bites only for self-defence	Eastern and southern coastal states of USA; Cuba; Mexico	Readio (1927)
Vescilnae			
Bescia minima		Brazil	Bequaert (1925)
Cimicidae			
Cimex lectularius		Cosmopolitan	Numerous
C. hemipterus		Tropical	Numerous

[a] Known vector of Chagas' disease.

Chandler's description for the triatomine bugs, which are all blood-suckers, is admirable.

The head of Triatomids is small and narrow. The slender beak bent back under the head is three-jointed and the long filamentous antennae are four-jointed [see Fig. 6.2]. The pronotum flares posteriorly and is usually fairly distinctly divided into an anterior and posterior lobe; the posterior angles of the latter may be rounded or pointed. Behind the pronotum is a triangular scutellum, which may have a posterior spine. The abdomen has flattened lateral margins, the connexivum, not covered by the wings. This and the leathery basal portion of the wing (corium) is usually marked with red or yellow, as is the pronotum.

To this could be added that the wings are folded across the back when walking. The diagram in Fig. 6.2 shows these features. Figures 6.3–6.8 illustrate these characteristics in a few of the more important species, including some predators. Accurate species identification requires the help of an experienced entomologist. Some common names for the reduviid bugs are shown in Table 6.5.

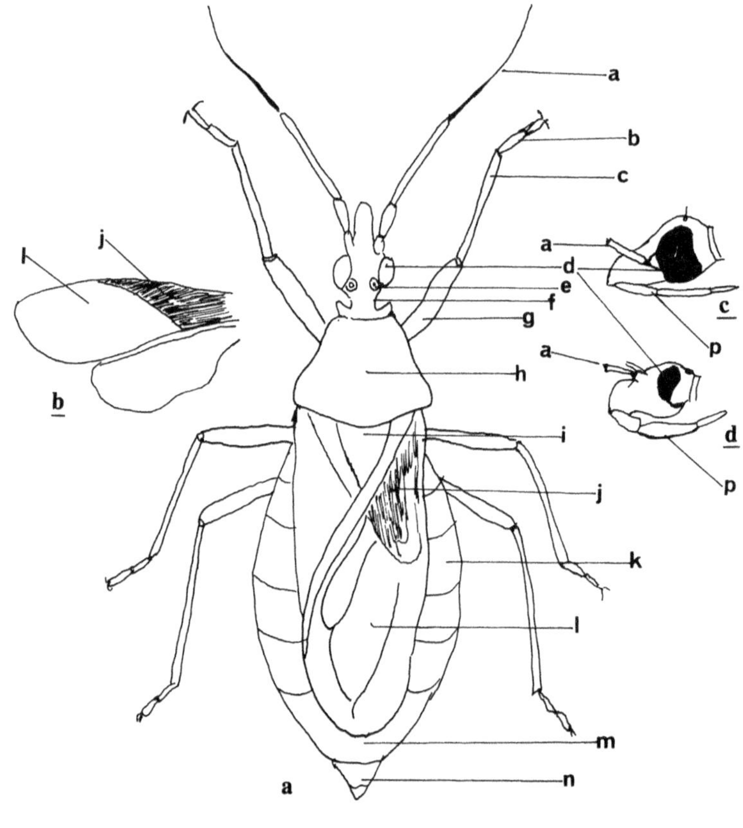

Fig. 6.2. a Outline drawing of *Triatoma rubrofasciata*. **b** Wing arrangement of Heteroptera. **c** Side view of head of *Panstrongylus mesgistus*, a triatomid blood-sucker. **d** Side view of head of *Melanolestes picipes*, a reduviid predator. **c** and **d** illustrate the position of the antennae and the proboscis. *a*, antenna; *b*, tarsus; *c*, tibia, *d*, eye, *e*, ocellus; *f*, neck; *g*, femur; *h*, pronotum; *i*, scutellum; *j*, hemielytron; *k*, connexivum; *l*, membranous portion of wing. **a** After Patton and Cragg 1913, by kind permission of the publisher. The Christian Literature Society for India; **c** and **d** after Chandler 1955, by kind permission of the publisher, John Wiley & Sons Inc.)

Table 6.5. Common names for some of the reduviid bugs

Common Name	Family	Species
Cone-nose bug	Reduviidae	Many
Kissing bug	Reduviidae	Many
Chinese bedbug	Triatominae	*Triatoma protracta*; *T. gerstaeckeri*
Bellows bug	Triatominae	*Triatoma protracta*; *T. gerstaeckeri*
Western blood-sucking corsair	Triatominae	*Triatoma protracta*; *T. gerstaeckeri*
Blood-sucking corsair	Triatominae	*T. sanguisuga*
Black corsair	Piratinae	*Melanolestes picipes*
Two-spotted corsair	Piratinae	*Rasahus biguttatus*; *R. thoracicus*
Assassin bug	Reduviidae	*Reduvius personatus*
Cannibal bug	Reduviidae	*R. personatus*
Wheel bug	Harpactorinae	*Arilus cristatus*

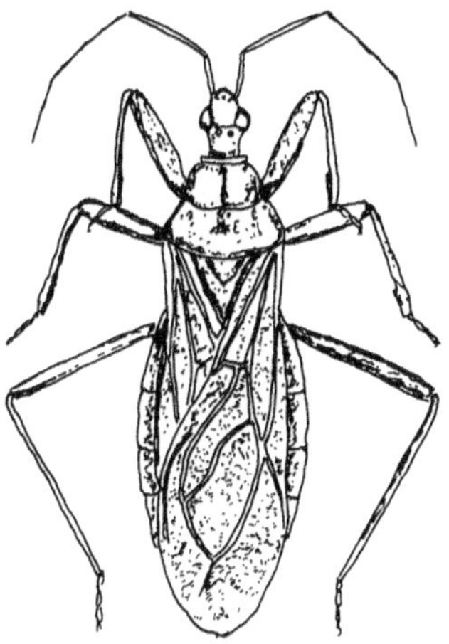

Fig. 6.3. *Reduvius personatus*, adult female. (After Readio 1927, by kind permission of the Editor of the *University of Kansas Science Bulletin*)

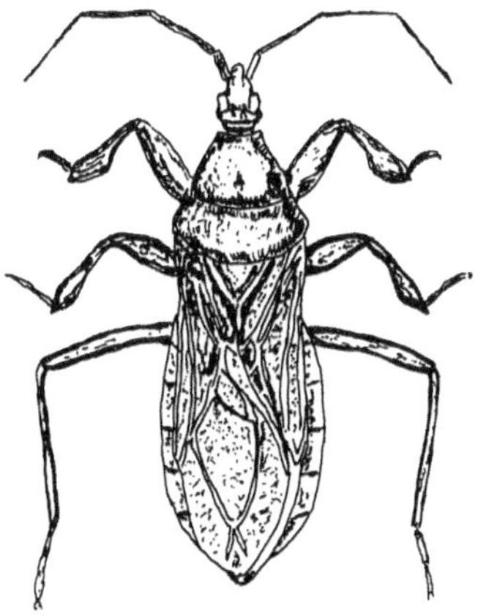

Fig. 6.4. *Melanolestes picipes*, adult female. (After Readio 1927, by kind permission of the Editor of the *University of Kansas Science Bulletin*)

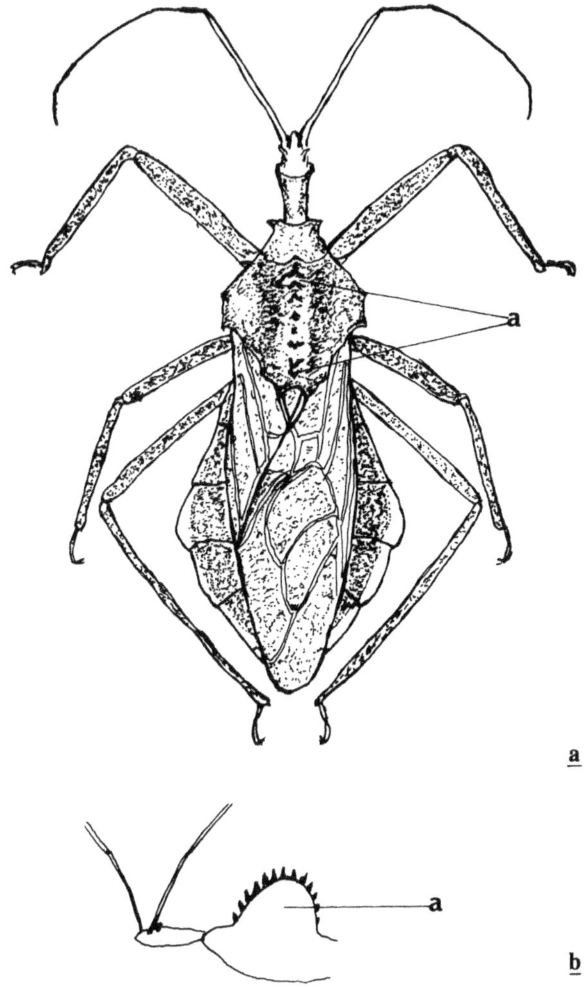

Fig. 6.5a, b. *Arilus cristatus*. **a** dorsal view; **b** sketch of profile of the crest (*a*). After Readio 1927, by kind permission of the Editor of the *University of Kansas Science Bulletin*)

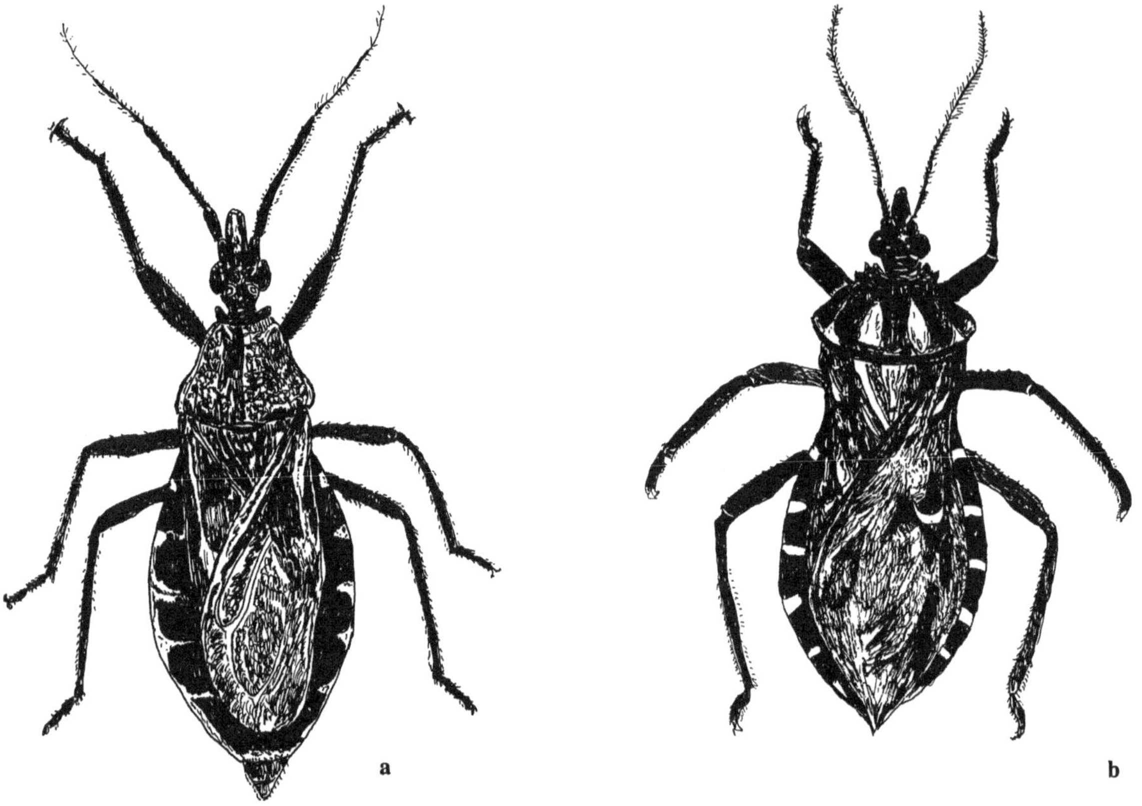

a b

Fig. 6.6. **a** *Triatoma rubrofasciata*; **b** *Panstrongylus megistus*. (After Patton and Cragg 1913, by kind permission of the publisher, The Christian Literature Society for India)

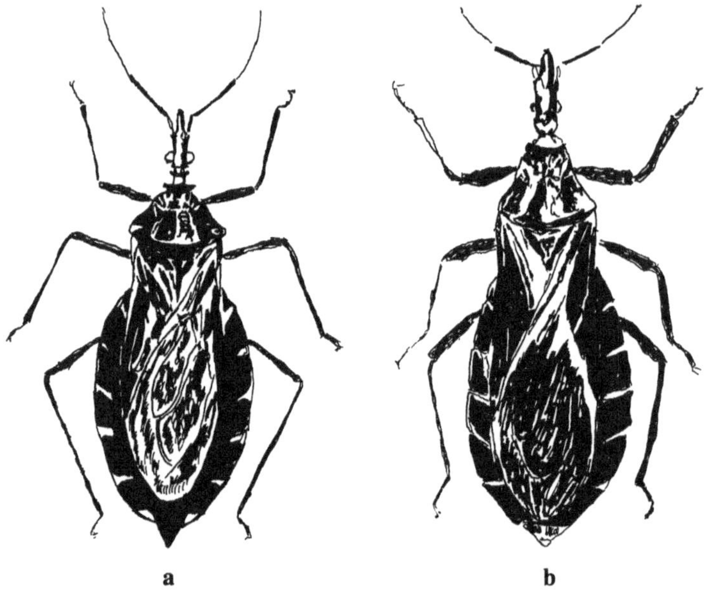

a b

Fig. 6.7. **a** *Triatoma gerstaeckeri* (Stal); **b** *Triatoma protracta* (Uhl)—both adults. [After Usinger RL (1944) The triatominae of North and Central America and the West Indies and their public health significance. US Public Health Services Bulletin No 288, by kind permission of the US National Health Information Clearinghouse]

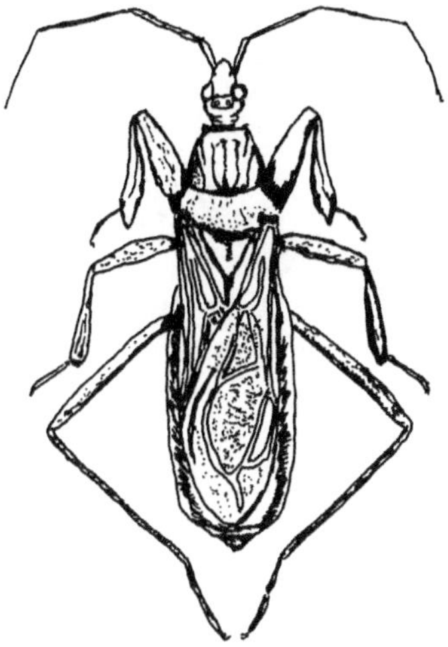

Fig. 6.8. *Rasahus biguttatus*, adult female. (After Readio 1927, by kind permission of the Editor of the *University of Kansas Science Bulletin*)

Life Cycle of Bugs

The life cycle of bugs of both the Cimicidae and the Reduviidae consists of egg, five nymphal stages and the adult. The duration of the cycle and the intervals between the various stages vary from species to species. Table 6.6 shows figures for *Cimex lectularius* taken from Patton and Evans (1929), whilst Table 6.7 gives figures for *Reduvius personatus* taken from Readio (1927) as an example from this family. The moult between each stage requires at least one blood meal, and sometimes more than one, in the case of all haematophagous bugs (see Table 6.6). The immature triatomid bugs rest for several days after the moult before feeding (Gordon and Lavoipierre 1962). The life span of the adult bedbug varies from 1 month to 1 year and for the reduviid bugs in general between 1 and 2 years (Gordon and Lavoipierre 1962). Readio (1927) reported the average life of the North American triatomids as between 210 and 260 days, giving about one brood annually. These times depend not only on ambient temperature and humidity but also on the availability of suitable hosts for food. Blood meals are essential for the normal development of haematophagous bugs but not for phytophagous or predator bugs. For this reason, whilst their normal habitat is often in the nests or burrows of small mammals such as rodents of various kinds, armadilloes or opossum, they can exist and multiply in the neighbourhood of human dwellings, providing there is a sufficiency of small mammals including domestic animals. They may then (in some species) become domesticated and live permanently in houses or huts occupied by humans. Bedbugs do not require the shelter of animals' burrows but live all the time in human habitations. In warmer or tropical climates bugs, especially the reduviid bugs, may be active all the year round but in cooler areas they may spend the winter in a relatively inactive state. Even in winter those which have become domesticated may show some activity; bedbugs do not undergo any period of quiescence in their habits but continue to be a nuisance all the year round. Different species of reduviid bugs spend the winter in different stages. For example, *Arilus cristatus* and *Acholla multispinosa* overwinter in the egg stage; *Reduvius personatus*, *Rasahus biguttatus* and *Apiomeris spissipes* overwinter, as nymphs; and *Melanolestes picipes* overwinters as an adult bug. *Triatoma sanguisuga* can go through the winter either as a nymph or an adult (Readio 1927). Immature forms of reduviid bugs are wingless but can crawl long distances (up to 60 m; Schofield 1979). Bedbugs are wingless for their whole life but can likewise crawl considerable distances in search of a blood meal. Many of the adult reduviid bugs can fly (Lehane and Schofield 1976) and so have access to buildings more than one storey high. One patient described by Goldman (1971) was bitten by *Triatoma sanguisuga* in his eighteenth floor apartment.

Table 6.6. Details of the life cycle of *Cimex lectularius* and the feeding requirements of the various stages. (After Patton and Evans 1929)

Stage	Period (days)	No. of feeds between
Incubation (egg)	6–17	—
Larva	3–14	1–3
First nymph	3–14	1–3
Second nymph	3–15	2–4
Third nymph	4–16	2–4
Fourth nymph	5–19	3–5
Total development range	24–95	9–19

Table 6.7. Life cycle of *Reduvius personatus*. (After Readio 1927)

Stage	Period (days)
Incubation (egg)	13–16
First instar	10–20+
Second instar	10–20+
Third instar	22–150
Fourth instar	10–78
Fifth instar	120–150
Total development range	188–434+

Feeding Habits

Bedbugs feed only on blood but can go long periods without a meal. According to Patton and Evans (1929), nothing but blood has ever been found in the digestive tract of bedbugs. Although they are nocturnal they will feed in the daytime. They have the habit of returning to feed even when they are already engorged. Reduviid bugs are also nocturnal but do not return to feed after engorgement and often feed only every 3 or 4 days. Bedbugs prefer to feed on exposed surfaces but will feed anywhere on the skin if they happen to get under the bedclothes. If disturbed they will bite again close to the previous bite, and their bites for this reason are often arranged in a linear fashion. Reduviid bugs as a general rule do not crawl on the skin but will do so if necessary. They also prefer the exposed surface of the skin, and some species feed with their hind legs firmly on the bed or bedclothes, reaching over to pierce the skin with their extended proboscis (Wood 1941). Wolf (1969) described this action rather picturesquely as "off-shore drilling". *Triatoma sanguisuga* and *T. gerstaeckeri* feed in this manner but others feed entirely on the skin surface, e.g. *Rhodnius prolixus* (Ebeling 1975). When the insects are very numerous they will crawl to find a feeding spot. When about to feed, the reflexed proboscis is erected forward and thrust into the skin. This action has been observed on many occasions since Darwin (1837) first described it, when one of his colleagues offered a finger to a bug (*Benchuca*, a species of Reduviidae, the "great black bug of the Pampas"), which obligingly inserted its proboscis in the above manner.

The technique of feeding by blood-sucking bugs has been studied in detail by Dickerson and Lavoipierre (1959) and by Lavoipierre et al. (1959) Briefly, the skin is pierced by the proboscis and the flexible maxillary portion finally pierces a blood vessel; blood is sucked up by the muscular movements of the insect's hypopharynx (*Rhodnius prolixus* in this instance), which are visible to the naked eye and gives the creature one of its common names, "the bellows bug" (Wood 1941). *Cimex lectularius* feeds in a similar way (Fig. 6.9). Neither feeds from the small microscopic haemorrhages but only from the actual vessel. Friend and Smith (1971) confirmed the pumping action and noted that a copious amount of saliva was produced throughout the feeding process. The first portion of saliva is deposited on the skin as the proboscis penetrates it, subsequently hardening to form a protective collar. The saliva of two other species of bug (*Platymeris rhadamanthus* and belostomatid

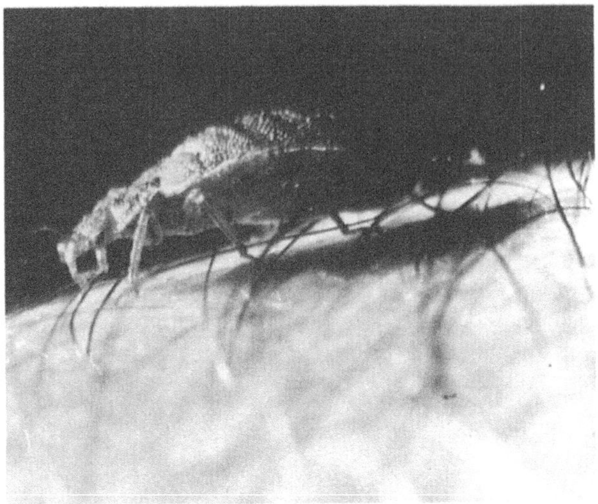

Fig. 6.9. *Cimex lectularius* (bedbug) feeding on human skin. (Courtesy of Rentokil Laboratories Ltd)

species) was shown by Edwards (1961) and Rees and Offord (1969), respectively, to contain highly active proteolytic enzymes together with hyaluronidase and other enzymes. These probably cause the severe pain quickly felt after defensive bites by predator bugs and by phytophagous bugs. The haematophagous bugs, on the other hand, need to feed for 10–20 min for full engorgement (Gordon and Lavoipierrre 1962). Their bites are painless and the salivary secretion much less irritating. Whilst itch is felt at once or very soon after the bite, most of the reactions are somewhat delayed and probably due to hypersensitivity to the protein content of the saliva (Chandler 1955; Dodge 1970). Myers (1929) observed that a phytophagous bug induced to feed on man did so for at least 1 h. None of the haematophagous bugs feed through clothing (Shields and Walsh 1956).

Characteristically all bugs defaecate after feeding, some immediately after and others after an interval. *Cimex lectularius* turns round during the process so that the puncture wound is contaminated. The importance of this action lies in the fact that some of the reduviid haematophagous feeders are vectors of Chagas' disease (see Tables 6.3 and 6.4) and carry *Trypanosoma cruzi* in their faeces. It can thus get inoculated directly into the puncture wound or rubbed into the skin through excoriation by the patient. The period between cessation of feeding and defaecation is then a matter of great practical importance. Bugs do not tarry on the skin after feeding. If there is a delay in defaecation, the faecal material (consisting of altered blood from the previous meal and sometimes *T. cruzi*) will be deposited not on the patient but on the bedclothes, night clothes, bed or walls of the room. In Brazil the vectors for Chagas' disease, chiefly *Panstrongylus megistus* and *Melanolestes picipes* and in the south *Triatoma infestans*, are all voracious feeders and defaecate readily on the skin surface. Chagas' disease is common. In the United States, on the other hand, the principal potential vectors are *T. sanguisuga*, which defaecates 30 min or so after feeding, by which time it will have left its victim, and *T. gerstaeckeri*, which is also disinclined to defaecate immediately after feeding. The chances of trypanosome infection are therefore reduced to almost nil, which is in line with the rarity of Chagas' disease in the United States (Woody et al. 1965).

Clinical Reactions to Bug Bites

The clinical picture resulting from bug bites is very variable, but in fact the different appearances are all part of the same basic spectrum influenced by two factors: the species of bug involved and, more important, the degree of sensitivity developed by the victim. Reference has already been made to the occasional attacks of some homopterous bugs and to bites from phytophagous species of the heteropterous group. Only the reactions to bugs of the Reduviidae and Cimicidae families will be considered here. The reactions to the bites of haematophagous and predaceous bugs differ in mode of onset and, to some extent, in their subsequent development. The predaceous bug bites to defend itself and its bite is invariably and immediately extremely painful. Haematophagous bugs, on the other hand, bite in order to feed. Their bite is painless and almost imperceptible, attention only being drawn to it by subsequent itching and other manifestations. The reaction to the bite of a predaceous bug is a response to the irritant character of the salivary secretion (or venom) injected by the insect together with any sensitivity developed against that secretion. With haematophagous bug bites almost the entire reaction is of a sensitivity nature. Sensitivity varies in degree according to the number of times the victim has been exposed to biting. Consequently the cutaneous reaction also varies in degree, which accounts for the considerable variance in the published descriptions of such reactions.

There are two classes of reaction: firstly, local and cutaneous, and, secondly, generalised and systemic. The reactions to haematophagous bites will be considered first. They are exemplified by the groupings given by Shields and Walsh (1956) for the lesions resulting from attack by *Triatoma sanguisuga*. No matter into which group a reaction falls the onset is similar. The patient is bitten in the dark, shortly after retiring to bed and is awakened sometime between midnight and 3 a.m. by itching, usually localised at first but often quickly generalised. The subsequent visible lesions can be of the following types:

1. Papular with a central punctum. There is a tendency to grouping, often in a linear fashion. Histologically there is a non-specific lymphocyte infiltrate. This represents a mild sensitivity reaction (see Fig. 6.10).
2. Groups of small vesicles clustered together in an area some 2–3 cm across but produced by a single bite. There is underlying erythema and moderate swelling. A central punctum is usually not seen. The appearance could easily be mistaken for a patch of contact dermatitis were it not for obvious bites in other areas.
3. Giant urticaria with weals up to 20 cm across and associated with a deep-seated brawny

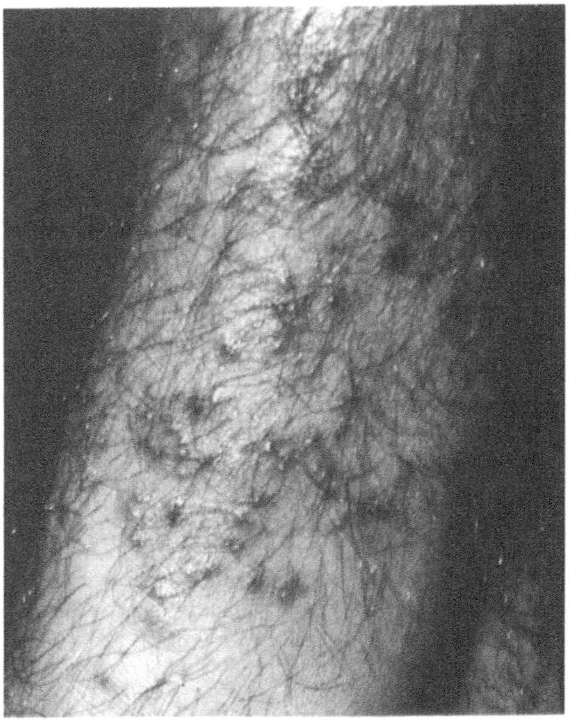

Fig. 6.10. "Bug" bites (species unidentified) on the upper arm of a Brazilian patient. The lesions on the lower part of the arm, just above the elbow and unobscured by hair, show a central punctum on an oedematous papule. (Courtesy of Prof. Sebasio Sampaio, Faculty of Medicine, University of Sao Paulo, Brazil)

oedema. A central punctum can sometimes be seen with this reaction.

4. Haemorrhagic nodular or bullous lesions of the hands and feet. These were said by Shields and Walsh (1956) to be characteristic of bites of *T. sanguisuga*. They resemble erythema multiforme but are unilateral.

The clinical changes in groups 3 and 4 are sometimes accompanied by lymphangitis and regional lymphadenopathy, uninfluenced by antibiotics. Additional to these cutaneous changes the patient may develop hypersensitivity and exhibit the features of the acute anaphylactic reaction. These features are enumerated in Table 6.8 and are based on Wood's findings.

The predominant clinical features vary with species. *Cimex lectularius* and *C. hemipterus* usually produce multiple bites in certain preferential areas, reported as follows: ankles, legs, buttocks, neck and shoulders (Allington and Allington 1954); the arms more often than the legs (Bartley and Harlan 1974): equally on limbs, trunk and face (Churchill 1930); the exposed areas as a rule, but elsewhere if the bugs accidentally get beneath the bedclothes (Patton and Evans 1929). These views suggest that the areas involved are to some extent dependent on the intensity of the infestation. Linear grouping is characteristic. Although feeding time is relatively short (3–5 min), and some think that one feed is sufficient and likely to be followed by several days without food (Canadian Ministry of Supply and Services 1980), others think that bedbugs feed several times in a night (Andrews and Domonkos 1971). Patton and Evans (1929) observed that whilst feeding time is indeed brief these bugs frequently return to feed again, although to all intents and purposes they are already fully engorged. These latter authors maintained that a central punctum and erythematous halo is not seen; however, not everyone agrees with them. Whether erythema is seen or not there is no doubt that red blotches which often go on to form large urticarial weals are frequent reactions to *Cimex* bites. The present writer sustained, at the age of 17, a single weal 20 cm in diameter, which developed within 20 min. Examination revealed a bug still firmly attached to the centre of the lesion. (This incidentally occurred in the daytime.) Multiple similar lesions can occur (Churchill 1930). Delayed weals appearing up to 48 h after bites have been reported (Bartley and Harlan 1974). Bullous lesions are not uncommon following bites from bedbugs, the best known example being the epidemic which occurred amongst women passengers on an infested Dundee tramcar in 1948 (Kinnear 1948). The lesions occurred in horizontal rows at the upper end of the calf where it had been in contact with a wooden seat harbouring the bugs. Many passengers were affected before the cause was discovered. According to Patton and Evans (1929) the furniture in Indian railway stations was also frequently infested, with similar results. Parsons (1955) has described an anaphylactic reaction to bedbug bites.

Triatoma sanguisuga may cause any of the four types of lesions described above. Anaphylactic reactions to this species are relatively uncommon but have been described (Patton and Cragg 1913; Shields and Walsh 1956; Mead 1965; Lynch and Pinnas 1978). The bites of *T. rubrofasciata* are followed by itching, which may have an intense burning character (Arnold and Bell 1944), and the bite site often has a central papule or vesicle (Gallardo 1940). Africa (1934) and Teo and Cheah (1973) both noted an anaphylactic response to *T. rubrofasciata*. *T. protracta* (sometimes associated with *T. gerstaeckeri*) has caused a great deal of trouble in the southwestern states of the United States, especially in southern California and Arizona, where it has attacked small communities very severely. Ebeling (1975) has observed that the tendency for people to build their homes in the wooded chaparral areas around the larger cities and in the Sierra Nevada foothills has increased the likelihood of their homes being infested by these bugs. Some mining villages of Arizona have been heavily infested with *T. protracta*. Apart from bites which quickly develop into painful swellings the outstanding feature of the reports from these areas has been the number of severe anaphylactic reactions, often requiring emergency medical care, amongst the permanent residents (Riley and Howard 1894; Wood 1941; Walsh and Jones 1962; Swezey 1963; Mansur 1975, this last instance being fatal) and also in holiday makers (Wood 1941). Wood (1975) has estimated on the basis of a questionnaire that between 5% and 15% of the population react to *T. protracta*; of the selected group questioned 25% reacted severely.

The species of reduviid bugs prevalent in South American, *T. infestans*, *Rhodnius prolixus* and *Panstrongylus megistus*, are all important vectors of Chagas' disease. (One of the diagnostic features of this disease is unilateral eyelid oedema "Romana's" sign; see Fig. 6.11.) However, they do not appear to give rise to such severe reactions as do those in the southern United States. All three species are common household pests. For example, 80% of the population (in an area not infested by *T. infestans*) showed an urticarial reaction of some

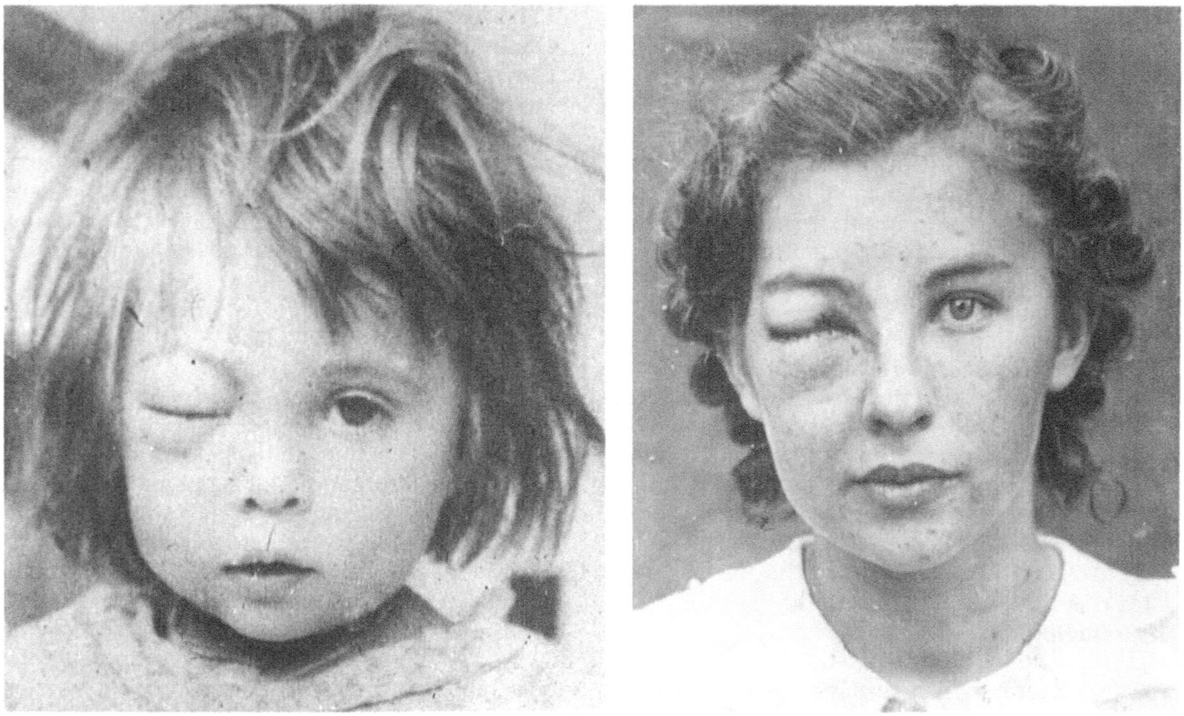

a b

Fig. 6.11. Romana's sign (unilateral eyelid oedema) in Chagas' disease, South American trypanosomiasis. **a** by courtesy of Prof. Dr. C. Andretta Jr, Faculty of Medical Science, Santos, Brazil; **b** by courtesy of Prof. Vincente Amata Neto, Faculty of Medicine, University of Sao Paulo, Brazil)

sort to its bites (used for xenodiagnosis), indicating either previous exposure to it or to a cross-reaction between it and the locally dominant species *P. megistus* (Mott et al. 1980). In either case the proportion of persons bitten by one or the other is very high, and yet the occurrence of anaphylactic reactions is not recorded in the literature cited for either species. Lapierre and Lariviere (1954) have noted such a reaction to *R. prolixus* bites.

Reaction to Predaceous Reduviid Bug Bites

Without exception the bites are defensive and very painful. *Melanolestes picipes* (Piratinae) is very common throughout the United States, is attracted by the lights of houses at night and bites readily if disturbed. Its bites are quite common. The pain was said by Readio (1927) to be worse than that of a bee sting and by McClure (1935) to be excruciating. It is almost instantaneous and is quickly followed by a small red spot, or even a vesicle. Considerable swelling rapidly ensues and may be accompanied by a feeling of numbness (Howard 1900; McClure 1935), which persists for several days. There are no sequelae.

The two species of *Rasahus* (*biguttatus* and *thoracicus*; Piratinae) cause similarly painful bites with swelling, which may proceed to blistering, ulceration, necrosis and scarring, probably as a result of cellulitis from secondary infection (Davidson 1897; Howard 1900). They are not so common as the bites due to *Melanolestes* and because of the ulceration have been mistaken for spider bites (Davidson 1897). The pain from the bite was described by Hoffman (1923) as like that of a scorpion sting. These two bugs feed on blood, but prefer it to be obtained indirectly by feeding on bedbugs (Howard 1900; Readio 1927).

Reduvius personatus (Reduviinae) is a common household pest in the northern and eastern and, to a less extent, the western states of the United States. Like *Rasahus* it feeds on bedbugs, and its immature forms, which are sticky, are concealed by adherent dust. Its bite was said by Blatchley (1926) and by Readio (1927) to be almost as severe as a snakebite. The site quickly swells and may remain so for a week. Some persons become sensitised (either directly or possibly by cross-sensititisation) and can develop anaphylactic symptoms (Matheson 1950). According to Readio (1927)

R. personatus may be fatal to weakly persons, but it is not clear whether he was referring to the bite or to the anaphylactic reaction.

Arilus cristatus, recognisable by its peculiar cog-wheel-shaped crest, preys on caterpillars and other insects (see Fig. 6.12) but bites viciously if handled. It seems generally accepted that its bite is more painful than that of any other insect. It may in some instances increase in intensity after initial pain, and persist for some hours (Glover 1876, cited by Readio 1927). The bite becomes swollen and inflamed and may involve a large area (Scott 1963). In the case reported by Barber (1919) the bite site became indurated as the result of secondary infection. In the instance described by Hall (1924) a papillomatous growth presented at the bite site and remained for 9 months. Scott thought that the saliva contained a haemolytic neurotoxic venom.

Immunology

Clinical reactions have clearly shown the development of sensitivity to bug bites. Nicholls and Green (1963) obtained positive skin reaction to *T. protracta* in all 12 patients tested, whereas the controls all gave negative results. Pinnas et al. (1978), using the radio-allergosorbent test (RAST) technique, obtained positive results with extracts of reduviid bug thorax and salivary gland. These results, they claimed, indicated IgE mediation of allergic activity.

A tangible result of the development of sensitivity is scratching, which, as Gordon (1958) pointed out, is important in the inoculation of *Trypansoma cruzi* from bug faecal material deposited on the skin.

Diagnosis

Single bites by predator species are obvious. With haematophagous bugs the appearance of a rash in the morning, preceded by itching for a few hours, is suspicious. Suspicion is greatly reinforced by finding the bugs. If they are not found then the presence of faecal or blood smears on the walls or bedding and the characteristic odour are additional evidence. In such circumstances parasites should always be sought, by inspecting the clothing, bedding, mattress, bed, furniture, upholstery, woodwork, walls and floor. Other members of the household may also have been attacked. The exposed parts of the body are mainly affected. Distinction from flea bites may be difficult, but with

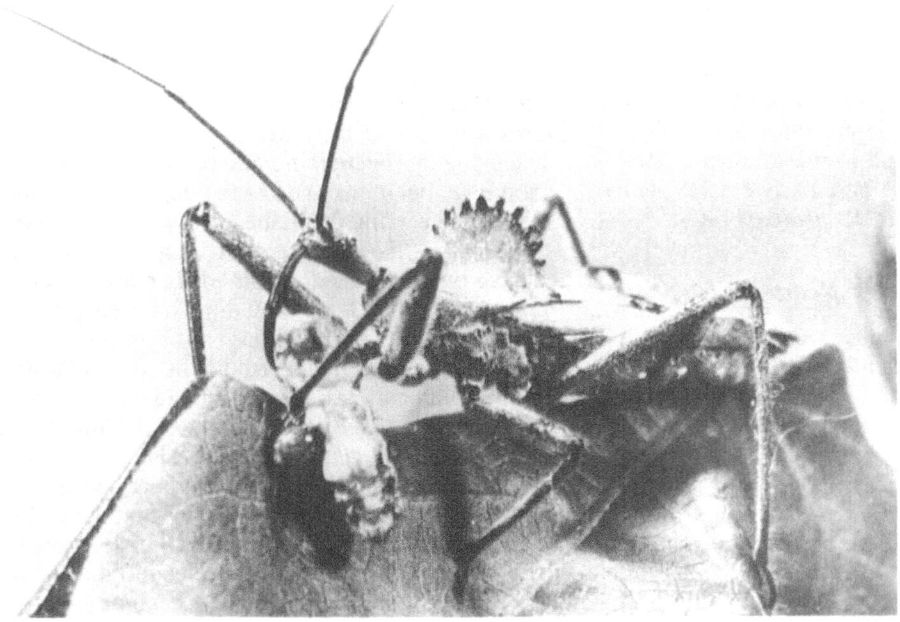

Fig. 6.12. *Arilus cristatus* (assassin bug or wheel bug) devouring its prey. Note the erected proboscis or beak, which has pierced the victim. Note also the "dinosaur-like" crest on the dorsum of the thorax, which gives the creature one of its popular names. (From Ebeling 1975, by kind permission of the author and the publisher, University of California, Agricultural Publications)

the latter the covered parts of the body are more frequently involved (see pp. 164–165). Infestation by lice may cause similar symptoms but of a more chronic nature; inspection of the patient's clothing should soon dispose of that possibility. Erythema multiforme is a symmetrical eruption usually of hands and feet, involving the oral mucosa and with systemic upset.

Anaphylactic reactions are usually of sudden and rapid onset with increasingly severe symptoms (Table 6.8). The association of insect bites and an urticarial reaction with dyspnoea, pallor, sweating, tachycardia, vomiting and collapse are strongly suggestive of this complication. In the absence of a rash and with no suspicion of insect bites the diagnosis is much more difficult but its occurrence in a district known for bug infestation should arouse suspicion, as should the rapidity with which the symptoms develop.

Table 6.8. Symptoms of anaphylactic reaction to bug bites in the order in which they commonly occur. (After Woods 1975)

1.	Generalised intense itch— may start on palms and soles
2.	Flushing erythema progressing to urticaria
3.	Local and generalised oedema
4.	Nausea
5.	Chills (rigors)
6.	Vomiting
7.	Fever
8.	Fainting—postural
9.	Partial paralysis
10.	Swelling of the tongue
11.	Tightening of the throat muscles
12.	Respiratory distress
13.	Severe abdominal cramp-like pains
14.	Unconsciousness

Treatment

The single bite of the predator species may not require any treatment, if pain is brief. If pain persists, oral analgesics are required. In the absence of inflammation local anaesthetic injected into the bite site could give instant relief; in the presence of inflammation 1% phenol in oily calamine lotion is very helpful. A topical corticosteroid/antibiotic combination might also help. If cellulitis should develop, avoid all corticoids and give oral antibiotics, combined with rest and support for the affected part. Smith et al. (1958) recommended magnesium sulphate compresses for *Arilus* bites. In the event of suppuration incision is required.

For urticarial reactions to haematophagous bugs symptomatic treatment with topical phenol and calamine lotion and oral antihistamines may be adequate. If the urticaria is severe, giving the antihistamine by intramuscular injection is often very effective (50 mg promethazine once or twice daily). Systemic corticosteroids are only justified in very severe cases.

Anaphylactic symptoms require urgent treatment. Slow subcutaneous injection of 0.5–1.0 ml of adrenaline hydrochloride is the single most important measure. Intramuscular promethazine (50 mg) should also be given, and, if the symptoms are severe or getting worse, intravenous hydrocortisone in a continuous saline infusion is indicated. Admission to hospital as soon as possible is also advisable.

Spread of Bugs

Bedbugs inhabit the dwellings where their source of food lives. In the main this means that they infest human habitations, but they may also be found in buildings housing poultry and other domestic animals upon which they can also feed. In houses they are most frequent in the sleeping quarters of the inhabitants, spending the hours of daylight hiding in cracks in woodwork, behind loose window frames and skirting boards, behind picture frames and other furnishings and loose wall paper, on beds and beneath mattresses and on furniture and upholstery. By choice they seem to prefer to rest on flat surfaces (Patton and Evans 1929). In other dwellings they infest similar places, and in public places they seem to have a predilection for hiding on the undersurfaces of seats (Patton and Evans 1929; Kinnear 1948). They are disseminated by carriage in second-hand furniture, bedding, possibly in luggage, but seldom if ever on the person. They are also, of course, capable of making their own way on foot to new quarters. Patton and Evans described this after observing old-fashioned bug traps—pieces of wood with holes bored into them for the bugs to hide in after feeding, which are placed on beds—being knocked out on the doorstep in the morning. The bugs immediately walked straight back into the house!

Reduviid bugs fly into houses at night, attracted by the light. In the later instar stages they can also walk in (Schofield 1979).

Control and Prevention

Swezey (1963) categorised the necessary measures under three headings: structure proofing, chemical proofing, and additional means. In the last category he included the use of bed nets at night and the encouragement of harmless predators. To this might be added education of the public, especially in developing countries.

Structural insect proofing involves checking all existing preventive screens over windows, doorways (including special entrances for cats and dogs) and fireplaces and installing them when necessary. It also involves inspection and, where necessary, repair of foundations, woodwork, plasterwork, window frames, and doorways. The destruction of rodent burrows, not only beneath houses but also in the immediate vicinity, is important where reduviid bugs are concerned. Schofield (1979) has pointed out that many of these precautions could be avoided by a great improvement in the housing standards of the rural and urban poor and the maintenance of these standards.

Chemical control of insects implies destruction of those in infested buildings. The measures recommended by the Canadian Ministry of Supply and Services (1980) seem admirable. The hiding and breeding places of the bugs should be sprayed with "residual" insecticides, i.e. ones which persist after evaporation of the solvent vehicle. For upholstery and bedding it is recommended that 0.5% malathion in a watery emulsion be sprayed on lightly with a continuous pressure apparatus as a fine "fan" or "cone" spray. For all other materials 2% emulsion is better. Flat surfaces should be sprayed with a fan or cone spray so as to wet them, whilst cracks, fissures and spaces behind boards should be attacked with a fine stream jet so as to penetrate adequately. Alternatively, 0.9% dichlorvos or 0.5% *d*-phenothrin could be used instead of malathion, and could also be used as dusts instead of sprays. If any bugs remain after 3–4 weeks the treatment should be repeated.

These chemicals should not be used for infants' bedding; instead pyrethrums should be used and repeated in 2 weeks. Powders should not be employed if children can get access to it. It is absolutely essential if a professional exterminator is not employed that all instructions be read carefully and adhered to accurately. Should any of the insecticides not be available, white kerosene can be sprayed on in the same manner, but care should be taken to minimise any fire risk. Where blocks of flats or office buildings are involved, professional exterminators should be employed to use gas fumigation with cyanide (Back 1937).

References

Africa CM (1934) Three cases of poisonous insect bite involving *Triatoma rubrofasciata*. Philippine J Sci 53: 169–178

Allington HV, Allington RR (1954) Insect bites. JAMA 155: 240–247

Andrews GC, Domonkos A (1971) Diseases of the skin, 6th edn. Saunders, Philadelphia

Arnold HL, Bell DB (1944) "Kissing bug bites" Hawaii Med J 3: 121–127

Back EA (1937) Bed bugs. US. Dept of Agricultive Leaflet No 146. US Govt Printing Office, Washington DC, pp 1–8

Banks CS (1919) The blood-sucking insects of the Philippines. Philippine J Sci 14: 169–189

Barber GN (1919) On the bite of *Arilus cristatus*. J Econ Entomol 12: 466

Bartley JD, Harlan HJ (1974) Bed-bug infestation; its control and management. Milit Med 139: 884–886

Becker GG (1918) *Empoasca mali* Le B. attacks man. Psyche 25: 101

Bequaert J (1925) Medical and economic entomology, Part II of medical report of the Hamilton Expedition to the Amazon in conjunction with the Department of Tropical Medicine of Harvard Univerity, 1924–1925. Contribution to the Harvard Institute of Tropical Biology and Medicine, No 4. University Press, Cambridge, Mass pp 184–185

Blacklock B (1923) Pyrrhocorid bug capable of biting man. Ann Trop. Med Parasitol 17: 337–354

Blatchley WS (1926) Heteroptera or true bugs of Eastern North America, vol 1. Nature Publishing Company, Indianopolis, p 116.

Brues CT (1972) Insects, food and ecology. Dover, New York

Canadian Ministry of Supply and Services (1980) Control of bugs. Publ No 1293. Information Services for Agriculture. Acland, Ottowa

*Chandler AC (1955) Introduction to parasitology with special reference to the parasites of man, 9th edn. Wiley, New York

Churchill TP (1930) Urticaria due to bed bug. JAMA 95: 1975

Costa CHN, Costa MJ, Weber JN, Gilks GF, Castro C, Marsden PD (1981) Skin reactions to bug bites as a result of xenodiagnosis. Trans R Soc Trop Med Hyg 75: 405–408

Crosby CR (1926) A leaf hopper becomes predaceous. J Econ Entomol 19: 812

Darwin C (1837) Journal of researches into the natural history and geology of the countries visited during the voyage of H.M.S. Beagle round the world. (Reprinted 1890.) Nelson, London

Davidson A (1897) So-called spider bites and their treatment. Ther Gazette Whole series 21; Third series 13: 80–83

de Bergevin E (1925) Les hemipteres suceurs de sang. Arch Inst Pasteur Alg 3: 28–41

*Dickerson G, Lavoipierre MMJ (1959) Studies on the method of feeding of blood-sucking arthropods II. The method of feeding adopted by the bedbug (*Cimex lectularius*) when obtaining a blood meal from the mammalian host. Ann Trop Med Parasitol 53: 347–357

Dodge NN (1970) Poison dwellers of the desert, 12th edn revised. Southwest Parks and Monuments Association, Globe, Arizona

Donovan C (1920) A frog-hopper as a blood-sucking insect. Br Med J I: 220

*Ebeling W (1975) Urban entomology. University of California, Division of Agricultural Science, Los Angeles, Cal

Edwards JS (1960) Insect assassins. Sci Am 202: 72–78

Edwards JS (1961) The action and composition of the saliva of an assassin bug *Platmyeris rhadamanthus* Gaerst. (Hemiptera: Reduviidae). J Exp Biol 38: 61–77

Essig EO (1926) Insects of western North America. Macmillan Company, New York

Ewing HE (1928) Observations on the habits and the injury caused by the bites or stings of some common North American arthropods. Am J Trop Med 8: 39–62

Ferreria L de C, Dean L (1938) Encontro de um nova hematophago do homen com habitos domiciliares. Brasil Med 52: 1137–1141

Foley H (1929) Sur divers arthropodes piqueurs observés au cours de la mission du huggar. Bull Soc His Nat Afr Nord 20: 47–54

Friend WG, Smith JBB (1971) Feeding in *Rhodnius prolixus*: mouth part activity and salivation and their correlation with change of electrical resistance. J Insect Physiol 17: 233–243

Gallardo VP (1940) Observations on the sting of *Triatoma rubrofasciate* DeGeer. J Philippine Med Assoc 20: 35–36

*Ghauri MSK (1973) Hemiptera (bugs). In: Smith KGV (ed) Insects and other arthropods of medical importance. Trustees of the British Museum (Natural History) London pp 373–393

Goldman L (1971) Reduviid bites in an arthropod reactor. Arch Dermatol 104: 407

Gordon RM (1958) The reaction to arthropod bites and its relation to arthropod-borne infection with special reference to filariasis. East Afr Med J 35: 393–400

Gordon RM, Lavoipierre MMJ (1962) Entomology for students of medicine Blackwell, Oxford

Gorgas Memorial Institute (1976) Trypanosomiasis. Gorgas Memorial Institute 47th annual report. House document No 94–353, 94th Congress, 2nd Series US Govt. Printing Office, Washington DC, pp 15–18

Hall MC (1924) Lesions due to the bite of the wheel bug *Arilus cristatus* (Hemiptera: Reduviidae). Arch Intern Med 33: 513–515

Hoffman WH (1923) Observaciones biologicas sobre la Reduviidae Cubana llamada *Triatoma flavida*. Rev Med Cubana 28: 299–305

Howard LO (1900) The insects to which the name "kissing bug" became applied during the summer of 1899. US Dep of Agriculture Bulletin No 22. US Govt Printing Office, Washington DC, pp 24–30

Howard LO, Schwarz (1901) The 145th meeting of the Entomological Society of Washington. Proc Entomol Soc Washington 4: 398

Illingworth JF (1916) *Clerada apicicornis* sucking blood (Hemip). Proc Hawaii Entomol Soc 3: 274

Imms AD (1938) Text book of entomology, 4th edn. Methuen, London

Judd WW (1959) *Sinea diadema* Fabr. (Hemiptera: Reduviidae) biting a human. Entomol News 70: 137

Keh B (1956) Cone-nosed bugs of California. Cal Vector Views 3: 47–49

Kinnear J (1948) Epidemic of bullous erythema on legs due to bed bugs. *Lancet II*: 55

Kinnear NB (1909) The blood-sucking propensities of a bug (*Nabis capsiformis*). J Bombay Nat Hist Soc 19: 534–535

Kofoid CA, Whittaker BG (1936) Natural infection of American trypanosomiasis in two species of cone-nose bugs, *Triatoma protracta* Uhler and *Triatoma uhleri* Neiva, in the western United States. J Parasitol 22: 259–263

Lapierre J, Lariviere M (1964) Réaction allergique aux piqûres de réduvide. (*Rhodnius prolixus*) Bull Soc Pathol Exot 47: 563–566

Lathrop GD, Ominsky AJ (1965) Chagas disease. Study in a group of individuals bitten by North American triatomids. Aero-Med Rev 9: 1–5

*Lavoipierre MMJ, Dickerson G, Gordon RM (1959) Studies on the methods of feeding of blood-sucking arthropods. I The manner in which triatomine bugs obtain their blood meal as observed in the tissues of the living rodent, with some remarks on the effect of the bite on human volunteers. Ann Trop Med Parasitol 53: 235–250

Lehane MJ, Schofield CJ (1976) Preliminary report on flight by some triatomine bugs. Trans R Soc Trop Med Hyg 70: 526

Lewis DJ (1958) Hemiptera of medical interest in the Sudan Republic. Proc R Entomol Soc Lond 33: 43–47

Lugger O (1896) Insects injurious in 1896. The bedbug. Univ Minn Agric Exp Station Bull 48: 222–227

Lynch PJ, Pinnas JL (1978) "Kissing bug" bites. *Triatoma* species as an important cause of insect bites in the Southwest. Cutis 22: 585–591

McClure HE (1935) The bite of *Melanolestes picipes* Herrick-Schiffe (Hemip: Reduviidae) Entomol News 46: 138–139

McKeown KC (1942) Australian insects XVII: The bugs. Order Hemiptera–Heteroptera. Aust Museum Mag 8: 27–31

Mansur GP (1975) Autopsy report 30/5/1975. Cited by Ryckman and Bentley (1979)

Matheson R (1950) Medical entomology, 2nd edn. Comstock, Ithaca, NY, pp 182–193

Mend FW (1965) The blood-sucking cone-nose. Florida Department of Agriculture, Division of Plant Industrial Entomology Circular No 33, pp 1–2

Misra CS (1924) Observations on some rhyncota from northern India. In: Report of the proceedings of the fifth entomology meeting, Pusa (1923), p 442

Mott KE, Franca JT, Barrett TV, Hoff R, de Oliveriera TS, Sherlock IA (1980) Cutaneous allergic reactions to *Triatoma infestans* after xenodiagnosis. Mem Inst Oswaldo Cruz 75: 3–10

Myers JG (1929) Facultative blood sucking in phytophagous Hemiptera. Parasitology 21: 472–480

Nicholls N, Green TW (1963) Allergic reactions to "kissing bug" bites. Cal Med 98: 267–268

Nuñez-Andrade R (1953) Nuñez-Andrade's diseases, In: Simons RDG (ed) Handbook of Tropical Dermatology and Medical Mycology. Elsevier, Amsterdam pp 901–907

Parsons DJ (1955) Bed-bug bite anaphylaxis misinterpreted as coronory occlusion. Ohio State Med J 51: 669

Patton WS, Cragg FW (1913) A Text-book of medical entomology. Christian Literature Society for India, Madras, pp 478–526

*Patton WS, Evans AM (1929) Insects, ticks, mites and venomous animals of medical and veterinary importance. Part I Medical. HR Grubb, Croydon

Picado CT (1936) Estudio experimental sobre o veneno de *Lethocerus delpontei* (De Carlo) Hemiptera: Belostomatidae) Mem Inst Butantan 10: 303–310

Pick F, Roubaud E (1954) Presence d'histamine chez les reduviides hematophages. CR Acad Sci (Paris) 239: 1076–1078

Pinnas JL, Chen TMW, Hoffman DR (1978) Evidence for IgE-mediation of human sensitivity to reduviid bug bite. Fed Proc 37: 1555

*Readio PA (1927) Studies on the biology of the Reduviidae of America north of Mexico. Univ Kansas Sci Bull 17: 5–291

Rees AR, Offord RC (1969) Studies on the protease and other enzymes from the venom of *Lethocerus cardofanus*. Nature 221: 675–677

Riley CV, Howard LO (1894) The blood-sucking cone-nose again. US Dep of Agriculture, Division of Entomology, Insect Life No 6. US Govt Printing Office, Washington DC, p 267

*Ryckman RE, Bentley DG (1979) Host reactions to bug bites (Hemiptera: Homoptera) A literature review and annotated bibliography. Cal Vector Views 26: 1–50

Schofield CT (1979) The behaviour of Triatominae (Hemiptera: Reduviidae). A review. Bull Entomol Res 69: 363–379

Scott HG (1963) How arthropod venoms affect man. Pest Control 31: 40–50
Shields TL, Walsh EN (1956) "Kissing bug" bite. Arch Dermatol 74: 14–21
Smith FD, Miller NG, Carnazzo SJ, Eaton WB (1958) Insect bites by *Arilus cristatus*, a North American reduviid. Arch Dermatol Syphilol 77: 324–330
Stys P, Daniel M (1957) *Lyctocoris campestris* (F.) (Heteroptera: Anthocaridae) as a human facultative ectoparasite. Acta Soc Entomol Czech 54: 88–97
Swezey RL (1963) "Kissing bug" bite in Los Angeles. Arch Intern Med 112: 977–980
Teo SK,Cheah JS (1973) Severe reaction to the bite of the triatomid bug (*Triatoma rubrofasciata*) in Singapore. J Trop Med 76: 161–162
Torre-Bueno JR de la (1931) Biting bugs. Bull Brooklyn Entomol Soc 26: 176
Townsend CHJ (1893) Notes on the coruco, a Hemipterous insect which infests poultry in Southern New Mexico. Proc Entomol Soc Washington 3: 40–42
*Usinger RL (1934) Blood-sucking among phytophagous Hemiptera. Can Entomologist 66: 97–100
Vanderplank FL (1958) The assassin bug *Platymerus rhadamanthus* (Hemiptera: Reduviidae) a useful predator of the rhinoceros beetles *Orytes boas* (F) and *Orytes monoceros* (Oliv) (Coleoptera: Scarabaeidae). J Entomol Soc S Afr 21: 309–314
Walsh JD, Jones JP (1962) Public health significance of the cone-nosed bug *Triatoma protracta* (Uhler) in the Sierra Nevada foothills of California. Cal Vector Views 9: 33–37
Wehrle LP (1939) Observation on three species of *Triatoma* (Hemiptera: Reduviidae). Bull Brooklyn Entomol Soc 34: 145–154
Wolf AF (1969) Sensitivity to *Triatoma* bite. Ann Allergy 27: 271–273
Wood SF (1941) New localities for *Trypanosoma cruzi* Chagas in Southwestern United States. Am J Hyg 34: 1–13
Wood SF (1942a) Observation on vectors of Chagas disease in the United States. 1. California. Bull South Cal Acad Sci 41: 61–69
Wood SF (1942b) Reactions of man to the feeding of reduviid bugs. J Parasitol 28: 43–49
Wood SF (1953) Cone-nose bug (*Triatoma*) annoyance and *Trypanosoma cruzi* in Southwestern national monuments. Bull South Cal Acad Sci 52: 57–60
Wood SF (1975) Reaction of man to the feeding of *Triatoma protracta* (Hemiptera: Reduviidae) Nat Pest Control Operators News 35: 19–21
Woody NC, Hernandez A, Suchow B (1965) American trypanosomiasis.. III The incidence of serologically diagnosed Chagas disease among persons bitten by the insect vector. J Pediatr 66: 107–109
Wray DL (1959) Hemipteron bites human. Proc Entomol Soc Washington 61: 71

7 Skin Eruptions Caused by Beetles (Coleoptera)

Beetles of various species, particularly those whose body fluids possess blistering properties, are liable to cause cutaneous problems in man. There are so many different species involved and the order Coleoptera is so large that any dermatologist or other physician who is not an expert in entomology can only be expected to recognise the insect concerned as a beetle. This is not particularly difficult as far as adults of the species are concerned, the characteristic elytra (the hard chitinised first pair of wings modified to form wing covers) being instantly recognisable. With larvae the problem is not so easy. Coleopterous larvae resemble those of Diptera and Lepidoptera but with certain characteristic differences, which are well summarised by Smith (1973). Beetle larvae have three pairs of thoracic legs, each ending in a claw. Each also has a head capsule. Lepidopterous larvae have, in addition, pseudopods on the third to sixth segments and on the tenth segment (except for Geometridae which have pseudopods only on the sixth and tenth segments). Dipterous larvae have no legs and an incomplete head capsule.

Beetles belonging to the following families can affect the human skin: Staphylinidae, Meloidae, Dermestidae, Oedemeridae, Tenebrionidae, Coccinellidae and Paussidae.

Paederus Dermatitis

The genus *Paederus* of the family Staphylinidae has been recognised as a cause of dermatitis since Da Silva (1912) first reported this condition from Brazil. A number of other reports from various other parts of the world implicating many species have also been published (see Table 7.1).

Clinical Features

Sporadic and epidemic examples of *Paederus* dermatitis have the same basic appearance. It is usually but not invariably contracted during the night, the patient awakening in the morning conscious of itching and burning sensations in one or more areas, although Dao (1964) declared from personal experience on two occasions that the symptoms start with the contact with the beetle but are almost imperceptible at first. The affected areas, which are discrete even if multiple, are usually on the nose, alae nasae, malar areas of the cheeks, eyelids or neck (Chapin 1926) and may also be found on the shoulders, upper trunk as far as the waistline and on the legs and thighs, and even on rare occasions on the scrotum. The palms and soles are rarely affected (Earle 1949). Kerdel-Vegas and Goiman-Yahr (1966) observed that contiguous areas of skin in close contact with one another (e.g. the inner surface of the thighs, the cubital areas or the axillary folds) may show "kissing" lesions, i.e. one surface is contaminated by the beetle fluid, which is then transferred to the contiguous surface, with the result that both surfaces develop lesions. These authors, who recorded 92 patients with this condition in Venezuela, listed the affected areas in order of frequency as follows: face (excluding the eyelids), neck, eyelids, thorax, arms, forearms, thighs, hands, legs, abdomen and ears.

The skin is reddened and then quickly becomes a little swollen. If the eyelids are involved the swelling may be enough to close the eye partially or completely. There may be associated oedema of the palpebral conjunctivae, much lacrimation and sometimes clouding of the cornea and iritis. Dao (1964) thought the eye lesions were due to indirect contamination by the involuntary rubbing of the eyes with contaminated hands. About 24 h after the initial appearance minute pinpoint vesicles appear on the reddened surface, which is still swollen and itchy. The vesicles are more pronounced when the redness is more noticeable. Over the

Table 7.1. The different species of *Paederus* beetles reported as having produced skin lesions in man, the regions where they have been active and some appropriate references

Species	Geographical locality	References
Paederus columbinus	Brazil; Venezuela	Da Silva (1912); Dao (1964)
P. goeldi	Brazil	Bequaert (1920)
P. peregrinosus	Java	Bequaert (1920), citing Jolivet
P. sabaeus	Belgian Congo	Rodhain and Houssiau (1915)
P. fuscipes	Southern Russia	Bequaert (1920), citing Netolitzky
P. crebripunctatus	Kenya	Ross (1916)
P. ruficollis (= *gemellus*)	Central Europe	Bequaert (1920), citing Netolitzky
P. limnophilus	Central Europe	Bequaert (1920), citing Netolitzky
P. litoralis	Central Europe (and UK)	Dallas (1936), citing Netolitzky
P. riparius	Central Europe	Dallas (1936), citing Netolitzky
P. amazonicus	Brazil	Gordon (1925)
P. irritans	Ecuador	Chapin (1926)
P. ornaticornis	Ecuador	Dallas (1934), citing Campos
P. albipilis	Russia	Dallas (1936), citing Pawlowsky
P. signaticornis	Guatemala	Dallas (1936), citing Bequaert (1932)
P. idae	China; Korea	Dallas (1936), citing Esak (1932)
P. brasiliensis	Argentina	Dallas (1934)
P. ferris	Argentina	Dallas (1934)
P. grandis	Arizona	Earle (1949)
P. femoralis	Lower California	Earle (1949)
P. littoreus	Georgia, USA	Earle (1949)
P. lactus	Central America	Earle (1949)
P. rubrothoracicus	France	Theodorides (1950)
P. melampus	Southern India	Andrews and Domonkos (1971)
P. cruenticollis	Australia	Millard (1954)

following day or two the blisters increase in size and number. Some may coalesce and even burst, giving rise to erosions with a weeping surface. Sometimes some of the vesicles may become purulent. After about the fifth day the itch begins to subside; the blister roof starts to dry, turning a yellowish brown, and feels somewhat thickened. A few days later it peels off by desquamation leaving a reddish spot which persists for a week or two. Eyelid lesions require a rather longer time to clear (Dao 1964). Secondary pigmentation is not uncommon and this has been known to persist for 6–8 weeks (Armstrong and Winfield 1968). Should secondary infection occur [not infrequent around the oil wells in Venezuela (Dao 1964)], the vesicular lesions become pustular and ulceration occurs. Normally there are no sequelae, but if secondary infection supervenes there may be some scarring. According to Maegraith (1967) these beetles are suspected of causing blindness in young children, but there does not appear to be any documentary proof of this.

There is no predilection for age, sex, social status or ethnic group, the determining factors according to Kerdel-Vegas and Goiman-Yahr (1966) being the patient's occupation and the insect's habits. This explanation is probably correct for those patients who contact the eruption as a result of working in an area where the environment is infested with the beetles, e.g. the Caracas valley in Venezuela, the oil rig camps around Guayaquil in Ecuador (Chapin 1926; Earle 1949), the Guarico and Anzoatequi regions in Venezuela (Dao 1964) or the agricultural country of the Bahia region in Brazil (Da Silva 1912). However, in other areas European settlers appear to be the victims much more often than the indigenous population, e.g. Leopoldville (Rodhain and Houssiau 1915) and Nairobi (Ross 1916; Roberts and Tonking 1935). There are two possible reasons for this:

1. The houses of Europeans are well illuminated at night, in contrast to those of the native populace, so that beetles are attracted to the former rather than the latter. This suggestion seems to have been borne out in the case of Meloidae in Gambia (Giglioli 1965).
2. The native population in these areas have less fear than Europeans of small beetles crawling

on their skin and do not molest them, whereas Europeans instinctively tend to swat the insects or to brush them off their skin. Either action results in subsequent eruptions.

Children may be more liable to dermatitis in some situations than adults because they play in the grass in gardens and fields. Grass pollens are the staple food of some species and they are therefore present in numbers when the children are playing (Roberts and Tonking 1935).

Morphology and Biology of *Paederus* Beetles

Da Silva first drew attention to the connection between the beetle *Paederus columbinus* and the typical skin eruption in the Bahia region of Brazil in 1912. The beetle was extremely common there

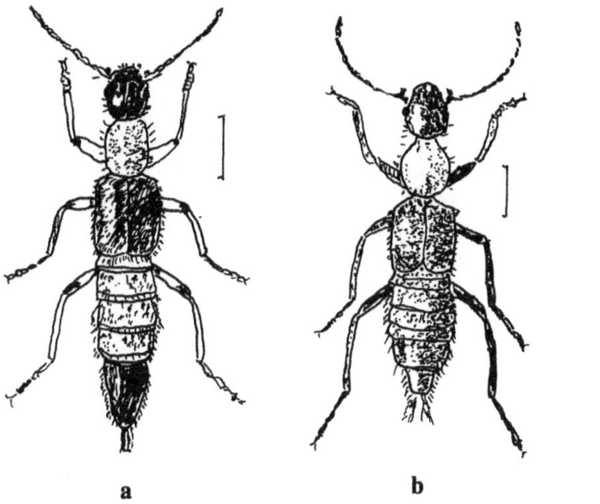

Fig. 7.2. **a** *Paederus fuscipes*; **b** *P. gemellus* (= *ruficollis*). (After Patton 1931)

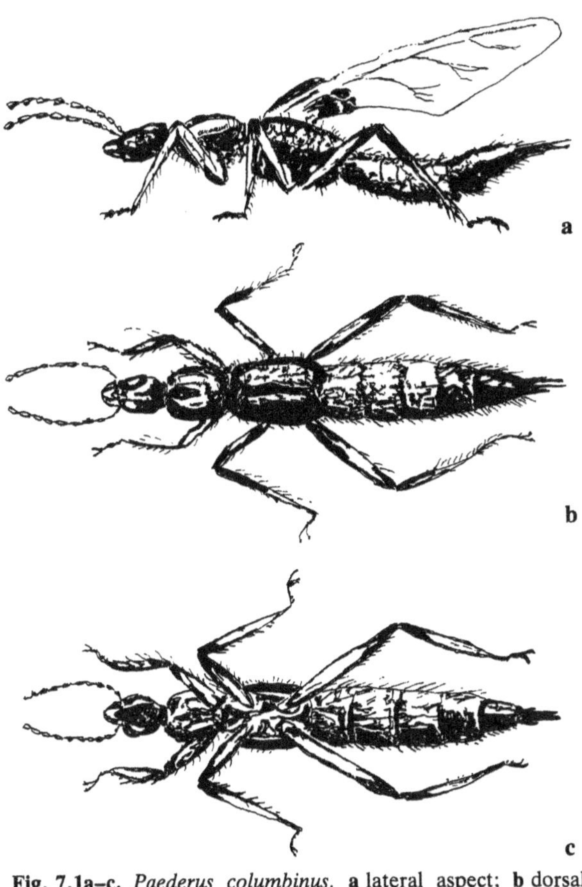

Fig. 7.1a–c. *Paederus columbinus.* **a** lateral aspect; **b** dorsal aspect; **c** ventral aspect. (After Kerdel-Vegas and Goiman-Yahr 1966, by kind permission of the publisher, the American Medical Association. Copyright 1966, American Medical Association)

and was a great nuisance to those working with potato, corn and bean crops, amongst whom it was known as *poto* or *trepa moleque*. Rodhain and Houssiau (1915) demonstrated that another species of the same genus, *P. sabaeus*, was the cause of the Leopoldville outbreak. The beetles of this genus have a narrow body, short elytra beneath which long membranous wings are folded and are often beautifully coloured (Fain 1966). The head and posterior end of the abdomen are usually black, the thorax and anterior portion of the abdomen are yellow or orange, whilst the elytra are metallic blue or green according to species. These beetles are said to resemble flying ants and have a curious habit of curling up the tip of the abdomen over the back (Figs. 7.1, 7.2).

The natural habitat of these insects is amongst decaying vegetable matter and beneath stones, bark or logs, preferably in sandy soil near water such as on river banks or in swamps (Earle 1949; Fain 1966). The life cycle is long, involving no less than seven instar stages between the egg and the pupa, followed by the emergence of the adult beetle. Only one generation is produced annually. The adults emerge in or, more usually, towards the end of the rainy season. The periodic seasonal appearance of these beetles is associated with the heat and humidity which occurs at these times. This obviously will vary in different localities depending on the latitude. Earle (1949) attributed this seasonal occurrence to the coincidental flowering of certain plants. The life cycle seems to be so arranged that the adults emerge just as their food supply (pollen) is appearing. Ebeling (1975) has indicated that the same occurs in other areas as well as in Ecuador. Fain (1966) and also Faust and Russell (1964) have noted that humidity is essential for the wellbeing of these beetles, thus giving added reasons for their natural habitat and seasonal appearance. Reduction in food supply and humidity with the approach of the dry season heralds the disappearance of the beetles (see also under Family Meloidae, p. 81).

Mechanism of the Production of the Lesions

Staphylinid beetles neither bite nor sting, but they contain a fluid which causes blistering on human skin. This vesiculating power was demonstrated by Rodhain and Houssiau (1915). They found that allowing the insects to run freely over the skin in a confined space, even after stimulation, caused no reaction whatever. Crushing a beetle on the skin and removing it with the finger and thumb resulted in no immediate lesions, but next day a red spot appeared where it had been crushed. This was followed in sequence by the development of a lesion with vesicles, proceeding to ultimate desquamation exactly like a naturally acquired lesion. A similar result was obtained by applying ground-up beetles to the skin of a guinea pig. These experiments were confirmed by various other workers (Strickland 1924; Pawlowsky and Stein 1927; Froes 1935; Roberts and Tonking 1935; Pickel 1940; Earle 1949; Theodorides 1950, with European species; Millard 1954; Kerdel-Vegas and Goiman-Yahr 1966). They all showed that the beetles were harmless when just running over the skin but if crushed by the flat of the hand or brushed off by wiping the hand over the skin they caused lesions—patches when crushed and linear streaks when brushed off. Their body fluids thus contained the vesicating principle. It had been thought by some that the beetle secreted the fluid but no such secretion was observed, except by Gordon (1925), who observed it, under the dissecting microscope, coming from the insect's mouthparts when the beetle was compressed. At no time was it ever seen coming from any other orifice or from the legs joints, as it apparently does from the Meloidae (Giglioli 1965). McKeown (1951) quoted Beebe as having seen it coming from the posterior end of female beetles, but this has not been confirmed.

The blistering fluid, at first thought to be cantharidin, was shown to differ from the latter mainly on account of the delay in the appearance of lesions (Netolitzky, cited by Bequaert 1920; Fain 1966; Armstrong and Winfield 1968). Armstrong and Winfield also noted that the two fluids have differing chromatographic patterns. Fain (1966) listed the differences in the clinical effect (see Table 7.2). Both act as primary irritants. To date no reports of allergy to these beetles have been published. Froes (1935) demonstrated that vesicating fluid is contained in *all* parts of the insect's body.

The distribution of the lesions seems to depend on purely physical reasons. The beetles fall onto the skin of victims when they are in bed or indoors in an adequately protected house, or standing around outside in a well-lit area, or when at work in an illuminated area at night (oil rigs for example), or when working with crops on which the beetle is feeding. Thus the exposed parts of the body are most likely to be affected (e.g. the face and neck of those who are in bed, and all the exposed areas of those indoors but not in bed). The exposed areas are often limited by collars or belts, but in the absence of such constricting garments the beetles may wander onto the shoulders or upper trunk and get crushed by the hand or clothing. Workers and children in the fields may be affected around the ankles, or on the legs.

Table 7.2. Differences between the lesions produced experimentally by cantharidin and by paederin. (After Fain 1966)

Feature	Cantharidin	Paederin
Delay between contact and onset of erythema	18–24 h	36–72 h
Character of erythema	Mild or symptomless	Marked and painful
Character of vesicle	Small, rapidly coalescing; clear fluid on a superficial base	Small or very small; clear fluid, becoming purulent; tendency to coalesce; deep base
Symptoms	Almost none	Pronounced itching and burning
Healing	By resorption or by blister bursting	Formation of a crust
Residual lesion	May be none; may be light transient pigmentation	Marked persistent pigmentation; itching may also be present

Histology

The only record comes from Kerdel-Vegas and Goiman-Yahr (1966), who took biopsies from volunteers after carrying out experimental tests. In the early stages subcorneal intraepidermal vesiculation occurred, the floor of the vesicle, which could be extensive, being formed by the basal layer of the epidermis. In the fluid content of the vesicles could be seen ghost epidermal cells and some invading polymorphonuclear cells. As a rule the basal layer was intact, but sometimes the dermo-epidermal junction could be disrupted. In the papillary dermis there was a perivascular mononuclear infiltrate intermingled with a few polymorphonuclear cells. There was some papillary oedema.

In the "full-blown lesion" similar but exaggerated features were seen with an increased number of polymorphonuclear cells invading the epidermis and also present in the dermal infiltrate, which was more intense. Healing occurred by regrowth of the epidermis from below with some acanthosis and pushing off the whole vesiculopustule as a dried crust. During the period of the beginning of recovery the appearance was said to resemble the spongiform pustule of Kogoj. This histological picture is not so much that of a contact eczema as a toxic epidermal effect caused by the toxic fluid.

Diagnosis

The clinical features are very like those of contact dermatitis of a primary irritant type, with its sudden onset, rapid and consistent development in all cases and equally regular recovery, leaving no traces except for residual staining. Several factors make diagnosis of paederus dermatitis easy for the experienced dermatologist or physician: (1) The occurrence in more than one member of the household simultaneously in the absence of an obvious chemical irritant, (2) the distribution and sometimes streaky appearance, (3) the onset after a night's sleep (in those in whom it occurs in bed) and (4) the seasonal association with the presence of small beetles in the house, which may or may not have been noticed on the skin. However, diagnosis may be difficult for those without previous experience. The condition could easily be confused with herpes simplex or zoster and has even been taken for dermatitis herpetiformis (Kerdel-Vegas and Goiman-Yahr 1966). The identification of the beetle and demonstration of its vesiculating powers is sufficient proof.

Treatment

Strickland and Roy (1939) advocated thorough washing with soap and water before the lesions appear, if the condition is suspected in time. This will prevent any lesion developing if it is done within an hour or two of contamination, and is helpful in minimising symptoms later. Roberts and Tonking (1935) noted that the painful burning and itching sensations could quickly be relieved by the application of soaks of saturated solution of magnesium sulphate. They suggested that in fact this remedy had a specific neutralising effect on the toxin apart from any astringent effect. It is very doubtful if any other treatment is necessary, except perhaps oily calamine lotion in the later stages. Topical antibiotics should be used (e.g. tetracycline or clioquinol, Vioform) if secondary infection is suspected. Topical or systemic corticosteroids are of no value (Fain 1966). Eye lesions require repeated bathing with water or isotonic saline. Dao (1964) recommended 5% magnesium sulphate compresses for the eyelid oedema.

Prophylaxis

Those at risk should be educated to flick off or blow off the beetles from the skin rather than to crush them or wipe them off. Men and women working in areas where the beetles are prevalent should have a good wash or even a shower bath immediately after a shift. Bathing the eyes is also probably a good precaution for these people to take. Control of the insects by chemical or other means has proved impractical. Repellent creams are of little value and the local use of DDT has ecological drawbacks. Fan and Chang (1967) have suggested that "in the season" the use of greasy application to the skin at night could lessen the risk of contact of blistering fluid with the skin.

Family Meloidae

Various members of this family are also known as "blister beetles" and were so known before *Paederus* species were incriminated for the same reason. The best known are listed in Table 7.3. The Spanish fly, *Lytta vesicatoria*, is the most well known. It is a large bright metallic green beetle with a rather unpleasant smell. The majority of the beetles in this group, like the *Paederus* species, only cause trouble when crushed on the skin but

Table 7.3. Species of the family Meloidae which are said to cause blistering of the human skin

Species	Remarks	Reference
Lytta vesicatoris	Spanish fly; Europe; bright metallic green	Patton (1931)
L. tenuicollis	Common in India; dark green	Patton (1931)
L. sidae	China	Patton (1931)
L. phaleratus	China	Patton (1931)
Epicauta maculata	Spotted blister beetle	Ebeling (1975)
E. cinerea	Clematis blister beetle; southwestern USA	Lehman et al. (1955); Ebeling (1975)
E. vittata	Striped blister beetle; eastern USA	Lehman et al. (1955); Ebeling (1975)
E. pennsylvanica	Black blister beetle; eastern USA and Mexico	Lehman et al. (1955); Ebeling (1975)
E. hirticornis	India	Smith (1973)
E. tomentosis	Sudan	Patton (1931)
E. sapphinina	Sudan	Patton (1931)
E. flavicornis	Senegal	Roubaud (1915)
E. vestita	Senegal	Roubaud (1915)
Mylabris cichorii	India	Smith (1973)
M. bifasciata	Nigeria	Browne (1960)
Cylindrothorax melanocephala	Gambia	Roubaud (1915); Giglioli (1965)
Psalydolytta substrigata	Gambia	Giglioli (1965)
P. fusca	Gambia	Giglioli (1965)

some may emit fluid if provoked, without necessarily being crushed. As a group they have a worldwide distribution.

Clinical Effects

The clinical effects are very like those caused by *Paederus*. A large blister quickly appears after contact with the insect. Although Lehman et al. (1955) noted slight tingling and burning within 10 min of contact with *Epicauta vittata*, there are as a rule no initial symptoms of pain or itch and none as long as the blisters do not rupture (Giglioli 1965). The blisters are normally larger than those which occur after rove beetle contamination but can also progress into a vesicular dermatitis. The areas commonly involved are the face, neck, chest, thighs and calves, and in children the buttocks. There is less tendency for meloid beetle rash to become purulent, and in 5 years Giglioli never saw eye involvement. Ebeling (1975) stated that the vesicular fluid from such a contact should itself produce secondary dermatitis. In the present writer's opinion this is extremely unlikely. It is much more probable that the reason for such so-called secondary eruptions is that they are in fact "kissing" lesions like those described by Kerdel-Vergas and Goiman-Yahr (1966) and due to transfer of some of the original toxic fluid from one skin surface to another. A short delay in the onset of the secondary dermatitis could be accounted for by the lower concentration of the noxious fluid.

This opinion is supported by the case recorded by Giglioli (1965), in which one man who had crushed a beetle on his back subsequently leant back to back with a friend on the verandah, both being without a shirt because of the heat. The friend also developed a blister dermatitis as a mirror image of that of the patient. Browne (1960) patch tested himself with blister fluid from a bulla from a patient with this dermatitis with negative result. Browne also recorded an instance of percutaneous absorption of cantharidin from blister beetles crushed on the skin. The cantharidin produced severe toxic effects on the kidney causing haematuria and strangury, which fully recovered in about a week after alkalinizing the urine. Burbach (1961) has shown that the blisters caused by cantharidin are acantholytic in structure.

Morphology and Biology

Meloid beetles have many of the same properties that staphylinid beetles have. They are attracted to light and may enter houses which are well lit. They are equally annoying to those trying to enjoy an evening in the tropical warmth near such houses but do not annoy the occupants of the less well-lit native dwellings. The majority of patients are to be found amongst the agricultural workers labouring in fields which are infested with the feeding beetles in daytime. Workers harvesting the potato crop in the United States are particularly liable to attack, as are children running about barefoot. Lehman and his colleagues (1955) reported an outbreak amongst soldiers on exercise in infested pastures.

Figures 7.3 and 7.4 illustrate examples of the genera *Lytta* and *Epicauta*. The principal difference between these and *Paederus* is that the elytra cover the whole abdomen as well as the thorax, except for the tip of the abdomen in some species.

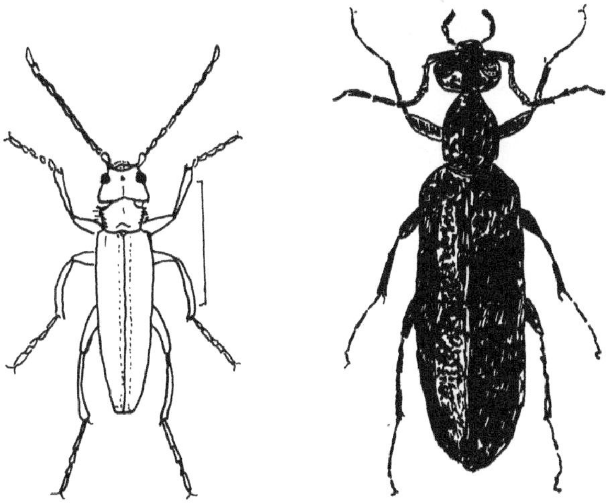

Fig. 7.3. **a** *Lytta vesicatoria*, the Spanish fly; **b** *L. tenuicollis*, a common blister beetle in India. (After Patton 1931)

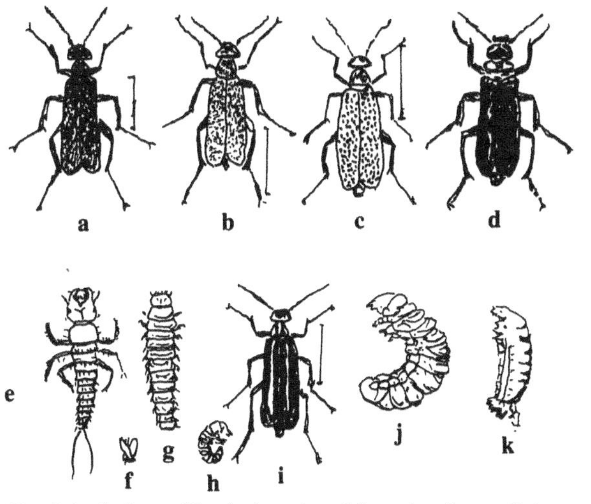

Fig. 7.4a–i. Some North American blister beetles. **a** *Epicauta pennsylvanica* (black blister beetle); **b** *E. cinerea* (grey blister beetle); **c** *E. maculata* (spotted blister beetle); **d** *Lytta nuttali* (western blister beetle); **e** "triangulin" (instar of *E. vittata*); **f** eggs of *E. vittata*; **g**, **h**, and **j** larval instars of *E. vittata;* **k** pupa of *E. vittata*; **i** adult *E. vittata*. (After Patton 1931)

Many are highly coloured. They all go through a similar complicated developmental cycle involving seven instar stages between egg and pupa. Each female beetle lays a large number of eggs because a high proportion never reach maturity. The first instar, the triangulins, have to search for grasshopper eggs or lie in wait for a solitary bee for their food. Many perish. However, Giglioli (1965) has noted that whenever there is such an occurrence as a visitation of a swarm of locusts to a region where these beetles flourish, there is a greater number of the latter the following year, which suggests that epidemics of these beetles depend not so much on the climatic conditions as on the larval food available.

The toxic fluid is contained in all parts of the beetle, as with *Paederus*, and the active principle is cantharidin. It is not secreted by any special gland. When the insect feels threatened it closes off all its tracheae and builds up internal pressure. The fluid then oozes out at exoskeletal joints if it is handled in any way. Thus when the beetle is brushed off the skin or crushed against the skin, fluid is deposited on the latter. According to Giglioli (1965), on very humid days the carcases of dead beetles retain some of this fluid and are just as likely to cause trouble as are live insects. Consequently, children sitting on the carcases are liable to develop lesions on the buttocks.

Family Oedemeridae

Fleisher and Fox (1970) recorded three patients with a blistering dermatitis due to the oedemerid beetle *Oxycopis vittata* (Fahr) in Puerto Rico, whilst Smith (1973) mentioned that *Sessinia collaris* (Sharp) and *S. decolor* (Fairm), coconut beetles, caused a similar condition in the Gilbert Islands.

Clinical Effects

All three patients in Puerto Rico, two workmen and one tourist, developed itching shortly after they had either brushed the beetles off their skin or killed them on their skin. Vesicles with associated surrounding erythema forming a halo quickly appeared in all three men. Lesions only occurred where the insects had been noted, on the right upper eyelid, arms and shins in one workman, on the legs in the second and around the ankles in the tourist, who had been sunbathing. All the lesions cleared in less than 1 week.

The authors noted that similar lesions could be produced by crushing the beetles on the skin, but not by allowing them merely to walk thereon. The beetles exuded a fluid when crushed.

Histology

Biopsy done in one patient 19 h after contact with the beetles showed an intact stratum corneum and a subepidermal blister with regenerating epithelium on its floor. The dermis showed a moderately severe perivascular round cell infiltrate. Although it was not specifically identified, the authors appeared to imply that the toxin in this instance was not cantharidin. This is probably correct, since the blisters were subepidermal and not acantholytic, as with cantharidin.

Morphology

The beetle *O. vittata* was described as having blue-grey elytra with a median yellow band. The ventral surface was yellow. It was about 1 cm long, not unlike some species of Meloidae, but with a large prominent coxa on leg II.

Family Dermestidae

Several species of the family Dermestidae are said to cause skin lesions. They are listed in Table 7.4, together with several species not mentioned so far but which have also been implicated at some time as causes of dermatitis.

Clinical Effects

Two reports of the so-called carpet beetle dermatitis have been published (Cormia and Lewis 1948; Ahmed et al. 1981). This is a papulovesicular dermatitis which is due to the larval form of certain carpet beetles. In the first case, the patient was a 47-year-old woman with lesions which started on the forearms and spread over the forearms to the adjacent surface of the chest and also to the legs. This eruption was of 3 weeks' duration when seen. In the second case, the patient was a man aged 22 years who had recurrent lesions on the arms and legs for 5 years. The lesions started in both cases as papules or weals and quickly progressed to papulovesicles with very slight discharge and the formation of tiny crusts (Fig. 7.5). Both patients itched considerably at night.

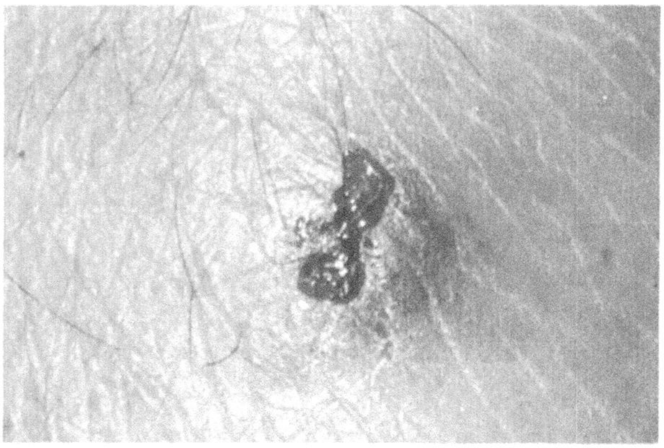

Fig. 7.5. Encrusted scratch mark in "carpet beetle dermatitis". (From Ahmed et al. 1981, by kind permission of the authors and the Editor of the *Journal of the American Academy of Dermatology*)

Table 7.4. Species of the Dermestidae family and others which may cause lesions on the human skin. (Cited by Ahmed et al. 1981, with some additional remarks taken from Patton 1931)

Species	Remarks
Anthrenus scrophulariae	Carpet beetle; the larva has urticating hairs
A. verbasci	Variegated carpet beetle
A. flavipes	Furniture beetle
Attagenus megatoma	Black carpet beetle
Dermestes frischii	Europe and North America; a pest of silkworms
D. undulatus	
D. lardarium	Larva has urticating hairs
Trogoderma ornatum	Pest of grain, nuts, tobacco and entomological collections
Necrobia rufipes	
N. ruficollis	
Tenebrio molitor	
Tribolium castaneum	Britain (Williamson 1964)

In the case of the woman, the floor of her house was found to be infested with the larvae of a beetle, *Anthrenus scrophulariae*, in the case of the young man, his bedroom contained two woollen rugs infested with the larvae of *A. verbasci*. The woman gave a negative patch test reaction to extract of the larva but an almost instantaneous positive reaction when the larva itself was used as the patch test (biting being excluded). Moreover, distant sites were reactivated. Results of intradermal tests of larval extracts were positive in the young man but negative in controls. Fumigation of the young man's room resulted in the disappearance of all the lesions without recurrence.

Histology

Biopsy from the woman patient of Cormia and Lewis (1948) showed slight acanthosis, dilatation and mild congestion of the blood vessels of the upper and mid-corium, with a perivascular infiltrate of lymphocytes, histiocytes and a few polymorphonuclear cells. The picture was regarded as one of mild toxic erythema. The clinical appearances were not due to irritant properties in the larvae, as with the adult blister beetles, but rather to a hypersensitivity to the larvae, as indicated by the appearance of lesions at a distance when the patch tests were applied.

Morphology and Biology of Larvae

Although listed as furniture beetles, these insects must not be confused with true furniture beetles of the *Anobium* species, which bore into the woodwork of furniture. The dermestid beetles are very small (about 3 mm long), and the adults live outdoors, feeding on flowers (Fig. 7.6). The larvae consume a variety of materials, the *Anthrenus* species specialising in upholstery, carpets, rugs and clothing. The adults are strong fliers and often fly against windows; they should be destroyed whenever possible. The larvae are very hairy (Figs. 7.6 and 7.7) and can be mistaken for lepidopterous larvae (but see p. 75). The hairs are of two kinds, one covered with multiple scale-like

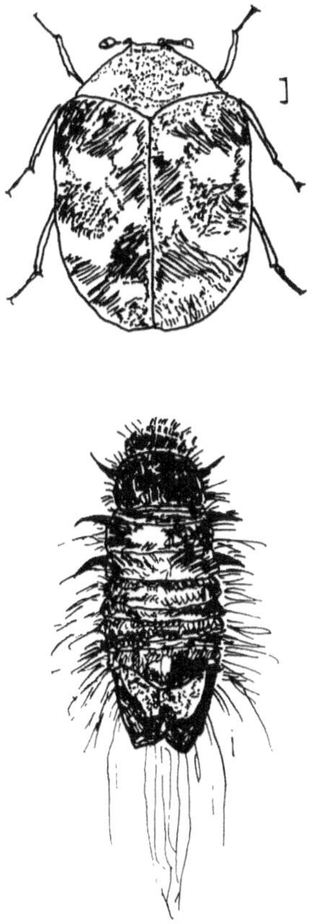

a

b

Fig. 7.6. *Anthrenus verbasci.* **a** adult; **b** full-grown larva. (After Patton 1931)

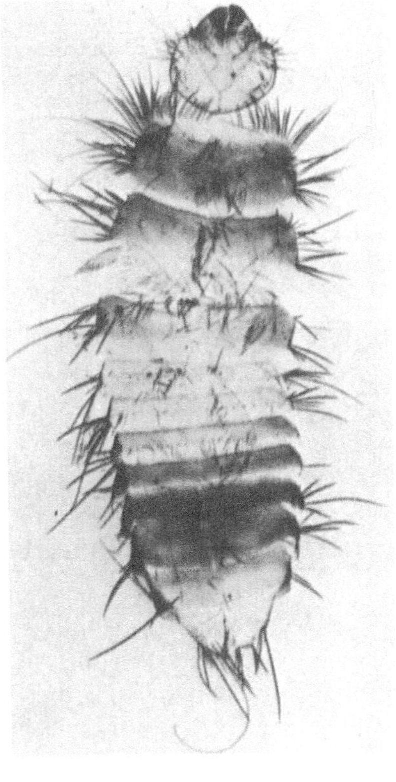

Fig. 7.7. Larva of *Anthrenus verbasci* taken from infested rug, showing the hairs. (From Ahmed et al. 1981, by kind permission of the authors and the Editor of the *Journal of the American Academy of Dermatology*)

barbs and the other slightly barbed with a spear-like tip (Fig. 7.8). They can easily escape notice in their habitat unless regular and careful inspections are made of carpets and rugs (which may necessitate lifting), upholstery and clothing in cupboards (Patton 1931). Apart from causing skin lesions, some have been incriminated as causes of asthma and rhinitis (Faust and Russell 1964; Ahmed et al. 1981).

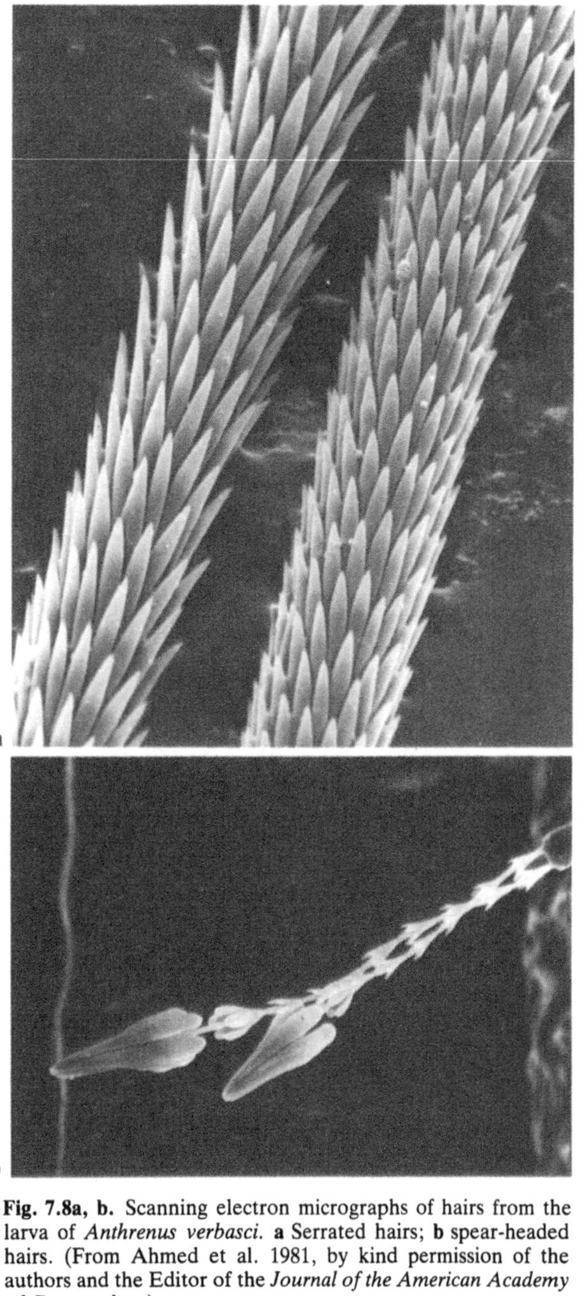

a b

Fig. 7.8a, b. Scanning electron micrographs of hairs from the larva of *Anthrenus verbasci*. **a** Serrated hairs; **b** spear-headed hairs. (From Ahmed et al. 1981, by kind permission of the authors and the Editor of the *Journal of the American Academy of Dermatology*)

Other Species which Cause Dermatitis

De Meillon (1937) reported that *Cerapterus concolor* Westm. (Paussidae), an inhabitant of ants' nests, can eject a blistering liquid when disturbed. Linear blistering can occur, especially in children.

Williamson (1964) noted an outbreak of severe itching with scratch marks amongst miners working with jute bags contaminated with *Tribolium castaneum*, the red rust flower beetle. The itching affected the trunk and limbs and cleared quickly once the source was removed.

References

*Ahmed AR, Moy R, Barr AR, Price Z (1981) Carpet beetle dermatitis. J Am Acad Dermatol 5: 428–432

Andrews CC, Domonkos A (1971) Diseases of the skin, 6th edn. Saunders, Philadelphia

Armstrong RK, Winfield JL (1968) Staphylinidae dermatitis on Okinawa. J Med Entomol 5: 362

Bequaert J (1920) À propos des Staphylinides vesicants du Bas-Congo. Ann Soc Belg Med Trop 1: 227–229

Browne SG (1960) Cantharidin poisoning due to a "blister beetle". Br Med J 2: 1290–1291

Burbach JPE (1961) Experiments on blister formation IV. The action of cantharidin. Dermatologica 123: 42–56

Chapin EA (1926) A new *Paederus* (Coleopt: Staphylinidae) causing vesicular dermatitis in man. Arch Schiffs Trop Hyg 30: 369–372

Cormia FE, Lewis GM (1948) Contact dermatitis from beetles with a report of a case due to the carpet beetle (*Anthrenus scrophularia*) NY State J Med 48: 2037–2039

Dallas ED (1934) Breve nota sobre dermatitis ocasionada por Coleopteros del genero *Paederus* (Staphylinidae) en la Rep. Argentina. Rev Chil Hist Nat 38: 168–169

Dallas ED (1936) Dermatitis causadas por coleopteros del genero *Paederus* (Staphylinidae). Rev Chil Hist Nat 39: 219–224

Dao L (1964) Dermatitis causadas por coleopteros *Paederus columbinus* en Venezuela. Dermatol Trop 3: 169–172

Da Silva MP (1912) Le *Paederus columbinus* est vesicant. Arch Parasitol 15: 431

De Meillon B (1937) A note on two beetles of medical interest in Natal. S Afr Med J 11: 479

Earle KV (1949) Fuetazo dermatitis. J Trop Med Hyg 52: 183–187

*Ebeling W (1975) Blister beetles (Meloidae). In: Urban entomology. University of California, Division of Agricultural Science, Los Angeles, Cal, pp 523–525

*Fain A (1966) Toxic action of rove beetles (Coleoptera: Staphylinidae). Simposio internationale sobre venenos animais. Mem Inst Butantan 33, Suppl comemorativo: 835–844

Fan J, Chang HS (1967) Paederus dermatitis. Dermatol Int 6: 203–206

Faust BC, Russell PF (1964) Clinical parasitology. Lea and Febiger, Philadelphia, pp 934–936

Fleisher TL, Fox I (1970) Oedemerid beetle dermatitis Arch Dermatol 101: 601–605

Froes HP (1935) Observations on Brazilian "blister beetles". J Parasitol 21: 124
Giglioli MEC (1965) Some observations on blister beetles, family Meloidae, in Gambia, West Africa. Trans R Soc Trop Med Hyg 59: 657–663
Gordon RM (1925) A note on two vesicant beetles belonging to the family Staphylinidae. Ann Trop Med Parasitol 19: 47–51
*Kerdel-Vegas F, Goiman-Yahr M (1966) Paederus dermatitis. Arch Dermatol 94: 175–185
Lehman CF, Pipkin JL, Ressmann AC (1955) Blister beetle dermatitis. Arch Dermatol 71: 36–38
McKeown KC (1951) Dermatitis apparently caused by a Staphylinid beetle in Australia. Med J Aust 2: 772–773
Maegraith BG (1967) Vesicant beetles. In: Adams and Maegraith: Clinical tropical diseases, 5th edn. Blackwell, Oxford, pp 382–383
Millard PT (1954) Whiplash dermatitis produced by the common rove beetle. Med J Aust 1: 741–744
*Patton WS (1931) Insects, ticks, mites and venomous animals of medical and veterinary importance. Part II Public health. HR Grubb, Croydon, pp 424–434
Pawlowsky EN, Stein AK (1927) The cutaneous poison of the beetle *Paederus fuscipes*. Trans R Soc Trop Med Hyg 20: 450–451
Pickel DB (1940) Dermatitis purulenta produzida por duas especies de *Paederus* (Col: Staphylinidae). Rev Entomol 11: 775–793
Roberts JS, Tonking HD (1935) Notes on an East African vesicant beetle *Paederus crebripunctatus* Epp. Ann Trop Med Parasitol 29: 415–420
Rodhain J, Houssiau J (1915) Dermatitis vésiculeuse saisonnière produite par un coléoptère. Bull Soc Pathol Exot 8: 587–591
Ross PH (1916) Dermatitis due to the secretion of a beetle in British East Africa. J Trop Med Hyg 19: 202
Roubaud M (1915) In discussion on Rodhain and Houssiau (1915)
Smith KGV (1973) Coleoptera and other insects (beetles, mayflies, caddis flies). In: Smith KGV (ed) Insects and other arthropods of medical importance. Trustees of the British Museum (Natural History), London, pp 413–416
Strickland C (1924) On spider-lick, a dermatozoosis. Indian Med Gazette 8: 385–387
Strickland C, Roy DN (1939) A simple means of preventing spider-lick. Indian Med Gazette 24: 285–286
Theodorides J (1950) Considérations sur les *Paederus* vésicants (Coleoptera: Staphylinidae) et assais de vésication avec les espèces de France. Bull Soc Pathol Exot 43: 100–113
Williamson DM (1964) Itching eruption in miners caused by a rare beetle (*Tribolium castaneum*). Br J Dermatol 76: 388–389

8 Cutaneous Myiasis

Patton (1921) defined myiasis as "The condition or conditions resulting from invasion of the tissues and organs of man and animals by all the stages of Diptera." In cutaneous myiasis this means invasion of the skin by the larvae of the Diptera concerned. The number of species capable of doing this is large and many invade other tissues as well. Involvement of other organs will only be mentioned when relevant to skin myiasis, although it should be remembered that the skin is not necessarily the only or even the principal organ attacked. Detailed reviews of myiasis in general can be found in the monographs by James (1947) and by Zumpt (1965).

Many species of flies must be considered individually here because their habits, mode of attack and clinical effects differ widely from one another. Moreover, the clinical appearances, especially when the patient is out of context geographically speaking, may not only be very puzzling but also recalcitrant to treatment, particularly if incorrectly diagnosed. Incorrect treatment may result in much tissue damage and even death. A further reason for presenting such details here is their absence from some larger textbooks of dermatology and tropical medicine (Peters and Kramer 1966).

Classification

A systematic consideration of myiasis is essential to avoid confusion. Two classifications have been evolved. Patton (1921) proposed three categories based on the parasitic habits of the species of fly involved (Table 8.1), whilst Bishopp et al. (1926) grouped the cases according to the tissues and organs involved. James (1947) adopted a modification of Bishopp's classification (Table 8.2). For the purposes of clinical description only James' groups 1, 7, 8 and 10 will be considered here. James gave a comprehensive list of all the species involved in each of Patton's groups, and those concerned with cutaneous myiasis will be described in accordance with this grouping. Other classifications, e.g. Dove (1937), Herms (1950), Zumpt (1965), which is based on the biological relationship between parasite and host, and Soulsby (1968), add little to the two mentioned. Zumpt, however, made the point that the term "accidental" should be avoided since it really refers to facultative parasitosis (or even psuedoparasitosis, when larvae are swallowed with food, do not live a parasitic existence but may cause allergic or toxic symptoms). Larvae which

Table 8.1. Entomological classification of myiasis according to the parasitic habits of the Diptera concerned, as proposed by Patton (1921)

Group	Remarks
1. Specific	Most of the Diptera in this group can cause cutaneous lesions
2. Semi-specific	Eggs are laid on diseased tissues of man and animals. The larvae may subsequently attack adjacent normal tissues. Wounds are occasionally attacked
3. "Accidental"	Larvae may be taken in with the food. Wounds are occasionally attacked

Table 8.2. Bishopp's classification of myiasis according to the tissues attacked, as modified by James (1947)

Group	Remarks
1. Traumatic (wound)	Includes cutaneous myiasis
2. Nose, mouth and sinuses	
3. Aural	
4. Ocular	
5. Anal and vaginal	
6. Urinary tract	
7. Furuncular	Cutaneous myiasis
8. Creeping:	Cutaneous myiasis
a) Dermal	
b) Subdermal	
9. Enteric	
10. Attack by blood-sucking larvae	Congo floor maggot

normally breed on carcases or food debris of animal or vegetable origin may occasionally develop on or be deposited on wounds. This should be regarded as facultative and not accidental.

Cutaneous "Wound" Myiasis in Man

"Wound" myiasis is caused by a variety of flies. The most important belong to the family Calliphoridae, which, in the United States are responsible for 86–90% of cases of myiasis (Schreiber et al. 1964), but whether these statistics include furuncular myiasis was not made clear. *Callitroga americana* (Fig. 8.1), the primary screwworm fly of the New World, which inhabits the region between latitudes 35°N and 35°S (Aubertin and Buxton 1934), is certainly the most important myiasis-producing fly in the New World (James 1947). Another calliphorid, *Chrysomya bezziana* (Fig. 8.1), the Old World screwworm fly is, after the tsetse fly, the most important dipterous pest in Africa (Zumpt 1965) and is also a serious cause of myiasis in India, Southeast Asia and Formosa (Patton 1920–1921; 1921–1922). Both species are obligatory parasites of wounds and diseased tissues of man and animals and, except under certain experimental conditions, do not penetrate unbroken skin (Laake et al. 1936). Other calliphorid flies—including *Callitroga macellaria* (the secondary screwworm) and a common cause of myiasis in Brazil (Da Silva 1912); *Phormia regina* (black blowfly); *Lucilia cuprina*, *sericata* and other species (greenbottles); *Calliphora vomitoria* and *vicina* (bluebottles); the muscid fly *Musca domestica* (housefly) (Fig. 8.1); and the sarcophagid, *Sarcophaga haemorrhoidalis* (Fig. 8.1)—can all be facultative parasites of the same tissues. Most of these flies breed on carrion or decomposing animal or vegetable material. All the species of Calliphoridae parasitise domestic animals, principally cattle

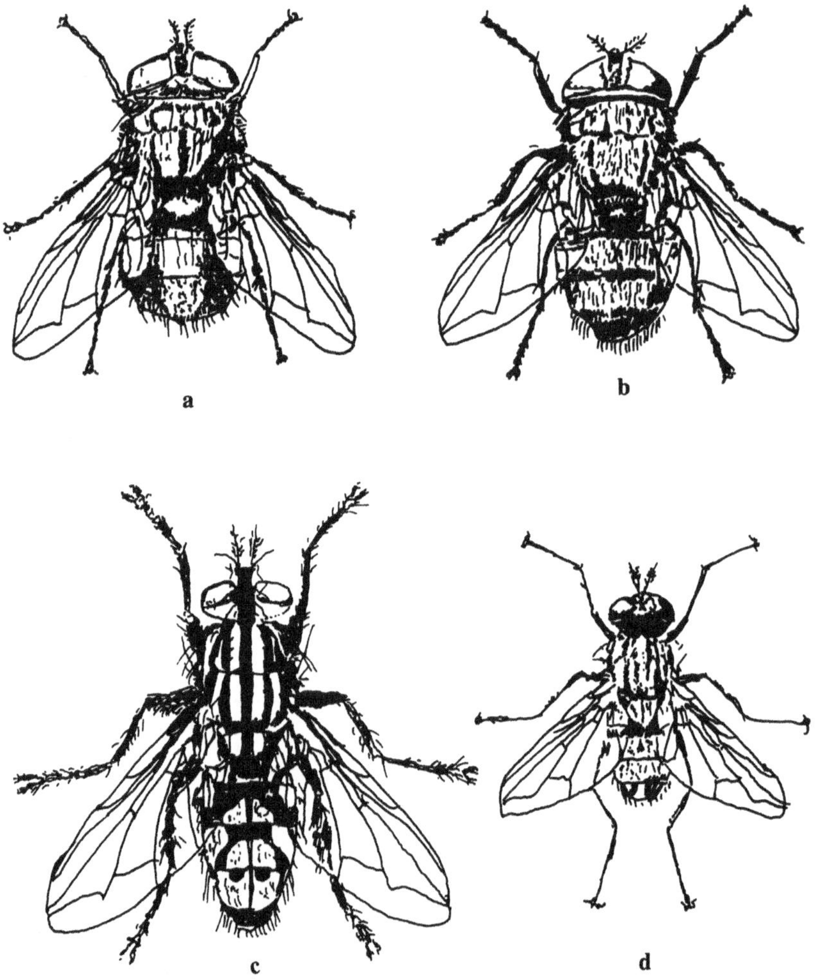

Fig. 8.1a–d. Some adult flies whose larvae cause "wound" myiasis in man. **a** *Callitroga americana*, female; **b** *Chrysomya bezziana*, female; **c** *Sarcophaga haemorrhoidalis*, male; **d** *Musca domestica*. (After James 1947, by kind permission of the author and the publisher, the US Department of Agriculture)

but also sheep, camels, horses and goats, but seldom wild animals (Zumpt 1965). (The *Lucilia* and *Calliphora* species parasitise sheep predominantly). It is important to stress the relationship between these flies and farm animals because the incidence of human infestation parallels that of animal incidence (Dove 1937; Hunter and Berrocal 1957). The economic effects of *C. americana* infestation can be very severe. Graham (1982) has pointed out that host animals such as young cattle can be killed within 1–2 weeks. In the late nineteenth century farmers often had to restock their herds completely because of its depredations (Baumhover 1966), whilst Turnley (1954) observed that uncontrolled attacks could wipe out whole herds of cattle, deer, hogs, sheep or goats. McCuiston et al. (1958) estimated the cost to Texan farmers between 1940 and 1944 to be US $14 million, whilst Baumhover (1966) said the annual cost to farmers in the southeastern states of the United States was US $20 million and between US $50 and 100 million in the southwestern states. Incidence figures are equally high. Dove (1937) noted that 1 300 000 animals were affected in the southeastern states of the United States in 1934. Even with careful husbandry the incidence was still 50 000 in 1962 (Baumhover 1966). The clinical effects on man can be very serious. Yount and Sudler (1907) recorded that only one of 12 patients seen by a doctor in Iowa had recovered. Aubertin and Buxton (1934) gave the overall mortality as 8%. None of the deaths were due to cutaneous myiasis, but were chiefly the result of infestation of nasal passages and sinuses. *Chrysomya bezziana*

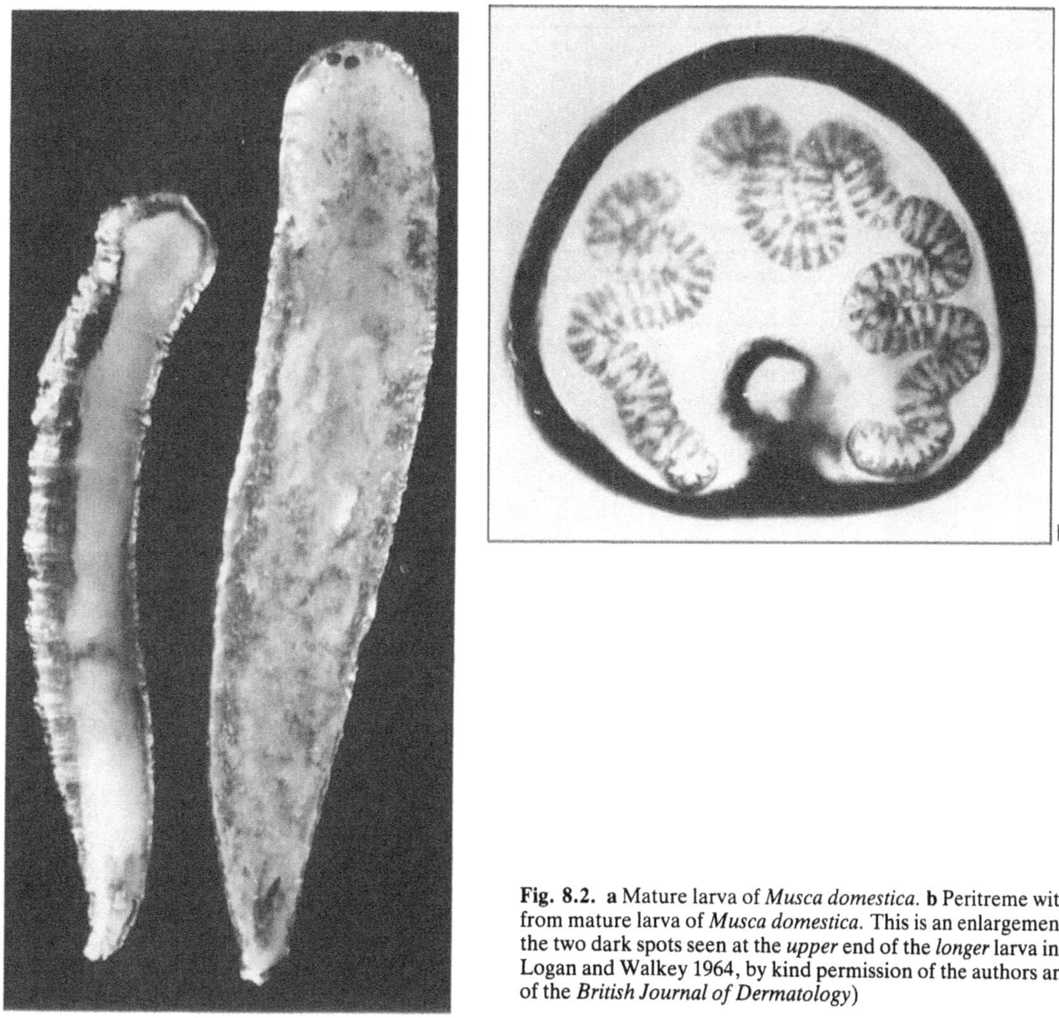

a b

Fig. 8.2. **a** Mature larva of *Musca domestica*. **b** Peritreme with spiracles from mature larva of *Musca domestica*. This is an enlargement of one of the two dark spots seen at the *upper* end of the *longer* larva in **a**. (From Logan and Walkey 1964, by kind permission of the authors and the Editor of the *British Journal of Dermatology*)

Table 8.3. Size and other macroscopic details of the adult flies (the most common species) causing "wound" myiasis. (Compiled from James 1947; Zumpt 1965)

Species	Length (mm)	Features of note
Callitroga americana	8–10	Head reddish to orange-brown with black parafrontal hair; body bluish-green
C. macellaria	6–9	Head orange with yellow parafrontal hairs; green body
Chrysomya bezziana	8–12	Head black above and orange below with green to greenish-purple body; posterior end black
Phormia regina	7–9	Black head; greenish-black or olive green body with orange hairs
Lucilia cuprina	6–8	Metallic coppery green body; occasionally bright green
L. sericata	6–9.5	Metallic green body with yellow or coppery sheen
Calliphora vomitoria	10–14	Head black above and yellow below; thorax black with grey pollen; abdomen blue
C. vicina	9–11	
Musca domestica	6–9	Thorax has hairy propleura; four black stripes; infuscated abdomen
Sarcophaga haemorrhoidalis	10–14	Thorax has three broad stripes; abdomen has chess-board pattern; genitalia reddish

Table 8.4. Biological details of various flies causing myiasis of the skin. The details are pertinent to the type of myiasis produced

Species	O or L	No. of ova/larvae	Incubation period	Larval period	Type of myiasis	Parasitic type
Callitroga americana	O	2850	11–21 h	$3\frac{1}{2}$–10 d	Wound	Obligatory
C. macellaris	O	25–1000	4 h	6–20 d	Wound	Facultative
Chrysomya bezziana	O	500–600	18–24 h	6 d	Wound	Obligatory
Phormia regina	O				Wound	Facultative
Lucilia sericata	O				Wound	Facultative
L. cuprina	O		1 d	4–6 d	Wound	Facultative
Calliphora vomitoria	O				Wound	Facultative
C. vicina	O	540–720	1 d	7 d	Wound	Facultative
Musca domestica	O				Wound	Facultative
Sarcophaga haemorrhoidalis	L	30–64		4 d	Wound	Facultative
Cordylobia anthropophaga	O	500+	2 d	8–9 d	Furuncular	Obligatory
Stasisia rodhaini	O	500+	2 d	12–15 d	Furuncular	Obligatory
Wohlfahrtia vigil	L			7–9 d	Furuncular	Obligatory
W. opaca	L			7–9 d	Furuncular	Obligatory
W. magnifica	L	124–168		6–7 d	Wound	Obligatory
Hypoderma bovis	O	laid singly	3–7 d	Months	Furuncular and migrating	Obligatory
H. lineatum	O	Laid in groups	3–7 d	Months	Furuncular and migrating	Obligatory
Dermatobia hominis	O	?	variable	7 w	Furuncular	Obligatory
Cuterebra spp.	O	1000	1–2 w	28–38 d	Furuncular	Obligatory
Gasterophilus haemorrhoidalis	O	50–200	2–4 w	Variable	Migrating	Obligatory

O, ovipositor; L, larvipositor; d, days; h, hours; w, weeks

has had equally profound effects on man and animals in the areas where it flourishes (Patton 1921–1922). *Lucilia cuprina* is the important sheep maggot in Australia (Watts 1974).

Infestation with *Callitroga americana* has a seasonal incidence starting usually in the late spring and early summer and continuing through to autumn. The actual time of year is related to the latitude (Laake et al. 1936; James 1947).

Some morphological details of various flies are shown in Figs. 8.1. and 8.2. Details of some of the more easily identifiable features are given in Table 8.3. Biological details of the life cycles of the common flies causing myiasis are summarised in Table 8.4, whilst the geographical distribution of the principal flies causing wound myiasis is shown in Table 8.5. Accurate identification is a matter for an entomologist, but the information given here adds interest to the subject for the physician. Figure 8.3 shows the essential features to be studied to identify larvae, although in most instances it is necessary to have the mature flies for complete identification of a particular species. The shape of the cephalopharyngeal skeleton, the appearance of the posterior surface of the terminal segment and the pattern of spiracles on the peritreme of this segment are features with individual characteristics for each species (see also Fig. 8.5).

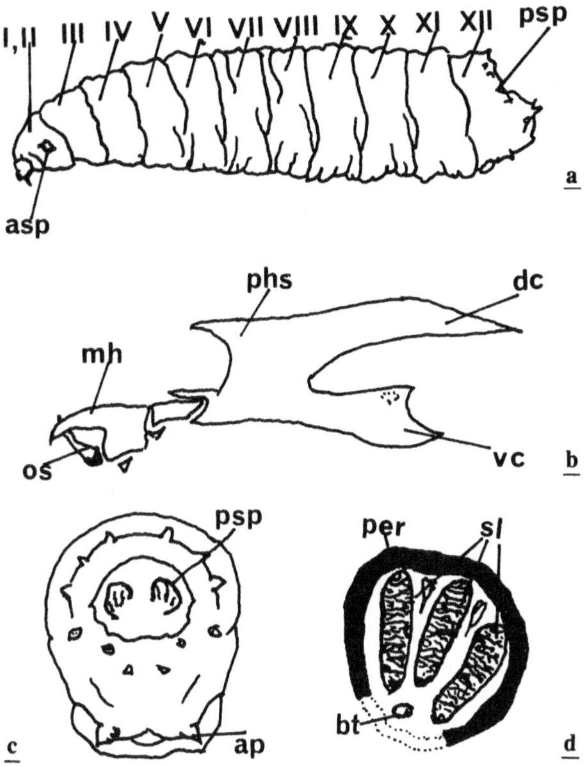

Fig. 8.3a–d. Third larval instar of a musciform fly. **a** lateral view; **b** cephalopharyngeal skeleton; **c** posterior view; **d** one posterior peritreme. *I–XII*, numbering of segments; *ap*, anal protuberance; *asp*, anterior spiracle; *bt*, button; *dc*, dorsal corona; *mh*, lateral sclerites or mouth hooks; *os*, oral sclerite; *per*, peritremal ring; *phs*, pharyngeal sclerite; *psp*, posterior spiracles; *sl*, slits; *vc*, ventral cornua. (After Zumpt 1965, by kind permission of the author and the publisher, Butterworth and Co.)

Table 8.5. Geographical distribution of flies commonly associated with wound (cutaneous) myiasis. (Compiled from James 1947; Zumpt 1965)

Species	Distribution
Callitroga americana	USA; Mexico; Costa Rica; Panama; Caribbean Islands; Colombia; Venezuela; Brazil; Uruguay; Chile; Argentina; Guyana and French Guiana
C. macellaria	Same, plus Quebec and New England states; Guatemala; Honduras; Surinam; Ecuador; Peru; Bolivia; Paraguay
Chrysomya bezziana	Ethiopan region of Africa; India; Ceylon; southeast Asia; Philippines; Formosa
Phormia regina	Europe; Russia; Canada; USA; Mexico; Hawaii
Lucilia sericata	Temperate areas of holarctic region; South Africa; Australia, New Zealand; Paraguay; Argentina
L. cuprina	Ethiopian region; tropical areas of Far East region; Australia; Pacific islands
Calliphora vomitoria	Holarctic region; northern India; northern and southern African coastal states; Hawaii
C. vicina	Worldwide in temperate region
Musca domestica	Almost worldwide

Mode of Infestation

Infestation always occurs out of doors (Yount and Sudler 1907). Oviposition takes place on damaged skin or in the immediate vicinity of a wound (Patton 1921–1922), the egg mass being glued to the surface (James 1947). Any discharging wound, nostril, ear or ulcer, or encrusted or even scaly area of skin will attract flies. For this reason Turnley (1954) advised those suffering from chronic sinus infection and others "not to sleep in the yard with the orifices open". He pointed out that the flies only required a few seconds to deposit their eggs. Macias et al. (1973) noted that all eight of their patients, seven of whom were girls, had pediculosis of the scalp with excoriations which attracted the flies. Certain categories of persons, with any of the conditions mentioned above, are more likely than average to be infested. These include mental defectives, the very young and the very old, and those whose personal hygiene is poor (McCuiston et al. 1958).

Clinical Features

The most serious cases are undoubtedly those involving the nasal cavity and sinuses, in which the most horrific damage can occur (Yount and Sudler 1907; Da Silva 1912; Dove 1937). Cutaneous myiasis caused by this group of flies was probably first recorded in 1823 in a man scalped by Red Indians (Dove 1937). The scalp is the commonest site to be attacked, especially when a seborrhoeic eczema is present (McCuiston et al. 1958; Schreiber et al. 1964), but in addition to pediculosis (see above), it has also been infested in the presence of a haematoma (Da Silva 1912; Hunter and Berrocal 1957). Leg ulcers are also not infrequently attacked (Da Silva 1912; Patton 1921; Lawton et al. 1957), whilst squamous carcinoma of the skin (Patton 1921; Dove 1937) and basal cell carcinoma (Schreiber et al. 1964) have also been complicated by larval infestation. Wounds in general, if unprotected, are easily infested, and Dove (1937) mentioned a fatal case in an infant with umbilical involvement.

The larvae quickly hatch from the eggs and commence feeding at once in a gregarious fashion. Except for the screwworm, the larvae feed on the surface, but they quickly consume necrotic debris and begin to attack normal tissue at the margins and base of the lesion causing much destruction (ulceration) and foul smell. *Callitroga americana* and *Chrysomya bezziana* bore into the tissues producing pocket-like sinuses (James 1947; Lawton et al. 1957; McCuiston et al. 1958; Schreiber et al. 1964) in the healthy surrounding skin. These sinuses may often be very large, resulting in a great deal of destruction. Patton (1921–1922) recorded the case of a small Indian boy whose penis was severely damaged by infestation following circumcision. Tissues infested by either of the primary screwworm flies can be damaged extremely quickly. Young and Sudler (1907) recorded an instance where, in spite of prompt treatment of an infestation of a skin abrasion, an underlying tendon was found to have been damaged. In the scalp infestation of one of the patients described by Schreiber and his colleagues (1964), the outer table of the skull was perforated. Lesions may be associated with burning pain (Dove 1937). Infested children may show a febrile reaction (McCuiston et al. 1958). Whilst secondary infection may occur, it usually subsides very quickly after the removal of the larvae.

Figure 8.4 shows the scars left after infestation on the buttock of a 74-year-old vagrant who was in a filthy condition and doubly incontinent. The invading larvae, present in hundreds, were those of *Musca domestica*, which had doubtless been attracted by the state of the patient's skin. They caused much superficial ulceration which resulted in the scarring shown, but tissue destruction was minimal (Logan and Walkey 1964). Patton and Cookson (1925) reported a case where similar larvae invaded a varicose eczema causing a chronic inflammatory reaction with a thickened moist surface apparently devoid of epithelium but raised into small elevations and intervening crevices (resembling the so-called elephantiasis nostrum without epidermis). The crevices were swarming with larvae, which caused no inconvenience to the patient and little or no secondary tissue destruction.

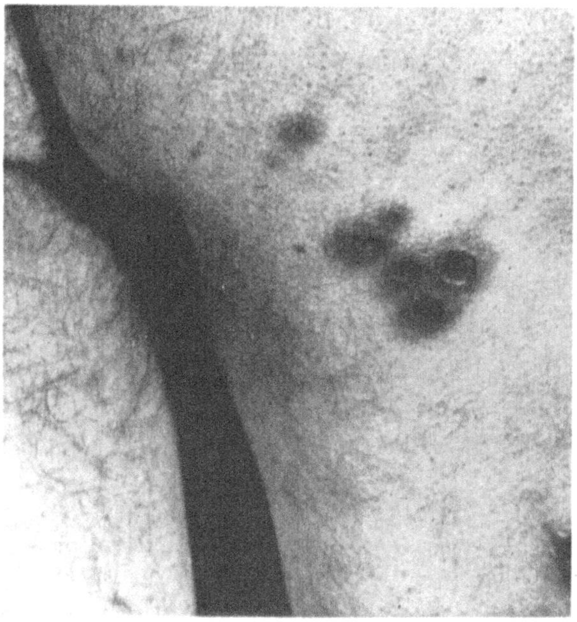

Fig. 8.4. Clinical appearance of lesions caused by the larvae of *Musca domestica*. (From Logan and Walkey 1964, by kind permission of the authors and the Editor of the *British Journal of Dermatology*)

Diagnosis

Making a diagnosis is easy as a rule, since the larvae can be seen, but sometimes they may have successfully bored in below the surface, as occurred in the third case reported by McCuiston et al. (1958). The diagnosis may then be delayed until the larvae mature and emerge to pupate. Sporadic cases are more difficult to diagnose in the absence of visible larvae. In the case of non-cutaneous lesions, Yount and Sudler (1907) stated that any patient with a foul-smelling serosanguineous nasal discharge should be suspected of having myiasis.

Treatment

The aim of treatment is to remove all the larvae. With facultative parasites all that this usually entails is debridement with irrigation. However, where the larvae have burrowed into the tissues and live in their own sinus pockets, more drastic measures are required. These generally involve irrigation with chloroform or ether under local or general anaesthesia. Such irrigation may have to be repeated daily for several days. For example, in the third case reported by McCuiston et al. (1958) initial irrigation with water removed about 100 larvae. Chloroform was then applied with a sponge, and over a period of 2 h a further 500 larvae were extracted from various pockets. Over the next 8 days yet another 100 were removed using daily chloroform irrigation. Simple antiseptic or sterile dressings are all that is needed after this treatment and healing is usually complete within a week of removal of larvae. The use of gamma-benzene hexachloride dressings is effective, but very risky in the very young.

Prophylaxis

In man prophylaxis depends on good nursing care of wounds and skin disorders. Wounds should be kept clean, free of infection and adequately covered. Encrusted skin lesions should have appropriate medicaments applied. If dressings are not recommended, patients should be advised to stay indoors until such time as there are no exudative lesions. Turnley's exhortation not to sleep out of doors should be heeded. Physicians should be alert to infestation in the season of fly activity in myiasis regions. The possibility of infestation by non-indigenous flies should be remembered now that air travel has made distant places easily accessible. Furthermore, a lesion acquired abroad can become infested at home. The first of two cases reported by Poindexter (1979) was an example of this, the patient having developed a leg ucler in West Africa, which became infested by *Callitroga americana* some time after returning home. The severe consequences of infestation by screwworms can be avoided by early diagnosis.

Animal prophylaxis is equally important for man. The incidence of cutaneous myiasis can be greatly reduced by good animal husbandry, which includes not only regular and meticulous inspection of livestock during the whole of the "fly season" but also the avoidance, where possible, of surgical procedures during the season. That is to say, cattle should not be castrated, branded, earmarked or dehorned at such times (Dove 1937). To this Herms (1950) added that the use of whips and dogs should be abandoned to avoid minor trauma. Dove (1937) also recommended control of ticks to prevent tick bites, which could be the foci of attention for flies. Herms advised the use of repellent creams on and around wounds. Since up to 13% of cases of myiasis in animals may involve facultative larval parasites (Knipling and Rainwater 1937), breeding grounds for these should be destroyed. They include carcases and decaying animal and vegetable refuse. Failure to take these precautions will lead to an increased incidence of myiasis with all that that entails.

Eradication of the Flies Responsible

The ideal way of dealing with the problem of myiasis is the eradication of the flies responsible. Spraying with insecticidal or larvicidal chemicals may be partially effective, but to cover an adequate area might well be ecologically inadvisable and possibly dangerous to the operator.

The method used to eradicate *Callitroga americana* in the United States is very important and may have far-reaching implications for similar circumstances involving other insects. The programme of eradication was undertaken by the US Department of Agriculture, Entomology Research Division (Baumhover 1966). Knipling (1937) had suggested that the release of sterile male flies might be used to control such pests. This form of population control is particularly applicable to *C. americana*, which mates only once (Chapman 1971). After a successful preliminary trial on the island of Curaçao the research team cultured *C. americana* by the billion, using, during the campaign, no less than 6.3 million pounds weight of whale meat as culture medium. The flies were sterilised by irradiation and the sterile males were released in very large but calculated numbers over at first an area covering 50 000 square miles in the southeastern states and then over a greater area in the southwestern states of the United States. Previous experiments had shown that a group of females mingled with a mixed group of fertile and sterile males produced sterile and fertile eggs in the same proportion as that of sterile to fertile males present. The release of huge numbers of sterile male flies into the indigenous fly population quickly reduced the number of that population and with it the incidence of screwworm myiasis. Over the period 1962–1965 the annual incidence fell from 50 000 to 5000 to 223 to 300 (the last figure in a hot summer favourable to the fly). The cost of the operation was US $15 million plus US $750 000 for research expenses. The saving was between US $140 and 275 million. Furthermore, at the end of the campaign all that was necessary was to maintain by the same means a suitably wide fly-free zone between the treated areas and neighbour countries where such a campaign had not been used. The cost of this was relatively very small.

The eradication programme has now been extended to clear other states in the United States and also in Mexico. It is proceeding satisfactorily with occasional reinfestations of some areas with a temporary increase in the number of animals involved, as in 1972 and 1976 when nearly 91 000 and just over 29 000 cases respectively were recorded (Spencer et al. 1980). The original testing ground in Curaçao became reinfested in 1971 after being completely free of flies since 1955. In 1975–1976 179 cases were recorded in dogs, sundry other cases in various domestic animals and 14 human patients were affected (Snow and Coppedge 1978). Constant vigilance and maintenance of control is necessary to avoid this.

Furuncular Myiasis in Man

Furuncular myiasis is caused by the larvae of several different species of fly. Since these not only inhabit different regions but also have differing biological behaviour they will be described individually. However, the furuncular lesions produced are very similar whichever fly is the cause. For this reason a detailed description of these lesions is given only for *Dermatobia hominis*. Any variations from this are mentioned in connection with the various flies concerned. The flies causing furuncular myiasis in man are *Dermatobia hominis*, *Cuterebra* (a related species), *Cordylobia anthropophaga*, *Stasisia rodhaini*, three species of *Wohlfahrtia* and two species of *Hypoderma*. The differential diagnosis of cutaneous myiasis in general and furuncular lesions in particular has been well set out by Peters and Kramer (1966). Figure 8.5 is from their paper.

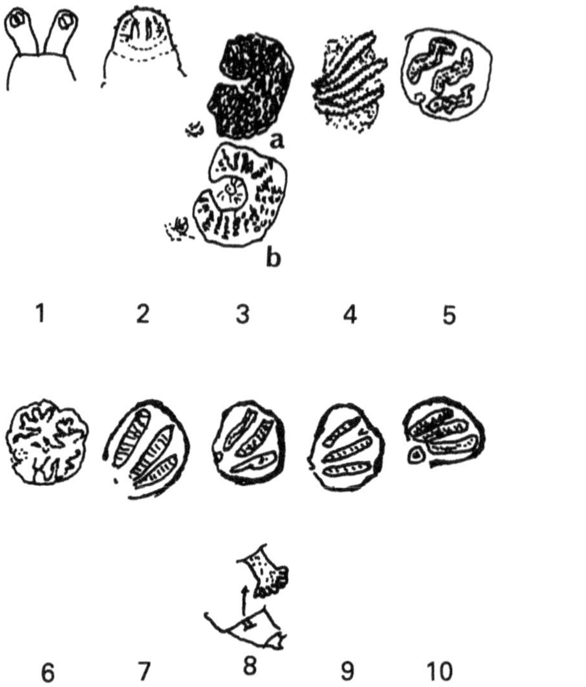

Fig. 8.5. Posterior spiracles of peritreme of third larval instar (except where stated) of **1** *Gasterophilus* (first instar); **2** *Hypoderman* (first instar); **3a** *H. bovis*, **b** *H. lineatum*; **4** *Dermatobia hominis*; **5** *Cordylobia anthropophaga*; **6** *Stasisia rodhaini*; **7** *Wohlfahrtia vigil*; **8** *Callitroga americana*; **9** *Chrysomya bezziana*; **10** *Wohlfahrtia magnifica*. (After Peters and Kramer 1966, by kind permission of the authors and the Editor of *Hautarzt*)

Infestation by *Dermatobia hominis*

The following description is based on that of Dunn (1930), who described the entire course of untreated lesions produced by *D. hominis* from personal experience of natural and experimental infestation. His lesions lasted from $46\frac{1}{2}$ to $54\frac{3}{4}$ days, with an average of just over 49 days. Patients, however, usually seek treatment much earlier because of pain. In man there are seldom more than four or five lesions, although Andersen (1960) pointed out that in cattle up to 1000 could be found in a single animal (see also Fig. 8.18). The distal parts of the limbs and the scalp (Dalmat 1955; Prasad and Becik 1969) are the areas most frequently affected, but lesions have been recorded on the ear (Kaye and Higgins 1964), the eyelid (Price 1937; Alessandro 1978), nipple area (Iannini et al. 1975), prepuce (Kleeman 1983) and upper back (Dunn 1934), although exposed areas are more commonly involved. There appears to be no predilection for age, sex or ethnic origin of the victim.

The newly hatched larva is deposited on the skin and penetrates it, without the patient being aware of the fact. After 24 h a small slightly reddened papule 2–3 mm in diameter appears. It itches slightly at intervals, especially at night and in the evening. It slowly enlarges over the next 3 weeks into an erythematous dome-shaped nodule more than 1 cm across with a rather ill-defined indurated inflammatory oedema extending for 1–2 cm around. It closely resembles a furuncle but may not be tender (Katz and Taylor 1971) or only slightly so (Hoben et al. 1966; Hubler et al. 1974). Dunn (1930) noted tenderness during moulting. After the first few days there is a serous or serosanguineous discharge, which comes from a tiny central punctum. As the lesion enlarges, this central pore increases to almost 3 mm in diameter and is easily visible. At times it appears to "point" like a boil (Dunn 1930) because it has a creamy- or pearly-coloured central "core", which is in fact the posterior end of a larva. The discharge increases and may sometimes contain a little pus or blood. It has a characteristically unpleasant smell (Huber et al. 1974). After approximately 14 days and again at about 28 days the discharge may contain portions of the cast larval skin following the first and second moults. From time to time the posterior end of the larva is protruded from the cavity, as much as 5 mm being visible (Sweet 1962; Fig. 8.6). Dunn (1930) reported that the end of the larva appeared to push out fluid and tiny bubbles at this time. When touched it retracts immediately. According to M. Bunney (1981, personal communication), the purpose of the protrusion is to gain room for manoeuvre by the larva inside its living quarters. Katz and Taylor (1971) noted that the larval movements, which are commonly observed, gave a pulsating character to the lesion but that this "pulsation" was not synchronous with the patient's arterial pulse.

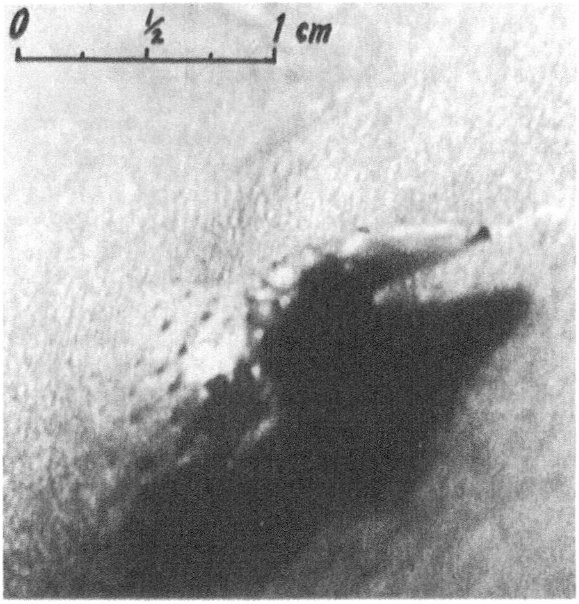

Fig. 8.6. *Dermatobia hominis* larva spontaneously protruding from the hole it has made in the skin. (From Field 1981, by kind permission of the author and the Editor of the *Medical Journal of Australia*. Photograph taken by the patient and reproduced by the University of New South Wales and Teaching Hospitals Department of Medical Illustration)

The appearance of the lesion is overshadowed by the symptoms. The intermittent itch continues throughout the course and was attributed by Dunn (1930) to allergy to the secretory and excretory products of the larva. In his case it was also associated with a papulovesicular sensitivity eczema of the surrounding skin and also of the hands. He also experienced smarting and stinging sensations, which he blamed on larval movements with consequent rasping of its body spines and oral hooks on the cavity wall. By far the most important symptom, however, is pain. This seems to begin around the time of the first moult towards the end of the second week, is intermittent, mainly but not exclusively nocturnal and has a sharp stabbing character. It persists for periods of a few minutes and, as the disorder progresses, it becomes increasingly severe, reaching an intensity which Dunn described as excruciating and nauseating. He considered this pain to be caused by the tearing of tissues by oral hooks during feeding. Ruch (1967) felt it was due to larval movements alone. Some attacks of pain are accompanied by bleeding.

The inflammatory reaction around the lesion may be accompanied by lymphangitis and regional lymphadenopathy. General symptoms such as lassitude, malaise and fever were noted by Dunn (1930) and by Hubler and his colleagues (1974); however, Iannini et al. (1975) noted the absence of such symptoms, and they have not been a feature of the recorded cases, possibly because the larvae were removed fairly early.

The infestation ends by the emergence of the larva to pupate. This is heralded by repeated protrusion of the posterior end of the larva through the central aperture as it attempts to escape. When it fails it retreats and has been observed rasping round the periphery of the hole with its body spines to enlarge it. When the hole is 5–6 mm in diameter the larva emerges, quite painlessly and often unobserved by the patient, in about 3 h. The wound heals rapidly and within a week only a small pigmented scar is visible.

Complications may occur. According to Curran (1939), if the larva dies in situ secondary infection may ensue because the protective larval secretion of urea has ceased. Such infection can occur in an active lesion (Dunn 1930). Harrell and Mosely (1942) observed penetration of a prepatellar bursa in their patient, whilst Dunn (1934) recorded fatal penetration of the left cerebral hemisphere by a larva in a child with a scalp lesion. Hubler et al. (1974) found leucocytosis with esosinophilia.

Histopathology

There is a polymorphous infiltrate of histiocytes, lymphocytes, plasma cells and eosinophils around the larva and its surrounding reactionary fibrous capsule (Everett et al. 1977; Hubler et al. 1974).

Diagnosis

Diagnosis of infestation with *D. hominis* depends on the history of onset and of exposure to infestation. It should not be forgotten that the condition may only present after the patient has returned home from a stay in an infested area (Sweet 1962; Price 1937; March 1964; Casner and Wiseman 1965; Schorr 1967; Field 1981; Kleeman 1983). The patient described by M. Bunney (1981, personal communication) was a Scottish soldier who had been on duty in Belize during the period of seasonal fly activity. The clinical resemblance to a furuncle with intermittent pain and the protrusion of the posterior end of the larva are highly suggestive of the diagnosis, which can be confirmed accurately by the identification of the larva. Distinction from other forms of furuncular myiasis depends upon the geographical origin of the exposure, the duration of the lesions and the identification of the larva.

Treatment

Attempts to express the larva by pressure on or around the lesions are fruitless and painful. Antibiotics and topical applications of an antiseptic nature are equally useless. The method, used by the indigenous inhabitants of endemic areas, of binding a piece of pork fat over the lesion for 24 h seems to be very effective in inducing the larva to evacuate its home (Ruch 1967; Fig. 8.7). Harrell and Mosely (1942) injected 10 ml of local anaesthetic into and around the lesion. This not only anaesthetises the area but also the larva, which can then easily be picked out after incising the lesion. The latter is then curetted and stitched if small, or left to granulate. It heals uneventfully within a week.

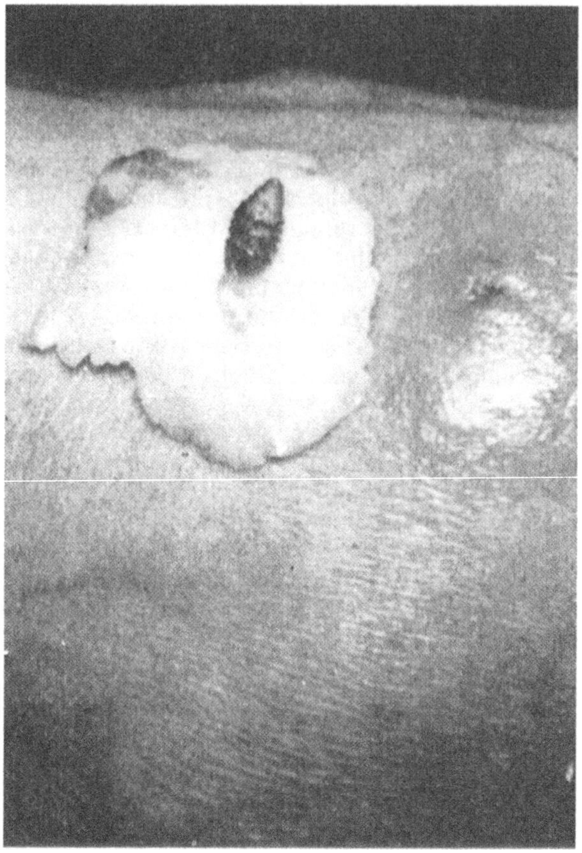

Fig. 8.7. Larva of *Dermatobia hominis* extracted from a furunculoid lesion of skin by means of the piece of pork fat upon which it is seen resting. (From Ruch 1967, by kind permission of the author and the publisher, the American Medical Association. Copyright 1967, American Medical Association)

Morphology and Biology

D. hominis is a medium-sized fly resembling a bluebottle. Full details of the adult and larval stages can be found in James' monograph (1947). Figures 8.8, 8.9, 8.10 and 8.11 illustrate its appearances. It is sufficient here to add that it has a mainly yellow head and legs, pale-brown wings, a dull-blue thorax and a metallic blue abdomen. The oral hooks of the larva are well depicted in Figs. 8.10 and 8.12. The larval body segments are armed with rows of spines (Figs. 8.10 and 8.13).

This fly, which is found only in the neotropical areas of the New World extending from southern Mexico to northern Argentina, is a serious economic pest in these Latin American countries. It causes growth retardation and even death in calves, a serious weight deficiency in adults, low milk production, partial or even total hide damage, acclimatisation difficulties and reduced commercial value for affected animals amounting to about US $260 million annually (Mateus 1978). As for human infestation, there is almost certainly a much higher incidence than the published examples would lead one to suppose. For example, Adams (1904) recorded that six out of a party of seven men became infested in Panama. He associated the high incidence to exposure of the skin to the attentions of the fly (he had no idea how the infestation was acquired) and noted that the only person to escape was the man who refused to remove his clothes for the entire stay.

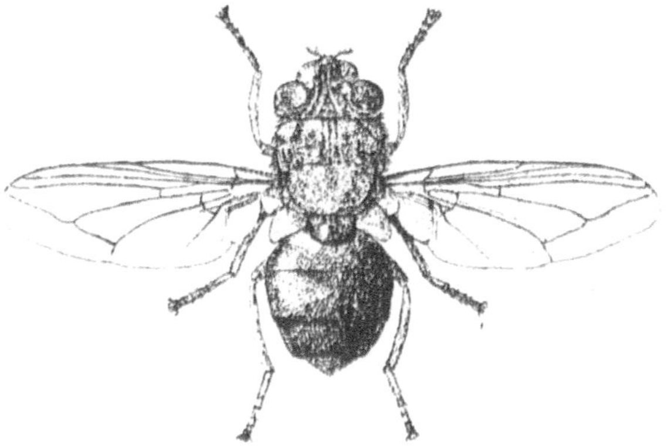

Fig. 8.8. Female adult *Dermatobia hominis*. (After Patton and Evans 1929)

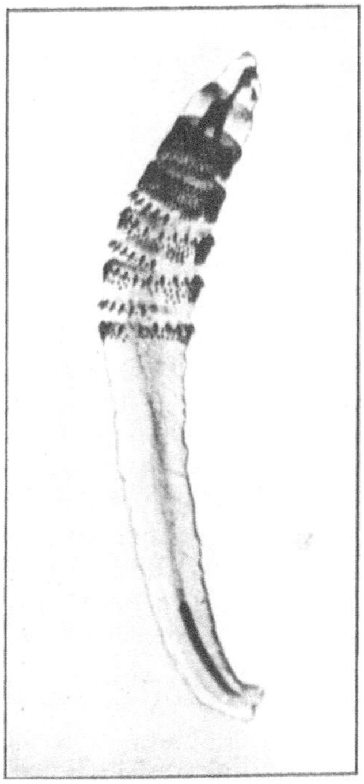

Fig. 8.9. First instar larva of *Dermatobia hominis*. (Courtesy of Dr. M. Bunney, Edinburgh)

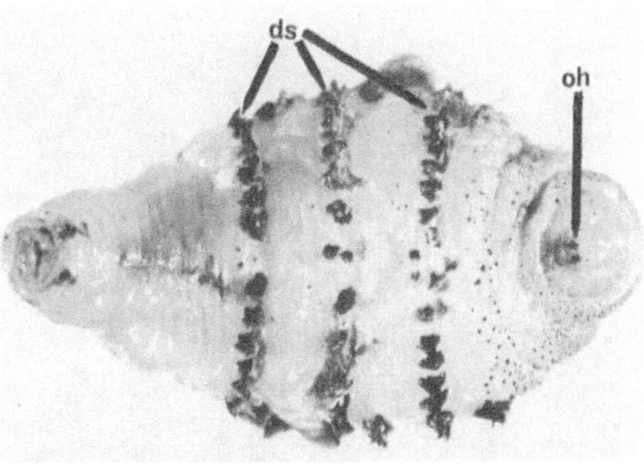

Fig. 8.10. Mature larva (third instar) of *Dermatobia hominis*. Note the two oral hooks (*oh*) and the girdle of spines (*ds*) on the body segments. (Courtesy of Dr. M. Bunney, Edinburgh)

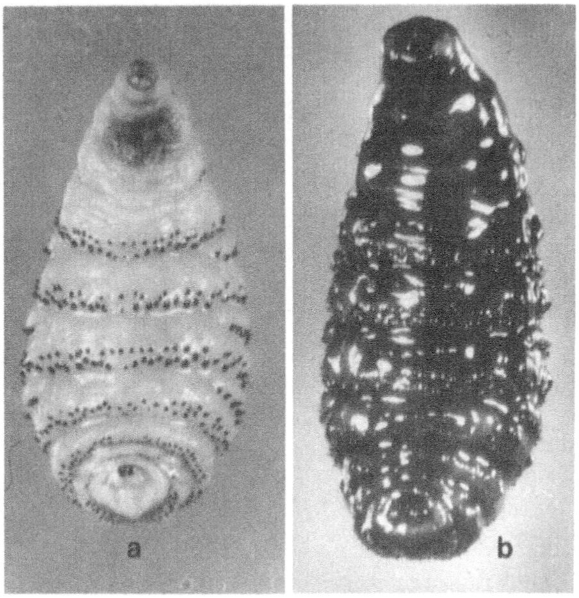

Fig. 8.11a, b. *Dermatobia hominis* from Colombian cattle. **a** third-stage larva; **b** fourth-stage larva. (Courtesy of Dr. M. Bunney, Edinburgh)

The life cycle of *D. hominis* is remarkable. It tends to live in shaded areas of pasture land, avoiding open fields. It does not deposit its eggs directly on the chosen host animal (usually cattle, dogs or men) but utilises other Diptera such as day-flying mosquitoes (*Psophora* species), *Stomoxys calcitrans*, *Synthesomyia* etc. or occasionally ticks (Dunn 1918) as vectors, a state of affairs

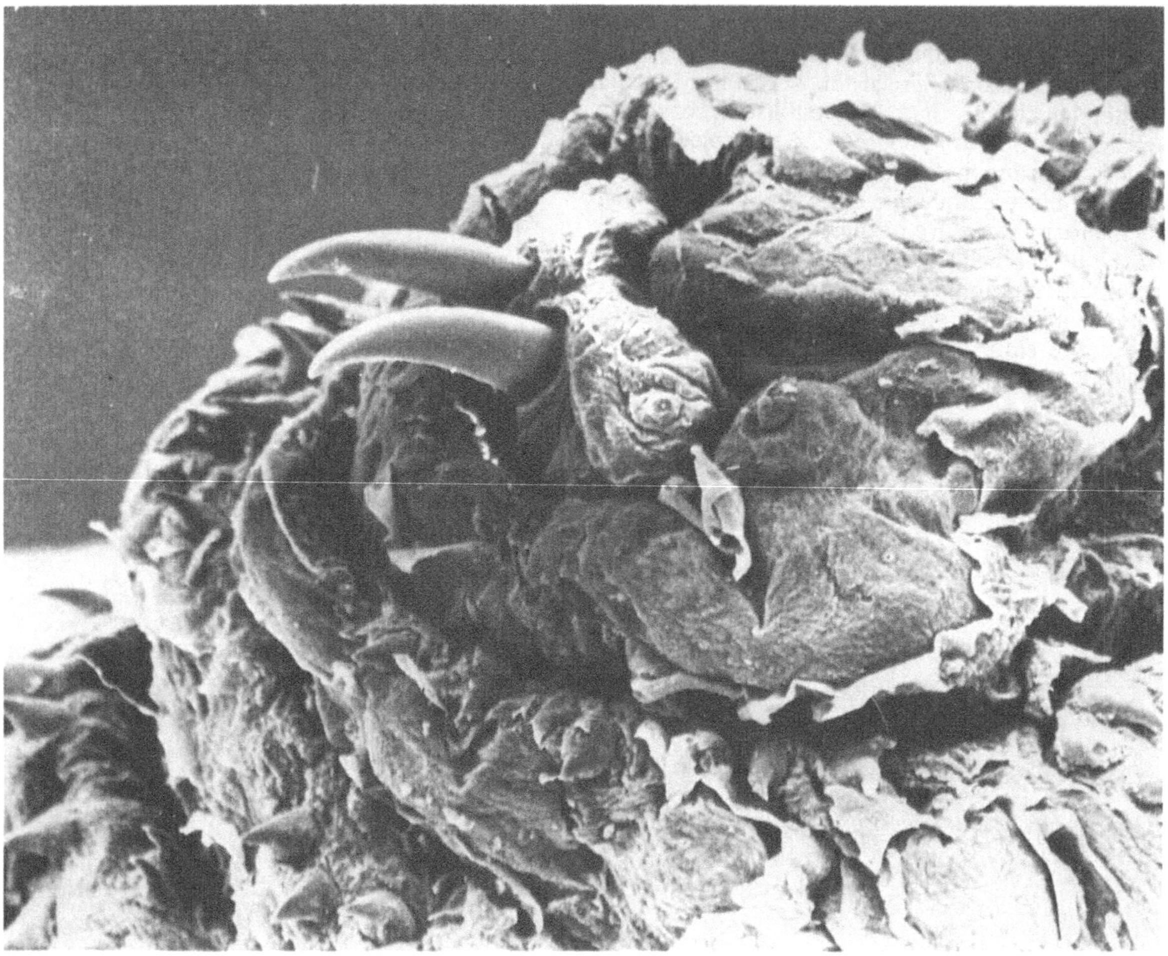

Fig. 8.12. Scanning electron micrograph of oral hooks of third instar of *Dermatobia hominis* larva. (Courtesy of Dr. M Bunney, Edinburgh)

known as phoresy. It tends to hover around the selected host or sits on the skin awaiting the arrival of the vector insect in search of a blood meal. The *Dermatobia* fly seizes its victim on the wing, grasping it firmly with its legs whilst hovering above the host. The vector insect is adjusted by the *Dermatobia*, which then quickly deposits its egg—about 12 or so within a minute (Bates 1943)—usually on the underside of the abdomen of the vector (Fig. 8.14). The number of eggs laid depends to some extent on the size of the vector. They hatch in about 4–6 days, the actual hatching process being accelerated at the last moment by the warmth of the intended host's skin when the vector insect lands. Whilst the latter is feeding the *Dermatobia* larvae hatch and crawl onto the skin of the host where they at once begin to dig in. This latter process is very efficient and is exactly similar to that used by the larva of *Cordylobia anthropophaga* (see Fig. 8.17).

Curran (1939) stated that in South America *D. hominis* could also lay eggs on the foliage of trees and shrubs and that cattle were attacked by the eggs falling onto their hide as they brushed the foliage on passing. The larvae hatched quickly and then crawled down the hair to the skin and penetrated it. James (1947) agreed that the fly used this method of disseminating its eggs if no suitable vectors were available. One female *D. hominis* can make use of several mosquitoes or other vectors. In a survey carried out by Bates (1943) the number of mosquitoes found to be carrying *D. hominis* eggs varied from 8.4% of *Psorophora ferox* to 2.2% of *Aedes seriatus*. The species chosen as carriers depended on their habits.

The pupal stage lasts from 20 to 120 days, depending on the environment, especially as regards humidity. The whole life cycle is about 3–4 months.

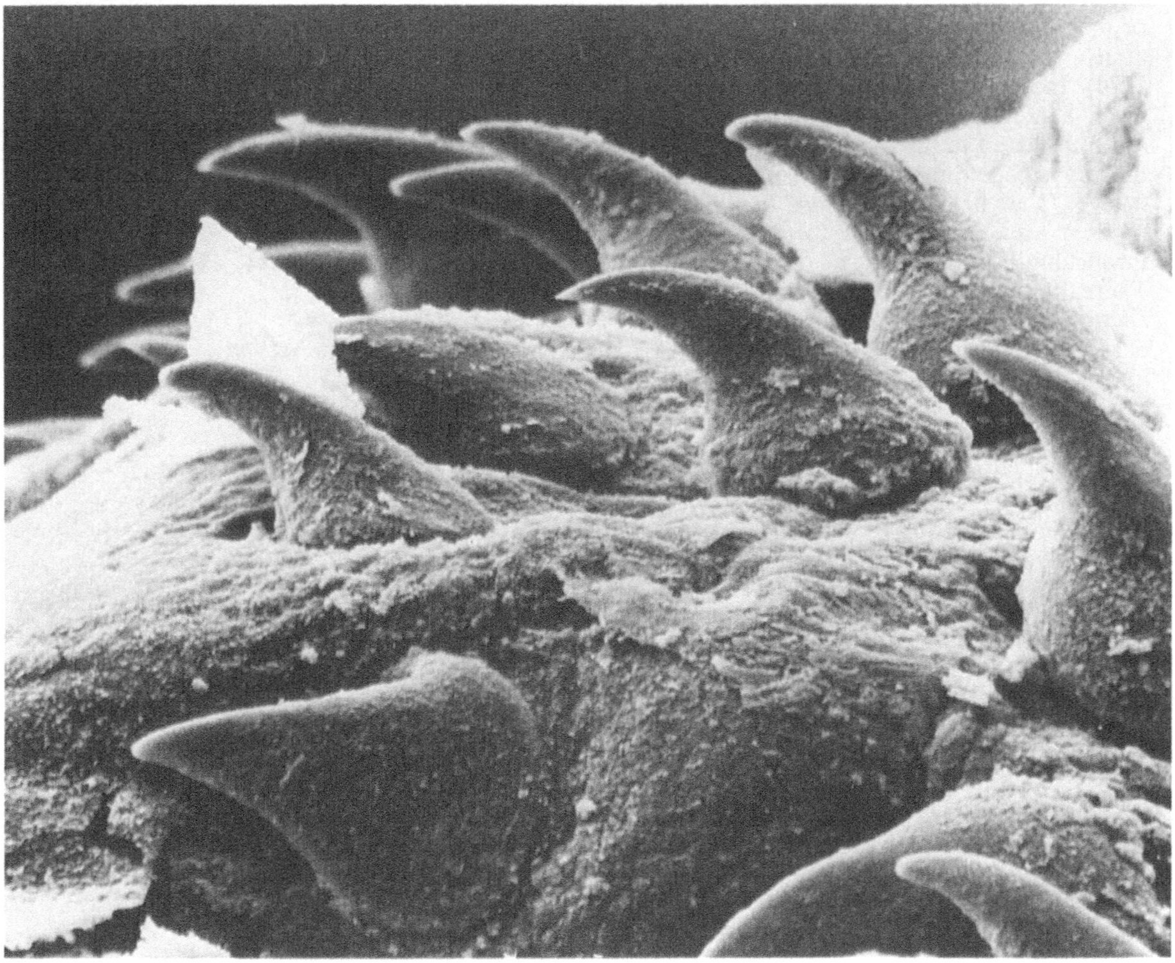

Fig. 8.13. Scanning electron micrograph of spines on the body segments of third instar larva of *Dermatobia hominis* (Courtesy of Dr. M. Bunney, Edinburgh)

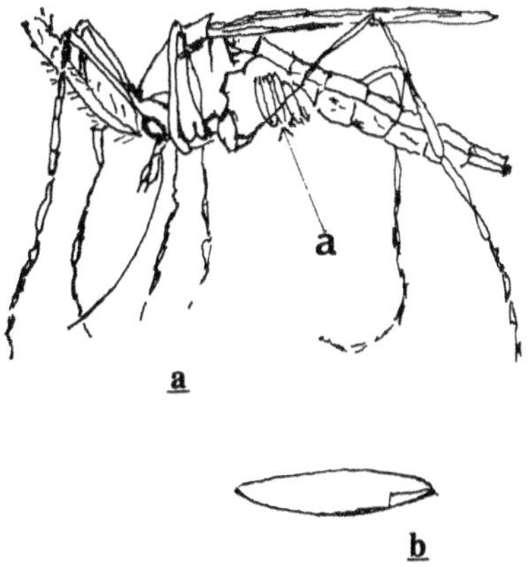

Fig. 8.14. **a** *Psorophora* mosquito carrying a load of *Dermatobia* eggs (*a*). **b** Egg enlarged. (After James 1947, by kind permission of the author and the publisher, the US Department of Agriculture)

Infestation by *Cuterebra* Species

There are some 20 species of the genus *Cuterebra*, which is zoologically related to *Dermatobia* (Salomon et al. 1970). These botflies are parasitic on rabbits and rodents and are indigenous to North America. Eleven cases of cutaneous infestation of man by the larvae of these flies have been recorded but only three or four have been described in detail. The reports originated in widely separated states of the United States (Hodges 1955; Scott 1964; Salomon et al. 1970). In only one case was the species identified as *C. cuniculi*, the rabbit bot (Scott 1964).

The eggs are laid in warm weather on leaves, stems and underbrush. In nature they hatch out under the influence of a sudden rise in temperature induced by the heat of a mammalian body lying on or near the infested plants and the larvae quickly attach themselves to the host (Salomon et al. 1970). In man the eggs probably become attached to the hands of those working in infested areas and are transferred to the face, where, after hatching, the larvae penetrate the mucosa of the mouth, nose or eye. Once below the surface they migrate to a random area of skin and form a subcutaneous furunculoid lesion with a surface perforation. Thereafter the larva behaves as in the furuncle of *Dermatobia* infestation, causing pain and discharge. The length of time spent in the lesion is not known. In nature in rodents the duration of the furunculoid lesion is 28–38 days (Catts 1967). The patient described by Salomon et al. (1970) had been troubled for 1 year, but this included the migratory period. The affected areas which have been recorded are the neck, chest and eyelid. All the patients have been adults, except the one described by Hodge (1955), who was a boy aged 11 months. The larvae may emerge spontaneously with or without encouragement (Hodges used Tinct. Benzoin Co.) or can be excised. Subsequent healing is rapid, and no sequelae have yet been observed.

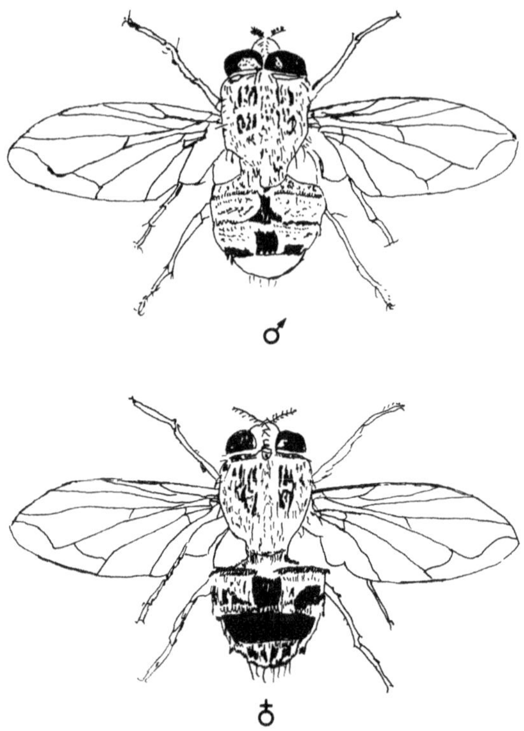

Fig. 8.15. Adult male and female *Cordylobia anthropophaga*. (After Blacklock and Thompson 1923, by kind permission of the Editor of the *Annals of Tropical Medicine and Hygiene*)

Infestation by *Cordylobia anthropophaga*

Morphology and Biology

The Tumbu fly *Cordylobia anthropophaga* and, in some areas, *Stasisia rodhaini* cause furuncular myiasis throughout west, central and east tropical Africa. It has also been recorded in southwest Africa (Namibia), southern Rhodesia (Zimbabwe) and the Transvaal and Orange Free State provinces of South Africa (Zumpt 1959). Gomez-Armario and Mira-Gutierrez (1976) reported a case which originated in the Congo, whilst Wildy and Glover (1982) described an instance in a visitor to the United Kingdom from Ghana and noted that the condition has been recognised in Southern Spain. The larva is the commonest maggot found in human tissues in Africa (Patton 1921).

Full details of the life cycle and morphology of *C. anthropophaga* can be found in the paper by Blacklock and Thompson (1923), from which most of the following description has been taken. It is a medium-sized, compact fly about 10 mm long with straw-yellow head, body and legs, the thorax and abdomen having blackish markings and the wings a brownish tint. Figures 8.15 and 8.16 depict the adult and larval stages. Like *Dermatobia hominis* the larva possesses two oral hooks which are part of the cephalopharyngeal "skeleton", which is the

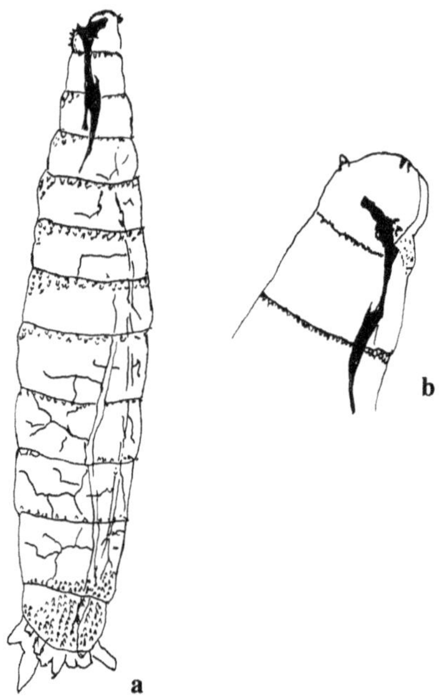

Fig. 8.16a, b. *Cordylobia anthropophaga*. **a** first larval instar; **b** head of first larval instar, lateral view. Note scaly spines on the body segments and also the cephalopharyngeal skeleton. (After Blacklock and Thomson 1923, by kind permission of the Editor of the *Annals of Tropical Medicine and Hygiene*)

key to the ability of these larvae to penetrate the skin of the host. It also has rows of chitinised spines on the body segments and specialised soft processes on the caudal segment. The adult flies seek shelter and are quickly killed by bright sunlight. They rest indoors at night and much of the daytime, being active only for short periods in the early morning and late afternoon. They feed on sugar and plant juices, pulped food, urine-soaked soil and decomposing animal matter. Oviposition occurs in darkened places, for preference on dry urine-soaked soil or sand. When bred in captivity they do not lay eggs on human clothing or animal skin, but Zumpt (1959) maintained that they preferred the dry portions of urine-soaked nappies. The eggs hatch in 1–3 days (Gunther 1971) depending on temperature and humidity. Immediately after hatching, the young larva, which is about 1 mm in length, "stands" on its caudal end, adhering to the ground by means of the soft processes on the caudal segment already mentioned. Its cephalic end reaches upwards seeking for a suitable animal host. In the wild this is the brown or black rat, but around human habitations the dog and man, especially small children, are common hosts. It can survive for 16 days while looking for a host (Gunther 1971). When it contacts the skin of a host it at once attaches itself by its oral hooks and then commences to penetrate the skin. This is accomplished by levering up horn cells of the epidermis with the oral hooks, using the clinging effect of the backward pointing body spines to give purchase to exert pressure with the hooks. The cephalic end is inserted below the raised epidermis and the process is repeated until the entire larva is below the surface (Fig. 8.17). In an area of soft skin this painless penetration may only take 25–60 s, but up to 30 min on the sole of the foot. Once below the surface the larva digs more deeply into the subcutaneous tissues to form a dwelling cavity.

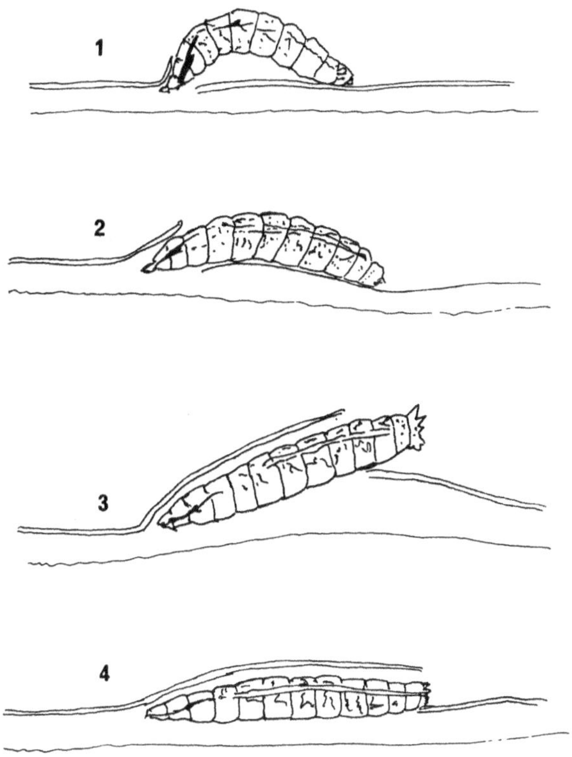

Fig. 8.17. *Cordylobia anthropophaga*. First larval instar penetrating the skin. (After Blacklock and Thompson 1923, by kind permission of the Editor of the *Annals of Tropical Medicine and Hygiene*)

Clinical Appearances

The clinical appearances are almost identical with those caused by *Dermatobia hominis*. Sometimes the painless penetration may give rise to a local reaction of anaphylactic type. Any part of the body may be attacked, but the feet, buttocks, genitalia and neck are common sites. Konotey-Ahulu et al. (1967) have pointed out that whereas the nodules are red in European skins, they are shiny in black skins. The course of infestation caused by *Cordylobia* is much shorter than that caused by *Dermatobia*, being completed in 14–16 days.

Treatment

Methods of treatment are similar to those used for *Dermatobia*, but with the use of liquid paraffin the subsequent expression of the larva is more easily achieved. Healing after excision under local anaesthesia is rapid, but healing after natural emergence of the larva is very slow and pigmented scars remain, which are visible up to 10 years later. Gomez-Armario and Mira-Gutierrez have noted that pouring water onto the aperture will induce the larva to emerge.

Konotey et al. (1967) have indicated that clothing should never be dried in a shady area, whilst Radcliffe (1972) recommended that all personal laundry should be ironed on both sides—an impractical suggestion for most potential victims.

Histology

Korting et al. (1971) reported that there is a fistulous track lined with pseudoepitheliomatous epidermis leading to the depths of the dermal cavity. Around this cavity, especially in the immediate vicinity of the larva, there is a dense infiltrate of eosinophils, plasma cells and histiocytes.

Differential Diagnosis

Stasisia rodhaini, a forest dweller (Zumpt 1965; Peters and Kramer 1966), was described as causing similar lesions in the Congo by Gedoelst (1905, 1908–1909). It was some years before this fly was identified in relation to the skin lesions because of the paucity of material available for laboratory examination. This serves to emphasise the necessity for referring as much fresh undamaged entomological material as possible to experts for examination and cultural investigation, which greatly facilitate accurate diagnosis. Zumpt has pointed out that the lesions caused by *Stasisia* are larger and more painful than those caused by *C. anthropophaga* because of the larger size of the larva. The limbs, trunk, neck, scalp and eyelids may all be the site of the infestation.

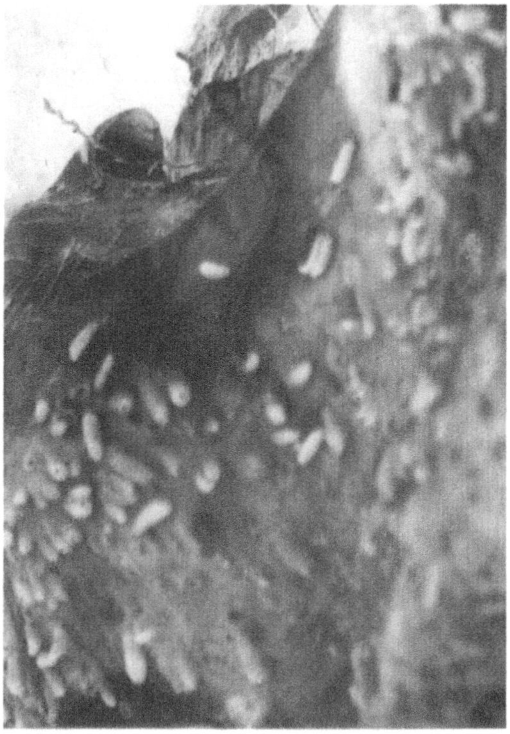

Fig. 8.18. Larvae of *Hypoderma diana* in the hide of a red deer. The picture shows numerous larvae (warbles) attached to the undersurface of the skin. [Postmortem picture by courtesy of Mr. D. J. Brown of Hawick, Scotland, and Prof. J. T. Baxter of the Royal (Dick) School of Veterinary Studies, University of Edinburgh.]

Fig. 8.19. Female flies of **a** *Hypoderma bovis* and **b** *H. lineatum*. (**a** After Zumpt 1965, by kind permission of the author and the publisher, Butterworth and Co.; **b** after James 1947, by kind permission of the author and the publisher, the US Department of Agriculture) ▷

Infestation by *Hypoderma* Species

Morphology and Biology

The larvae of *Hypoderma lineatum* (the heel fly) and *H. bovis* (warble fly) have been known since Roman times to cause lesions in cattle (Bishopp et al. 1926). A similar fly (*H. diana*) attacks reindeer (Fig. 8.18). The egg-laying activity of *H. lineatum* around the ankles of cattle induces panic in those attacked, and may even cause them to stampede. They find protection by standing ankle deep in water, preferably in the shade. *Hypoderma* species are abundant in Europe and North America and are also found in South Africa and more recently in Australia. In the United Kingdom *H. bovis* is by now the most predominant species; *H. lineatum* is found only in small numbers, except in the Hebrides (Tarry 1982). In those areas where these flies are active the economic loss is severe and similar in type and magnitude to that caused by *Dermatobia* in Latin America (see pp. 96–97). Man can also be affected, children proportionately more than adults (Nicholson et al. 1954).

A detailed account of the life cycle, morphology and clinical effects of these flies has been given by Bishopp and his colleagues (1926), although some of their findings on the larval stages have been modified by Patton (1936). Figures 8.19 and 8.20 depict the principal morphological features of the fly and its larva. The adult is a large buzzing, bee-like fly. It is believed not to feed, having sufficient reserves of its own to last its brief lifetime, which is 1 week in warm weather and 3 weeks in cooler weather, according to Patton. In Europe it is seen from July until early September, whilst in Texas the season is December to March, in the central United States from March to May and in the northern United States from April to June. *H. bovis* tends to be a little later in appearance than *H. lineatum*.

Fig. 8.20a–d. *Hypoderma bovis*. **a** first larval instar, dorsal view; **b** first larval instar, ventral view; **c** first larval instar, posterior view of the caudal segment; **d** third larval instar. The scale marking refers to the third larval instar only. (After Zumpt 1965, by kind permission of the author and the publisher, Butterworth and Co.) ▷

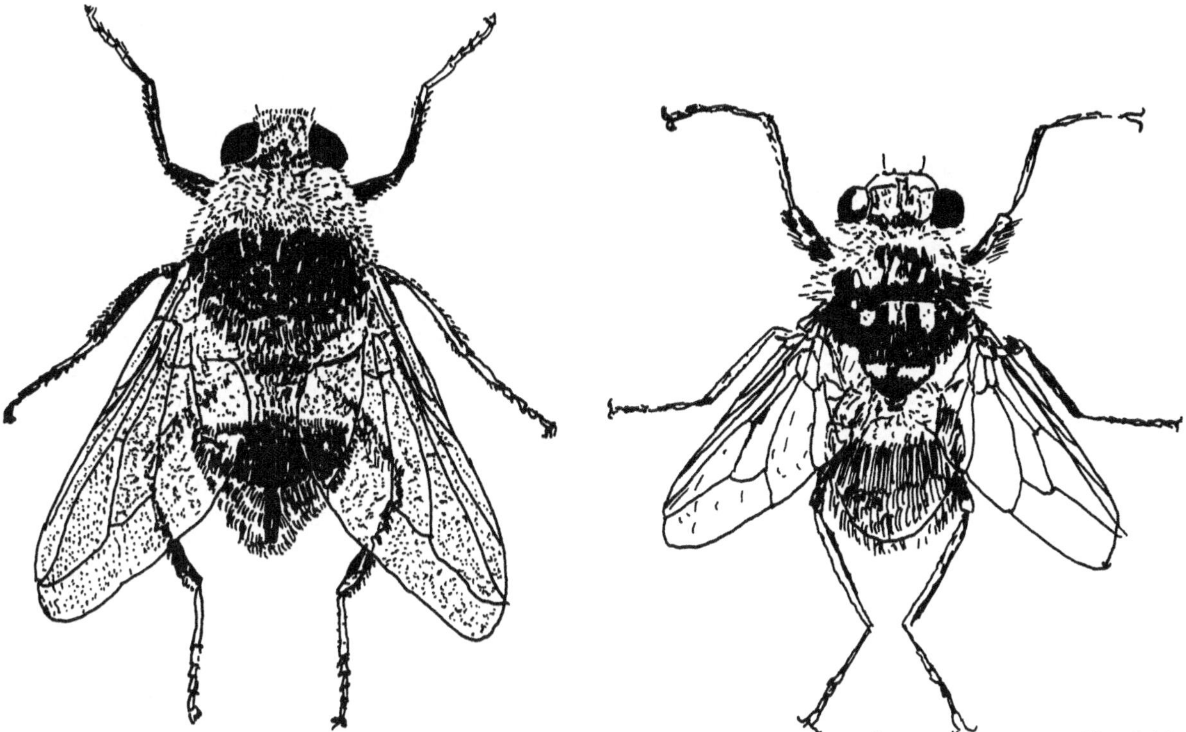

a b Fig. 8.19.

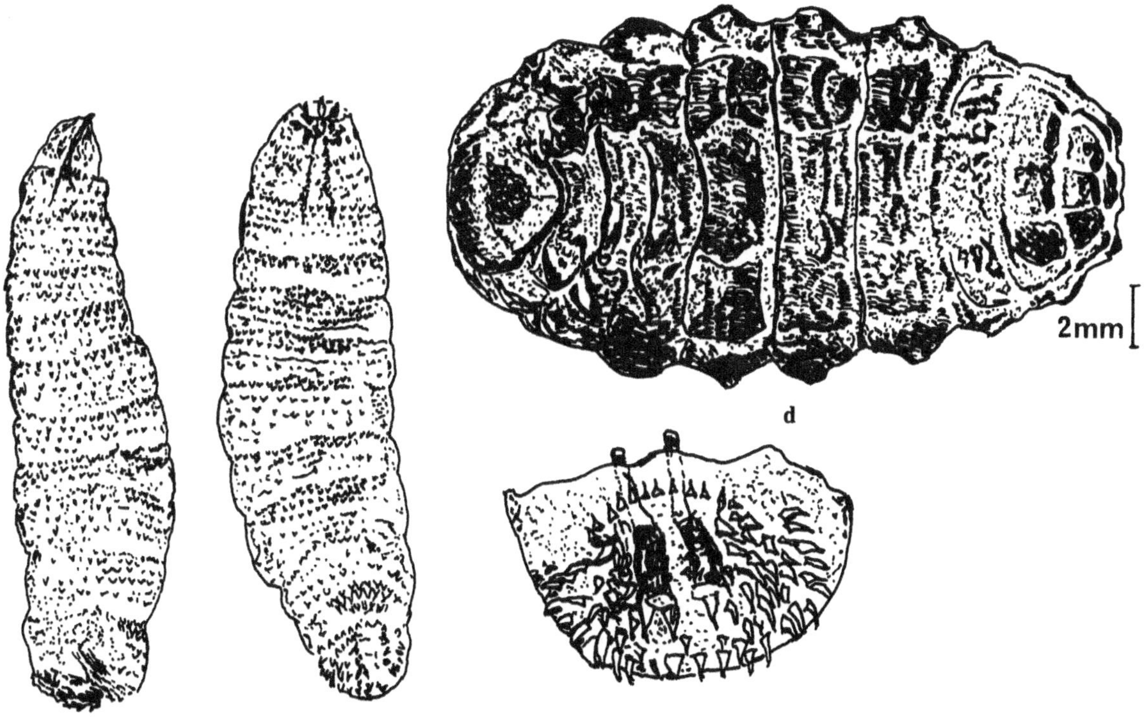

a b c Fig. 8.20.

Oviposition is usually completed in 24 h. *H. lineatum* lays its eggs in rows on the hairs of the ankles in cattle standing in bright sunlight. *H. bovis* oviposits whilst the cattle are lying down, choosing the hair around the root of the tail, over the ischial area and on the udder. Its eggs are laid singly on hair (Fig. 8.21). Oviposition on man has not been observed, but Bishopp et al. (1926) suggested that the probable sites were the head, legs and clothing. The eggs hatch in 2½–6 days, and the young larvae crawl to the base of the hair to reach the skin, which they penetrate within 6 h, causing much annoyance to the animal (Patton 1936). The next immediate stage has yet to be clarified, but it is known that the larvae appear some time later in a body cavity, usually beneath the oesophageal mucosa. After remaining there for some months they migrate to the back of the animal, where, after moulting to the final instar, they appear in the subcutaneous tissues, thus causing warbles, between late February and early May in Europe—some 7–8 months after the initial infestation. The larva contained in each warble penetrates the skin to form a breathing aperture and remains in situ for 70–80 days, the lesion closely resembling the furunculoid lesion of *Dermatobia* infestation. According to Patton (1936), warbles have been found in cattle in Scotland as late as August before the larvae finally emerge to drop off and pupate.

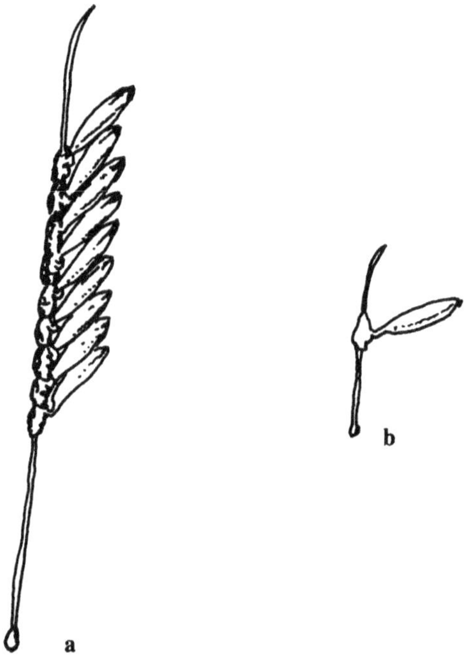

Fig. 8.21. Eggs of **a** *Hypoderma lineatum* and **b** *H. bovis*, showing the multiple attachment to the same hair with *H. lineatum* and the single attachment of *H. bovis*. (After Zumpt 1965, by kind permission of the author and the publisher, Butterworth and Co.)

Clinical Features

Man is an abnormal host for *Hypoderma* and the larvae do not mature fully (Bishopp et al. 1926; Nicholson et al. 1954), although Morgan et al. (1964) mentioned that infestation by *Hypoderma* in man was commoner than is generally accepted. The clinical course is rather different from that in cattle. It occurs chiefly but not exclusively in persons associated with cattle. Symptoms first occur in the winter months and usually present as painful subcutaneous or deeper swellings which persist for a few days, disappear for a week or more and reappear elsewhere, this migration continuing for some months. These lesions may also be multiple, and the migration has been noted by all observers to be in a general upward direction towards the head and shoulders. Hunter (1966) has pointed out that the migration tends to be against gravity in cattle, and therefore man's upright posture may disorientate the larvae, which tend to wander in a very haphazard manner, although in a general upward direction. Sometimes the presenting feature may be a localised or even widespread lymphadenopathy, often associated with a temporary subcutaneous swelling.

The migratory swellings finally terminate in one from which the contained larva perforates the overlying skin to produce a breathing hole, thus forming a characteristic furunculoid lesion, from which the larva eventually emerges, occasionally spontaneously but usually by surgical excision under local anaesthesia. Bishopp et al. (1926) quoted one instance where each of several such lesions was preceded for 24 h by toxic symptoms of malaise, abdominal pain, fever, bradycardia, coldness of the hands and drowsiness. The patient, a child, also developed a somewhat persistent peripheral neuritis of the lower legs, which was considered to be due to larval penetration of the spinal canal. A fatality was also reported by these workers, resulting from a warble involving the root of the tongue and the lower jaw around the back. Nicholson et al. (1954) noted leucocytosis with a pronounced eosinophilia in two of their patients, one of whom had an orbital lesion, which ultimately subsided. These authors stated that such lesions could lead to loss of sight. Morgan et al. (1964) also observed eosinophilia in two of their cases.

Infestation by *Wohlfahrtia* Species

Wohlfahrtia vigil and *W. opaca* are exclusively North American species causing furuncular myiasis, whilst *W. magnifica* occurs in southeastern Europe, southern and Asiatic Russia, the Middle East and North Africa, areas with semi-nomadic populations (James 1947), and invades through wounds, at times causing much tissue damage. According to Stabler et al. (1962) *W. vigil* predominates in the eastern states of the United States and *W. opaca* in the western states. Their effects are identical.

New World Species

Morphology and Biology. *W. vigil* was first described as attacking man by Walker (1921), who gave the morphological features of this fly in that paper and two others (1922, 1937). The condition is well known in Canada (e.g. Brady 1923) and the United States (Sanders 1928; Silverthorne and Brown 1934; Israels and Shuman 1949) and is apparently commoner than the reported cases indicate (Strickland, cited by Lewis 1947; O'Rourke 1954). The adult flies are relatively inconspicuous. The sun-loving male is most active between 10 a.m. and 4 p.m. but the female seeks shade and is only seen outside these hours in the early morning and late afternoon (Ford 1933). Both are flower feeders, especially on caraway, and do not feed on carrion (Ford 1933). They frequent railway tracks, near to which many of the victims have lived, and it was suggested by Ford (1936) that the trains were responsible for their spread to nearby towns. Both species are larvipósitors and in nature enter the burrows of small mammals such as the rabbit, ferret or mink to deposit larvae on the very young animals. Human infestation is similarly almost confined to very young babies, which are infested whilst lying in their prams in shady places out of doors. Only four times has an infestation been noted as occurring indoors (Walker 1921; Chown 1924, species unconfirmed; Lewis 1947; Stabler et al. 1962). Morphological details of these flies and their larvae are shown in Figs. 8.22 and 8.23.

Larviposition occurs on the cheeks in the vicinity of the oral, nasal or conjunctival mucosae, the larvae being deposited in a few seconds in a rapid stream and quickly dispersing thereafter (Ford 1933). They tend to seek the shelter of the skin folds at the point where clothing reaches (Lewis 1947). They start penetrating the skin straight away and are often invisible an hour or two later. That they are unable to penetrate the tougher skin

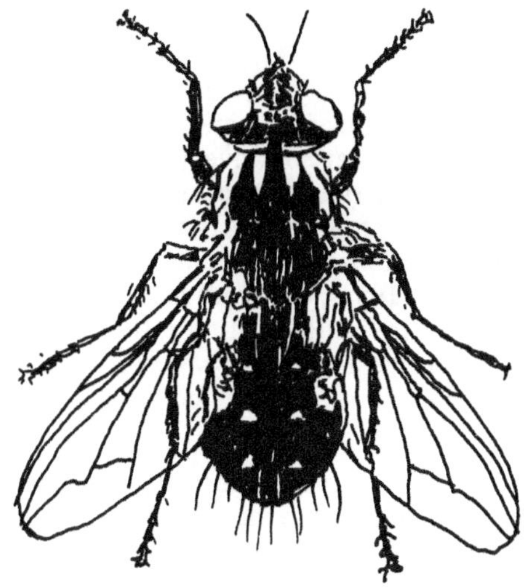

a

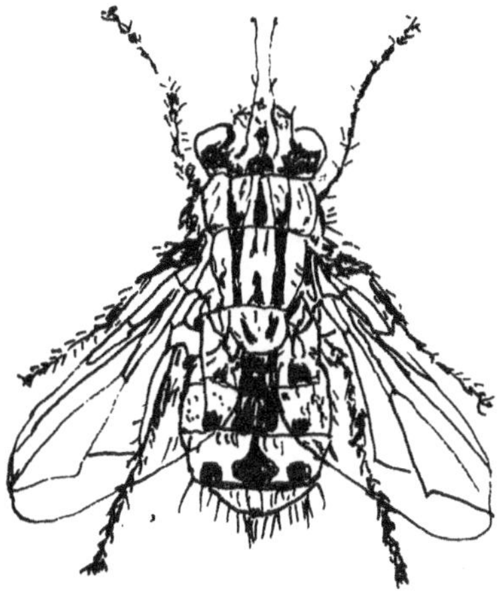

b

Fig. 8.22a, b. Adult female flies of *Wohlfahrtia*. **a** *W. vigil* and **b** *W. magnifica*. (After James 1947, by kind permission of the author and the publisher, the US Department of Agriculture)

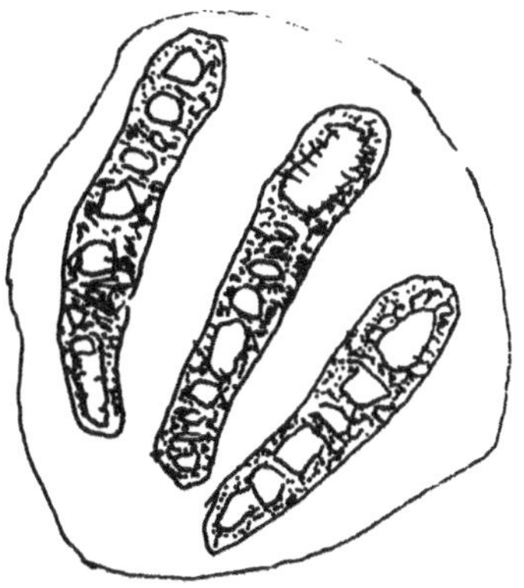

Fig. 8.23. Peritreme with posterior spiracles of third instar larva of *Wohlfahrtia vigil*. (After Walker 1922, by kind permission of the Editor of the *Journal of Parasitology*)

of adults was shown by Ford (1936). This was attributed by O'Rourke (1954) to the inadequate strength of the oral hooks. There is no evidence to support the suggestion by Lewis (1947) that penetration is aided by larval salivary secretions. It is interesting that the only two cases recorded in persons older than infants were both males, one aged $4\frac{1}{2}$ years (MacKenzie 1946) and the other, 24 years (Stabler et al. 1962), and both had furuncular lesions on the soft preputial skin. Another unconfirmed case in a 79-year-old man was recorded by Wohlrabe (1957).

Clinical Features. Unlike most of the other furunculoid-producing larvae the penetration of the infant skin by numbers of larvae simultaneously causes considerable irritation, which makes the child cry, refuse food, become restless and febrile, these symptoms persisting until the larvae are removed. If this is delayed for more than a day or two the affected infant may become dehydrated and quite ill. It is noteworthy, as Ford (1933) has pointed out, that between 5 and 20 such lesions in young animals can be fatal. The furunculoid lesions are identical in appearance to those caused by *Dermatobia* but are of much shorter duration. Their development is therefore more rapid. The initial tiny, bright-red papule becomes what appears superficially to be a pustule; however, close inspection reveals the pustular tip to be in fact the posterior end of a larva. The latter also appears to pulsate, due partly to its movements and also perhaps to its feeding activities (Lewis 1947; Stabler et al. 1962; DeGuisti and Zackheim 1963). Gertson et al. (1933) observed that physicians tend to belittle claims made by mothers that they have seen movement in the lesions. The lesions grow rapidly: Walker in 1923 observed three larvae, each measuring between 7 and 9 mm, reach a length of 17 mm in a further 48 hours. Some lesions may contain several larvae and the breathing aperture in such cases may be as large as 5 mm in diameter (Ford 1933). The lesions are commonly multiple, the average number being 12–14, but as many as 40 can occur in one patient (James 1947). Leucocytosis but no eosinophilia was recorded by Lewis 1947.

Treatment is usually requested in the early stages because of maternal alarm. Larvae may be seen on the surface and can be brushed off, but should be kept for examination; others may have only partially buried themselves and can be picked out; others may easily be expressed by pressure. Unlike other forms of furunculoid myiasis, expression of larvae in *Wohlfahrtia* infestation seems to be easy, relatively painless and uncomplicated. Removal under local anaesthesia does not seem to be required. The administration of suitable antibiotics for secondary infection results in complete healing without sequelae in a few days.

Mothers should be warned to protect babies with fly-proof netting when putting them outside in the pram. Both Ford (1933) and O'Rourke (1954) have pointed out that infestation has nothing to do with a lack of cleanliness.

Old World Species

Morphology and Biology. W. magnifica is an Old World fly with the distribution given above. It was first described by Wohlfahrt, a surgeon who removed one from a patient's eye in 1770 (Portschinsky 1916). The following information is from Portschinsky's paper. The adult flies are flower feeders living in fields and orchards, active in the brightest time of the day and rarely entering houses. Portschinsky warned about the dangers of sleeping out of doors between 10 a.m. and 4 p.m. Carrying up to 168 eggs, which mature simultaneously, the fly deposits the young larvae on the skin of the sleeping host (man or domestic animals). The larvae at once seek the shelter of skin folds or burrow into injured or diseased tissues of the nasal sinuses, eyes or ears. They do not penetrate unbroken skin but may enter the mucosa. They are gregarious feeders and very voracious, grow rapidly and have matured with two moults in 5–7 days. During this period they cause much tissue destruction but do not produce furuncular lesions.

Treatment. Portschinsky (1916) recommended wound irrigation and, where necessary, washing out cavities with chloroform beforehand. As a preventive measure he advocated the removal and destruction of all larvae by frequent inspection of livestock and early treatment of any lesions found.

Creeping Eruption

The form of migratory cutaneous myiasis known as "creeping eruption" is caused by *Gasterophilus* larvae, which wander intradermally rather than subcutaneously. Several species can penetrate the skin (see Table 8.6); however, two which are commonly included in this group (*G. nasalis* and *G. intestinalis*; Fig. 8.24), whilst prominent causes of equine nasal and gastric myiasis, were shown by

Table 8.6. Relevant biological details of species of *Gasterophilus* capable of causing cutaneous myiasis (creeping eruption) in man. (Compiled from data in Chereshnev 1954; Zumpt 1965. For details of *G. intestinalis* see text)

Species	Number of eggs laid	Oviposition	Incubation period in days	Remarks	Distribution
Gasterophilus pecorum	1300–2425	In batches on plant stems	12–21	Man infested by passing moist hand over infested grass	Widespread in Africa, Europe and palaearctic Asia
G. nigricornis	330–350	Attached singly to hairs	3–9	Able to penetrate skin; rare cause of creeping eruption	China; Mongolia; Russia and Roumania around Black Sea
G. haemorrhoidalis	50–200	Attached singly to hairs	2	Hands infested when handling mouths of horses. Female fly lays eggs within 2 h of emergence	Worldwide but a rare cause of cutaneous myiasis in Australia (Lee 1968)
G. inermis	320–360	Attached singly to hairs	Nil	Common cause of summer dermatitis in horses; causes creeping eruption occasionally	Palaearctic region and parts of South Africa

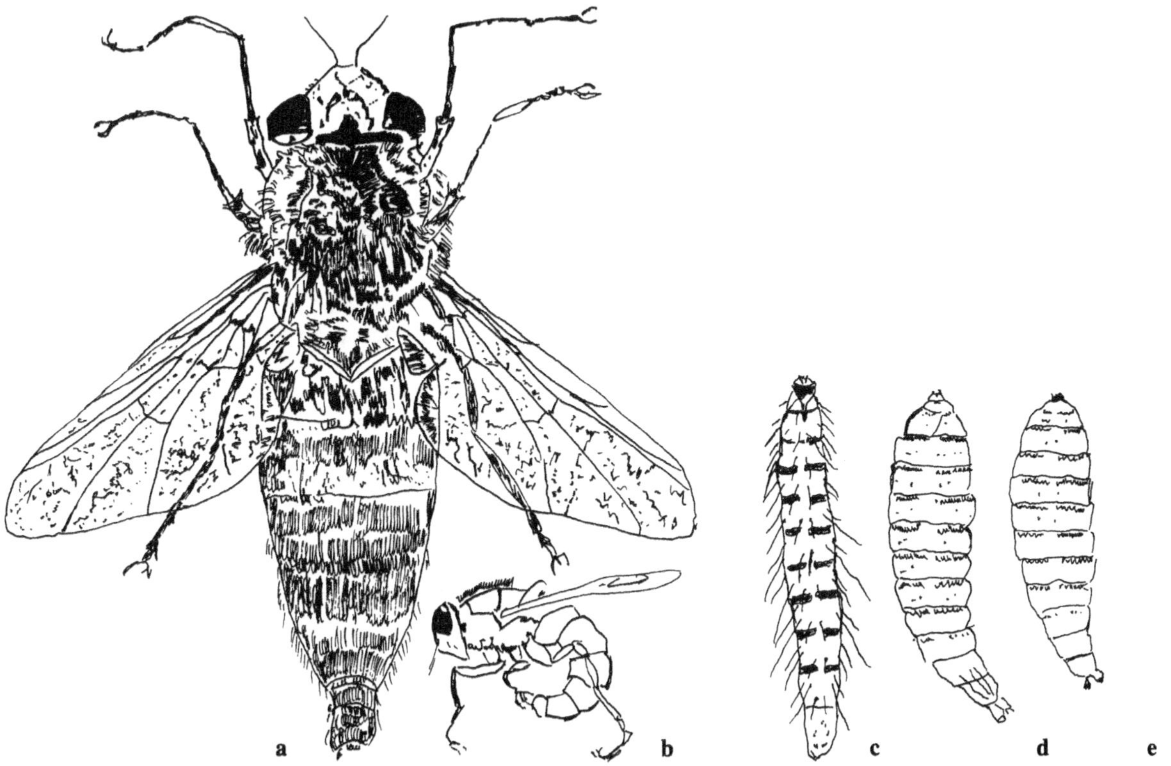

Fig. 8.24. a Adult female fly of *Gasterophilus intestinalis*. **b** Lateral view of the same. **c** Larva of *G. nasalis*. **d** Larva of *G. intestinalis*. **e** Larva of *G. haemorrhoidalis*. (After James 1947, by kind permission of the author and the publisher, the US Department of Agriculture)

Chereshnev (1954) to be incapable of penetrating human skin. Suter et al. (1972) recorded an instance where the eggs of *G. intestinalis* were found on a young woman's leg but no skin lesions, whilst the lesions in the cases reported by Kandratev (1934) were identified as being caused by *G. intestinalis* in each instance. Patton (1921) declared that *G. intestinalis* could cause skin lesions in man, but Zumpt (1965) concluded that where creeping eruption had been held to be caused by either of these two species the entomological diagnosis was mistaken. The adult flies resemble hive or bumblebees in form and colouring (Fig. 8.24; Cogan 1973).

Creeping eruption was first described by Lee (1874) in Britain, but it was (and possibly still is) commoner in Russia. Pawlowsky and Stein (1924) noted that it almost always occurred in those who handled horses (see also Suter et al. 1972), although Kandratev (1934) recorded two cases in which the victims had been picking raspberries and walking in a quarry, respectively. In horses the larvae are swallowed directly after hatching or after removal from their cutaneous burrows by the animal's teeth, tongue or lips. Development is subsequently completed in the stomach. In the skin (of man or horse) the larva has never been shown to develop beyond the first instar (Pawlowsky and Stein 1924). Patton (1921) considered that its aimless wandering was in search of the alimentary tract of the host (as it was indirectly in the horse), but because man was an unnatural host the larva perished in situ after days, weeks or even months of tunnelling. It has characteristic backward pointing spines on its body segments, which would undoubtedly prevent any movement except in a forward direction. According to Chereshnev (1954), it can penetrate skin in a matter of minutes. Further biological details, as well as distribution details, are shown in Table 8.6.

Clinical Features

Commencing as a small itching papule, within a day or two a thin (1.5-mm wide) red, slightly raised, often tortuous line appears, which extends daily at an average of 1.5 cm, but may reach up to 30 cm daily (Austmann 1926). Austmann stated that this line was devoid of vesicles, but both Hunter (1966) and Rook (1979) agreed that the distal end terminated in a small vesicle. Kandratev (1934) reported that the distal end was a solid pink inflammatory papule with a dark spot beyond it. Activity and itching are most marked at night. The proximal parts of the lesion fade and disappear progressively (Fig. 8.25).

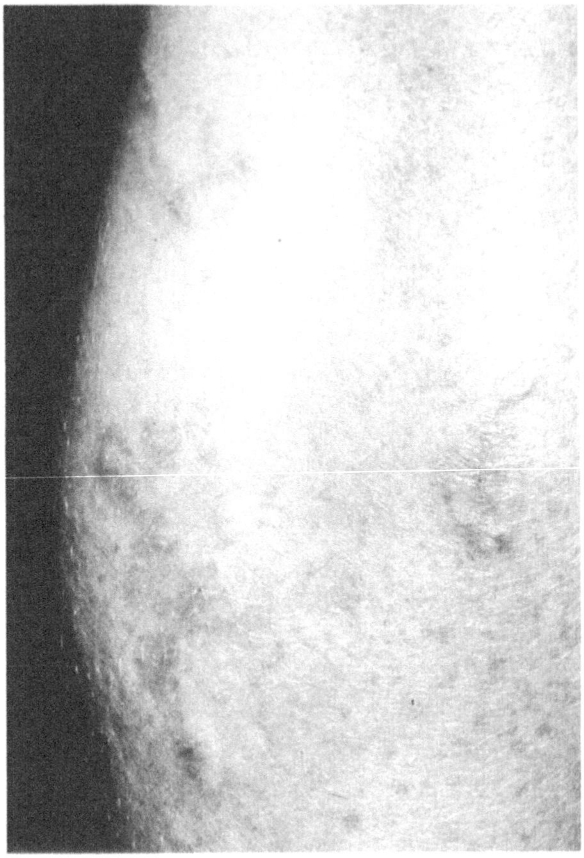

Fig. 8.25. Cutaneous myiasis, creeping eruption. (Photograph of patient of the late Dr. A. G. Fergusson, by courtesy of Mr. P. S. Waldie, the Department of Medical Illustration, Stobhill Hospital, Glasgow)

Histology

Pawlowsky and Stein (1924) showed that the lumen of the tunnel occupied almost the entire thickness of a rather acanthotic epidermis, with the roof formed by the stratum granulosum (stratum lucidum on the palms). The cells of the roof and the side walls of the tunnel were compressed, often without nuclei, the cells beyond being oedematous with vacuolated nuclei. The papillae were also oedematous and a leucocytic infiltrate containing many eosinophils penetrated between the fibrous bundles. A little of this infiltrate invaded the lumen itself.

Diagnosis

The epidermis can be made translucent by placing on it a drop of machine oil (Lombard's technique for demonstrating skin capillaries; Austmann 1926).

As Austmann demonstrated, the larva can be visualised with the aid of a lens and shows black transverse rows of segmental spines. The caudal end lies immediately beyond the distal end of the red linear lesion and the head of the larva beyond that. In Austmann's patient the head was 13 mm beyond the end of the visible lesion. Under observation it advanced painlessly 8 mm in 4 h. The diagnosis can be conjectured almost on sight, and if the geographical origin can be established the cause can also be ascertained with some accuracy. Austmann stated that *Gasterophilus* infestation occurred north of the fortieth parallel of latitude and usually north of the fiftieth parallel, and generally inland. The other cause of creeping eruption, nematode larvae (*Ancylostoma brasiliense*), originates in more tropical climates near to lakes or the seashore. Accurate diagnosis can only be achieved by laboratory identification of the parasite involved. Confusion may rarely be caused by linear migratory lesions which are produced by penetrating *hairs* and not larvae (Schamberg and Strauss 1961).

Treatment

Various measures, including freezing, the use of the hyfrecator (Kingsley 1961), cutaneous injection of larvicides and surgical excision, have all been advocated. However, Austmann (1926) stated that once the position of the *Gasterophilus* larva had been established it was a very simple matter to pick it out with a sterile needle painlessly in much the same manner as the *Sarcoptes* mite is removed from its burrow. Any other treatment is unnecessary.

Congo Floor Maggot

Although not strictly a cause of myiasis, the Congo floor maggot is traditionally included in this group because it is a dipterous, blood-sucking larva of man with intermittent activity of a parasitic nature.

Morphology and Biology

The fly, *Auchmeromyia luteola* occurs throughout tropical Africa south of the Sahara (Garrett-Jones 1951). It lives in the dark shade in native huts, where its pale-yellow colour renders it almost invisible as it sits motionless on the straw walls, except for brief activity in the early morning and late afternoon (Patton and Evans 1929). The female (9–13 mm) is less numerous than the male (8–11 mm) (Schwetz 1914). It lays up to 300 eggs in batches of about 50 each, but each egg is deposited individually in the sandy soil of the floor (Zumpt 1965). According to Gordon and Lavoipierre (1962), they hatch in 1–3 days, but this period varies with temperature and relative humidity (Patton and Evans 1929).

The larvae (Fig. 8.26), which lie buried in the soil in the daytime, emerge at night hungry and are guided by the warmth of the human body to the victim's skin (Roubaud 1913). Schwetz (1914) noted that if man sleeps in the daytime the larva adapts to this new schedule, although, as he also showed, in the absence of food the larvae are inherently nocturnal. They are also regarded as

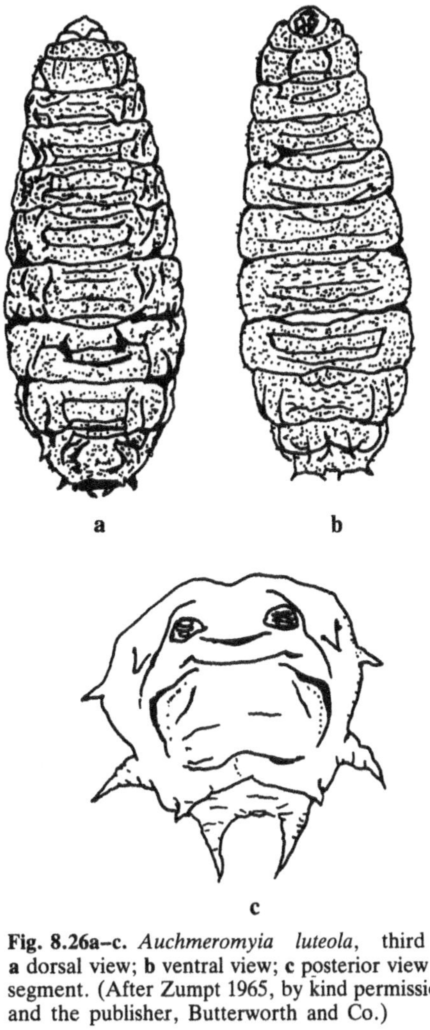

Fig. 8.26a–c. *Auchmeromyia luteola*, third larval instar. **a** dorsal view; **b** ventral view; **c** posterior view of the caudal segment. (After Zumpt 1965, by kind permission of the author and the publisher, Butterworth and Co.)

obligatory parasites of man, but Zumpt (1965) claimed to have found them in the burrows of small mammals 30 miles away from the nearest human habitation. In order to feed, the larvae attach themselves initially to the skin by their mouth hooks (Fig. 8.27) and, according to Garrett-Jones (1951) they subsequently scarify it. They then apply the free margin of the postcephalic segment closely to the skin and forcibly retract the head to create a partial vacuum. Blood flows into this vacuum cup and is ingested into the larval body by intermittent bodily contractions (Roubaud 1913). After 10–20 min of this syringe-like suction of blood they drop off engorged and burrow into the soil again.

The larvae usually feed three or four times weekly, never more than once per 24 h and moult after 2 and 6 days in normal circumstances, although they are quite capable of fasting for 3 weeks, or even, in dry conditions, for up to 2 months (Roubaud 1913). Schwetz (1914) observed that pale larvae were unfed and red larvae engorged with fresh blood, assuming a black colour as the blood altered with digestion. Small pale larvae never pupated, whilst large red ones were the most likely to complete the life cycle, which is about 10 weeks (Zumpt 1965). Garrett-Jones (1951) noted that moulting is weight related and that at least two meals are required between moults.

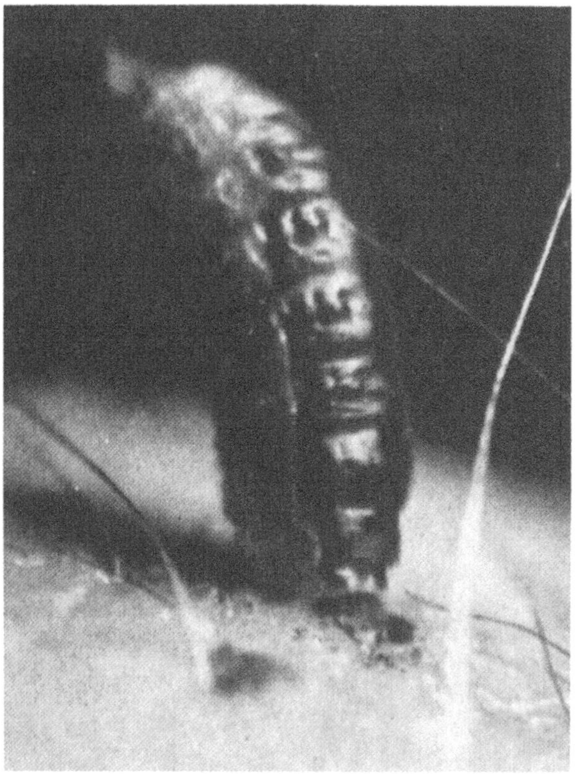

Fig. 8.27. The Congo floor maggot, *Auchmeromyia luteola*, attached to the human skin. (Courtesy of the Wellcome Museum of Medical Science)

Clinical Effects

Clinically the larva is regarded as more of a nuisance than a serious pest, although multiple bites can disturb sleep. The bites are trivial as a rule, but Garrett-Jones (1951) stated that at times patients found them painful with residual itch and burning sensations for up to 4 days. Any part of the skin within reach of the larvae may be attacked. There are no sequelae. Prevention can be achieved by sleeping at least 1 cm from the floor out of reach of the larvae. Roubaud (1913) considered that this nuisance will disappear with progress towards civilisation.

Immunity in Myiasis

Blacklock and Thompson had observed in 1923 that a form of immunity seemed to develop in those persons whose skin was invaded by *Cordylobia anthropophaga*. This infestation was common in the young indigenous inhabitants or in newcomers of any age, but older natives who had been attacked when young did not subsequently suffer. Zumpt (1959) confirmed that larval invasion of such persons always resulted in the death of the larva within a few days. Blacklock and Gordon (1927) showed experimentally in guinea pigs that such an immunity was acquired following previous infestation and was not just due to aging. Moreover, they showed that the immunity was locally acquired, i.e. cell mediated rather than by the development of circulating antibodies This locally acquired immunity was at first confined to the immediate areas of skin invaded by the parasite. The longer the latter remained in situ the larger the area to become immune, the immunity ultimately spreading beyond the invaded area. With multiple infestation of numerous areas of skin, immunity finally involved the whole skin. The result of this was the death in a few days of any larva subsequently invading the skin. These workers showed that the serum, on the other hand, had no deleterious effect on larvae. This immunity was independent of eosinophilia. Gunther (1967) noted that rats did not seem to develop immunity.

Clinically, apart from the protective effect of the immunity, Blacklock and Thompson (1923) also noted that there was no immediate reaction of the skin to a first infestation but subsequent invasion by larvae produced an immediate inflammatory oedematous reaction. This they showed to be a reaction to larval salivary secretion, akin to an acute contact reaction following a previous sensitisation.

In their original experiments Blacklock and Gordon (1927) found no precipitin or complement fixation reaction in the serum to *Cordylobia* infestation. Later, however, in collaboration with Fine and Watson (1930), they showed that precipitin reactions to certain larval enzymes, to haematocoele fluid and to larval excreta could be detected. These, they felt, offered a possible opportunity for the early diagnosis of infestation by *Hypoderma*. If testing for precipitin reactions could detect infestation before the development of cutaneous lesions it would have considerable economic and veterinary benefits.

References

Adams JL (1904) Tropical cutaneous myiasis in man. JAMA 42: 947–949

Alessandro AD (1978) Comparative experience with Dermatobia in Latin America. Centro Internacional de Agriculture Tropical. Workshop on the ecology and control of external parasites of economic importance on bovines in Latin America, August 25–30, 1974. Series CE13, pp 125–126

Andersen EH (1960) Biology, distribution and control of *Dermatobia hominis*. Vet Med 55: 72–78

Aubertin D, Buxton PA (1934) *Cochlyomyia* and myiasis in tropical America. Ann Trop Med Parasitol 28: 245–254

Austmann EJ (1926) Creeping eruption. Report on first case from Manitoba. JAMA 87: 1196–1200

Bates M (1943) Mosquitoes as vectors of Dermatobia in Eastern Colombia. Ann Entomol Soc Am 36: 21–24

*Baumhover AH (1966) Eradication of the screwworm fly. JAMA 196: 150–158

*Bishopp FC, Laake EW, Brundett HM, Wells RW (1926) The cattle grubs or ox warbles, their biologies and suggestion of control. US Dept of Agriculture Technical Bulletin No 1369. US Govt Printing Office, Washington DC, pp 1–119

Blacklock DB, Gordon RM (1927) The experimental production of immunity against metazoan parasites and an investigation of its nature. Ann Trop Med Parasitol 21: 181–224

Blacklock DB, Thompson MG (1923) A study of the Tumbu fly, *Cordylobia anthropophaga* Grinberg in Sierra Leone. Ann Trop Med Parasitol 17: 444–510

*Blacklock DB, Gordon RM, Fine J, Watson M (1930) Metazoan immunity, a report on recent investigations. Ann Trop Med Parasitol 24: 5–54

Brady (1923) Cutaneous myiasis in an infant. Arch Pediatr (NY) 40: 638–640

Casner SW, Wiseman JS (1965) Human botfly infestation in the United States. Tex State J Med 61: 411–413

Catts EP (1967) Biology of a California rodent botfly *Cuterebra latifrons* Coquillett (Diptera: Cuterebridae). J Med Entomol 4: 87–101

Chapman RF (1971) The insects; structure and function. English Universities Press, London, p 321

Cheresnev NA (1954) Subcutaneous myiasis in man caused by first stage larva of the gastric gadfly (Fam. Gasterophilidae) (in Russian). Rep Acad Sci USSR 99: 661–664

Chown G (1924) Report of a case of cutaneous myiasis in an infant. *Wohlfahrtia vigil* (Walker) infection. Can Med Assoc J 14: 967–968

Cogan BH (1973) Cyclorrhapha of minor medical importance. In: Smith KGV (ed) Insects and other arthropods of medical importance. The Trustees of the British Museum (Natural History), London, pp 279–287

Curran CH (1939) The human botfly—How did this extraordinary insect develop the habit of forcing a mosquito to deposit its eggs for it? Natural Hist 66: 45–48

Dalmat HT (1955) Cutaneous myiasis of the scalp due to *Dermatobia hominis* Linnaeus Jr. O (Diptera: Cuterebridae) Am J Trop Med Hyg 4: 334–335

Da Silva MP (1912) Nouveaux cas de myiase dus à *Chrysomia macellaria* Fabricius à Bahia. Arch Parasitol 15: 425–430

DeGuisti DL, Zackheim H (1963) A first report of *Wohlfahrtia vigil* (Walker) myiasis in man in Michigan JAMA 184: 782–783

Dove WE (1937) Myiasis of man. J Econ Entomol 30: 29–39

Dunn LH (1918) The tick as a possible agent in the collocation of the eggs of *Dermatobia hominis*. J Parasitol 4: 154–158

*Dunn LH (1930) Rearing the larvae of *Dermatobia hominis* Linn. in man. Psyche 37: 327–342

Dunn LH (1934) Prevalence and importance of the tropical warble fly *Dermatobia hominis* Linn. in Panama. J Parasitol 20: 219–226

Everett ED, DeVillez RL, Lewis CW (1977) Cutaneous myiasis due to *Dermatobia hominis*. Arch Dermatol 113: 1121

Field AS (1981) Myiasis in an Australian abroad. Med J Aust 1: 581–582

*Ford N (1933) Observation on the behaviour of the Sarcophagid fly *Wohlfahrtia vigil* (Walker). J Parasitol 19: 106–111

*Ford N (1936) Further observations on the behaviour of *Wholfahrtia vigil* (Walker) with notes on the collecting and rearing of the flies. J Parasitol 22: 310–328

Garrett-Jones C (1951) The Congo floor maggot, *Auchmeromyia luteola* (F), in a laboratory culture. Bull Entomol Res 41: 679–708

Gedoelst L (1905) Contribution à l'étude des larves cuticoles de muscides Africaines. Arch Parasitol 9: 568–592

Gedoelst L (1908–1909) *Cordylobia rodhaini* nova species; Diptere Congolais à larve cuticole. Arch Parasitol 13: 538–547

Gertson GD, Lancaster WEG, Larson GA, Wheeler GC (1933) *Wohlfahrtia* myiasis in North Dakota. Report of two cases. JAMA 100: 487–488

Gordon RM, Lavoipierre MMJ (1962) Entomology for students of medicine. Blackwell, Oxford, p 196

Gomez-Armario JM, Mira-Gutierrez J (1976) Una zoodermatosis tropical lesiones producidas por la "*Cordylobia anthrophaga*". Actas Dermosifiliogr 67: 543–546

Gunther S (1967) Furuncular Tumbu fly myiasis of man in Gabon, Equatorial Africa. J Trop Med Hyg 70: 169–174

Gunther S (1971) Clinical and epidemiological aspects of the dermal Tumbu fly myiasis in Equatorial Africa. Br J Dermatol 85: 226–231

Harrell WB, Mosely V (1942) The surgical treatment of subdermal myiasis due to *Dermatobia hominis*. South Med J 35: 720–723

Herms WB (1950) Medical entomology, 4th edn. Macmillan Company, New York, pp 372–385

Hoben WP, Gregory GA, Karlsberg RC (1966) Furuncular

dermal myiasis from *Dermatobia hominis*. JAMA 195: 787–788
Hodges FJ (1955) Cutaneous *Cuterebra* myiasis. Am J Dis Child 90: 202–204
Hubler WR, Rudolph AH, Dougherty EF (1974) Dermal myiasis. Arch Dermatol 110: 109–110
Hunter GW (1966) Medically important arthropods. In: Hunter GW, Frye WW and Swartzwalder JC (eds) A manual of tropical medicine, 4th edn. Saunders, Philadelphia, Chap XI, pp 774–777
Hunter GW, Berrocal CM (1957) A case of human myiasis in Texas caused by the primary screwworm *Callitroga hominovorax* (Coqueral). Tex Rep Biol Med 15: 378–380
Iannini PB, Brandt D, Laforce FM (1975) Furuncular myiasis. JAMA 233: 1375–1376
Israels S, Shuman B (1949) Myiasis dermatosis in infancy. Paediatrics 4: 665–669
*James MT (1947) The flies that cause myiasis in man. Miscellaneous Publication No 631. US Dept of Agriculture, Washington DC, pp 1–175
Kandratev VI (1934) Two cases of gastrophylomyiasis in man (in Russian). Med Parazitol (Mosk) 3: 349–350
Katz SI, Taylor R (1971) Cutaneous myiasis. South Med J 64: 759–760
Kaye HDL, Higgins RP (1964) Human botfly infestation in the United States. JAMA 189: 650
Kingsley HJ (1961) Larva migrans; an effective treatment. Arch Dermatol 83: 510
Kleeman FJ (1983) *Dermatobia hominis* comes to Boston. N Engl J Med 308: 847–848
Knipling EF (1955) Possibilities of insect control or eradication through the release of sexually sterile males. J Econ Entomol 48: 459–462
Knipling EF, Rainwater HJ (1937) Species and incidence of dipterous larvae concerned in wound myiasis. J Parasitol 23: 451–455
Konotey-Ahulu FID, Frimpong M and Dodu SRA (1967) Myiasis from *Cordylobia anthropophaga*. Ghana Med J 6: 10–12
Korting GW, Denk, Sundhausen (1971) Myiase de Tumbu. Bull Soc Fr Dermatol Syphiligr 78: 233–234
Laake EW, Cushing EC, Parish HE (1936) Biology of the primary screwworm fly *Cochliomia americana* and a comparison of its stages with those of *C. macellaria*. US Dept of Agriculture Technical Bulletin No 500. US Govt Printing Office, Washington DC, pp 1–24
Lawton AH, Dexter MW, Warren LO (1957) Double infestation of varicose ulcer with screwworm and house fly maggots. Am J Trop Med Hyg 6: 336–338
Lee DJ (1968) Human myiasis in Australia. Med J Aust 1: 170–173
Lee RJ (1874) Case of creeping eruption. Trans Clin Soc Lond 8: 44–45
Lewis L (1947) Cutaneous myiasis occurring in Western Canada. Can Med Assoc J 56: 319
Logan JCP, Walkey M (1964) A case of endemic cutaneous myiasis. Br J Dermatol 76: 218–222
McCuiston CH, Schoch EP, McKee R, Wiseman JS, Eads RB (1958) Human myiasis. Tex State J Med 54: 796–799
MacKenzie EA (1946) Phimosis from the flesh fly *Wohlfahrtia vigil*. Can Med Assoc J 54: 52
Macias EG, Graham AJ, Green M, Pierce AW (1973) Cutaneous myiasis in south Texas. N Engl J Med 291: 1239–1241
March CH (1964) A case of "ver du Cayor" in Manhattan. Arch Dermatol 90: 32–33
Mateus G (1978) Ecology and control of *Dermatobia hominis* in Colombia. Centro Internacional de Agriculture Tropical. Workshop on the ecology and control of external parasites of economic importance in bovines in Latin America, August 25–30, 1974. Series CE13, pp 117–124
Morgan RJ, Moss HB, Honska WL (1964) Myiasis. Arch Dermatol 90: 180–184
Nicholson BH, Smith PE, Desch WH (1954) Human hypodermal myiasis. J Okla Med Assoc 47: 161–162
O'Rourke FJ (1954) Furuncular myiasis due to *Wohlfahrtia vigil* (Walker) Can Med Assoc J 71: 146–149
Patton WS (1920–1921) Some notes on Indian Calliphorinae. Part I. *Chrysomya bezziana* Villeneuve, the common Indian calliphorine whose larvae cause cutaneous myiasis in man and animals. Indian J Med Res 8: 17–29
*Patton WS (1921) Notes on the myiasis producing diptera of man and animals. Bull Entomol Res 12: 239–261
Patton WS (1921–1922) Some notes on Indian Calliphorinae. Part VII. Additional cases of myiasis caused by larvae of *Chrysomya bezziana* Vill. together with some notes of the diptera which cause myiasis in man and animals. Indian J Med Res 9: 654–682
Patton WS (1936) Studies on the higher diptera of medical and veterinary importance. The warble flies of the genus *Hypoderma*. Ann Trop Med Parasitol 30: 453–468
Patton WS, Cookson HA (1925) Cutaneous myiasis in man caused by *Musca domestica*. Lancet I: 1291
*Patton WS, Evans AE (1929) Insects, ticks, mites and venomous animals of medical and veterinary importance. Part I Medical. HR Grubb, Croydon
Pawlowsky EN, Stein AK (1924) Die Gastrophilus Larve als Gastparasit in der Menschenhaut. Parasitology 16: 32–43
Peters H, Kramer S (1966) Zur Differentialdiagnose der Myiasis cutanea in der ärztlichen Praxis. Hautarzt 17: 195–210
Poindexter HA (1979) Cutaneous myiasis. Arch Dermatol 115: 235
*Portschinsky IA (1916) *Wohlfahrtia magnifica* Schin. and allied Russian species. The biology of this fly and its importance to man and domestic animals (in Russian). Mem Bureau Entomol Sci Comm Min Agri 11 (9): 108. Summarised in Rev Appl Entomol (Series B) 4: 88–89
Prasad C, Beck AR (1969) Myiasis of the scalp from *Dermatobia hominis*. JAMA 210: 133
Price AS (1937) The warble fly *Dermatobia hominis* Linn. Report of two imported cases from Costa Rica. NY State J Med 47: 1503–1505
Radcliffe W (1972) Tumbu fly. Br Med J II: 164
Rook A (1979) Skin diseases caused by arthropods and other venomous or noxious animals. In: Rook A, Wilkinson DS and Ebeling FJG (eds) Textbook of dermatology, 3rd edn. Oxford, Blackwell pp 911–954
Roubaud E (1913) Études biologiques sur les Auchmeromyies. Bull Soc Pathol Exot 6: 128–130
Ruch DM (1967) Botfly myiasis. Arch Dermatol 96: 677–680
Salomon PF, Catts EP, Know WG (1970) Human dermal myiasis caused by rabbit botfly in Connecticut. JAMA 213: 1035–1036
Sanders HC (1928) Myiasis dermatosa. N Engl J Med 199: 38
Schamberg L, Strauss PE (1961) Bristle migrans. Arch Dermatol 83: 663
Schorr WF (1967) Tumbu fly myiasis in Mushfield Wisconsin. Arch Dermatol 95: 61–62
Schreiber MM, Schuckmell N, Sampsel J (1964) Human myiasis. JAMA 188: 828–829
Schwetz J (1914) Quelques observations preliminaires sur la morphologie et la biologie de la larve, de la nymphe et de l'image de l'*Auchmeromyia*. Ann Trop Med Parasitol 8: 497–507
Scott HG (1964) Human myiasis in North America (1952–1962 inclusive). Fla Entomologist 47: 255–261

Silverthorne N, Brown A (1934) Cutaneous myiasis in infants. Arch Dis Child 9: 339–342

Snow JW, Coppedge JR (1978) The screwworm *Cochliomyia hominovorax* (Diptera: Calliphoridae) reinfests the island of Curaçao, Netherlands Antilles. J Med Entomol 14: 592–593

Soulsby EJL (1968) Helminths, arthropods and protozoa of domesticated animals (formerly Mönnig's veterinary helminthology and entomology), 6th edn. Baillière Tindall, London

Spencer Jp, Snow JW, Smith FE (1980) Effectiveness of the screwworm (Diptera: Calliphoridae) eradication program during 1978 in the United States and Mexico. US Dept of Agriculture APHIS; VS 172. US Govt Printing Office, Washington DC, pp 1–7

Stabler RH, Nelson MR, Lewis BL, Berthrong M (1962) *Wohlfahrtia opaca* in man in Colorado. J Parasitol 48: 209–210

Suter I, Brown D, Hansman D (1972) Horse botfly (*Gasterophilus intestinalis*) eggs laid on human hair. Med J Aust 2: 609–610

Sweet RD (1962) A clinical occasion provided by a larva of *Dermatobia hominis*. Br J Dermatol 74: 141–143

Tarry DW (1982) Cattle warble flies and the eradication scheme. In: Ectoparasites of veterinary and medical importance in temperate areas. Proceedings of a symposium held on 5 Nov 1982 at Royal Army Medical College, Millbank, London, pp 68–69

Turnley WH (1954) Screwworm infestation in humans. J Fla Med Assoc 40: 733–736

Walker EM (1921) *Wohlfahrtia vigil* (Walker) as a human parasite (Diptera: Sarcophagidae). J Parasitol 7: 1–7

Walker EM (1922) Some cases of cutaneous myiasis with notes on the larvae of *Wohlfahrtia vigil* (Walker). J Parasitol 9: 1–5

Walker EM (1937) The larval stages of *Wohlfahrtia vigil* (Walker). J Parasitol 23: 163–174

Watts J (1974) Cutaneous myiasis "blowfly strike". Aust J Dermatol 15: 31

Wildy GS, Glover SC (1982) Myiasis due to Tumbu fly larva. Lancet I: 1130–1131

Wohlrabe JC (1957) Primary cutaneous myiasis. Minn Med 41: 323

Yount CE, Sudler MT (1907) Human myiasis from the screwworm fly (*Compsomyia macellaria*, Fabr). JAMA 49: 1912–1916

Zumpt F (1959) The Tumbu fly *Cordylobia anthropophaga* (Blanchard) in Southern Africa. S Afr Med J 33: 862–865

*Zumpt F (1965) Myiasis in man and animals in the old world. Butterworth, London

9 Reactions to Dipterous Biting Flies

The blood-sucking dipterous flies are composed of several distinct families, which are shown in Table 9.1. The common feature of this group is the requirement of a blood meal for the proper development of eggs and their deposition. The biting techniques vary with the different species. Their mouthparts are developed accordingly and are depicted for some species in Fig. 9.1.

The mosquito has a long slender proboscis composed of sharp-pointed and paired maxillae and mandibles, together with a tubular hypopharynx and a supporting labium. The palps are also part of the proboscis but take no part in the biting procedure. When the insect bites it inserts its sharp maxillae and mandibles along with the hypopharynx through the epidermis into the corium, where a blood vessel is sought. Meanwhile the labium remains resting on the surface; it bends as the piercing parts are thrust deeper and serves as a supporting stay for the whole structure. When a vessel is found it is pierced. Blood may be sucked direct from the vessel or from the pool of blood

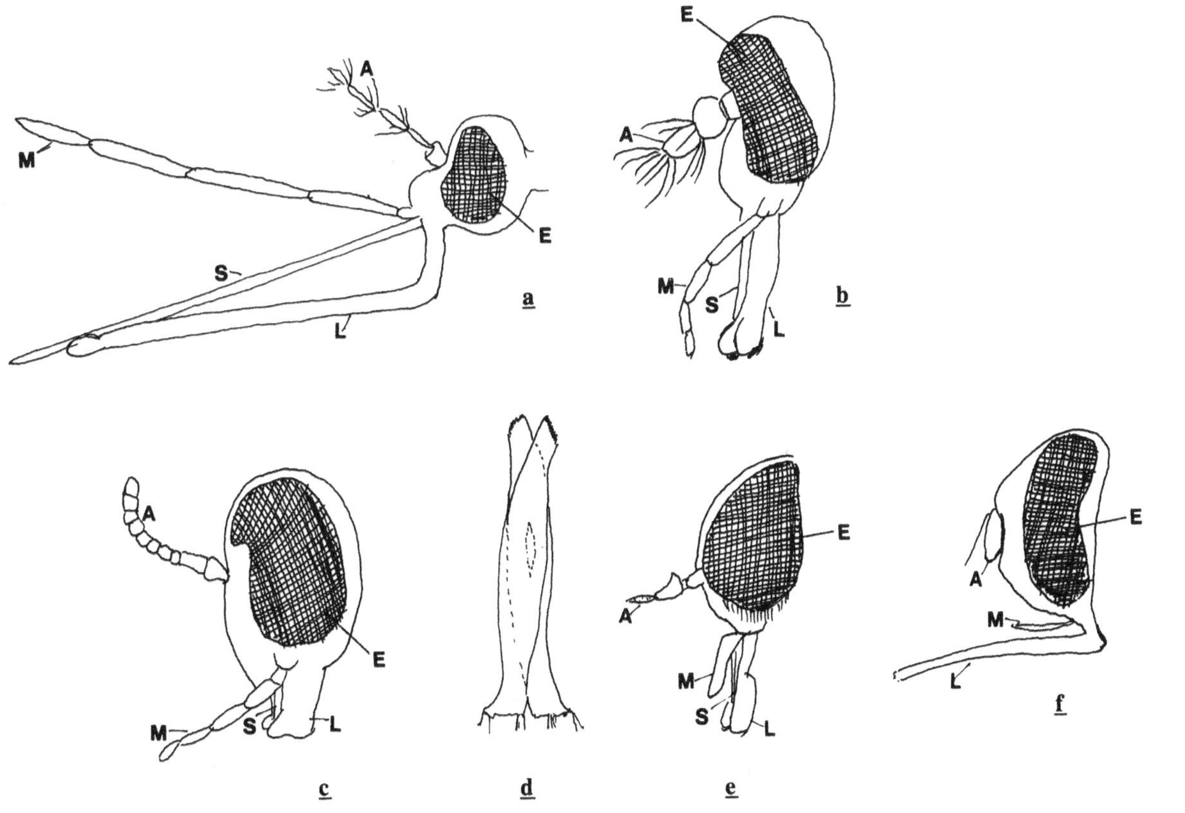

Fig. 9.1a–f. Heads of some biting flies, all viewed from the left side. **a** anopheline mosquito; **b** *Culicoides*; **c** *Simulium*; **d** mandibles of *Simulium* enlarged to show scissor-like action; **e** *Tabanus*; **f** *Stomoxys*. *A*, antenna; *E*, compound eye; *L*, labium; *M*, maxillary palp; *S*, stylets (mandibles and maxillae). (After Busvine 1966, by kind permission of the author and the publisher, Methuen)

which collects around (Gordon and Crewe 1948). *Phlebotomus* flies feed similarly although their mouthparts are much shorter. *Glossina* acts similarly but is mainly a pool feeder. *Chrysops* and other tabanids, the simuliids and hippoboscids, as well as *Stomoxys calcitrans*, all obtain blood after inserting their mouthparts by cutting and slashing the tissues and so damaging blood vessels that haemorrhage results; they then feed from the pool of blood.

In this section the different groups will be considered individually; they are sufficiently diverse in their structure, biology, habitat and habits to warrant this. Although the lesions and general pattern of eruption they produce have many similarities, there are sufficient differences to make separate descriptions also worthwhile. Treatment for the most part is merely palliative, the greatest benefit being derived from prevention of bites and control of the arthropods.

With Simuliidae and Hippoboscidae the number of species which cause annoyance to man are few enough to warrant listing only the principal species responsible. With the other groups the numbers are enormous, and since there are many specialised works in which the species are enumerated in full it would be superfluous to do so here. The reader who requires more information should consult these works.

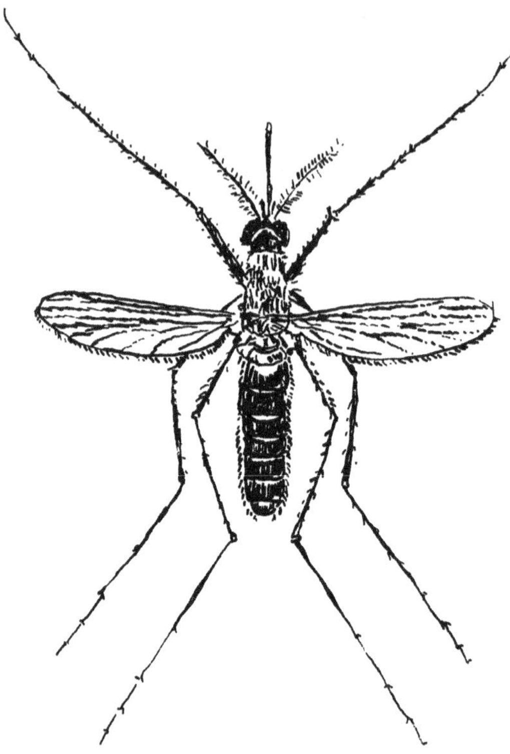

Fig. 9.2. *Culex fatigans*. To show the general appearance of a mosquito. (After Patton 1931)

Culicidae

Mosquitoes are probably one of the commonest biting insects and certainly those about which most research has been done. They have a cosmopolitan distribution. There are about 2500 or more species, a large number of which can and do bite man. Table 9.1 gives a very broad division into three important categories. Culicine mosquitoes do not carry malaria but are the vectors of diseases caused by an innumerable number of arboviruses and of *Wuchereria bancrofti* and other filariae. *Aedes aegypti*, a culicine with special importance, carries yellow fever virus and many others, whilst anophelines are the carriers of malaria as well as arboviruses. Other genera of mosquitoes also carry arboviruses. Mattingley et al. (1973) have given a comprehensive list of the diseases for which mosquitoes are vectors.

Morphology

Mosquitoes are delicate Diptera with a well-defined head, thorax and abdomen (Fig. 9.2). The head has very large compound eyes and long filiform antennae of 14 or 15 segments, which arise between and in front of the eyes. The male antennae are densely plumose, but those of the female are adorned with much shorter and fewer hairs (pilose). The mouthparts are complex and have already been described in discussion of the biting mechanisms (see Fig. 9.1). One of the distinguishing features between culicine and anopheline adults is the relationship between the palpi and the antennae. In culicines the palps are half as long as the antennae, but in anophelines they are the same length (James and Harwood 1969). The thorax is relatively strong and very slightly humped, but not noticeably so. It gives support to the wings and legs. The wings have a fairly standard venation arrangement, but the veins are coated with scales which may be light or dark and thus give rise to a variety of patterns which are characteristic for each species. The legs are similarly adorned. The abdomen is long and slender but may be distended after engorgement (in females). The external male genitalia are ornate and prominent. They are used in classification. A special atlas is required to compare the appearances of these structures in the different species (James and Harwood 1969). Such

Table 9.1. The various groups of blood-sucking Diptera which bite man. There are very many genera of mosquitoes, which are therefore indicated only by broad groups. Many but not all of the species in this table are vectors of infectious or parasitic diseases. (Compiled from James and Harwood 1969 and Mattingley et al. 1973)

Species or group	Remarks
Culicidae	
Culex pipiens complex	Includes house mosquitoes; active late at night; very widespread. *C. p.* and *C. p. fasciatus* are vectors of filariasis
Culex spp. other than *C. p.*	
Culiseta (*Theobaldia*) spp.	
Aedes complex	
1. Salt marsh species	
2. Flood-water species	
3. Tree-hole species	
4. Snow pool species	
5. *A. aegypti* varieties	Very important vectors of yellow fever dengue, chikungunya encephalitis etc. Very susceptible to environmental changes
Psorophora spp.	Some vicious biters; carry *Dermatobia hominis* eggs
Anopheles spp.	Vectors of malaria; many species with varying habitats
Psychodidae	
Phlebotomus spp.	Vectors of cutaneous and visceral leishmaniasis; Old World species
Lutzomyia spp.	Vectors of South American leishmaniasis and bartonellosis
Simuliidae	
Simulium spp.	Vicious biters; vectors of onchocerciasis in Africa and Central and South America
Ceratopogonidae	
Culicoides spp.	
Tabanidae	
Chrysops spp.	Vectors of loiasis
Tabanus spp.	Vectors of tularaemia and anthrax
Haematopota spp.	Vicious painful biters
Muscidae	
Stomoxys calcitrans	A painful biter
Glossinidae	
Glossina spp.	Vectors of African trypanosomiasis
Hippoboscidae	
Lipoptena cervi	Deer ked

illustrations can be found in the useful work by Mattingley et al. (1973). Much of the above information about morphology has been obtained from Gordon and Lavoipierre (1962).

Biology

A few days after the blood meal the eggs are deposited in water, or at least in damp surfaces. Most species lay their eggs whilst resting on the surface of the water, but a few may drop them whilst hovering over the surface. Any number up to about 300 may be deposited at a time. The water usually has to be of the stagnant type, but the sites where the eggs are laid depends on the attractions for the female of. materials in the vicinity. In the arctic regions eggs laid in summer and autumn hatch out the following spring, when the snow has melted. That is to say there is one generation annually (James and Harwood 1969). The eggs usually hatch in 2–3 days, but this period may lengthen if the weather is cold. The aquatic larvae behave characteristically in the water. They all have to breathe through spiracles, which are situated in the eighth segment. They must therefore be attached to the water–air interface by this segment. Culicines hang downwards from this attachment, but anophelines hold on by other segments as well and also by the thorax and head so that they lie parallel to the surface. The larval stage lasts through four instars. Pupation results in the pupa floating free in the water until the adult is ready to emerge. At this stage the pupa floats to the surface, and the imago escapes, dries out and flies off. The average life cycle, depending on the temperature, varies between 10 days and 1 month.

Whilst the above description holds good in general for the life cycle, conditions vary greatly. As Table 9.1 shows, for example, *Aedes aegypti* can breed in a variety of situations, but water is required for all. The possible variations are enormous, and reference should be made to specialised sources, such as James and Harwood (1969) or Mattingley et al. (1973).

Clinical Picture

The progression of lesions caused by mosquito bites (and other dipterous biting flies) is described in the section on immunology (pp. 129–131). Figures 9.13–9.17 illustrate some of the possible types. Persistent papular lesions may be seen frequently (see Fig. 9.14). At other times tiny punctate haemorrhages with or without a halo also occur (see Fig. 9.15). Sometimes multiple lesions appear with both these types and with weals (see Fig. 9.13). In severe sensitisation the weals may be very large and confluent with gross surrounding oedema, whilst eczematisation may occasionally result (see Fig. 9.17). Bullae, when they arise, usually appear surmounting weals or papules but very rarely on apparently normal skin, as in Fig. 9.16. All of these lesions itch severely and may be heavily scratched, resulting in secondary infection. Anaphylaxis is rare but can occur.

Treatment

For mild lesions palliative antipruritic creams or lotions are adequate. Hydrocortisone with an anti-infective agent may be needed if there is much scratching, whilst stronger topical or even systemic corticosteroids may be required. For anaphylactic reactions adrenaline and other measures will be required. Full details of this emergency are given in Chapter 10 (see p. 149).

Prevention

Repellent creams containing *N,N*-diethyl-*m*-toluamide (DEET) (see Chap. 26, pp. 404–406) or dimethylphthallate are very useful. Netting of suitable mesh in necessary in infested areas for screening the doors and windows of dwellings and for covering the beds of sleeping persons.

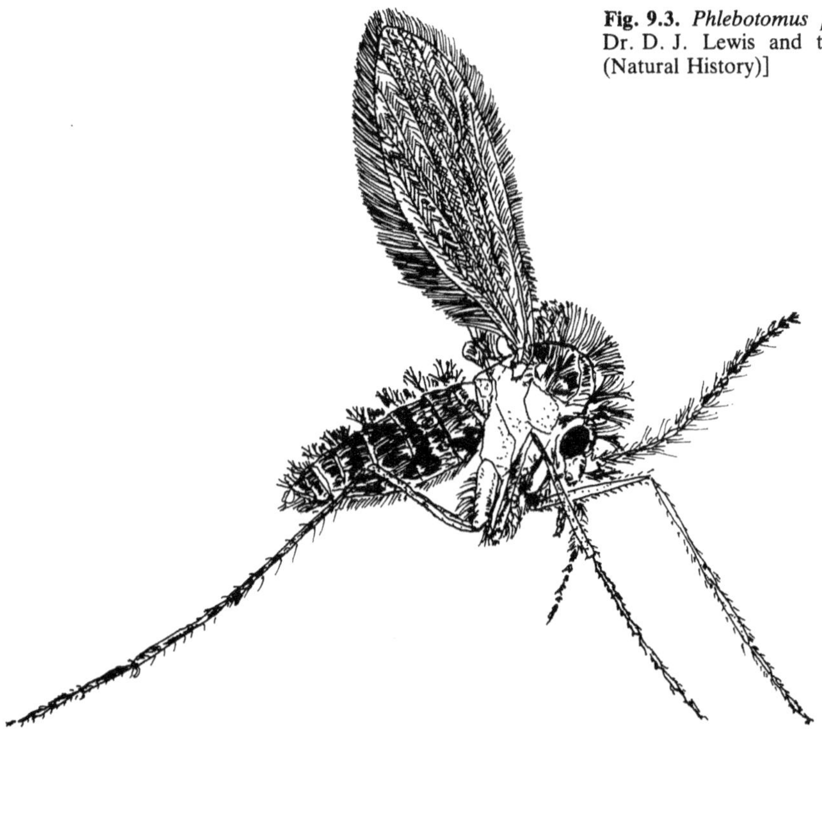

Fig. 9.3. *Phlebotomus papatasii,* adult female. [Courtesy of Dr. D. J. Lewis and the Trustees of the British Museum (Natural History)]

Control

Drainage of stagnant pools, proper street drains in towns and villages and the clearing out of breeding places are just some of the measures which can be taken, directed principally against larvae. Insecticidal spraying of these breeding places and the haunts of the adult mosquitoes is also necessary.

Psychodidae

Principal species are *Phlebotomus* for the Old World and *Lutzomyia* for the New World. There are over 400 species (Lewis 1971). They are known in Europe, North Africa and the Middle East as "sandflies," justified by their colour (Patton 1931); however, in view of the fact that this name is used for two other species in the United States and Australia respectively, it would be better to refer to them as phlebotomid flies. Their prime importance rests on the fact that they are vectors for several very important diseases. *Phlebotomus* is the vector for cutaneous and visceral leishmaniasis in the Old World, whilst *Lutzomyia* species perform the same function in the New World. Additionally *Phlebotomus* is the vector for sandfly fever and *Lutzomyia* for bartonellosis. Apart from these diseases the phlebotomid flies can cause unpleasant skin lesions in man. They inhabit a wide stretch of the globe from latitude 40°S to about 45°N and have been found at an altitude of up to 2743 m (9000 ft) in Ethiopia and the Andes (Minter 1982).

Morphology

Phlebotomid flies are very small, being 2–3 mm long (Fig. 9.3). They have a delicate slender appearance with characteristically erect lanceolate wings, slender bodies and very long legs. The head has large compound eyes. The antennae, with 16 segments, are long and hairy with an enlarged pedicellar base. The head is attached to the thorax at almost a right angle. The thorax bears a pair of pear-shaped wings with pointed apices. The long legs hang downwards and give the appearance as if the insect is dancing (Patton 1931; Lewis 1973).

Biology

Minter (1982) described the life cycle as follows: The eggs hatch within 1–2 weeks. There are four larval instars, the whole development of which can be encompassed in as little time as 3 weeks but usually spans from 4 to 12 weeks or more. Busvine (1980) has pointed out that the life cycle varies according to where it takes place. For example, in Malta it is 47 days, in Uzbekistan, 44–53 days and in Tiflis, 45–129 days.

About 15–40 eggs are laid singly in moist soil, in cracks and crevices of walls or on the ground, in rubbish heaps or debris. All the sites chosen are protected to some extent. The larvae crawl in caterpillar fashion amongst the debris feeding on organic matter. They like moist soil, or damp, well-sheltered corners or debris, and especially rodent burrows.

The adult flies readily enter houses. They proceed in a series of short hopping flights but are capable of covering a distance of up to 1 km. They tend to remain within a small compass of about 150 m, preferably in a shaded area. They feed indiscriminately on man and other mammals. They are crepuscular and nocturnal feeders both indoors as well as outdoors. Lewis (1971) notes that persons who sleep out of doors in Iraq are liable to be badly bitten.

Clinical Features

Phlebotomid bites cause a condition which has been called *Harara* in Israel and the surrounding countries. First described by Dostrovsky (1953) in 1925, it has become uncommon in this area of the Middle East since the control of the phlebotomids by insecticides. However, a similar condition is still seen in those places where the population of these flies is large. The eruption closely resembles papular urticaria. Dostrovsky pointed out that those most affected were newcomers to the district, neonates and non-immunised persons. Only exposed areas of skin are involved. Itching begins a few days after arriving in the region and is sufficient to cause insomnia. Painful impetiginised crusted lesions can develop from scratching. The initial lesions are firm red papules of variable size with associated scratch marks. Clear or haemorrhagic vesicles can occur with a red halo. These tend to occur only in sensitised persons. Often, but not always, urticarial weals are present. At first only a few lesions are seen but the number steadily increases. The areas chiefly affected are the dorsa of the hands, volar aspect of the wrists, dorsal surface of the forearms and the upper arms. The cubital and axillary fossae are spared. On the legs, the feet, ankles, achilles tendon area and lower legs are affected in that order of severity. The thighs are seldom involved. Many lesions occur on the face but only a few on the neck and thorax. After several weeks the condition begins to subside.

These clinical appearances were exactly reproduced experimentally by Theodor (1935) in previously unexposed volunteers. His findings indicated the progress of the immunisation phenomenon, as later defined by Mellanby (1946) (see under Immunology, p. 129). He emphasised that the reaction could be delayed for up to 34 days so that the connection between the lesions and the original bite became forgotten or overlooked. In fact the reaction might appear during or shortly after a subsequent attack, thus giving a false impression. Nevertheless, Theodor noted that in general the delay was usually about 4 days. These lesions could persist for 2–3 weeks with residual pigmentation and were often reactivated by subsequent bites elsewhere. There was at first no local immunity so that a bite area could produce a fresh lesion if bitten again. The intensity of the reaction steadily increased up to the stage of gross oedema with lymphangitis and lymphadenopathy, usually after about three to five biting sessions. Within about 1 year complete immunisation could be achieved in the same manner as described by Mellanby (1946) and by Gordon (1950). The long initial period before the appearance of the delayed reaction had given rise to the opinion that the bites were painless. When blisters occurred they were regarded by Theodor as an exaggerated response. The immune status is only temporary if further biting ceases for a while. Reference to Chapter 11 will show the resemblance to papular urticaria.

Treatment

Palliative antipruritic lotions or creams are used for symptomatic treatment. If the reaction is severe it may even be necessary to have recourse to brief courses of systemic corticosteroids, but this may be very uncommon.

Repellent insecticidal creams or lotions are the same as for mosquitoes. DEET or dimethylphthallate are the best. Sandfly nets to protect sleepers and to keep the flies out of houses are of much finer mesh than those for mosquitoes. They are essential for protection at night in infected areas.

Control

Removal of all debris and refuse where the flies may breed is an important part of control. Cracks and crevices should be filled in. Other breeding places such as rodent burrows should be treated by fumigation. Residual insecticides (see Chap. 26), against adult flies are important because of their "hopping" flights and propensity to land frequently. The construction of dwellings tends to destroy their breeding places (Lewis 1973).

Simuliidae

The family Simuliidae, popularly known as "black flies" or "buffalo flies", comprises over 1000 species (Crosskey 1973). They have a cosmopolitan distribution; in the northern temperate and subarctic zones they are active in the spring and early summer (White 1982), whilst in the tropics, where they are the vectors of onchocerciasis in Africa and America, as many as five or six generations may occur in a season (Gudgel and Grauer 1954). Table 9.2 shows some of the commoner biting species. They are fierce biters and will attack any exposed surface and are capable of causing great inconvenience quite apart from their role as vectors. Crosskey noted that their effects, caused principally by the huge numbers which bite simultaneously, are especially disturbing at seasonal peaks of their population, when they may seriously interfere with forestry and tourism and can reduce the milk yield of cattle and the egg production of poultry. In Australia cattle have been killed by their attentions, through a combination of toxaemia, anaphylactic shock and blood loss (James and Harwood 1969).

Morphology

As the name "buffalo flies" implies, they resemble miniature buffaloes with their characteristic humped thorax, the similarity being enhanced by their relatively short legs and horn-like antennae (Fig. 9.4). They are from 1 to 5 mm long. The head is held low relative to the thorax and faces slightly downwards. The compound eyes are large; they meet in the midline (holoptic), in the male but are separated (dichoptic) in the female. The antennae are short and point upwards and outwards. The female mouthparts (see Fig. 9.1c, d) consist of two lanceolate maxillae and a hypopharynx. The thorax is arched, which causes the humped appearance, and has three pairs of short stout legs. The wings are broad, colourless and with pronounced anterior venation, but the other veins are ill-defined. The abdomen is short and squat and "sessile" in its attachment to the thorax, having no waist. (Gordon and Lavoipierre 1962).

Table 9.2. Some of the common Simuliidae which bite man

Species	Notes
Simulium damnosum[a]	Africa
S. naevei[a]	Africa and Central America
S. ochraceum[a]	Central and South America; vicious biter
S. metallicum[a]	Guatemala
S. callidum[a]	Guatemala
S. venustum	USA and Canada; area breeder
S. vittatum	North America; very abundant
S. meridionale	
S. (*?Boophtora*) *erythrocephalum*	Europe
S. arctium	Saskatchewan; river breeder; vicious biter
Prosimulium mixtum	Canada and New York State; area breeder
P. rufipes	European
P. fuscum	North America
Eusimulium equinum	Japan
Cnepha pecaurum	Southern USA; the southern buffalo gnat; not a nuisance since the Mississippi levees were built

[a] Vector of onchocerciasis.

Biology

Simuliidae breed in running water such as mountain streams or waterfalls, whether man made or natural (Van den Bosch 1978). The eggs are laid in masses of 300–400 and quickly hatch. White (1982) put the hatching time as 1–2 days, but Crosskey (1973) said that it was about 5 days in warm weather. The larvae are entirely aquatic. There are six to eight instars (White 1982) over a period which may vary from 3 to 10 weeks. Pupation is also aquatic, this stage being passed in a silken cocoon for from 2 to 10 days. Air collects in the pupal case, which splits. The adult emerges and floats to the surface inside the air bubble and then takes flight. The adult flies tend to head towards open grassland or woodland glades, although they are frequently found along the banks of rivers and can also be seen in housing areas. They never enter buildings (Gudgel and Grauer 1954).

Simuliids bite man freely on any exposed surface of his skin, large numbers often biting simultaneously. Only the females bite and only in the daytime, especially after rain. Gudgel and Grauer

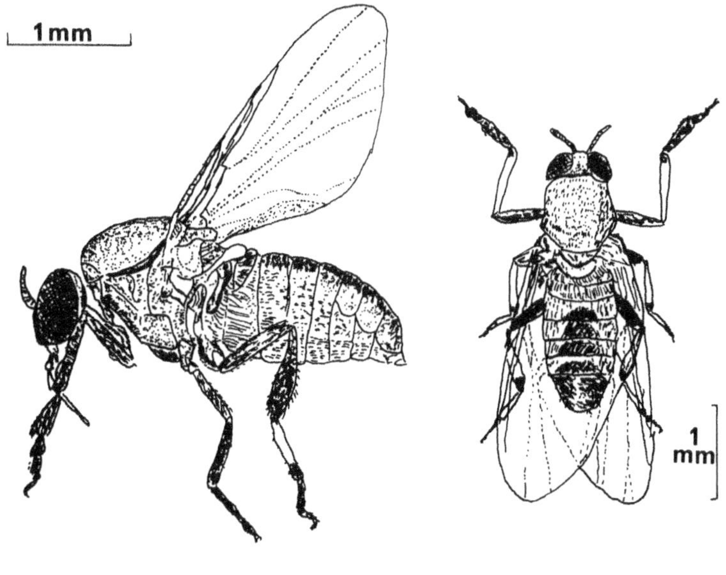

Fig. 9.4. *Simulium damnosum*, a black fly. Note the "buffalo hump". [After Crosskey 1973, by kind permission of the author and the Trustees of the British Museum (Natural History)]

(1954) found that most biting activity took place early in the morning or late afternoon. Biting is done by the maxillae and hypopharynx piercing the skin and slashing or tearing at the underlying tissues, causing them to bleed. The fly feeds from the pool of blood so formed (Rothschild and Clay 1952; Gordon and Lavoipierre 1962). This blood meal is essential for egg laying.

In some seasons conditions are very favourable for simuliids and vast numbers appear causing an epidemic of bites. One such was reported from Bratislava by Jedlicka (1982) and by Farkas (1982), when 81 cases of simuliosis were seen at one clinic.

Clinical Features

The eyes, ears, nostrils, wrists and other areas are commonly attacked, although in Japan the legs (and uncovered heels in those who wear sandals) are most frequently involved (Gudgel and Grauer 1954). The eruption is a mixture of lesions (see under Immunology, p. 129). According to Gudgel and his colleague, the actual bites are painless because the saliva contains a local anaesthetic as well as an anticoagulant. James and Harwood (1969), however, considered them to be very painful. The first sign of an attack may be a tiny drop of blood, the bleeding being regarded as large for such a small insect. This gives place to a tiny blood crust and sometimes causes ecchymotic discolouration around the bite. Within a few hours a small itching papule appears which may persist for several days but then disappears without trace. Erythematous weals up to 1 cm across may also occur. It is not uncommon with multiple *Simulium* bites for a whole affected area to swell markedly. A leg may double in volume (Gudgel and Grauer 1954) or the face become severely oedematous (James and Harwood 1969). Such swelling, which is probably a hypersensitivity reaction, occurred quite frequently in the patients at Bratislava (Farkas 1982). Some of these patients also showed erosions and central necrosis of the lesions with accompanying lymphadenopathy. Iijima (1949) described a patient who developed prurigo nodularis following bites from *Eusimulium equinum*, with a recurrence caused by the same species the following year.

Treatment

Local treatment is palliative to relieve itch. Simple oily calamine lotion or a hydrocortisone ointment with an anti-infective agent should be adequate. For severe reactions with systemic symptoms oral antihistamines and adrenaline may be needed (see treatment of reactions to Hymenoptera stings, Chap. 10, p. 149). Immunisation is impractical and would be very expensive.

Prevention

Repellent insecticidal creams may give some protection for a few hours. Dimethylphthallate or DEET are probably the best, although Travis et al. (1951) reported fairly good results with Rutgers 612 and Indalone. More recently Noamesi (1970) claimed that a preparation made from extracts of three local tropical plants, the active ingredients of which had not been identified, gave 100% protection for 12 h after application against *Simulium damnosum*. If the effectiveness of this treatment is confirmed, it should prove valuable.

Control

Since the eggs and pupae of *Simulium* are immune to insecticides, control is not easy. Adult flies are best dealt with by aerial insecticide sprays in the form of a fog, provided that the operator and inhabitants of the infested area are not likely to be harmed. However, this is likely to have only a temporary effect because of the emergence of the next generation of adults from the pupal stage. Antilarval measures probably provide the best opportunity to control the black fly population and involve using insecticides in the water in which they breed. Expert entomological opinion should be sought to estimate the best dosage and time of use. The insecticides will be carried downstream by the currents. If breeding occurs over a wide area the application should be done by aerial spraying, but otherwise spraying from the ground is adequate. DDT and dieldrin were used at one time, but for ecological reasons (damage to the environment) are now likely to be replaced by organophosphorous compounds. Reiter (1982) has pointed out that whatever insecticide is used it is important to choose one of optimal particle size to have maximum effect and this must be decided locally by an expert, taking into account all the factors which may influence its uptake by the flies.

Ceratopogonidae

This group contains all the biting midges belonging to the genera *Culicoides*, *Lasiohelea* and *Leptoconops*. There are a large number of species (over 800 in *Culicoides* alone) and very many are vicious biters of man. They have many common names including "midges", "gnats", "pinkies", "no-see-ums" etc., and may cause considerable upset by the sheer effect of their vast numbers. They tend to occur in swarms, which may appear suddenly and even contain males and females of more than one species. When this happens they will attack any mammal in their vicinity (Patton 1931). They seriously interfere with agricultural work, especially amongst crofters in Scotland. They can also damage the tourist trade of any area where they appear in large numbers. Their distribution is cosmopolitan and their effect correspondingly widespread.

Morphology

Culicoides species are very small (Fig. 9.5) being from 1 to 4 mm long. The head has a pair of compound eyes and 14- or 15-segmented antennae,

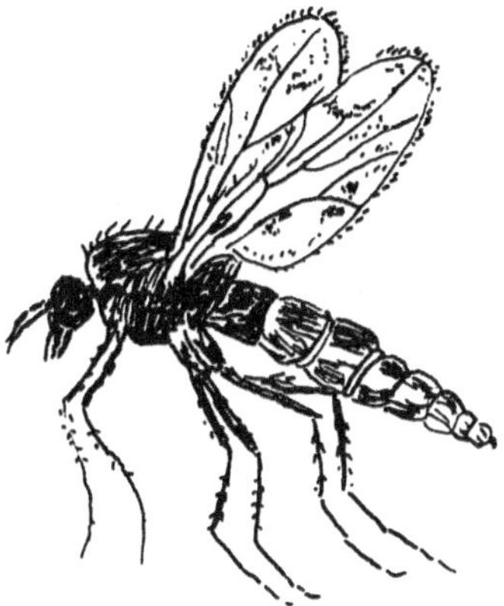

Fig. 9.5. *Culicoides pulicaris*. (After Patton 1931)

which are hairy in the female (Busvine 1966) and directed forwards and upwards. The wings, which are usually speckled with pigment and not scales as with mosquitoes (White 1982), lie folded over one another when the insect is at rest. The biting mouthparts resemble those of the mosquito but are much shorter (see Fig. 9.1). The thorax is relatively stout, slightly humped but less than in Simuliidae. There are characteristic slit-like pits on the thorax at the anterolateral border. There are three pairs of slender legs, which are also short compared with mosquitoes. The abdomen is short. The external male genitalia are prominent and used by taxonomists in classification (Gordon and Lavoipierre 1962; Freeman 1973). The breeding places are variable. They are commonly found in Scotland, for example, on rush and bog moors, but elsewhere in swamps, mud at the edge of pools and in salt marshes.

Biology

The life cycle varies from 70 days to $10\frac{1}{2}$ months, according to whether the climate is tropical or temperate. In tropical climates these flies breed all the year round but in colder countries there are one or two generations per year. Eggs are laid in moist places, preferably semisubmerged by water, in clusters or rows. However, if only mud is available, they may be scattered indiscriminately (Gordon and Lavoipierre 1962). Up to 120 may be laid. The incubation period, which varies with environmental temperature and humidity, is from 2 to 8 days. If the weather turns very cold the egg may not hatch until the following spring. The emerging larvae are relatively large (5–6 mm long), creamy or pale brown in colour, with a darker rather conical head. There are four larval instars, which require variable times to reach pupation. In the tropics the whole cycle is about 3 weeks, but, according to Gordon and Lavoipierre (1962), the larva may overwinter in the third or fourth instar stage for as long as 6 or 7 months. Pupation occurs in drier ground, the pupa being 3–4 mm long. Different species are buried at different levels in the soil. Busvine (1980) gives several examples of this. The adult emerges after 3–8 days, again governed by temperature. After a brief drying-out period they swarm, mate in flight and the females search for a blood meal. Their flight is short but they are capable of flying in light rain and slight breezes. They are daytime feeders as a rule and mostly crepuscular, but some feed in the early morning. Most authorities assert that they are exclusively outdoors species and never enter houses, but Gordon and Lavoipierre noted that two species, *C. austeni* and *C. grahami*, do enter buildings and bite at night. Feeding is rapid, the mouthparts being inserted in the same manner as for mosquitoes. They do not carry any human disease but are vectors for animal filariasis and oncherciasis (Freeman 1973). Several species are vicious biters and can drive their victims indoors.

Clinical Features

The biting midges cause minute papular lesions which may persist for several days. There is usually a slight halo of erythema. The whole lesion may only be 2–3 mm in diameter. In some persons (e.g. the present writer) the lesions do not itch, but the majority of people find them intolerable because of their numbers (see Fig. 9.18). Exposed areas only are attacked, especially the forearms and ears. Some species are said to have a predilection for special parts of the body. For example, *C. tristriatulus* attacks the head, whilst *C. furens* prefers the legs (Busvine 1980). Weals may occur in sensitised persons (James and Harwood 1969). Secondary infection can occur but is not common.

Treatment

Simple antipruritics (oily calamine lotion or hydrocortisone with added anti-infective agents) are all that is required.

Prevention

Freeman (1973) considered larval insecticide control impractical except in important holiday resorts where money is available. For special events temporary aerosol "fogs" of insecticides may be used (e.g. dichlorvos or methyl parathion) before the arrival of those participating in the event. The fogs should be allowed time to settle. DDT and dieldrin are not now used for ecological reasons. Repellent creams containing materials like DEET, which are effective against mosquitoes, might help for short periods only, but it must be remembered that what repels one species may not have the same result with another. Readers are advised to consult local entomologists.

Tabanidae

The family Tabanidae of the suborder Brachycera contains about 3000 species. Only three genera are important to man: *Chrysops* ("deer flies"), *Tabanus* "horse flies") and *Haematopota* ("clegs"). They are robust, fairly large flies, *Chrysops* and *Haematopota* being about 1 cm long and the horse flies reaching 2.5 cm in length. Only females suck blood, the males being flower feeders. The eyes are often brilliantly coloured in life (Oldroyd 1973). In the females they are dichoptic (separated in the midline) but in the males holoptic (meeting in the midline). The biting mouthparts are blade-like, sharp cutting implements (James and Harwood 1969; Figs. 9.6, 9.7 and 9.8).

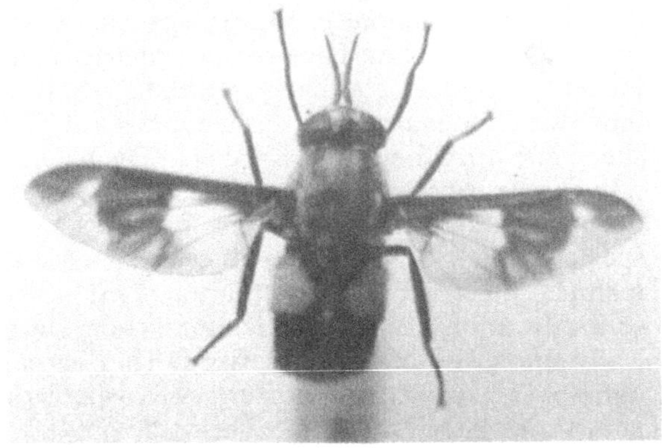

Fig. 9.6. *Chrysops calateus*. (Courtesy of the Curator of the Scottish Natural History Museum)

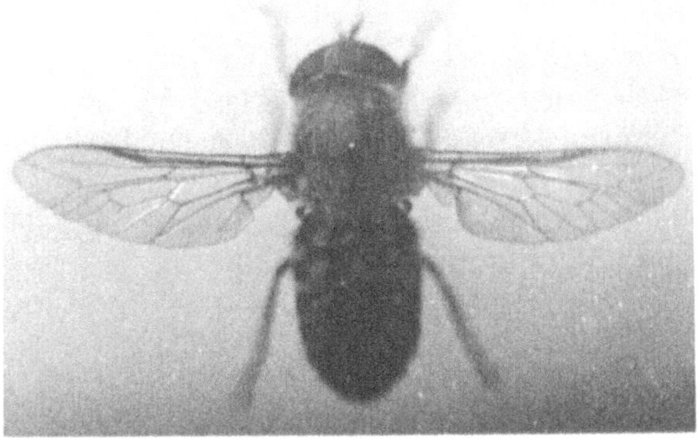

Fig. 9.7. *Tabanus brumpti*, the horse fly. (Courtesy of the Curator of the Scottish Natural History Museum)

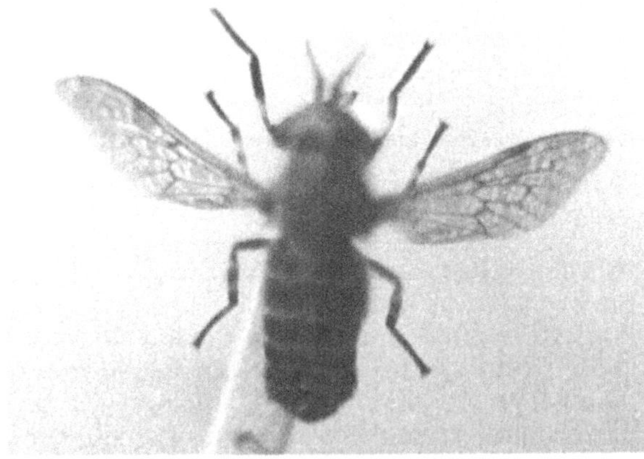

Fig. 9.8. *Haematopota pluvialis*, the cleg. (Courtesy of the Curator of the Scottish Natural History Museum)

Eggs are laid in moist or semi-aquatic ground in large sticky batches of up to 1000 (Busvine 1980). The number laid varies with the species. The eggs, about 1–2 mm long, hatch within 7 days. The emerging larvae fall to the bottom of the water or mud in which the egg was laid, where they feed off organic debris of both animal and vegetable origin (Gordon and Lavoipierre 1962; James and Harwood 1969). There are up to nine larval instars spanning some two to three seasons before pupation occurs in drier soil. The adult emerges 5–21 days later. The females are strong fliers and have a speed in excess of 30 mph and a range of several miles (Busvine 1980).

The adults prefer open woodlands or savannah type of country, but this covers a wide spectrum of places. They are common around farms, where there is stagnant water of any kind. They constitute a nuisance, to say the least, to visiting picnickers. Flies in this group tend to follow and attack moving animals and people and will therefore be more likely to bite those who are walking, riding, cycling or even travelling in a vehicle.

Clinical Features

The bites are deep and very painful. The victim's attention is therefore quickly drawn to the attack and feeding is interrupted. This implies repeated attempts to feed. Although individually these flies are not gregarious and often attack singly, they tend to emerge from the pupal state *en masse*, and people may thus be bitten by several flies simultaneously (Oldroyd 1973; personal experience). This is particularly the case with *Haematopota*. This fly is mainly a European species, although the whole family is thought by Oldroyd to be of South American origin in a palaeontological sense. The bite itself frequently becomes secondarily infected and, because it is deep, often causes a severe cellulitis out of all proportion to the size of the orginal wound. It usually appears on the lower legs and ankles although any exposed part can be bitten. There may be associated lymphangitis, lymphadenopathy and fever.

The attack of these flies can interfere with the efficiency of both man and his animals. The flies can act as mechanical vectors of disease, e.g. anthrax, on account of their size and feeding habit of flitting from animal to animal. Their capacious mouthparts enable them to transport infectious material direct from one animal to the next (Oldroyd 1973). They are also true vectors of animal trypanosomiasis, tularaemia and some forms of loiasis (Calabar swellings).

Treatment

Local lesions are treated symptomatically. For uninfected bites simple oily calamine lotion with perhaps 1% of either phenol or menthol is usually adequate; however, in the event of cellulitis developing, nearly always of staphylococcal origin, the appropriate antibiotic in suitable dosage must be given systemically together with comforting dressings such as 10% ichthammol in glycerine soaks. Analgesics may be needed for a day or two. It is also advisable to rest the affected part.

Prevention

Repellent insecticides may be tried. It seems likely that pyrethroids may be helpful (see Chap. 26, p. 403, and the notes below on the prevention of *Stomoxys* bites). Control is difficult (Busvine 1980) because of the density of the larval population and the extensive areas involved. Spraying of pastures with insecticides and clearing shrubs (insect resting places) in the pastures may help livestock, as may temporary flooding of the tabanid breeding places.

Stomoxys calcitrans

Morphology and Biology

The muscid *Stomoxys calcitrans*, popularly known as the "stable fly", is very common and has a cosmopolitan distribution. It closely resembles the housefly, *Musca domestica*, in its general appearance (Fig. 9.9) although somewhat lighter in colour. The chief difference is in the mouthparts (see Fig. 9.1). Those of the housefly are of a telescopic nature and used for surface feeding by suction

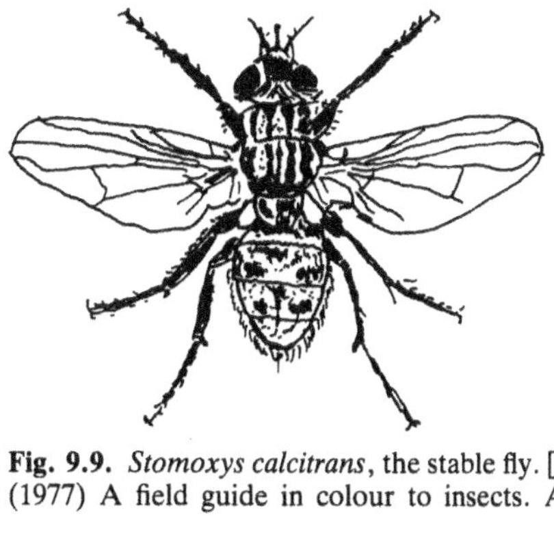

Fig. 9.9. *Stomoxys calcitrans*, the stable fly. [After Zahradnik T (1977) A field guide in colour to insects. Artia, Prague]

only. Those of *Stomoxys* are adapted for blood sucking and are pointed, slender and rigid. The proboscis projects in front of the fly's head and is non-retractable. For feeding purposes it is thrust through the host's epidermis to a depth of about one-third of its length (Gordon and Lavoipierre 1962).

Eggs are not laid until some days after partaking of a blood meal (both sexes suck blood). They are deposited in dung or other farmyard refuse and hatch in 1–4 days. The subsequent larval development takes between 10 and 30 days, depending on the ambient temperature. Pont (1973) stated that the life cycle (presumably in the tropics) could be as short as 12 days. The feeding ground for the larvae must be moist. They then leave for drier ground, dig into the soil and pupate. The pupal stage lasts from 1 to 3 weeks. In temperate zones breeding occurs only in the warm seasons, the colder months being spent in the larval or pupal state. Breeding takes place all the year round in the tropics.

Biting (i.e. feeding) usually but not always occurs out of doors. *Stomoxys* is a diurnal feeder, except in cold weather, when it does not feed at all. It can insert its proboscis through the thickest stocking and bites equally well on exposed and unexposed skin. Pont maintained that it seldom bit the former, preferring to feed through clothing, but this is contrary to the present writer's personal experience. It penetrates the skin with a rasping movement (Busvine 1966). The bite itself is quite painful; the victim is well aware that he is being bitten and will take steps to drive the fly off. It is persistent, however, and will repeatedly return to bite until it has fed sufficiently. If undisturbed, Busvine noted that this fly would feed for 15 min. In spite of the painful bite, *Stomoxys* is not so annoying as those flies which attack in swarms, although in tropical countries this species is plentiful. Lloyd and Dipeolu (1974) collected large numbers of *Stomoxys* from a tethered bull in northern Nigeria, its frequency being second only to *Musca domestica*. It is commonly found around farm and village buildings, especially in the vicinity of livestock and manure heaps.

Clinical Features

The bite seldom causes much trouble. There are never more than three or four and often only a single bite. A tiny evanescent papule arises which quickly fades. The only real risk is from secondary infection, which may be a problem because of the fly's habitat and habits. Treatment is palliative.

Control

Although *Stomoxys* is not a vector of any human disease, it carries helminths to livestock and its attentions may disturb cattle and reduce milk yield (Busvine 1980). Control is therefore necessary for agricultural reasons. This can be effected by good husbandry in dealing with forage storage and avoiding wet stacks and also by applying contact insecticides to refuse heaps and dung piles. Roberts and Peers (1982) have shown that the numbers of *S. calcitrans* or of *Haematobia irritans* (the cattle horn fly) attacking cattle can be greatly reduced by the use of sprays of cypermethrin and ear tags impregnated with this pyrethroid insecticide.

Hippoboscidae

There are some 120 species in the family Hippoboscidae. None normally bites man but at least 13 have been recorded as doing so (James and Harwood 1969; Table 9.3). *Melophagus ovinus*, the sheep ked, may cause much discomfort to those engaged in sheep shearing and wool packing and constitutes an occupational hazard.

Table 9.3. Some of the commonest Hippoboscidae which are said to bite man

Species	Notes
Hippobosca rufipes	
H. equina	Horse ked
H. camelina	Camel ked
H. variegata	
H. longipennis	
Melophagus ovinus	Sheep ked; very widespread
Lipoptena cervi	Deer ked
Crataerina pallida	A parasite of swifts
Pseudolynchia canariensis	Pigeon fly

Morphology

Taking the deer ked, *Lipoptena cervi*, as an example (Fig. 9.10), both sexes are seen to be winged, although they lose these quickly when they have found a host. They are flattened dorsoventrally and have a tough leathery consistence. The head is sunk into an emargination of the thorax. The palps of this species are rigid and ensheath the proboscis. The latter, which is hidden when retracted, can be projected forwards for biting. The body as a whole is squat, with powerful legs and strong claws.

The females are viviparous. The larvae are pale and immobile and pupate early (Imms 1938).

Clinical Features

The bite has been declared by Imms to be painless; however, James and Harwood (1969) and Cogan (1973) have stated that it is painful, although Cogan added that its persistence is more distressing to the patient than the bite. Shortly after biting, small reddish-brown papules appear, which itch severely (Fig. 9.11). They recur with each succeeding new exposure (Reunala et al. 1980). They are very persistent for up to 12 months (Rantanen et al. 1982).

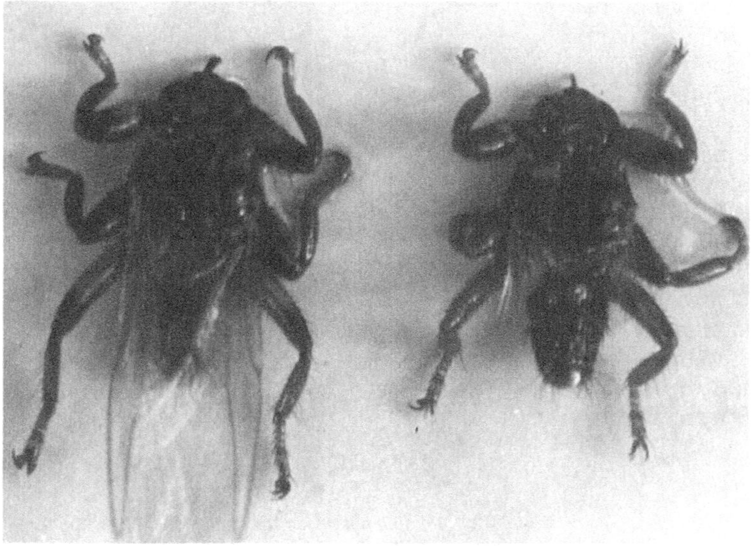

Fig. 9.10. *Lipoptena cervi*. The deer ked. Winged and wingless stages. (Courtesy of Dr. T. M. Reunala, Helsinki)

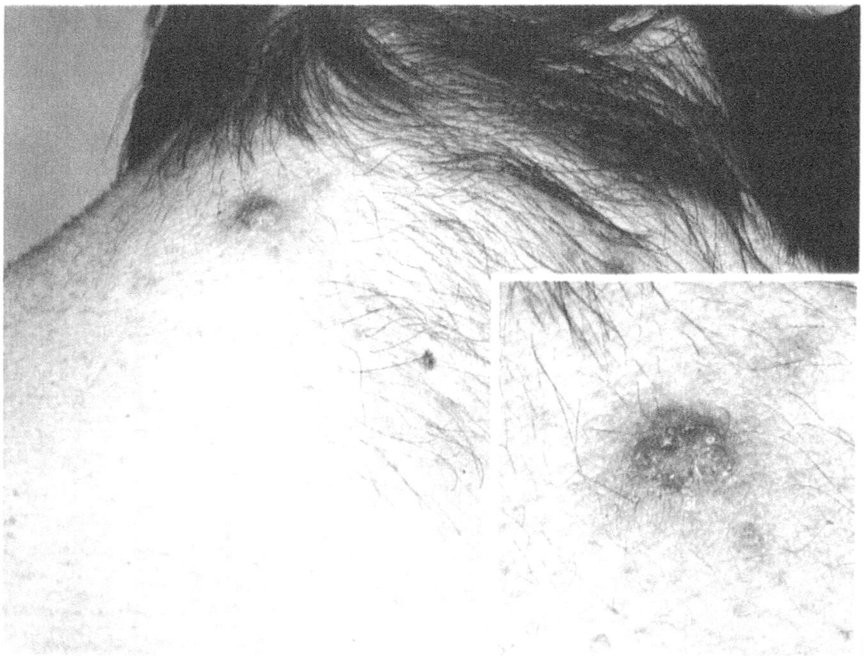

a b

Fig. 9.11a, b. Papular oedematous lesions at nape of the neck resulting from the bite of *Lipoptena cervi*, the deer ked. **a** showing the whole area; **b** close-up of the central lesion. (Courtesy of Dr. T. M. Reunala, Helsinki)

Histology

The papules of the Finnish patients described by Rantanen et al. showed a "typical insect bite" reaction, but no retained mouthparts were seen in sections. Direct immunofluorescence revealed deposits of C_3 in the dermal blood vessels. Skin tests gave positive immediate and delayed reactions and the IgE level was raised in the serum of 10 of 19 patients. These findings suggested to Rantanen et al. that IgE and complement were involved in a cell-mediated immune response. The bites of the Finnish patients occurred when walking in forests. (From 10 to 200 keds attacked at a time.)

Nelson and Bainborough (1963) described the development of immunity in sheep. This involved marked arteriolar vasoconstriction in the deep dermis, which in turn deprived the superficial dermal capillaries of their blood content. Consequently, keds which tried to feed on these immune sheep found no sustenance and fell off. On the other hand, if they fed on susceptible sheep which had not developed this "immunity", they were able to engorge satisfactorily.

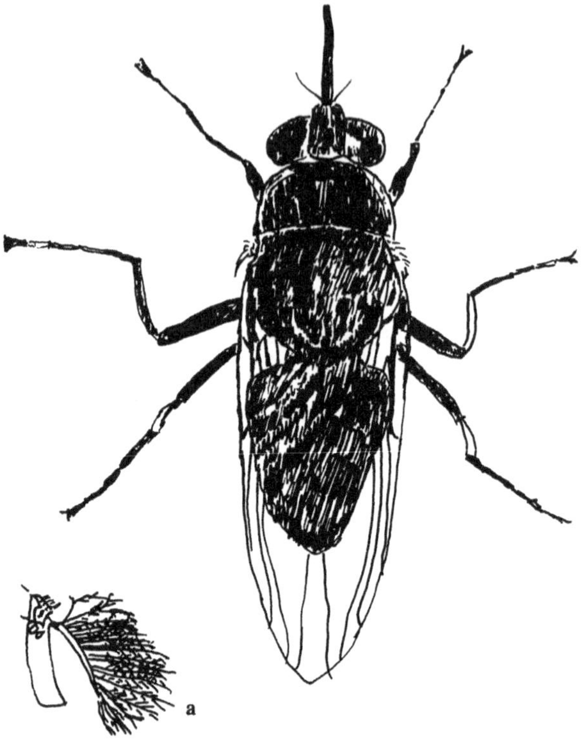

Fig. 9.12. *Glossina palpalis*, the tsetse fly. Note the pointed mouthparts. **a**, antenna. (After Gordon and Lavoipierre 1962)

Glossinidae

There are 22 species of tsetse (the African name means "fly destructive to cattle"), all of which feed exclusively on vertebrate blood, usually mammalian. Many species are vectors of human and cattle trypanosomiasis (Potts 1973). They are confined to Africa between latitudes 15°N and 20°S (30°S on the east coast), although isolated specimens have been found in Brazil (Gordon and Lavoipierre 1962) and Australia (James and Harwood 1969), probably as accidental aeroplane passengers.

Morphology

Tsetse flies are moderately large, reaching 15 mm in length. They are yellowish to very dark brown. The head has large lateral eyes separated anteriorly. The paired antennae are three segmented, the large terminal banana-shaped segment bearing a characteristic arista at its base, which is covered on its dorsal surface with branching hairs (Fig. 9.12). The forward-projecting proboscis is composed of two palps, a hypopharynx, a labrum and a labium. The last three together form a piercing stylet. There are no mandibles or maxillae. Traversing the length of the hypopharynx is a fine salivary duct. The stout thorax supports three pairs of legs and two wings. The latter are folded longitudinally over one another at rest. On the dorsal thoracic surface there are dark stripes and spots. The abdomen may be uniformly coloured or show alternate light and dark bands. The posteriorly situated external genitalia are easily distinguished in the two sexes, those of the male comprising an elaborate, folded, chitinous plate, the details of which are used by taxonomists for differentiating species (Gordon and Lavoipierre 1962). Potts (1973) gives full details of all the species.

Biology

Unusually for muscids, the tsetse fly is viviparous. The larva emerges from the egg after 3–4 days and matures through three instars over the next 8–10 days, all within an insect uterus. The larva feeds from specialised "milk" glands. The mature larva extricates itself backwards in a few minutes. It is creamy white, about 1 cm long, active and with a pair of characteristically dark, functionless "polypneustic" lobes posteriorly (Potts 1973). In the soft, shaded debris in which it is deposited it quickly buries itself 2–5 cm deep and is rapidly transformed into a rather smaller barrel-shaped pupa.

About 1 month later (up to 100 days at low temperatures, according to Potts 1973) the adult emerges and begins to feed a day or two later.

The feeding habits and skin reaction have been described in detail by Gordon and Crewe (1948) and by Gordon (1950). The stylet of the proboscis is directed ventrally and inserted into the skin. Repeated probing inside the dermis lacerates the tissues and induces a relatively profuse haemorrhage, from which the fly feeds avidly. This haemorrhage has been shown experimentally to permeate even underlying muscle. Invasion of the area within 48 h by histiocytes quickly results in involution of the reaction. Gordon and Crewe showed that the severity of the haemorrhage is dependent on the presence of salivary secretion, which presumably contains an anticoagulant.

Tsetse flies prefer warm, damp, shady places in which to live and breed and are therefore found in pockets where these conditions exist throughout the region of their occurrence. Different species tend to favour slightly different general conditions, but one species can readily spread to an area cleared of another species unless suitable control is maintained (Jordan 1978).

Clinical Features

Little is recorded about the actual bites, nearly all the attention being devoted to the trypanosomiasis which is transmitted. White (1982) observed no lesions resulting from the bites. However, an uncomplicated bite must show at least a tiny punctate haemorrhage. Apart from this, Gordon and Crewe (1948) stressed that the only clinical reactions were those of sensitisation of salivary content. Gordon (1950) stated that a person would not react to the initial bite and if subsequently exposed continuously and regularly to these bites he would not develop sensitivity; however, if the exposure was irregular, then sensitivity would occur. The clinical appearance of such lesions is the same as those of mosquito bites.

Treatment and Control

Treatment is palliative and the same as that for mosquito bites. Prevention depends on destruction of the tsetse fly. Local eradication can be achieved by insecticides such as organophosphorous compounds to which these flies are particularly susceptible (Busvine 1980). Large-scale eradication may cause problems. Biological techniques have not yet been adequately developed for economic use in Africa. Clearance of breeding grounds has ecological disadvantages, as has the killing off of wild ungulate hosts (Potts 1973). Jordan (1978) has indicated that discriminatory application of insecticides to certain parts of selected trees and shrubs has been effective in Nigeria with relatively little ecological upset.

Immunology

The apparently chaotic reactions to the bites of mosquitoes and other dipterous biting flies, some persons showing little or no effect, some evanescent irritating weals, some persistent papular lesions and others being almost incapacitated by the severity of their response, were reduced to order by Mellanby (1946). He carried out experiments on 25 volunteers, who had never been outside the United Kingdom and therefore probably never been bitten by *Aedes* mosquitoes. They were repeatedly exposed to controlled biting by these insects. The initial bites in each case showed no response beyond a minute red punctum at the bite site. With subsequent bites after about 24 h a marked delayed reaction occurred consisting of a central weal about 1 cm in diameter with a red halo up to 3 cm in diameter around. This lesion itched irregularly for several days. After repeated bites for about 1 month the reaction changed. An immediate weal appeared at the bite site with a halo and itch. This disappeared within 2 h to be followed by the delayed reaction as usual. With further exposure the immediate reaction appeared but not the delayed response. The volunteers did not go beyond this stage, but Mellanby noted that persons who had received thousands of bites showed no response at all.

Accordingly he tabulated his results (excluding the non-reaction with the first bite) as shown in Table 9.4. In stage 4 the person was said to have developed immunity to the bites. This did not mean that they would not get bitten but that they would not react. Gordon and Crewe (1948) confirmed this and pointed out that the development

Table 9.4. Different stages in the development of immunity to mosquito bites. (After Mellanby 1946)

Immunological Stage	Immediate	Delayed
Stage 1	Negative	Positive
Stage 2	Positive	Positive
Stage 3	Positive	Negative
Stage 4	Negative	Negative

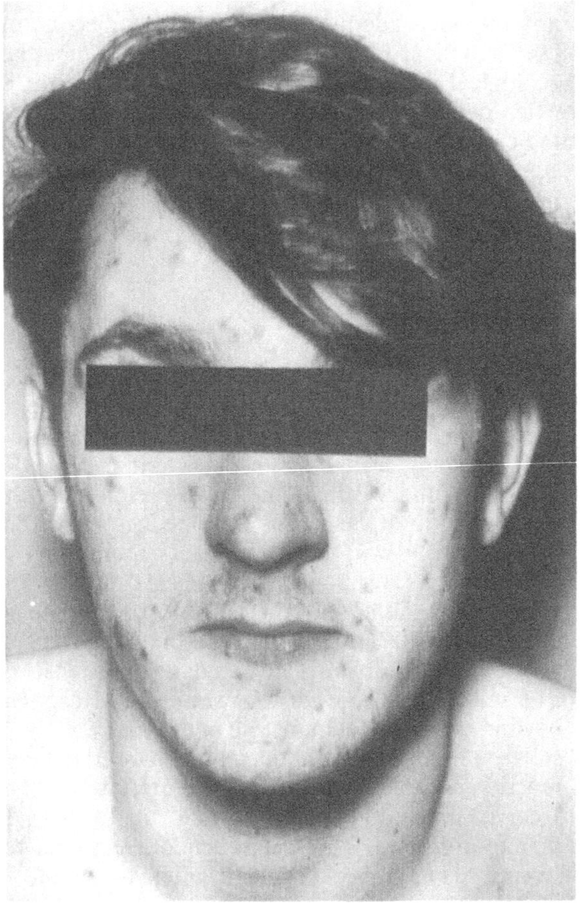

Fig. 9.13. Multiple "insect" bites, possibly from mosquitoes or *Simulium* spp. History too vague to be absolutely certain which species responsible. Note the central punctum visible in some of the oedematous papules.

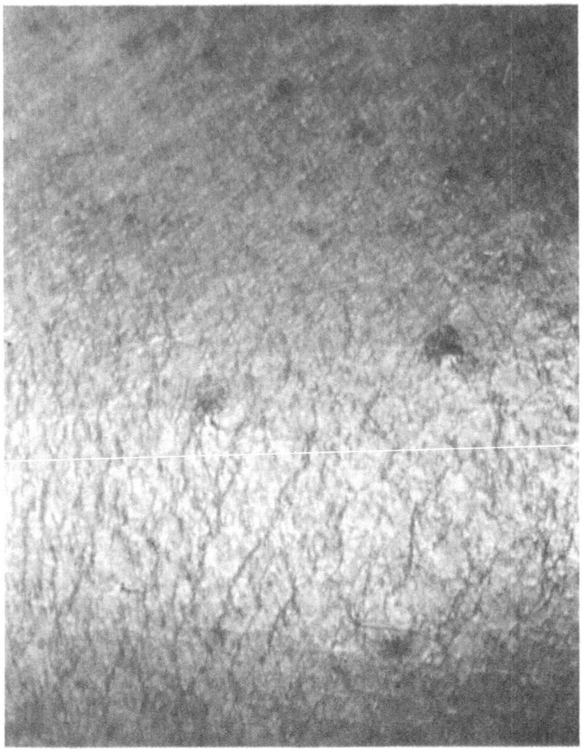

Fig. 9.14. Mosquito bites. (Courtesy of Prof. Ney Romiti of Sao Paulo, Brazil)

of these reactions up to stage 3 depended on continued irregular bites. Only if biting was continued regularly was the immune stage 4 reached. They added that this accounted for the immunity of native inhabitants of a mosquito-infested region and this immunity was thus seen to be acquired and not racial. They thought the delayed reaction was due to a slow-acting substance in the insect saliva, but since this stage occurs in all arthropod sensitisation it is more likely to be part of the immunising process.

Heilesen (1949) confirmed these general findings and pointed out that the delayed reaction could sometimes present as an Arthus phenomenon, as recorded by Brown et al. (1938). Even more severe reactions could occur. Suzuki et al. (1976) reported a reaction which, apart from skin lesions, included fever, hepatosplenomegaly, hypergammaglobulinaemia and pancytopenia. Specific antibodies to mosquito antigens were found. Both types I and IV and possibly III skin reactions were present. Siegel et al. (1954) described thrombocytopenic purpura following mosquito bites. All these very severe reactions occurred in children aged 3 years and all were probably immunologically abnormal.

Benson (1936) succeeded in partially "desensitising" three out of four patients with marked skin sensitivity to mosquito bites, using whole body extracts of mosquitoes. He concluded that the antigen responsible for the sensitisation process in the first place was a heat-resistant protein present in the mosquito body. (See Chap. 10, pp. 146–149, for a full discussion of this subject.) It was noted in Chap. 2 (p. 3) that Gordon (1950) had postulated four possible stimuli from arthropods to which man might react. One of these was sensitivity, and Gordon had concluded that the sensitising antigen was in the saliva of the biting arthropod, a suggestion which was supported by Hudson et al. (1960). They showed that there was no reaction to mosquito bites if the insect's salivary ducts were cut.

Immunotherapy is possible, as demonstrated by Benson (1936), but is really impractical because of the number of persons involved, the difficulties in producing the salivary extracts and especially the cost. Moreover, it would not prevent the mosquitoes from biting and therefore transmitting whatever disease they might be vectoring. Prevention involves the use of repellent insecticides, protective clothing and nets and the destruction of breeding places of the insects concerned.

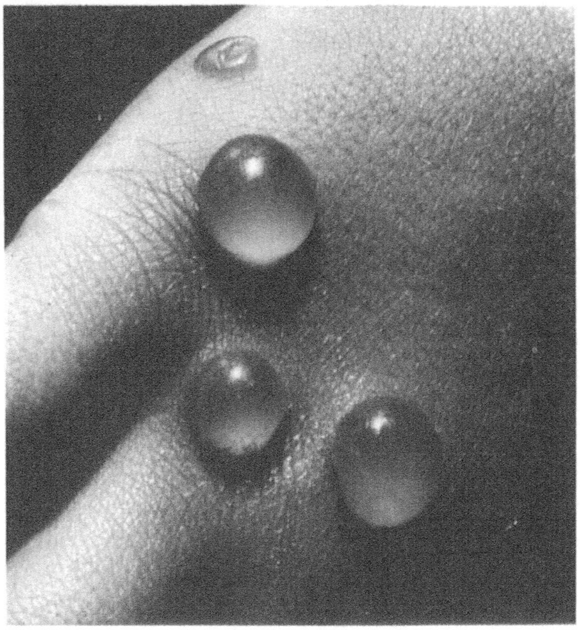

Fig. 9.16. Bullous "insect" bites. Species responsible not known. (Courtesy of Dr. A. Lyell, Glasgow)

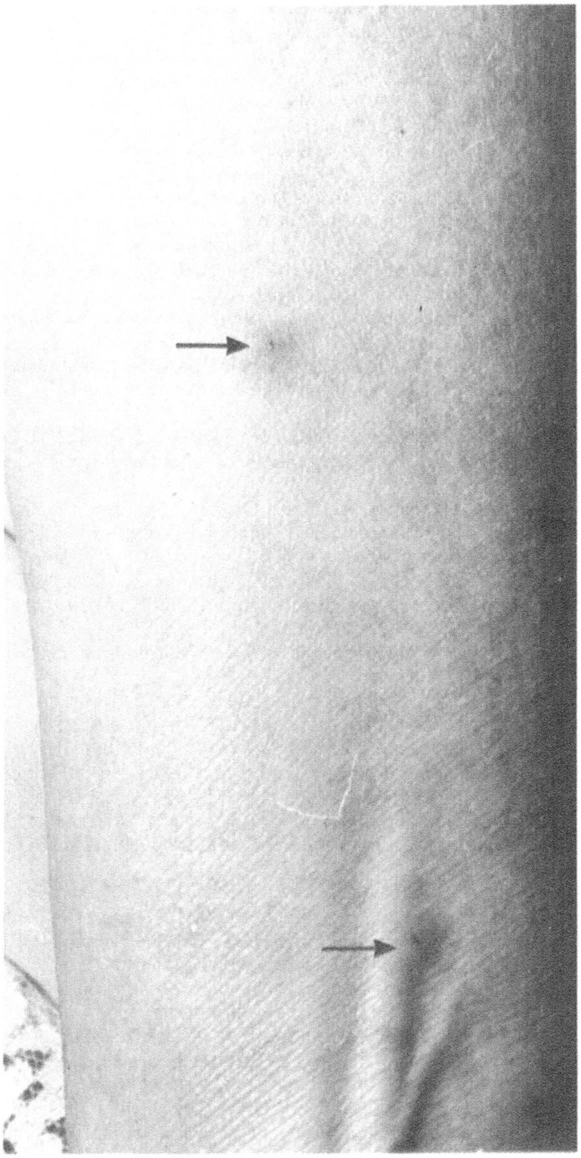

Fig. 9.15. Two "insect" bites on the forearm. Note tiny central punctum, which is haemorrhagic in the lower bite. Note also the red halo. Insect unidentified. (Courtesy of Dr. A. Lyell, Glasgow)

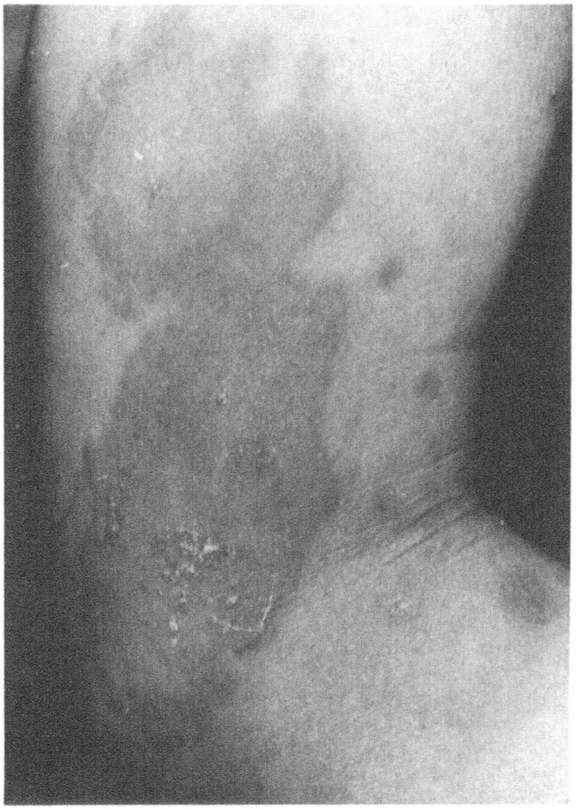

Fig. 9.17. "Insect" bites from unknown species with severe reaction becoming eczematised. (Courtesy of Dr. A. Lyell, Glasgow)

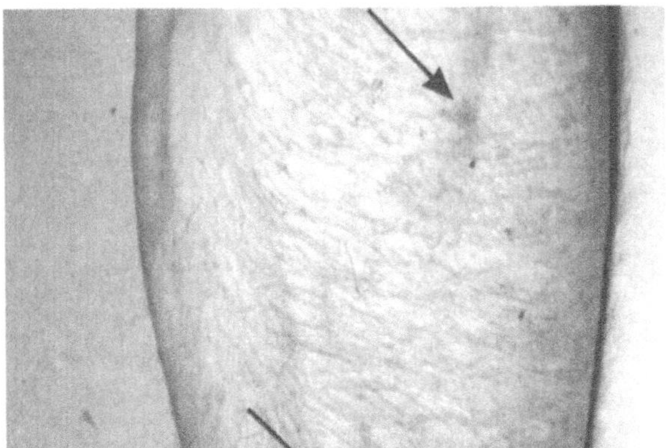

Fig. 9.18. "Midge" bites on the foream of the writer after an evening's mowing of the lawn. (Photographed by W. Towler)

References

Benson RL (1936) Diagnosis and treatment of sensitisation to mosquitoes. J Allergy 8: 47–59

Brown A, Griffiths THD, Erwin S, Dyrenforth LY (1938) Arthus phenomenon from mosquito bites. South Med J 31: 590–596

Busvine JR (1966) Insects and hygiene, 2nd edn. Methuen, London

*Busvine JR (1980) Insects and hygiene, 3rd edn. Chapman and Hall, London

*Cogan BH (1973) Cyclorrhapha of minor medical importance. In: Smith KGV (ed) Insects and other arthropods of medical importance. The Trustees of the British Museum (Natural History), London, pp 279–287

*Crosskey RW (1973) Simuliidae (black flies; German, Kriebelmucker) In: Smith KGV (ed) Insects and other arthropods of medical importance. The Trustees of the British Museum (Natural History), London, pp 109–153

Dostrovsky A (1953) Urticaria multiforme endemica (Harara) In: Simons RDG (ed) Handbook of tropical dermatology and medical mycology. Elsevier, Amsterdam, pp 889–894

Farkas J (1982) On the mass incidence of simuliosis. Skin manifestation after a sting by mites from the order Simuliidae in summer 1981 in Bratislava (in Czech). Cesk Dermatol 57: 324

Freeman P (1973) Ceratopogonidae (biting midges, "sandflies", "punkies"). In: Smith KGV (ed) Insects and other arthropods of medical importance. The Trustees of the British Museum (Natural History), London, pp 181–187

Gordon RM (1950) Reactions produced by arthropods directly injurious to the skin of man. Br Med J II: 316–318

*Gordon RM, Crewe W (1948) The mechanisms by which mosquitoes and tse-tse flies obtain their blood meal, the histology of the lesions produced and the subsequent reaction of the mammalian host together with some observations on the feeding of *Chrysops* and *Cimex*. Ann Trop Med 42: 334–356

Gordon RM, Lavoipierre MMJ (1962) Entomology for students of medicine. Blackwell, Oxford

Gudgel EF, Grauer FH (1954) Acute and chronic reactions to black fly bites (*Simulium* fly) Arch Dermatol Syphilol 70: 609–615

Heilesen B (1949) Studies on mosquito bites. Acta Allergol (Kbh) 11: 245–267

Hudson A, Bowman L, Orr CWM (1960) Effects of absence of saliva on blood feeding by mosquitoes. Science 131: 1730–1731

Iijima S (1949) Prurigo nodularis. Tohoku J Exp Med 51: 284

Imms AD (1938) A general textbook of entomology, 4th edn. Methuen, London

*James MT, Harwood RF (1969) On various groups of dipterous flies. In: Herms's medical entomology, 6th edn. London, Macmillan pp 147–277

Jedlicka L (1982) Simuliosis and some aspects of the medical importance of black flies (Diptera: Simuliidae) (in Czech). Cesk Dermatol 57: 325–332

Jordan AM (1978) Principles of the eradication or control of tse-tse flies. Nature 273: 607–609

*Lewis DJ (1971) Phlebotomid sandflies. Bull WHO 44: 535–551

*Lewis DJ (1973) Phlebotomidae and Psychodidae (sandflies and moth-flies). In: Smith KGV (ed) Insects and other arthropods of medical importance. The Trustees of the British Museum (Natural History), London, pp 155–179

Lloyd DH, Dipeolu OO (1974) Seasonal prevalence of flies feeding on cattle in northern Nigeria. Trop Anim Health Prod 6: 231–236

Mattingly PF Crosskey RW, Smith KGV (1973) Summary of arthropod vectors. In: Smith KGV (ed) Insects and other arthropods of medical importance. The Trustees of the British Museum (Natural History), London, pp 497–532

*Mellanby K (1946) Man's reaction to mosquito bites. Nature 158: 554

Minter DH (1982) Phlebotomine sandflies. In: Manson-Bahr PEC and Apted FIC (ed) Manson's tropical diseases, 18th edn. Baillière Tindall, London, pp 743–759

Nelson WA, Bainborough AR (1963) Development in sheep of resistance to the ked *Melophagus ovinus*. III Histopathology of sheep skin as a clue to the nature of resistance. Exp Parasitol 13: 118–127

Noamesi GK (1970) Preliminary report on a new repellent "Simco" against blackflies and other biting insects. Ghana Med J 9: 39–43

Oldroyd H (1973) Tabanidae (horse-flies, clegs, deer-flies etc.) In: Smith KGV (ed) Insects and other arthropods of medical importance. The Trustees of the British Museum (Natural History), London, pp 195–202

*Patton WS (1931) Insects, ticks, mites and venomous animals of medical and veterinary importance. Part II Public Health. HR Grubb, Croydon

Pont AC (1973) Muscidae (house flies, stable flies etc.) In: Smith KGV (ed) Insects and other arthropods of medical importance. The Trustees of the British Museum (Natural History), London, pp 251–269

Potts WH (1973) Glossinidae (tse-tse flies). In: Smith KGV (ed) Insects and other arthropods of medical importance. The Trustees of the British Museum (Natural History), London, pp 209–249

Rantanen T, Reunala T, Vuojolahti P, Hackman W (1982) Persistent pruritic papules from deer ked bites. Acta Derm Venereol (Stockh) 62: 307–311

Reiter P (1982) Insecticide particle size in *Simulium* tests. Ann Trop Med Parasitol 76: 235–237

Reunala T, Rantanen T, Vuojolahti P, Hackman W (1980) Deer ked (*Lipoptena cervi* L) causes chronic dermatitis in man (in Finnish). Duodecim 96: 897–902

Roberts SH, Peers RA (1982) Fly control on cattle in S. Wales. In: Ectoparasites of veterinary and medical importance in temperate areas. Proceedings of a symposium held on 5 Nov 1982 at the Royal Army Medical College, Millbank, London, pp 60–63

Rothschild M, Clay T (1952) Fleas, flukes and cuckoos. Collins, London, pp 211–223

Siegel JM, Brown HC, DiLeo LW (1954) Purpura as a result of insect allergy. Treatment with cortisone. Postgrad Med 15: 46–49

Suzuki S, Nesishi K, Tomizawawa S, Shirasaki M, Kuroume T, Matsumura T (1976) A case of mosquito allegy: immunological studies. Acta Allergol (Kbh) 31: 428–441

*Theodor O (1935) A study of the reactions to phlebotomus bites with some remarks on "Harara". Trans R Soc Trop Med Hyg 29: 273–284

Travis BV Smith AL, Madden AH (1951) Effectiveness of insect repellents againsts black flies. J Econ Entomol 44: 813–814

Van den Bosch H (1978) Chemotherapy of parasitic infection. Nature 273: 626–630

White GB (1982) Midges, blackflies, buffalo gnats, horse flies and gad flies. In: Manson-Bahr PEC and Apted FIC (eds) Manson's tropical diseases, 18th edn. Baillière Tindall, London, pp 788–791

10 Hymenoptera Stings

This large order of over 100 000 species (Davies 1967) includes a wide variety of species, most of which are harmless to man. Table 10.1. shows the main subdivisions of the order. Only the Aculeata class contains species which are injurious to man. All ant species and many wasp and bee species have a social organisation which is often highly developed, but many other bees and wasps live a solitary existence. Some of the solitary forms may attack man, but most assaults, whether accidental or deliberate, come from the social forms. A very great deal has been written about these creatures, especially honeybees. Only a bare outline of morphology is given here, together with those features of biology, habits and habitat which may be relevant to the production of lesions. For an excellent account of Hymenoptera and their association with man in one way or another the reader is referred to Ebeling (1975).

Hymenoptera (so named from Gk. *hymenopteras*, membrane-wing) have two pairs of membranous wing fastened together on each side during flight by a row of tiny hooklets. The mouthparts are adapted for biting, chewing or lapping. The antennae are angled, often showing a distinct elbow. The thorax and abdomen of most species of bees, wasps and ants are joined together by a very narrow petiole (the first one or two abdominal segments). Also in these groups the ovipositor is modified, in some for the purpose of piercing the integument of plants or insects to deposit an egg, in others, especially the social forms, as a stinger (Imms 1938).

Beyond recognising bees, wasps and ants as such and perhaps distinguishing between honeybees and bumblebees, little further identification is usual by the vast majority of those who are stung by them. The gross similarity between the species renders accurate identification, especially with a mobile buzzing insect, more or less impossible. Expert opinion is necessary. The same applies to ants, which are usually only noted by colour and size. The failure of identification in relation to all three groups has implications for immunotherapy (see p. 147). On the other hand, any observations of the habits and nesting propensities are often helpful in narrowing down possible choices of identity.

Both the honeybee (Apidae) and the bumblebee (Bombidae) stings, but the former does so more frequently and often with more serious consequences. In most countries honeybees are imported domesticated species bred for the honey

Table 10.1. The main subdivisions of Hymenoptera, with emphasis on the Aculeata group, which contains all the species which may attack man

Hymenoptera			
Hymenoptera	Apocrita	Parasitica: 4 superfamilies, all parasitic on insects or plants	
		Aculeata	Bethyloidea—solitary predators
			Scolioidea—solitary predators
			Formicoidea—social (ants)
			Pompiloidea—solitary predators
			Sphecoidea—solitary predators
			Vespoidea—social and solitary (wasps)
			Apoidea—social and solitary (bees)
	Symphata: 6 superfamilies, all parasitic on plants.		

they produce, but wild colonies are frequent in Africa and South America. Their general appearance is rather similar. All social bees have three classes: queens, drones, or males, and workers. The workers are 10–15 mm long, drones 15–17 mm long and queens 15–20 mm long. They are covered with fine hairs, which are most abundant on the thorax and less so on the dorsal aspect of the abdomen. Biery (1977) has pointed out that the bee hairs are individually "feathered", whereas wasp hairs are smooth. Bees in general are dark brown to black, the head, thorax and legs being rather darker than the abdomen. Bumblebees are larger than honeybees—up to 3 cm long and much broader (Fig. 10.1). They are characterised by their brighter colour, being striped black and various shades of orange or orange-yellow. They are also much more hairy than honeybees.

Wasps are divided into four superfamilies (Vespoidea, Sphecoidea, Bethyloidea and Scolioidea). However, for all practical purposes, those species which commonly sting man belong to the Vespoidea and principally to the family Vespidae or paper wasps, so called because of the papery nests

Table 10.2. Classification of Hymenoptera (excluding Formicoidea) recorded as having attacked man. (Compiled from details in Perlman 1955; McCormick 1963; James and Harwood 1969; Maschwitz and Kloft 1971; Ebeling 1975; Biery 1977; Richards and Davies 1977; Richards 1980. The superscript letters indicate references in the footnotes)

Species	Remarks
Vespoidea; Vespidae; Vespinae	Paper wasps
Vespa crabro L	European hornet; introduced into North America
V. c. germana (Christ)	Giant hornet; Europe and Northeastern America
Vespula maculata L	Bald-faced hornet; most dangerous species in USA[a]
V. vulgaris (L)	Holarctic distribution
V. germanica (F)	
V. pennsylvanica (Saussure)	Yellow jacket; severe pest in California[b]
V. atropilosa	All *Vespula* and *Dolichovespula* species are common in California[b]
V. maculifrons (Brysson)	Hornet
V. squamosus (Drury)	
V. vidna (Saussure)	
V. sulphurea (Saussure)	
Dolichovespula arenaria (F)	
D. maculata (L)	
Polistinae	Umbrella wasps; very numerous. Spindle-shaped abdomen Infests buildings and fruit areas[b]
Polistes pallipes	
P. fuscatus (F)	Several varieties; very abundant in California[b]
P. apachus (Saussure)	Fruit-growing areas; very aggressive[b]
P. dorsalis californicus R. Bohm	
P. exclamans exclamans Viereck	Very painful sting but not aggressive[b]
P. e. arizonicus Snelling	Citrus orchards; very painful sting[b]
Sphecoidea	Predacious on Diptera and others[c]
Sphecidae species	Mud dauber wasps; sting rarely[b] but sting can be painful and cause hypersensitivity[a]
Pompiloidea; Pompilidae	Predacious wasps[c]
Pepsis formosa (Say)	Tarantula wasp; has caused severe local swelling[d]
Bethyloidea; Bethylidae	Parasitic on lepidopterous and coleopterous larvae[c]
Epyris californicus (Ashmead)	Numerous cases reported from California[d]
Cephalonomia gallicola (Ashmead)	Found where coleopterous larvae infest stored products; can attack man[b,d]
Scleroderma domesticum Latreille	Same occurrence as *C. gallicola*; caused multiple stings and severe anaphylactic-type reactions
Apoidea; Apidae; Apinae	
Apis mellifera	Domestic honeybee; worldwide distribution
A. m. adansoni	Wild African honeybee; introduced South America
A. dorsata	Giant bee; Indian species; sting very painful
A. indica	Indian bee } stings mild
A. flora	India } stings mild
A. cerana	Japanese or Chinese bee
Bombidae	
Various species	Bumble bees; worldwide distribution[d]
Scolioidea; Mutillidae	
Dasymutilla occidentalis (L)	A hazard for bathers on the shores of Lake Erie[d]

[a] Biery (1977); [b] Ebeling (1975); [c] Richards and Davies (1977); [d] James and Harwood (1969).

which they construct. Solitary wasps of Sphecoidea can sting, but seldom do. Morphologically wasps are medium-sized insects with an average length of 10–20 mm, although the European hornet (*Vespa crabro*) can reach a length of 35 mm (Zahradnik 1977). In *Vespula* species (Fig. 10.2) the queens are 25% longer than workers or drones, but in *Polistes* all three castes are the same size. Wasps are usually distinguishable by their black and yellow striped abdomens, the shapes and patterns of the stripes having characteristic species differences. Facial markings are also helpful distinguishing features. Table 10.2 gives a list of some of the commonest stinging Hymenoptera (excluding ants, which are discussed separately in the latter portion of this chapter).

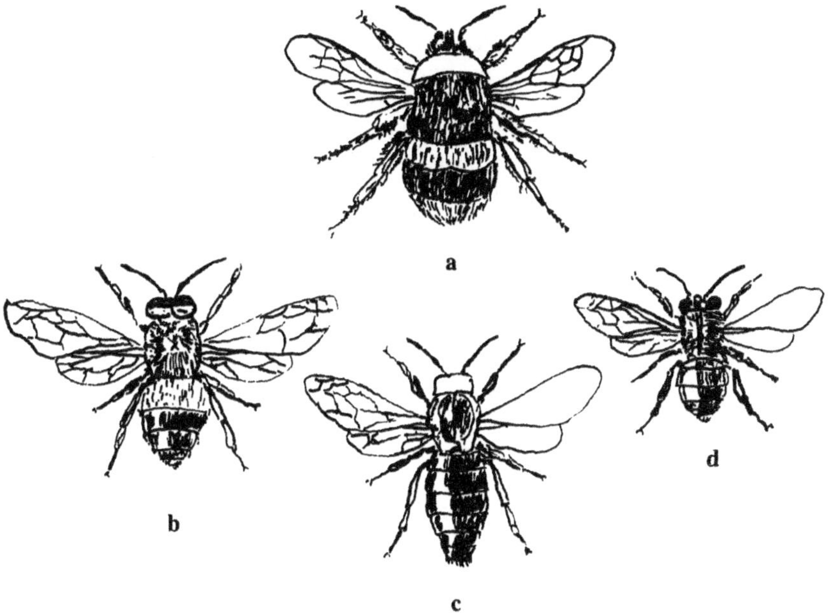

Fig. 10.1a. Bumblebee (*Bombus lucorum*) × $1\frac{1}{4}$. **b** Honeybee (*Apis mellifera*) drone × $1\frac{1}{2}$. **c** Honeybee (*Apis mellifera*), queen × $1\frac{1}{2}$. **d** Honeybee (*Apis mellifera*), worker × $1\frac{1}{2}$. [After Chinery C (1976) Field guide to the insects of Britain, 2nd edn. Collins, London]

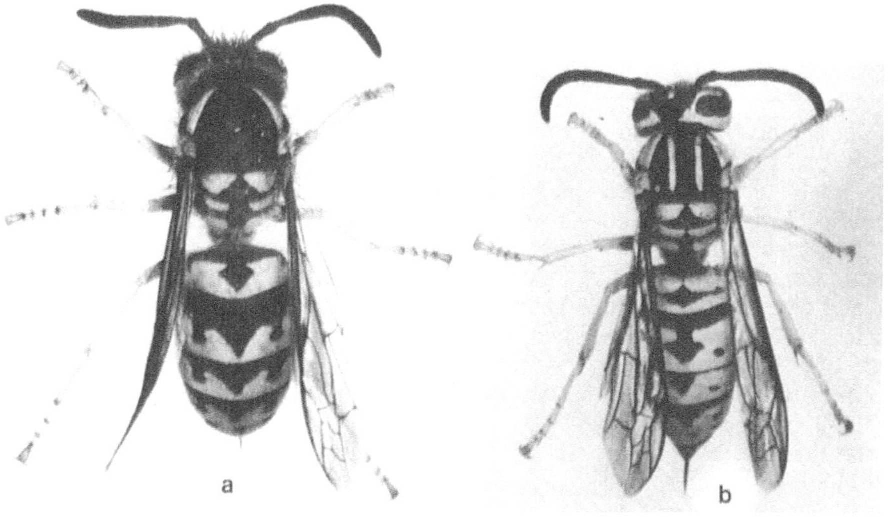

Fig. 10.2a, b. Wasps. **a** *Vespula pennsylvanica* (Western yellow jacket); **b** *V. vulgaris*. (From Ebeling 1975, by kind permission of the author and the publisher, University of California, Agricultural Publications)

Bees and Wasps

Biology

The biology of the honeybee has probably been studied more than that of any other insect. The queen mates once during flight and thereafter returns to the nest to lay up to 2000 eggs daily, one to each comb cell. After hatching, the larvae are fed by the workers and reach maturity in 15–16 days for queens (requiring special royal jelly food in an enlarged cell), 21 days for workers and 24 days for drones. The workers arise from fertile eggs and the drones from infertile eggs. The queens can live up to 5 years, although they may take flight and form another swarm during that period. The worker's life is about 3 months and that of the drone 3–4 months (Ebeling 1975).

Domesticated bee colonies were originally imported Italian strains of *Apis mellifera.* (see Fig. 10.1) Wild African bees of the variety *A. m. adonsonii* Latreille which were inadvertently imported into Brazil have now multiplied there and spread rapidly over most of South America, where the climate is suitable. It is estimated that they are moving northwards at about 200 miles per annum (Ebeling 1975). They have had a reputation for being very aggressive and attacking *en masse.* However, Ebeling avers that this aggressiveness has been exaggerated and that as the result of interbreeding with domestic bees they are in fact much the same as the latter in their habits and activities. It may well be that their "aggressive" behaviour has been a response which domestic bees would have made under similar circumstances. Bees are on their best behaviour on warm sunny days, which is when their hives should be inspected. On dull rainy days they are irritable because their food is less easily accessible, and consequently they are easily provoked to attack man. They are also more likely to attack as a result of sudden movements such as waving the arms about to ward off a suspected attack. They are attracted by flower-scented cosmetics, bright-coloured, loose clothing and sweet foods and drinks out of doors (Frazier 1966). If they are disturbed they will attack, and if their nest is threatened they will not only attack but release signal pheromones to summon other workers to assist them in combating the threat.

Bumblebees (see Fig. 10.1) are very widespread in distribution but relatively more frequent in temperate climates. According to Ebeling (1975), they can be found in Arctic latitudes and at elevations up to 396 m (1300 ft) in temperate regions. The bumblebee queen must hibernate after fertilisation, in a protected place such as a hole in the ground or in a tree. In the spring a nest is made, a store of honey is installed and the eggs are laid in cells. These hatch in 3–5 days, feed on the store of food supplied and further maternal supply by the queen. The emerging workers then take over, continue nest building and tending the larvae hatched from further eggs. Eventually further queens and then drones appear and the cycle starts again for the next year, with the current year's workers, queens and drones all dying.

Bumblebees attack for similar reasons to those given for honeybees, except that whereas a threat to the nest evokes a vigorous attack, the further away from the nest they are the less aggressive they become (Ebeling 1975).

Social wasps have many biological similarities to honeybees. Their nests are constructed of a papery material made by masticating wood fibre into a pulp. Wherever the nest is constructed it is still composed of this material. *Vespula* species (yellow jackets) (see Fig. 10.2) nest in holes in the ground, in between stones in walls or in tree roots. They are often found in orchards, where they form an increased hazard by becoming intoxicated by fermenting fruit juice (Lawson Tait 1893; Frazier 1966). According to Edery et al. (1978) the stimulus to aggressive defence of the underground nest is the vibration of footsteps close to the nest, and the numerical response is in proportion to the extent of the disturbance. The defence flight is brief, lasting from $1\frac{1}{2}$ to 5 min and confined to a radius of about 7 m around the nest. Only wasps of Vespinae produce alarm pheromones. Hornets (*Vespa* species) build large spherical nests hanging from the branches of trees. There may be up to 12 000 in a colony, which defend their nest aggressively and can be dangerous to man (Edery et al. 1978). *Polistes* species tend to nest in buildings, beneath the eaves, in attic space and under window sills. Their nests hang from the supporting structure and have a population of up to several hundred. (Frazier 1966). (Escaped honeybees may also build their nests in attics and similar enclosed spaces. They are much larger structures with broad base and a curved outer free wall. The present writer has found three such old nests on his premises. One was 90–120 cm across and about 45 cm deep.)

Stinging Apparatus

The stinging apparatus of bees and wasps is a modified ovipositor, which itself is a modified

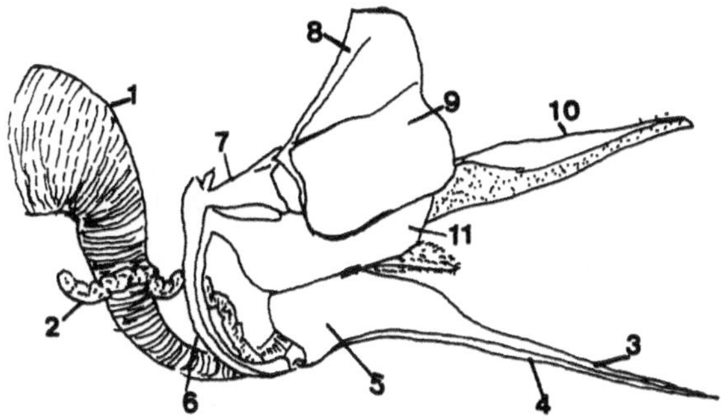

Fig. 10.3. Stinger apparatus from the honey bee (*Apis mellifera*). *1*, Poison reservoir; *2*, alkaline gland; *3*, stylet (second gonapophysis); *4*, lancet (first gonapophysis); *5*, bulb; *6*, rami of gonapophyses; *7*, gonangulum; *8*, apodeme; *9*, tergum (quatrate plate); *10*, gonoplac; *11*, second gonocoxa. (From Snodgrass 1935, by kind permission of the publisher, McGraw Hill)

eighth abdominal segment and consists of three parts (Fig. 10.3). The actual piercing section or stinger is a complicated structure composed of a dorsal sharp stylet and two ventrolateral barbed lancets. Together these enclose the venom canal, which communicates posteriorly with the poison sac. The skeletal support for the apparatus is comprised of chitinised plates. The actual poison apparatus consists of a pair of coiled glands which discharge through a common opening into the poison sac. Also discharging into this sac is the secretion of the alkaline gland. The function of the latter is unknown, but Chapman (1971) suggests it may have a lubricating action. The mixed gland secretions constitute the venom.

The bee stings by gripping the victim's skin with its claws and jabbing the stinger sharply into the skin. The barbed tip of the lancets give purchase for the stylet to be driven in deeper and deeper. At the same time compression of the venom sac injects venom through the stinger canal into the victim. Because the barbs prevent the stinger from being withdrawn from human skin (it can be withdrawn from insect victims; Ebeling 1975), the whole apparatus is torn out of the bee when it flies away and it subsequently dies. The retained stinger continues to penetrate and to pump in more venom automatically unless removed (by scraping with a fingernail or knife-edge, but not by seizing with forceps, which will only squeeze more venom into the wound). The wasp, on the other hand, can withdraw its stinger and sting again because it has either very small barbs or none at all at the tip of its lancet.

Venom

Venom has been collected from bees in a variety of ways (Benson and Semenov 1930; Loveless and Fackler 1956; O'Connor et al. 1963; Benton et al. 1963). Only the techniques of the latter two groups produce pure venom. The most productive is that of Benton and his colleagues, who, by electrical stimulation, induced large numbers of bees in hives to deposit venom through a sheet of nylon material onto glass or the undersurface of the nylon. In this way they were able to "milk" whole hives. It required 20 hives to provide 1 g of pure venom. The chemical contents of venom have been listed and discussed in great detail by Habermann (1971) and by O'Connor and Peck (1978) and Edery et al. (1978). The details compiled from their papers are summarised in Tables 10.3 and 10.4. Edery et al. thought that the initial pain was probably due to serotonin, although kinins may account for much pain in wasp stings. Ebeling (1975) has suggested that the pain of bee and wasp stings is due to formic acid, but there is no evidence that this is present in the venom of these insects. A considerable amount of the clinical effects of stings by bees and wasps must be due to histamine. It is not only present in the venom but there are several constituents—mellitin, mast cell degranulating peptide, phospholipase A (indirectly through its active product lysolecithin)—which all cause histamine release from the victim's own cells. Added to this is the histamine releasing effect of hypersensitivity reaction following repeated stings, many of the venom ingredients having antigenic properties or acting as haptens for the same purpose. Foubert and Stier (1958) showed by gel diffusion that there were antigens common to honeybees, yellow jackets, wasps, yellow and black hornets but with varying potency. Experimentally they demonstrated that homologous antigen caused fatal anaphylactic shock in sensitised guinea pigs, whereas heterologous antigen caused less shock or none at all. Hoffman (1977) has confirmed that some of these constituents are antigenic by showing that sera react by radioallergosorbent tests (RAST) to several of them. Hoffman and Shipman (1975) noted that 14 out of 15 sera tested reacted with phospholipase A. They also separated other antigens (Hoffman and Shipman 1976) which were immunologically distinct from hyaluronidase and in some instances from phospholipase A. Sobotka et al. (1976b) concluded that phospholipase A was the main allergen of honeybee venom. Aukrust et al. (1982) by crossed radioimmunoelectrophoresis identified phospholipase A, acid phosphatase, hyaluronidase and

Table 10.3. Constituents of the venom of bees, wasps and hornets and their pharmacological effects. The percentage figures refer to percentage of dried venom. (After Habermann 1971; Edery et al. 1978; O'Connor and Peck 1978)

Biochemical group	Bee venom	Wasp venom[b]	Hornet venom[b]	Pharmacological effects
Biogenic amines	Histamine 0.9–1%	Histamine	Histamine	Vasodilatation; ICP; pain; smooth muscle stimulant
	—[a]	Serotonin	Serotonin	Pain
	—	—	Acetylcholine	
Peptides and small proteins	Apamin 2%	—	—	CNS stimulant
	Mellitin 2%	—	—	Pain; ICP; cell damage; direct haemolysis; circulatory; neuromuscular and smooth muscle stimulant; ganglion synpase blocker releases histamine; synergistic with phospholipase A; antigenic
	MCD peptide 2%	—	—	Releases histamine and heparin
	—	Wasp kinin	Hornet kinin	Hypotensive effect; smooth muscle stimulant; pain possibly
	Protease inhibitor			
Enzymes	Phospholipase A 12%	Phospholipase A	Phospholipase A	Indirect haemolysis; slow smooth muscle contraction; hypotensive; conjunctival irritant retards blood coagulation; cellular respiratory enzyme inhibitor; releases histamine; antigenic
	—	Phospholipase B	Phospholipase B	
	Hyaluronidase	Hyaluronidase	Hyaluronidase	Increases spread of tissue fluids and substances in solution; antigenic
	Esterases			
	Phosphatases			

[a] Serotonin, dopamine and noradrenaline all said to be present, but not in dried venom (O'Connor and Peck 1978).

[b] See Table 10.4.

Table 10.4. Showing in more detail than Table 10.3. the pharmcological content of the venoms of Vespidae. (Compiled from Edery et al. 1978)

Pharmacological substances	Remarks
Low molecular weight material	
Acetylcholine	*Vespa* spp.
Histamine	*Vespa* spp.; *Vespula* spp., some *Polistes* spp. Histamine content of *Vespa crabro* and *Vespula vulgaris* is higher than that of any other arthropod venom
Dopamine	Not in *Polistes*
Noradrenaline	Not in *Polistes*
Kinins	Not in *Vespula maculata*. Wasp kinins are of various groups, differ somewhat from other kinins and are a principal cause of pain from stings
Serotonin	In all except *Vespula maculifrons*. Also an important cause of pain from stings
Enzymes	
Cholinesterase	Not in *Vespa orientalis*
Histidine decarboxylase	In *Vespula* spp.
Phospholipase	In *Vespa* spp.
Acid, alkaline or neutral DNA-ase	In *Vespa orientalis*
Hyaluronidase	In all species
Protease	In *Vespa* spp. and *Vespula* spp.
Poly- and disaccharidases	In *Vespa orientalis*

mellitin in bee venom, confirming their antigenicity, and proposed that they should be regarded as a group of similar antigens.

Clinical Effects

Stings by bee and wasp are so common as to be an almost universal risk wherever these arthropods exist and in the appropriate season in temperate climates. *Polistes* wasps are house dwellers; if conditions are suitable in cold weather, they may become active and can thus sting at any time of year (Mueller 1971). However, some persons are more vulnerable than others, e.g. those with constant outdoor occupations such as agricultural workers, builders, road workers etc. Women attract these insects because of cosmetics and bright-coloured clothing. Jensen (1962) said that children were seldom stung, but this view would seem to be contrary to general experience. Frazier (1966) indicated that a sting-prone child is one who is between 5 and 8 years, plays on the lawn near flower beds, in bare feet and clad in coloured clothing of rough material. Sportsmen and women may also be targets for bees and wasps because of their constant or sudden movements (e.g. during the Wimbledon Championships, 1982).

Settipane and Boyd (1970) and Abrashami et al. (1971) found the incidence of bee sting allergy in some thousands of Boy and Girl Scouts to be 0.4% and 0.35%, respectively, that for boys being later modified to 0.8% by Settipane et al. (1972). In a survey of 3705 allergic patients Chaffee (1970) found that 14 (0.38%) gave a history of severe systemic reaction to Hymenoptera stings. Three of the 14 were aged between 10 and 19 years and the rest between 40 and 59 years. Analysing 88 recorded fatalities O'Connor et al. (1964) noted that whilst one was aged under 21 years, nearly 80% were over 40; 74% were males. The majority recorded as dying of this cause came from the southern states of the United States. Yet of 71 of known ethnic origin only 8 were not Caucasoid, although there was a high proportion of Negroids in the population. This does not necessarily mean that Negroids are stung less often, although it may be so.

The clinical features are similar for bee and wasp stings, but in specific instances there may be special features. The reactions are local and systemic and each may have a toxic or a hypersensitive mechanism. Jensen (1962) described an "ordinary local reaction" (i.e. usually caused by the first sting experienced and occurring subsequently in those who did not develop sensitivity) as comprising a burning pain quickly followed by swelling and itching of the part stung. A central white spot marked the sting site (with the additional presence of stinger and venom sac in the case of honeybee stings), the whole surrounded by an erythematous halo and occupying a total area of a few square centimetres (Figs. 10.4, 10.5). Such a reaction appears within 2–3 minutes and represents a toxic manifestation of the injected venom.

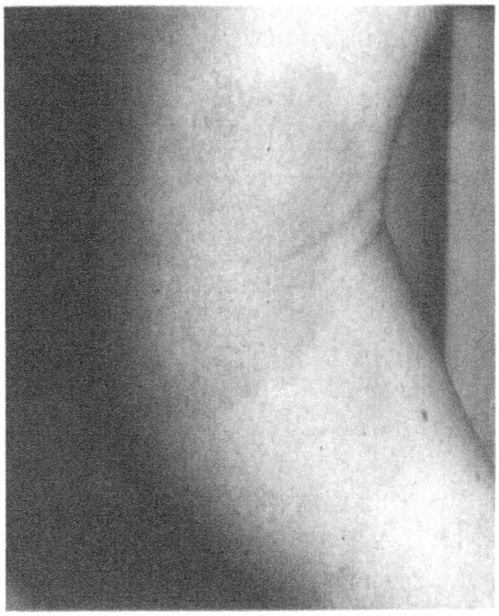

Fig. 10.4. Bee sting showing general oedema with giant urticarial reaction. (Courtesy of Prof. Ney Romiti, Sao Paulo, Brazil)

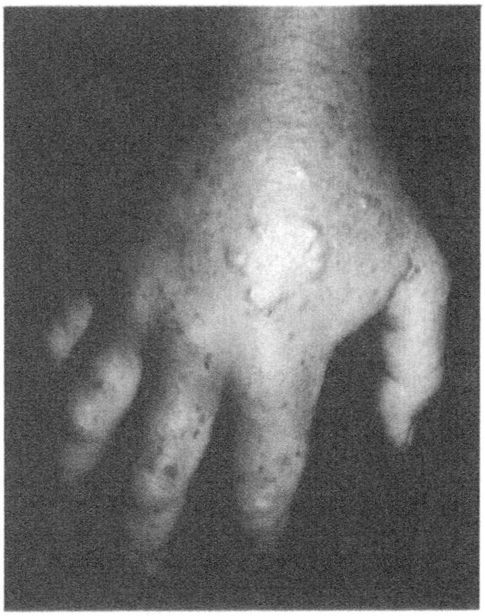

Fig. 10.5. Wasp sting showing general swelling of the hand with a bullous reaction around the centre of the lesion. (Courtesy of Dr. R. A. Fulton, Limavady, Northern Ireland)

All other appearances can be regarded as Jensen's "extraordinary local and general reactions". The actual clinical features recorded are listed in Table 10.5, compiled from papers by Derrick (1932), Jex-Blake (1942), Obermayer (1945), Reed (1946), Perlman (1955), Jensen (1962) and Barr (1974). There is no standard clinical picture which can be described as typical. From the numerous reports and classifications based on the predominant allergic features (Barnard 1966), some on clinical severity (Mueller 1959), some on timing, number and type of features (Bladek 1968), some on symptoms in increasing order of rarity and severity (Thomson, cited by Jensen 1962) and some on general grounds such as toxicity and local and general reactions (Frazier 1966), it seems preferable to outline a few of the different types of reaction recorded. Although the list of signs and symptoms in Table 10.5 is formidable, there may be only a very few in an individual patient, whilst another may experience a whole range of consecutive effects following a single sting.

An example of an acute toxic reaction probably caused by histamine is illustrated in Table 10.6.

Table 10.5. Local and general symptoms and signs of bee and wasp stings (see text for references)

Local	General
Symptoms	*Symptoms*
Pain, sharp	Pain, burning and spreading
Itch	Itch, may be intense
	Paraesthesiae; areas of anaesthesia or numbness (e.g. of lips)
	Headache; malaise
	Muscle weakness; uncontrolled spasms
	Transient paralysis including ocular
	Tonic and clonic convulsions
	Recurrent neuritis
	"Inability" to breathe; tightness of chest and pharynx; dyspnoea; wheezing
	Nausea and vomiting; diarrhoea
	Abdominal cramps
	Polyuria—occasional oliguria
	Incontinence
	Severe anginal type of praecordial pain
	Anxiety and sense of impending disaster
Physical signs	*Physical signs*
Erythema	Generalised erythema; urticaria; papular urticaria (rare)
Weals	Giant urticaria
Spreading swelling from oedema	Oedema (e.g. facial) irrespective of sting site
	Generalised "goose-flesh"
Petechial haemorrhage may spread	Pallor; cyanosis; cold, sweating skin
	Pulse may be impalpable
Blisters, delayed, rare	Tachycardia; hypotension
	Muscle hypotonia
Secondary infection with cellulitis	Mild pyrexia
	Regional lymphadenopathy
Gangrene, rare	Petechial haemorrhages
Bleeding at sting site, uncommon	Shivering and trembling
Retained bee stinger	

Table 10.6. Acute toxic reaction to a bee sting. (Compiled from Derrick 1932)

Time (min)	Features
0	Sting behind left mastoid process
2	Itching of "eyes", spread to scalp. Face flushed; eyes bloodshot; spreading redness; "gooseflesh" of shoulders, spreading to trunk
10	Anxious, shivering and trembling
15	Bright universal erythema; no urticaria. Swelling (2.5 cm) diameter at sting site. Pulse rate 90
25	Flush beginning to fade from arms
35	No evidence of any reaction. No other symptoms; felt well throughout

The effects on this young man aged 19 years were described by Derrick (1932). A much more dramatic and remarkable case with a similar cause was described by Murray (1964), in which a man of 30 was attacked without warning by a swarm of bees in the African bush. He felt an intense burning sensation all over, became momentarily unconscious and then found himself standing in the river with uncontrollable diarrhoea and vomiting and a severe headache, but with no respiratory difficulty. He was forced to remain submerged except for a breathing aperture and had to bite and swallow the bees which entered his mouth. He was rescued $4\frac{1}{2}$ hours later when the bees had departed at dusk; 2243 stings were removed, including 221 from his eyelids, lips and tongue. He was shocked, cold and exhausted, with a rapid thready pulse, and his face was oedematous. Emergency treatment gave immediate partial relief and in 5 days he recovered uneventfully. Murray noted that the effects of histamine overdosage were rapid fall in blood pressure, general vasodilatation, severe headache, vomiting, diarrhoea and shock. Intense smooth muscle stimulation was indicated in this case by the rapid passage of swallowed bees through his alimentary tract.

It was postulated by Derrick that his patient might have had the venom injected intravenously—O'Connor and Peck (1978) have noted that bee venom is significantly more toxic injected intravenously than subcutaneously—a suggestion which has been advanced by others to account for rapid onset or sudden death from Hymenoptera stings. However, this suggestion has rightly been rejected for lack of evidence by Jex-Blake (1942) and by Jensen (1962). Rapid absorption could easily occur from a very vascular area such as a finger tip or lip. Rapid onset could also be due to hypersensitivity. This was probably the explanation for the reaction in the patient described by Reed (1946), who developed facial flush and headache within 2–3 min followed by oedema of nasal mucosa and asthma and then urticaria which persisted, with temporarily relief by subcutaneous adrenaline, and was followed next day by nausea and vomiting. Histamine, initially from the venom and later released by the allergic reaction, could account for most of the symptoms. The rapid onset in this instance was compounded by the patient rubbing his affected ear and compressing the venom sac and sting simultaneously.

A quite different series of events occurred in the patient described by Obermayer (1945; Table 10.7) and were attributed by him to an allergic reaction.

Sometimes a coronary infarction can be imitated, as in the case of a 44-year-old man stung by a wasp, who, within a few moments, became unconscious, cyanosed and developed convulsions. His blood pressure fell sharply and the temperature and pulse rate were elevated. After emergency treatment he recovered; subsequent ECG showed that the apparent coronary symptoms were due to anoxia (Frazier 1966). On the other hand, severe reactions can be delayed in onset. Busse et al. (1975) described how a woman aged 25 years developed rhinorrhoea, angio-oedema, coughing, tightness of the chest and generalised itch 2 h after being stung, on two separate occasions in successive summers; the second reaction was more severe than the first.

Not all reactions end favourably. Schenken et al. (1953) recorded the case of a young man aged 21 years who had developed severe abdominal cramps, nausea, vomiting and diarrhoea after a sting at the age of 18 and with no previous sting history. In the absence of treatment the symptoms had persisted for 4 days. Two years later he had suffered exactly the same reaction to a sting, except that the onset occurred within seconds of the sting and again persisted. A third sting caused the same symptoms plus shock, cyanosis and gasping respiration. He died within 25 min.

Table 10.7. Sequence of events in patient stung on left big toe. (After Obermeyer 1945)

Time	Features
0	Stung on left big toe. Immediate sharp pain on plantar surface
10 min	Tingling and stiffness of *palms*, followed by numbness and oedema of lips and tingling on scalp, axillae and genitalia. No itch but a compulsion to touch the affected area. Generalised "gooseflesh" then developed
40 min	Malaise; abdominal cramps; angio-oedema of the eyelids and lips. Sharply demarcated dusky erythema around nasolabial folds, perioral region and chin
70 min	Urticaria in bathing trunk area (with preputial oedema) spreading to whole trunk. Intense itch; tightness of chest; abdominal cramps increasing. Oedema of left big toe and anterior part of foot. Pinhead puncture on left sole.
2–3 h	Relapse after alleviation with adrenaline
24 h	Cleared completely

Shilkin et al. (1972) described two cases, one fatal, in which the patients suffered local swellings after multiple hornet stings. After 24 h the symptoms of generalised aches and pains, nausea and vomiting had progressed to oliguria, rise in blood urea, hyperkalaemia and greatly increased serum phosphokinase enzymes. Autopsy in one patient and muscle biopsy in the other confirmed severe striated muscle damage with myoglobulinuria and secondary damage. The second patient was saved by peritoneal and renal dialyses based on knowledge of the pathology gained from the first patient.

Tauphaichitr and Tuchinda (1982) recorded an unusual case where a 6-year-old Thai girl developed a severe generalised toxic thrombocytopenic purpura 36 h after two bee stings. In addition to generalised purpura the sting sites were ecchymotic. No platelets were seen in the blood film on admission to hospital but quickly reappeared within 7 days with systemic corticosteroid therapy.

These case reports indicate the wide spectrum of reaction which can occur following the various Hymenoptera stings. Leaving aside those with special features, Mueller's (1977) grouping of the general reaction of allergic type (see Table 10.8) appears to have some merit in assessing the seriousness of a particular case and the likely treatment required.

Pathology

There is very little published material concerning the histological picture of a simple uncomplicated bee or wasp sting, as biopsies are rarely done; however, according to Mann and Bates (1960), it is much the same as any insect bite. There is rapid dermal oedema with neutrophil and lymphocyte infiltration. As the oedema subsides lymphocytes increase in number, especially around blood vessels and skin appendages. Eosinophils, plasma cells and histiocytes appear later, but the whole evanescent lesion subsides in a day or two. When allergic reactions occur, the corresponding histological appearances are present (see Chap. 2, p. 5). The more detailed pathology of serious reactions is revealed in a study of the autopsy reports on some of the fatalities recorded (in Europe and North America principally). A list of the various pathological changes encountered is detailed in Table 10.9 (Thomas 1958; Mann and Bates 1960; Barnard 1962; Day 1962; Jensen 1962; McCormick 1963; O'Connor et al. 1964).

Most writers regarded respiratory tract oedema as the immediate cause of death in the majority of cases. Jensen (1962) considered cardiopulmonary symptoms aggravated by shock to be the usual cause. The general tendency has been to attribute the deaths to anaphylactic shock (Jex-Blake 1942; Mann and Bates 1960; Day 1962; Barnard 1967) or severe hypersensitivity reactions (Jex-Blake 1942; Shenken et al. 1953; Barnard 1967). The clinical effects from these two causes could be indistinguishable (Jex-Blake 1942). O'Connor and his colleagues (1964), however, felt that such a conclusion was based only on the fact that death had occurred in many instances within a few minutes of being stung. Whilst conceding that 25% of the 88 cases of wasp sting deaths they analysed could be unequivocally attributed to anaphylactic shock, they suggested that in many other cases the shock syndrome had precipitated a fatal outcome because of pre-existing atherosclerosis or other heart disease: (The sudden steep fall in blood pressure induced by the shock has a profound effect on those conditions.) Of the 88 patients 13 had a history of cardiac disease and 13 "some sort of heart failure". Against this opinion must be placed Barnard's (1967) observation that some patients with marked atherosclerosis in fact died of respiratory failure. Jensen (1962) found that only four of 34 European patients who died from Hymenoptera stings had pre-existing disease which was shown at autopsy to

Table 10.8. Grading of sensitivity reactions to Hymenoptera stings. (After Mueller 1977)

Grade	Reaction	Features
I	Slight general	Generalised urticaria; itchy; malaise; anxiety
II	General	Any of I plus two or more of: generalised oedema; constriction of the chest; wheezing; abdominal pain; nausea; vomiting; dizziness
III	Severe general	Any of I or II plus two or more of: dyspnoea; dysphagia; hoarseness or blurred speech; confusion; feeling of impending disaster
IV	Shock	Any of I, II, or III plus two or more of: cyanosis; hypotension; collapse; incontinence; unconsciousness

Table 10.9. Principal pathological findings in patients dying from bee or wasp stings

System	Reaction	Frequency
Skin	Petechial haemorrhage	F
Respiratory		
Epiglottis and larynx	Oedema	F
Trachea and bronchial tree	Frothy, blood-stained mucus	F
	Oedema	F
	Petechial haemorrhage	F
Lung tissue	Oedema	F
	Emphysema	O
Pleura	Petechial haemorrhage	O
Cardiovascular system		
Heart	Dilatation	O
	Hypertrophy	O
	Patchy fibrosis	O
Coronary vessles	Atherosclerosis	O
	Occlusion	R
Pericardium	Haemorrhage	R
Central nervous system	Cerebral oedema	F
	Petechial haemorrhage	O
	Massive haemorrhage	O
General visceral congestion and patch oedema		

F, frequent; O, occasional; R, rare.

have played a significant part in the death. Mosbech (1983) noted that there were 26 deaths in Denmark over the period 1960–1980 which were the result of wasp and bee stings. He attributed death to anaphylaxis or allergy in 80% of the cases, including 15% in which death was caused by suffocation from laryngeal oedema. The remainder of the patients were already suffering from such conditions as arteriosclerosis or heart disease, and death was precipitated by the sting. Rubinstein (1982) claimed that underlying coronary atherosclerosis appeared to be the principal mechanism of death in recorded cases, but the published evidence scarcely supports this statement. Further evidence concerning hypersensitivity is given below, but it is probably true to say that a severe reaction to bee or wasp stings, with or without a previous history of such reaction, could precipitate a fatal outcome in persons with pre-existing atherosclerosis. The odd case might also succumb to a superimposed infection such as pneumonia. Barnard (1967) also observed that some severe allergic reactions could present with haemorrhagic or central nervous system features. Hatzel and Herrera (1962) described an instance in an alcoholic with poor liver function in whom thrombocytopenia was precipitated after a bee sting. Bruising and petechiae followed, then confusion and disorientation and, about 10 days after, death from massive cerebral haemorrhage.

There seems little doubt, however, that in a significant number of cases death has been due entirely to genuine anaphylactic shock (i.e. with no previous history of any severe reaction), and in a larger number of cases of patients who have previously had one or more increasingly severe reactions, death has been due to hypersensitive reactions with very similar symptoms. The remarkable uniformity of the clinical features in many of these patients and the respiratory tract findings cannot be overlooked in this respect. Parrish (1959) has remarked on the fact that fatal Hymenoptera stings always kill with alarming rapidity. Death from the toxic effects of the venom are very rare but can occur after multiple stings (Parrish 1963).

Diagnosis

For stings with only local reactions there is seldom any difficulty in diagnosis, a history being sufficient. Small children cannot give an adequate history and they must be examined for a local lesion. The presence of a bee stinger is proof, and capture of the offending insect is valuable evidence. For systemic reactions, however, it is important to make a careful but rapid examination of the skin for a local lesion or stinger and also to make assessment of the patient's general state. The blood pressure must always be recorded, and the heart, lungs, reflexes and pupils must always be examined. It is also advisable to search for a Hymenoptera sensitisation warning card in case the patient carries one. An ECG should be arranged at the earliest convenience. If a Hymenoptera sting is suspected, any necessary emergency treatment (see p. 149) should be given first, and a detailed history and observations about the offending insect, if possible, can be obtained later. A blood sample for immunological survey and a urine specimen to test for protein, haemoglobin and myoglobin should be obtained. Only in patients whose respiration has ceased should emergency treatment precede a rapid examination.

Differential diagnosis include (1) coronary infarction, which may require an ECG to distinguish from acute sensitisation reaction; (2) cerebral vascular accident; and (3) food or drug poisoning. If nausea and vomiting have occurred the presence of a diffuse erythema suggests a possible histamine reaction and could mean an acute sensitisation in the absence of multiple stings.

Immunology

The immunological basis for the human reaction to Hymenoptera stings and the resultant prophylactic treatment have evolved over the past 50 years or so. The terms "desensitisation" and "hyposensitisation" should be abandoned in favour of "immunotherapy" and "immunisation" (Perlman (1955); Lessoff et al. 1978). At first all very severe reactions were regarded as anaphylaxis, but Jex-Blake (1942) pointed out that such reactions might be either hypersensitivity or true anaphylaxis; these are not the same but at times can have indistinguishable clinical features. Benson and Semonov (1930) recognised that many of the clinical features resembled histamine overdosage. They showed that these patients reacted strongly by skin testing to the water-soluble moiety of bee protein from the body and stinging apparatus, which they considered to be the antigen responsible. They succeeded in immunising against bee stings using these water-soluble protein extracts. Jex-Blake (1942) suggested using as an immunising agent the bee venom introduced into the United Kingdom for the treatment of rheumatism.

McCormick (1963) first demonstrated a specific antibody to wasps in the serum of a fatal case. Reisman et al. (1974), using the RAST technique for IgE antibodies, concluded that phospholipase A was the principal sensitising agent in bee venom, an opinion originally expressed by Habermann (1971) and confirmed by Sobotka et al. (1974b), by Busse et al. (1975) and by Sobotka et al. (1976b). The last group also noted that mellitin had very little antigenic activity and hyaluronidase and apamine none at all. Reisman et al. were also able to identify species-specific IgE antibodies for various Hymenoptera, a useful diagnostic identification confirmed by Sobotka et al. (1976a), in 32 of 36 patients. The four with negative results were associated with low total IgE levels, but positive results were obtained using the histamine release test. Muller et al. (1978), however, were not so certain about the specificity of some IgE antibodies to Hymenoptera, there being some cross reactivity between bees and wasps by RAST. Nevertheless, they did find that clinical hypersensitivity to wasps correlated with the IgE antibody against yellow jackets. Sobotka et al. (1974a) could demonstrate only a limited cross reactivity between honeybee and wasp venoms, whilst Sobotka et al. (1974b) noted that sensitivity to both groups seldom occurred simultaneously. Loveless and Fackler (1956) had originally observed some cross reactivity among different wasp species in the serum of patients stung. Reisman and his colleagues also considered RAST to be an excellent means of measuring hypersensitivity.

Settipane et al. (1972) confirmed a previous finding by the Insect Allergy Committee of the American Academy of Allergy (1965) that the incidence of Hymenoptera reactions was equally common in atopics and non-atopics.

Perlman (1955) had noted the high reaginic (IgE) antibody titres in pollen-sensitive patients but that immunisation with pollen antigens (injections at intervals of 1 week or more) produced specific IgG blocking antibodies. (This was in contrast to the exhaustion of specific IgG antibody in sensitive patients by repeated injection of the corresponding antigen at very short intervals—true desensitisation.) Using the RAST technique Busse et al. (1975) demonstrated an increase in similar specific IgG blocking antibody and a reduction in IgE titre after immunisation with pure venom (confirmed by Urbanek et al. 1978). Sobotka et al. (1976b) found IgG blocking antibodies to bee venom to be present only in the serum of bee keepers and those who had been immunised with venom. IgE antibody to phospholipase A was found in the serum of these patients. Sobotka et al. (1976c) showed that passive immunisation with a preparation of human antiphospholipase A IgG antibody raised the recipient's specific IgG blocking antibody level some two to three times, but active immunisation with phospholipase A raised it by 20 to 150 times. Lessoff et al. (1976) noted that temporary passive immunisation with IgG blocking antibody did not impair the patient's ability to develop his own specific IgG antibody as a result of active immunisation. Immunisation with venom raised the IgG antibody by only two or three times but was sufficient to provide good clinical protection against bee stings in patients who had previously suffered life-threatening reactions. This finding was confirmed by Sobotka et al (1976a). Valentine et al. (1976) indicated that specific IgE antibody rose initially at the same time but fell later during the immunisation process. They also found that they could estimate the amount of free antigen remaining after a sting, and this allowed them to assess the quantity of antibody required for clinical protection. Lessoff and his colleagues (1976) also observed that there was no relationship between the levels of specific IgE antibody and the clinical reaction to venom. It is interesting to note that Hoveler et al. (1983) found 55 of 200 persons to have "silent sensitisation" to bee or wasp venom by demonstrating positive IgE/RAST reactions to one or other of these venoms. Only 9 of the 55 had positive IgG blocking antibodies, the remaining 46 IgE positive patients having neither blocking antibodies nor symptoms.

Loveless (1962b) had said that, although she had become sensitive to wasp stings whilst collecting specimens for their venom, under no circumstance would she consent to receiving injections of whole body extract (WBE) or be skin tested by it. Her opinion was vindicated when Hunt et al. (1978a, b) pointed out that immunisation with WBE gave rise to repeated clinical reactions akin to the serum sickness syndrome (and that these reactions did not recur when the WBE injections were discontinued), and that specific IgE antibodies to WBE proteins not present in venom developed. Patients who were sensitive to Hymenoptera venom but not immunised with WBE showed no such antibodies. Immunisation with venom caused no symptoms but gave protection. Muller et al. (1978) had shown by RAST inhibition tests that the IgE antibodies detected for WBE were in fact directed against the venom component of WBE.

Immunotherapy

Many workers have preferred to use mixed WBE for immunisation because they considered that it rather than venom contained the responsible antigen (Mueller 1959) and because the offending insects were accurately identified in only 10% of cases (Mueller 1962). The Insect Allergy Committee (1964, 1965) agreed and found that WBE immunisation caused diminished reaction to test stings in 89% of patients (10% in non-immunised controls). Although 3% were worse off, nevertheless they recommended WBE immunotherapy for *all* patients who had experienced systemic reactions. Frazier (1964, 1977) concurred, arguing that immunised patients were undoubtedly better off than the non-immunised. Mueller (1971, 1977) said that WBE immunotherapy was still effective, that the results were dose related and should continue to be used because modern substitutes were not yet fully established. On the other hand, Torsney (1973) cited eight fatalities from Hymenoptera stings in persons immunised with WBE (some, admittedly, inadequately). Other workers are against the use of WBE because it produced other antibodies in the recipients (see above) and are against immunising all who have had systemic reactions. They would confine immunotherapy to persons who have had life-threatening reactions (Loveless 1962a; Valentine et al. 1976; Urbanek et al. 1982). Rubenstein (1980a, b, 1982) would agree with the latter groups since he criticised the blanket recommendation of the Insect Allergy Committee and did not see how it was possible to predict future lethal reaction, particularly since some of the recorded deaths had occurred in persons with no previous history of stings.

The identification and qualification of specific IgE antibody and blocking IgG antibody recently achieved now offers an in vitro method of identifying many (but not all) possible future victims. Moreover, the objection of ineffectiveness and the production of marked side-effects levelled at WBE immunotherapy does not hold for pure venom immunisation, and if phospholipase A becomes freely available for immunotherapy it can be given in an accurately measured dose as can dried venom. However, these preparations are not yet commercially available on an adequate and economic scale; until then WBE may still have a place in immunotherapy, rather than give no protection in spite of the risks. Rubenstein's argument against this, that even one death due to treatment shows a higher mortality rate than the disease it is purporting to prevent, is false, since, in spite of the percentages and rates per million quoted, the fact remains that some 40 persons die annually in the United States from Hymenoptera stings, whereas the total number of recorded deaths directly as a result of immunisation by whatever means is probably no more than two or three.

Immunisation with WBE

Mueller's (1959) technique started by assessing the minimum reaction dose (MRD) by intradermal testing. The initial dilution for the tests was always 1 in 100 000 000. The MRD on average was 1 in 10 000 and 0.5 ml was injected subcutaneously, the dose being increased weekly until a dilution of 1 in 100 was reached or a local reaction exceeding 3 cm diameter was seen. Further injections at gradually lengthening intervals were given until a final dose level of 0.2–0.3 ml of 1 in 10 extract was achieved. This gave adequate clinical protection. Thereafter maintenance doses of the same strength were given at 3-monthly intervals more or less indefinitely. By 1977 Mueller had modified this to annual booster doses with better effect. He noted that no patient receiving injections of 0.2 ml of 1 in 10 extract had any reaction to stings during the resting phase. Coleman et al. (1974) used a similar regimen with intervals between injections of 1, 2 and 3 months respectively in the first, second and third years. The results did not seem as good as those obtained by Mueller. Ordman (1965) had 9 failures in 59 patients immunised. In his opinion subsequent stings in some immunised patients appeared to reduce the immunity that had been acquired. This is curious in view of Loveless' experience (see below).

Frazier (1966) stressed the precautions required during immunotherapy, which apply to all forms of this procedure. For convenience they are listed in Table 10.10. Tourniquets are used in this procedure to slow blood flow rather than to stop it completely.

Immunotherapy with Venom

Loveless (1962b) started immunotherapy in 1946 using lyophilised extracts of bee stinging apparatus and later WBE from yellow jackets. Venom extracts of wasps' stingers were introduced by Loveless and Fackler (1956), from which Loveless (1962a, b) progressed to using fresh venom extracted from the stingers of *Polistes* wasps. This venom was found to protect against the stings of other species, but the reverse did not hold. She treated nine patients, who had had alarming immediate reactions, by a single subcutaneous repository injection of 1.2 ml of an emulsion of venom with aracel and petrolatum. Each injection contained the equivalent of the venom from six *Polistes* sacs. There were no side-effects. Protection was shown to be adequate by subsequent, periodic, controlled test stings, which served at the same time as maintenance booster doses and were continued regularly. In a review of her experience, Loveless (1978) confirmed the success of her technique in over 400 patients since 1953. An anonymous reviewer (1981) also confirmed the value of specific dried venom extract for both bee and wasp stings, although using a different dosage schedule over a 2-year period. The cost of the material alone was over £250 for bee stings (and more for wasp stings) for a 2-year course. Valentine et al. (1976) treated 10 patients, all with previous life-threatening episodes, of whom 4 were WBE failures. Each was immunised by a specific venom selected by histamine release tests, the injections being started with the MRD and increased until the patient tolerated twice the amount of one sting.

Table 10.10. Precautions to be taken during immunotherapy. (After Frazier 1966)

Feature	Precautions
Injections	Always subcutaneous Always on a limb Always under the supervision of the physician
Dosage	Maximum starting dose = MRD as ascertained by skin testing Next dose not to be increased if the reaction exceeds 3 cm diameter
Reactions	Watch every injection for a reaction Keep patient in vicinity for 30 min after injections Always have tourniquet and adrenaline to hand Always treat any untoward reaction as necessary: e.g. Mild reaction—oral antihistamine or isoprenaline Severe reaction—adrenaline, intramuscular antihistamine, corticosteroids, oxygen, plasma, etc. as required
Patient self-help	If reaction occurs after leaving surgery, return at once Always carry sublingual isoprenaline or oral antihistamine Always carry card warning of possible systemic reaction to bees and wasps

This was achieved in 10 weeks in one patient by a rush technique. There was only one minor reaction to subsequent test stings. The specific IgG antibody rose in all the patients. Specific IgE antibodies also rose initially but fell subsequently, whilst the blocking IgG antibody titre continued to rise. Clinically immunisation was very effective. Golden et al. (1981) noted that the efficacy of venom therapy was dose dependent: 50 μg of dried venom, equivalent to the dry weight of one honeybee sting gave 79% protection, whereas 100 μg gave 96–100% protection. Moreover, specific IgG blocking antibody levels rose significantly higher with 100 μg than with 50 μg.

Treatment of Reactions

Bee stings should be removed by scraping (see p. 139). If the sting is in a limb and an unusual reaction is developing, a tourniquet should be applied and released every few minutes. Local reactions of a non-allergic type seldom require treatment, although Spencer (1968) has noted that the injection of 0.3 ml of 1% xylocaine with 1 in 100 000[1] adrenaline beneath each wasp sting will instantly and permanently relieve the pain of the sting. An application such as calamine lotion is probably all that is ever needed. For the more massive oedematous reactions, which are usually associated with systemic symptoms of varying severity, topical applications of corticosteroid creams may help, together with oral antihistamines such as promethazine 25 mg (Phenergan), repeated in an hour if necessary. Topical antihistamines have been recommended but they have no antihistaminic effect when applied topically, although they may have a mild anaesthetic action. If swelling is severe intramuscular antihistamines can be used (e.g. promethazine 50 mg).

Systemic reactions, after a preliminary examination (as indicated under Diagnosis, p. 145), require subcutaneous or intramuscular adrenaline given slowly at the rate of one minim (= 0.06 ml) per minute up to a total of 0.3 ml. This may have to be repeated for very severe reactions. Intravenous hydrocortisone 100 mg in a fairly rapid drip infusion of normal saline followed by oral prednisolone (40 mg daily) may be required. Shock may necessitate oxygen or a plasma transfusion, whilst respiratory embarrassment from oedema may indicate a tracheostomy. Diuretics to reduce pulmonary and other oedema may be needed (e.g. frusemide 40 mg intramuscularly). Transfer to hospital should be arranged as quickly as possible but should not delay prompt treatment. Biery (1977) gave some very useful schedules, to which reference should be made.

[1] Present writer believes this should read "1000".

Emergency Kit

Patients likely to develop or having previous experience of attacks should always carry emergency kits on their person. They and one or two close and reliable relatives (e.g. spouse or parent) should be carefully instructed in the correct use of these kits, especially in the administration of adrenaline. The first signs of an attack, such as flushing, wheezing, coughing, dyspnoea or severe headache following a sting, are indications of need for treatment. Sublingual isoprenaline, or inhalations of adrenaline or cromoglycate may be sufficient. If the symptoms increase, subcutaneous adrenaline is required. A tourniquet should be applied if the sting is on a limb, and the patient should be made aware of the necessity for its periodic release. The patient should lie down because of hypotension. Samples of urine should be taken and any insect captured if possible. Detailed contents of an emergency kit are listed in Table 10.11.

Table 10.11. Contents of emergency kit for persons hypersensitive to Hymenoptera stings. (Based on Frazier 1966)

Tourniquet
Antiseptic adhesive dressings
Mediswabs
Syringes: Two each of 1 ml capacity; disposable.
Needles: Four hypodermic size; disposable.
Oral drugs:
Three antihistamine tablets[a]
Three isoprenaline sublingual tablets, 10 mg each
Isoprenaline nebuliser. *Warning*: Do not overuse
Injections:
Adrenaline hydrochloride 1 in 1000 for subcutaneous use
Two ampoules of 0.5 ml each containing 1 mg per ml
Two antihistamine ampoules[b] for intramuscular use

[a] One of the following: promethazine 25 mg each; diphenhydramine 50 mg each; chlorpheniramine 4 mg each.

[b] One of the following: promethazine 50 mg in 2 ml; chlorpheniramine 10 mg in 1 ml.

Instructions should also be included in each kit.

Avoidance of Stings

Frazier (1966) listed measures which would help to avoid exposure to stings (see Table 10.12). He indicated that repellent applications were effective against Hymenoptera. Edery et al. (1978) have noted that 2,4-hexadienyl butyrate is a specific attractant for yellow jackets. Thousands can be trapped if it is used as bait.

Table 10.12 Measures to be taken to avoid unnecessary exposure to stings. (After Frazier 1966)

1. Keep doors and windows effectively screened during summer
2. Keep backyard and disposal bins and bags for rubbish clean and tidy
3. Avoid orchards during the fruit season, especially when fruit ripening
4. Wear light but not bright clothing out of doors
5. Small children should always wear shoes or boots when out of doors
6. Avoid perfume and scented hair sprays out of doors
7. Inspect premises each spring and summer for fresh nests
8. If you are sensitive to stings, hire a professional to deal with any nests on the premises

Ants

Ants comprise the superfamily Formicoidea (see Table 10.1). This group is subdivided into two complexes, Myrmecioid and Poneroid (Wilson 1971), the subfamilies in each of which are shown in Table 10.13. Apart from the Myrmeciinae, which are almost exclusively Australian, some genera of other subfamilies are to be found in almost every part of the world. Those species which have been recorded as particularly affecting man are enumerated in Table 10.14. There are doubtless very many more species which can or have attacked man (his skin particularly), but the literature consulted says very little regarding either their identification or the damage they can cause.

Morphologically, ants conform to the general structure of Hymenoptera. The demarcation between the head, thorax and abdomen is particularly well marked (see Figs. 10.6, 10.7, 10.8). The head varies greatly in size and shape, not only from species to species but also in the different forms in the same colony. The males and females are winged for the nuptial flight but otherwise ants are wingless. The males have compound eyes and three ocelli. The females and workers of Ponerinae, Dorylinae and Myrmeciinae all have powerful sting apparatus and are carnivorous, but all the other families are vegetarian and the sting apparatus is atrophic or vestigial.

Cavill and Robertson (1965) enumerated ten different groups of secreting glands in ants. The most important of these, from man's point of view, are given in Table 10.15, along with the primary function of these secretions. The chemicals produced vary widely and have quite different effects, which are set out in broad general terms in Table 10.16. Those species with proteinaceous components in the venom are potentially capable of inducing sensitisation reactions similar to those caused by bees and wasps. Other reactions include

Table 10.13. Subdivision of superfamily Formicoidea (After Wilson 1971)

Formicoidea

Myrmecioid complex	Poneroid complex
Subfamilies	*Subfamilies*
1. Myrmeciinae	6. Ponerinae
2. Pseudomyrmecinae	7. Cerapachynae (sometimes included in 6)
3. Formicinae	8. Leptanillinae
4. Dolichoderinae	9. Dorylinae
5. Aneuretinae (sometimes included in 4)	10. Myrmicinae

Table 10.14. List of ants known to sting man. Mostly from North America. (Compiled from various sources, notably James and Harwood 1969; San Martin 1971)

Species	Remarks
MYRMECIOID COMPLEX	
Myrmeciinae	Contains many species of aggressive stinging ants
Myrmecia gullosa	Australian red bull ant
M. pyriformis	
Pseudomyrmecinae	
Pseudomyrmex pallidus	
Formicinae	
Formica occidentalis Forel	
F. obscuripes Emery	
F. haemorrhoidalis Emery	
F. pilicosus Emery	
F. fusca L	Silky ant
F. exsectoides Forel	Allegheny mountain ant
F. rufa	
Dolichoderinae	
Iridomyrmex humilis Mayr	Argentine ant; a vicious biter.

Table 10.14. (*continued*)

Species	Remarks
PONEROID COMPLEX	
Ponerinae	
Paraponera clavata	Brazilian species; causes severe pain.
Dorylinae	
Eciton spp.	Army ants
Myrmicinae	
Myrmica rubra	British species; can sting freely[a]
M. ruginodes Nylander	
Solenopsis geminata (Fabr)	Common fire ant[b]
S. saevissima richteri Forel	Imported fire ant; South American species introduced into USA
S. geminata rufus	Hawaiian fire ant; not aggressive[c]
S. xyloni	Southern fire ant[b]
S. invicta	Imported fire ant
S. arirea	Seldom stings in the USA[c]
Pogonomyrmex barbatus (F. Smith)	Red harvester ant
P. californicus (Buckley)	Californian harvester ant
P. occidentalis (Cresson)	Western harvester ant; widespread in North America[b]
P. badius (Latreille)	Florida harvester ant; the only harvester ant east of the Mississippi[d]
P. rugosus Emery	
Monomorium bicolor	A widespread genus in India and Africa[e]
Monomorium spp.	

The superscript letters indicate the following references:
[a] Bolton and Collingwood (1975); [b] Ebeling (1975); [c] Arnold (1957); [d] Biery (1977); [e] Patton and Evans (1929).

histamine effects, either from the venom of hundreds of stings or through the effect of sensitisation, and also the local necrotic effect produced by the amino acid content of *Solenopsis* venom. Histamine effects have been observed especially with *Myrmecia forficata*, an Australian ant, the venom of which contains 2% of histamine. (De la Lande et al. 1963) and a histamine-releasing substance

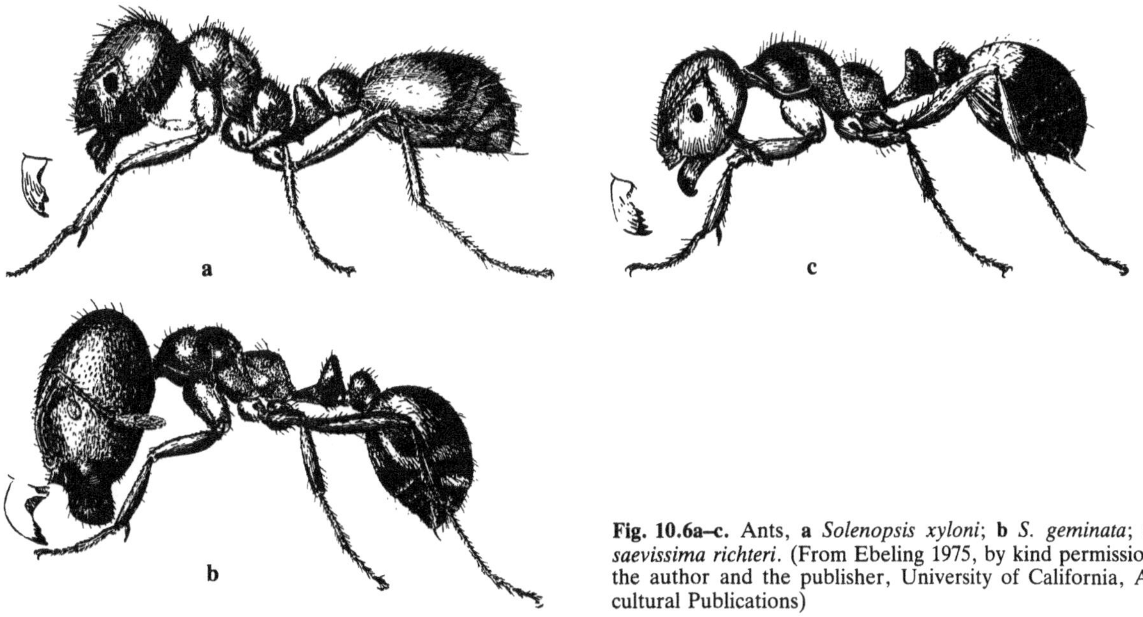

Fig. 10.6a–c. Ants, **a** *Solenopsis xyloni*; **b** *S. geminata*; **c** *S. saevissima richteri*. (From Ebeling 1975, by kind permission of the author and the publisher, University of California, Agricultural Publications)

(De la Lande and Lewis 1966). In the Formicinae the venom contains formic acid in varying concentrations, which, in the absence of a stinger, is sprayed onto the skin and can thus have a primary contact irritant effect. Some of the many chemicals secreted for trail laying or as defensive repellents may also have a contact irritant effect on human skin. These include isomers of citronellal and geraniol, which are contained in the perfumes of many cosmetics and can cause contact dermatitis. They include the various terpenoid derivatives produced by the Dolichoderinae (Cavill and Robertson 1965). At least one species of the group *Iridomyrmex humilis*, the Argentine ant, now introduced into the United States, is a known "vicious stinger" and has caused reactions which could be of a contact nature. The relationship between all these chemical attractants and repellents and the human skin has not been studied in any detail, one reason being the difficulty of obtaining the pure secretions. Ants cannot yet be "milked" in the same manner as can bees and wasps.

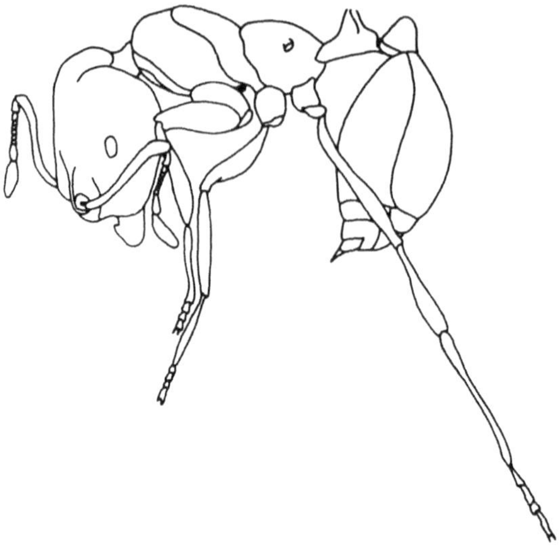

Fig. 10.7. *Solenopsis* ant. Note the humped attitude, the sharp stinger at the tip of the abdomen and the laterally directed antennae. (Courtesy of Dr. V. J. Derbes, Tulane University School of Medicine, Louisiana, USA)

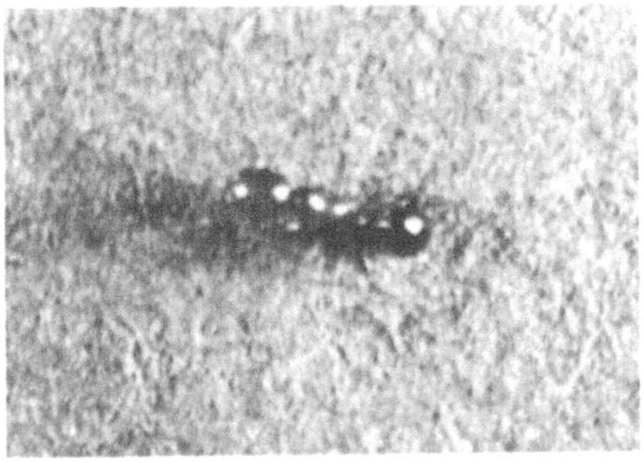

Fig. 10.8. *Solenopsis* ant. (Courtesy of Dr. V. J. Derbes, Tulane University School of Medicine, Louisiana, USA)

Table 10.15. Glandular secretions of ants, which could affect man's skin. (Compiled from Cavill and Robertson 1965)

Source	Primary function
Pharyngeal gland	Digestive
Mandibular gland	Alarm substances
Venom gland	Offensive and defensive
Dufour's gland	Stinger lubricant; trail odour
Anal gland	Defensive
Pavan's gland	Trail odour

Table 10.16. Broad division of the nature of venom and other ant secretions which could affect man. (Compiled from Cavill and Robertson 1965; Maschwitz and Kloft 1971; Blum and Hermann 1978)

Secretory content	Subfamily	Remarks
Protein (including hyaluronidase; phosphlipase A)	Ponerinae Myrmeciinae Pseudo-myrmecinae Myrmicinae Dorylinae	Potential sensitisers
Histamine	*Myrmecia* spp. *Myrmica* spp.	Histamine effects
Other amines (including 2,6-dialkyl piperidine)	*Solenopsis* spp.	Insecticidal and haemolytic properties
Formic acid	Formicinae	Involuted stinger; venom sprayed; contact reaction possible
Terpenoid derivatives	Dolichoderinae Formicinae	Complex of citral derivatives; alarm and trail laying; potential cause of contact reactions

Nests of ants vary with species and locality. They may be below the ground level, in various shaped mounds above the ground (Fig. 10.9), beneath rocks, logs, in hollow trees or even suspended from the trees. In cases of attack on man a knowledge of the type of nest involved may help in identification, which is, however, a matter for an expert.

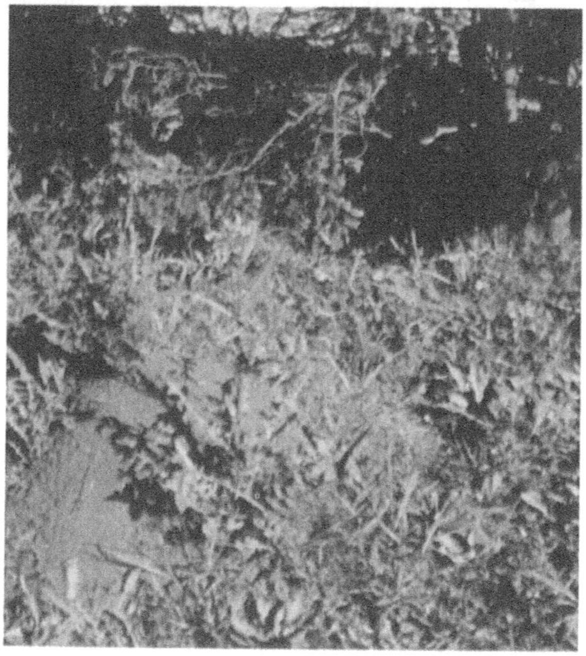

Fig. 10.9. *Solenopsis* ant mound. (Courtesy of Dr. V. J. Derbes, Tulane University School of Medicine, Louisiana, USA)

Clinical Effects

The clinical effects of ant stings are dependent on the method of using the stinger, on the venom content and whether the reaction is local or has added systemic features. The first action of the ant, whatever its species, is to fix itself to the skin by its powerful mandibles. This enables it to use the stinger in the manner appropriate to its genus.

Solenopsis Stings

Skin reactions to the sting of *Solenopsis saevissima* (the fire ant) were vividly described by Caro et al. (1957). The individual lesions were reproduced on volunteers. Their progression and appearance have been delineated in Table 10.17 (see also Figs. 10.10, 10.11). Solenopsis ants tend to sting several times without letting go with the mandibles. To do this the body rotates around the head, the stinger being re-inserted several times. The lesions thus appear characteristically in small clusters

Table 10.17. Sequence of events in development of the lesion caused by stings by *Solenopsis* spp. (Adapted from Caro et al. 1957)

Solenopsis stings	
Immediate erythema ↓	2.5–5.0 cm diameter
Central weal ↓	2–10 mm diameter. Persists up to 1 h
½–2 h: Small papule ↓	
4 h: Vesicle ↓	may rupture and dry
8–10 h: Pustules (sterile) ↓	
24 h: Umbilication	with narrow red halo or more commonly oedematous patch beneath cluster of pustules
3–10 days: Rupture forming crust	Heals leaving pigmented macule or scar

(Fig. 10.11). The mandibular bite may be marked by two tiny haemorrhagic puncta which may leave faint residual pigmentation. Although Ebeling (1975) considered the bite to be painful, most authorities thought it was imperceptible. Schmid (1977) held that this was the reason why the apparent first attack presented with severe systemic symptoms, the initial sensitising bites and accompanying stings on the feet having passed unnoticed.

The characteristic symptom of the sting is a burning itch. The features of the hypersensitivity reaction can be very marked. They are of the immediate type and may increase in severity with successive attacks (Brown 1972; Schmid 1977). A severe, rather persistent generalised itch is felt by most patients almost immediately, although in some it may take the form of tingling (Caro et al. 1957) and in others pain (Frazier 1974). Accompanying the itch an urticarial eruption spreads to involve the whole body but usually fades again within 24 h. An acute facial erythema independent of the urticaria also appears together with angio-oedema of the eyelids, tongue and oral mucosa. Laryngeal oedema may occasionally occur at any time from 1 to 12 h after the stings. Acute conjunctival injection (Brown 1972) and giant urticaria (Kennedy 1957) have also been recorded. Marked central chest pain associated with a feeling of apprehension, sometimes bordering on panic (Schmid 1977), dyspnoea and palpitation may occur within minutes of the onset or within the first hour but subside after 2 h. Simultaneously the patient may feel the effects of marked hypotension such as weakness, dizziness, a tendency to faint

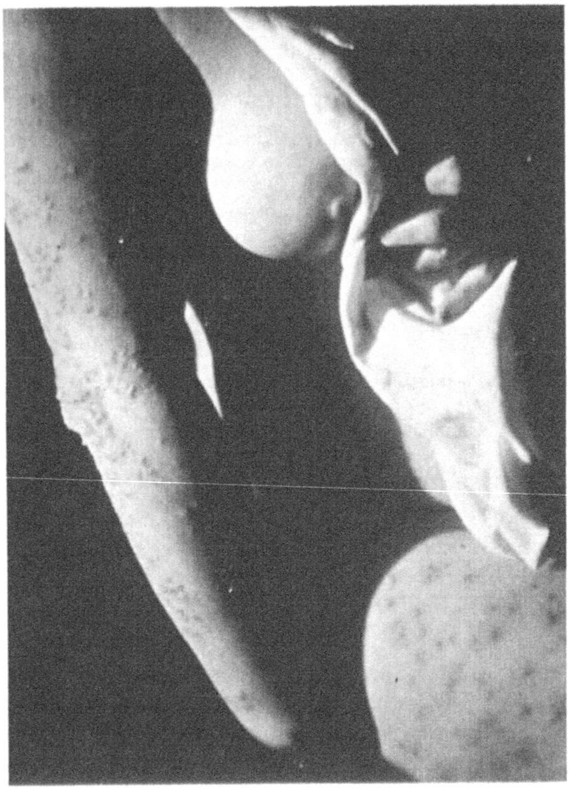

Fig. 10.10. *Solenopsis* ant stings. Note the distribution mainly on the limbs (arm and thigh), but sparing the trunk, which was protected to a great extent. (Courtesy of Dr. V. J. Derbes, Tulane University School of Medicine, Louisiana, USA)

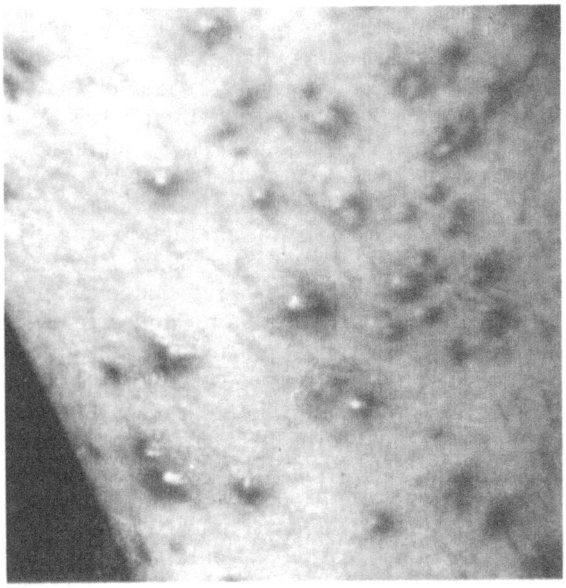

Fig. 10.11. *Solenopsis* ant stings. Note their pustular character and the large number of discrete lesions arranged in small clusters of four or five. (Courtesy of Dr. V. J. Derbes, Tulane University School of Medicine, Louisiana, USA)

when trying to stand or walk and blurring of vision. This hypotension, confirmed by examination, also recovers quickly (Brown 1972). Other recorded symptoms include wheezing, nausea, vomiting, abdominal cramps and faecal and urinary incontinence, as well as shock. Rhoades et al. (1974) analysed the incidence of these symptoms in 49 patients and found urticaria and/or angio-oedema in 33, wheezing in 10, chest tightness in 14, anaphylactic shock in 6 and nausea in 7; 15 patients were atopic and 4 had allergies to other insects. Schmid (1977) collected 325 instances of systemic reaction to *Solenopsis* stings in his own practice. The reaction seldom lasted longer than 24 h, although the skin lesions took up to 10 days to heal. Smith and Smith (1971) observed some eight to ten patients annually, all heavy drinkers, with severe *Solenopsis* sting reactions. Returning home after a drinking bout they would sleep off their imbibitions in a convenient field or yard infested with these ants, even occasionally selecting an ant heap for their pillow. They would be found next morning covered with ants, showing the characteristic pustular eruption. They felt neither itch nor pain and recovered quickly. Death has been recorded (Blum et al. 1958) but is very rare, although it is always a possibility on account of anaphylactic shock (Brown 1972). In general Ebeling (1975) estimated that up to one million persons are stung annually by *Solenopsis geminata* in the southeastern United States. Schmid's (1977) figures of 325 severe reactions would seem to support this estimate, taken in conjunction with his added remark that the vast majority of stings were uncomplicated. Secondary infection seems to occur only in very small children.

Histology. The histological changes in the skin due to *Solenopsis* stings were described in detail by Caro et al. (1957). Table 10.18 shows their findings in convenient form (see also Fig. 10.12). It was generally agreed that the picture was unlike that of any other "insect", bite although Winer (1957) remarked that, but for the absence of a lymphocytic infiltrate, it was not unlike the reaction to a tick bite. Lobitz (1957) pointed out that the initial reaction of weal, axon reflex flare and "gooseflesh" suggested a cholinergic reaction rather than a histamine effect, which might perhaps explain the non-response to antihistamine drugs.

Effects of Other Ants

Pogonomyrmex species sting in a similar manner to *Solenopsis*, but the effects are not localised. The venom apparently spreads along the lymphatics

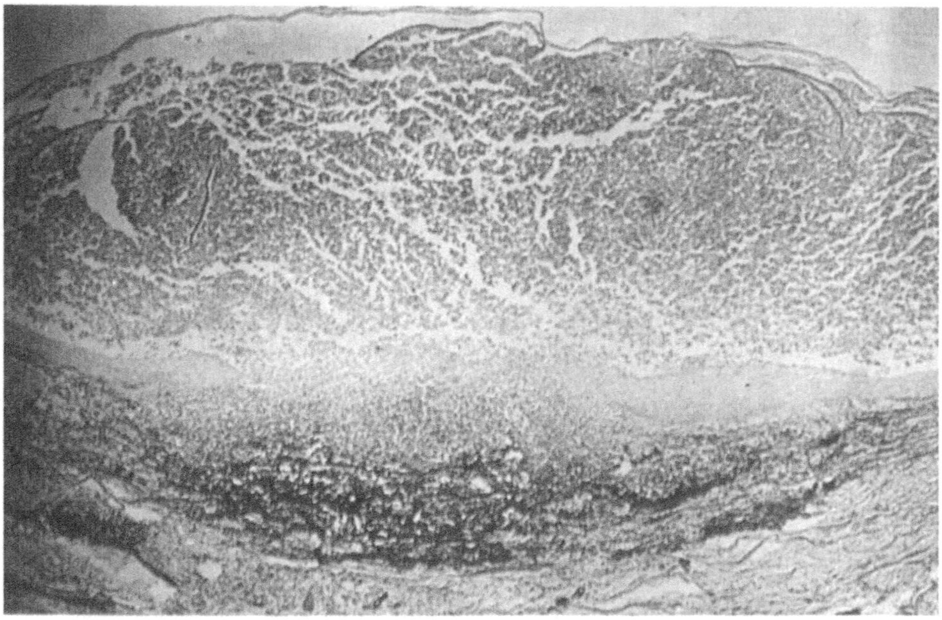

Fig. 10.12. *Solenopsis* ant sting. Low-power histological picture showing a superficial necrotic pustule. (Courtesy of Dr. V. J. Derbes, Tulane University School of Medicine, Louisiana, USA)

Table 10.18. Histology of *Solenopsis* sting reaction. (Based on Caro et al. 1957)

Time after sting	Epidermis	Corium
6 min	No change	Oedema of upper layer. Narrow perivascular cuff of L and H
30 min	Oedema, mostly intracellular; BL intact but oedematous	Superficial blood vessels dilated. Perivascular infiltrate of L, H. and Pc. Early necrosis in upper layer. Collagen fibres amorphous and poorly stained
24 h	Thin-roofed superficial pustules; sides rounded, containing many pyknotic PMN and L	Floor of pustule densely packed with necrotic collagen. Beneath floor diffuse infiltrate of PMN, L and pyknotic nucleated cells
72 h	Pustule still intact; very thin roof. Contents: E, Pc as well as PMN and L	Floor oedematous epidermis (? regrowing), except in centre where it is necrotic tissue, and inflammatory cellular infiltrate extending laterally and deeply

BL, basal layer; L, lymphocyte; H, histiocyte; Pc, plasma cell; PMN, polymorphonuclear; E, eosinophil.

(Ebeling 1975). Thus, apart from pain at the sting site, which quickly subsides, there is later aching in the corresponding regional lymph glands. *P. californicus* leaves its stinger in situ and causes severe pain.

Monomorium species (Pharaoh's ants), which are common in tropical regions of India and Africa and occur in the United Kingdom as introduced species, infest houses and attack persons in bed (Patton and Evans 1929). They cause eyelid oedema and sometimes urticaria (Chalmers and Marshall 1918). They may leave the whole head attached to the skin if disturbed during biting (Patton and Evans 1929).

Myrmica rubra is a British species which tends aphids for honeydew. These ants will sting freely and cause a localised urticarial reaction like "nettlerash" (Bolton and Collingwood 1975).

Maschwitz and Kloft (1971) regarded *Paraponera clavata*, which occurs in Brazil, as a dangerous species capable of causing painful inflammation. It is known in the Amazon basin as *viente-cuatro hora hormiga* because it is believed to kill man in 24 h. It is particularly aggressive to intruders and has a proteinaceous venom used by South American Indians to treat rheumatism (Hermann and Blum 1966). Spruce (1908), a botanist, described the effects of stings from this species. Multiple stings on the feet, legs and thighs caused him agonising burning pain, aggravated by heat and cold water, which persisted for 10 h with two exacerbations during this period. There was associated trembling of hands and feet, severe sweating and nausea. Laudanum gave some relief. Pain had subsided within 12 h, but the urticarial inflammation persisted for 30 h. Varying reactions have been reported. Weber (1939) described one sting (in the country then known as British Guiana) resulting in temporary paralysis, whereas a sting by the same species (in Panama) caused a large evanescent weal and halo with a burning pain which subsided in a few hours.

Maschwitz and Kloft (1971) noted that *Myrmecia* species could cause severe reactions because the venom contains protein, hyaluronidase and histamine, and is thus able to produce reactions as severe as bee stings.

Morhouse (1949) described an attack by an unspecified form of ant in which huge numbers were involved. "Bites" began on the forearms, quickly followed by itch, swelling of the eyelids and collapse. The entire body became covered with urticaria and there was acute, severe respiratory distress with stertorous breathing and frothy mucous expectoration. The patient was cyanosed and shocked. He recovered with intramuscular adrenaline and intravenous procaine together with oral antihistamine. It was thought that the symptoms were due to hypersensitivity to injected venom protein causing histamine release.

Treatment

Topical applications of antipruritic shake lotions such as 0.5%–1% phenol in oily calamine lotion may give relief, as may 1% hydrocortisone cream (Smith and Smith 1971). Caro et al. (1957) noted that volunteers with fire ant stings obtained no relief from fludrocortisone, antihistamines or antibiotics. Analgesics such as pethidine may be needed for severe pain. Glyceryl trinitrite did not relieve one of Caro's patients of praecordial pain, but Morhouse's (1949) patient was relieved instantly by the injection of intravenous procaine.

Systemic therapy may be necessary, mainly for histamine release effects and shock. Most patients recover within 24 h, but the regimen recommended for severe reaction to bee and wasp stings is advisable. It includes 1 in 1000 adrenaline solution—Biery (1977) recommended 0.2–0.5 ml for adults and 0.1–0.3 ml for children—subcutaneously; oral or intramuscular antihistamines, not always effective; and oral prednisolone or intravenous hydrocortisone. Specific antivenom therapy is not available and antidotes for the venoms are not known.

Control

Ebeling (1975) has advised using chlordane for domestic purposes (with appropriate precautions *carefully* observed as regards protection and dosage). In the field he suggested using microencapsulated mirex (2%) in oil drops because it is attractive to fire ants and persists on the ground. For heavy agricultural infestation application by aircraft of mirex bait (0.3% in a base of 85% corn cob grit and 14.7% soya bean oil) on three occasions will eliminate ants. Injection of calcium cyanide into the soil around individual nests is also very effective against fire ants (Ebeling 1975).

References

Abrishami MA, Boyd GK, Settipane GA (1971) Prevalence of bee sting allergy in 2010 Girl Scouts. Acta Allergol (Kbh) 26: 117–120

Anonymous (1981) Immunisation against bee and wasp stings. Drug Ther Bull 19: 47–48

Arnold HL (1957) In discussion of Caro et al. (1957). Arch Dermatol 75: 486

Aukrust L, Einarsson R, Ohman S, Johansson SGO (1982) Cross radioimmunoelectrophoretic studies of bee venom allergens. Allergy 37: 265–271

Barnard JH (1962) In: Siegal S, Barnard JH, Loveless MH, Mueller HL, Walzer EH, Hatzel G and Herrera N. Insect sting allergy (Report of a panel discussion.) State J Med 62: 3560–3572

Barnard JH (1966) Severe hidden delayed reaction from insect stings. NY State J Med 66: 1206–1210

Barnard JH (1967) Allergic and pathologic findings in fifty insect sting fatalities. J Allergy 40: 107–114

Barr SE (1974) Allergy to hymenoptera sting. JAMA 228: 718–720

*Benson RL, Semenov H (1930) Allergy in its relation to bee sting. J Allergy 1: 105–116

Benton AW, Morse RA, Stewart JD (1963) Venom collection from honeybees. Science 142: 228–229

Biery TL (1977) Venomous arthropod handbook. Disease Surveillance Branch, Epidemiology Division, USAF School of Aerospace Medicine. US Govt Printing Office, Washington DC, 1–49

Bladek R (1968) Bee and wasp stings. Appl Ther 10: 402

*Blum S, Hermann HR (1978) Venoms and venom apparatus of the Formicidae, Myrmeciinae, Ponerinae, Dorylinae,

Pseudomyrmecinae, Myrmicinae, Formicinae, Dolichoderinae and Aneuretinae. In: Bettini S (ed) Arthropod venoms. Springer, Berlin Heidelberg New York, pp 801–869, 871–894 (Handbook of experimental pharmacology, vol 48)

Blum MS, Walker JR, Callahan PS, Novak AF (1958) Chemical, insecticidal and antibiotic properties of fire ant venom. Science 128: 306–307

Bolton B, Collingwood CA (1975) Hymenoptera; Formicidae. Handbook for the identification of British insects, vol VI, pt 3(c). Royal Entomological Society of London, London pp 1–33

Brown LL (1972) Fire ant allergy. South Med J 65: 273–277

Busse WW, Reed CE Lichtenstein LM, Reisman RE (1975) Immunotherapy in bee sting anaphylaxis. Use of honeybee venom. JAMA 231: 1154–1156

*Caro MR, Derbes VJ, Jung R (1957) Skin responses to the sting of the imported fire ant (*Solenopsis saevissima*). Arch Dermatol 75: 475–488

*Cavill GWK, Robertson PL (1975) Ant venoms, attractants and repellents. Science 149: 1337–1345

Chaffee FH (1970) The prevalence of bee sting allergy in an allergic population. Acta Allergol (Kbh) 25: 292–293

Chalmers AJ, Marshall A (1918) Notes on minor cutaneous affections seen in the Anglo-Egyptian Sudan. J Trop Med 21: 197–200

Chapman HR (1971) The insects: structure and function, 2nd edn. English Universities Press, London

Coleman M, Barnard J, Barr S, Brown H, Levin M, Mueller H (1974) Prolonged interval therapy in Hymenoptera sensitive patients. J Allergy Clin Immunol 53: 111–112

Davies RG (1967) Insects (Class Insecta) In: Larousse encyclopedia of animals. Hamlyn, London, pp 147–153

Day JM (1962) Death due to cerebral infarction after wasp stings. Arch Neurol 7: 184–186

De la Lande IS, Lewis JC (1966) Constituents of the venom of the Australian Bull ant, *Myrmecia pyriformis*. Mem Inst Butantan. Simposio internacionale sobre venenos animais. 33, Suppl comemorativo: 951–955

De la Lande IS, Thomas DW, Tyler MJ (1963) Pharmacological analysis of the venom of the "Bulldog ant" *Myrmecia forficata*. In: Proceedings of the second international pharmacological meeting, Prague, 20–23 Aug 1963, vol 9. Pergamon, Oxford, pp 71–75

Derrick E (1932) A striking general reaction to a bee sting. Med J Aust 1: 833

*Ebeling W (1975) Urban entomology. University of California, Division of Agricultural Sciences, Los Angeles, Cal, pp 346–375

Edery H, Ishay J, Gitter S, Joshua H (1978) Venoms of Vespidae. In: Bettini S (ed) arthropod venoms. Springer, Berlin Heidelberg New York, pp 690–771 (Handbook of experimental pharmacology, vol 48)

Foubert EC, Stier RA (1958) Antigenic relationship between honeybees, wasps, yellow hornets, black hornets and yellow jackets. J Allergy 29: 13–23

Frazier CA (1964) Allergic reactions to insect stings; a review of 180 cases. South Med J 57: 1028–1034

Frazier CA (1966) Insect allergy and its management. West Va Med J 62: 99–108

Frazier CA (1974) Cutaneous manifestations of allergy. Cutis 13: 1038–1047

Frazier CA (1977) Defence of whole body extract in hyposensitisation to insect venom. Cutis 19: 789–791

Golden DBK, Sobotka KA, Valentine MD, Lichtenstein LM (1981) Dose dependence of Hymenoptera venom immunotherapy. J Allergy Clin Immunol 67: 370–374

*Habermann E (1971) Chemistry, pharmacology and toxicology of bee, wasp and hornet venoms. In: Bücherl N and Buckley EE (eds) Venomous animals and their venom. vol II Venomous invertebrates. New York, Academic, pp 61–93

Hatzel G, Herrera N (1962) In: Siegal S, Barnard JH, Loveless MH, Mueller HL, Walzer EH, Hatzel G, Herrera N Insect sting allergy. (Report of a panel discussion.) NY State J Med 62: 3560–3572

Hermann HR, Blum S (1966) The morphology and histology of the hymenopterous poison apparatus. I *Paraponera clavata* (Formicidae). Ann Entomol Soc Am 59: 397–409

Hoffman DR (1977) Allergy to bee venom; *In vitro* diagnosis and identification and isolation of allergen. Cutis 19: 763–767

Hoffman DR, Shipman WH (1975) Allergenic analysis of bee venom fractions. J Allergy Clin Immunol 55: 73

Hoffman DR, Shipman W (1976) Higher molecular weight allergens in honeybee venom. Fed Proc 35: 673

Hoveler H, Pullmann H, Gottmann-Luckerath I (1983) Latente Sensibilisierung auf Bienen- und Wespengift. Z Hautkr 58: 61–170

Hunt RJ, Sobotka AK, Valentine MD, Yunginger JW, Lichtenstein LM (1978a) Sensitisation following Hymenoptera whole body extract therapy. J Allergy Clin Immunol 61: 48–53

Hunt KJ, Valentine MD, Sobotka AK, Benton AW, Amodio FJ, Lichtenstein LM (1978b) A controlled trial of immunotherapy in insect hypersensitivity. N Eng J med 299: 157–161

Imms AD (1938) A general textbook of entomology, 4th edn. Methuen, London pp 544–615.

Insect Allergy Committee of the American Academy of Allergy (1964) 1963 Report. J Allergy 35: 181–187

Insect Allergy Committee of the American Academy of Allergy (1965) Insect sting allergy. Questionnaire study of 2606 cases. JAMA 193: 115–120

*James MT, Harwood RF (1969) Herm's medical entomology, 6th edn. Macmillan, London, pp 390–398

Jensen OM (1962) Sudden death due to stings from bees and wasps. Acta Pathol Microbiol Scand 54: 9–29

Jex-Blake AJ (1942) Bees. East Afr Med J 19: 73–86

Kennedy CB (1957) In discussion of Caro et al. (1957). Arch Dermatol 75: 486

Lawson Tait (1893) In JAMA 75 years ago. JAMA 206: 2413–2414

Lessoff MH, Sobotka AK, Lichtenstein LM (1978) Effects of passive antibody in bee venom anaphylaxis. Johns Hopkins Med J 142: 1–7

Lobitz WC (1957) In discussion of Caro et al. (1957). Arch Dermatol 75: 486

*Loveless MH (1962a) Immunization in wasp sting allergy through venom-repositories and periodic insect stings. J Immunol 89: 204–215

Loveless MH (1962b) In: Siegal S, Barnard JH, Loveless MH, Mueller HL, Walzer EH, Hatzel EH and Herrera N Insect sting allergy. (Report of a panel discussions) NY State J Med 62: 3560–3572

Loveless MH (1978) "Once-in-a-lifetime" venom injection therapy in bee allergy. Fed Proc 37: 1555

Loveless MH, Fackler WR (1956) Wasp-venom allergy and immunity. Ann Allergy 14: 347–366

McCormick WF (1963) Fatal anaphylactic reaction to wasp sting. A review with immunologic studies of a fatal case. Am J Clin Pathol 39: 485–491

*Mann GT, Bates HR (1960) the pathology of insect bites; a brief review and report of eleven fatal cases. South Med J 53: 1399–1406

*Maschwitz UWJ, Kloft W (1971) Morphology and functions of the venom apparatus of insects—bees, wasps, ants and caterpillars. In: Bücherl W, Buckley EE (eds) Venomous animals and their venoms. Vol III Venomous invertebrates Academic, New York, pp 1–60

Morhouse CH (1949) Unusual reaction to ant bites. JAMA 141: 193
Mosbech H (1983) Death caused by wasp and bee stings in Denmark 1960–1980. Allergy 38: 195–200
Mueller HL (1959) Further experiences with severe allergic reactions to insect stings. N Engl J Med 261: 374–377
*Mueller HL (1962) In: Siegal S, Barnard JH Loveless MH, Mueller HL, Walzer EH, Hatzel EH and Herrera N Insect sting allergy. (Report of a panel discussion.) N State J Med 62: 3560–3572
Mueller HL (1971) Insect allergy. In: Samta M, Alexander HL (eds) Immunological disease, 2nd edn. Little, Brown, Boston, pp 893–902
Mueller HL (1977) Maintenance of protection in patients treated for stinging insect hypersensitivity; a booster injection program. Pediatrics 59: 773–777
Muller U, Roth A, Yman L, Patrizzi R (1978) Use of RAST technique in wasp hypersensitivity. Allergy 33: 197–202
Murray JA (1964) A case of multiple bee stings. Central Afr J Med 10: 249–251
Obermeyer ME (1945) A severe systemic reaction to a bee sting. Arch Dermatol Syphilol 51: 396–397
O'Connor R, Peck ML (1978) Venoms of Apidae. In: Bettini S (ed) Arthropod venoms. Springer, Berlin Heidelberg New York, pp 613–659 (Handbook of experimental pharmacology, vol 48)
O'Connor R, Rosenbrook W, Erickson RW (1963) Hymenoptera; pure venom from bees, wasp and hornets. Science 139: 420
O'Connor R, Stier RA, Rosenbrook W, Erickson RW (1964) Death from "wasp sting". Ann Allergy 22: 385–393
Ordman D (1965) Desensitisation against the effects of bee stings. Transactions of the College of International Allergy, 6th symposium, London, March 1965. Int Arch Allergy Appl Immunol 28: 25
Parrish HM (1959) Deaths from bites and stings and venomous animals and insects in the United States. Arch Intern Med 104: 198–207
Parrish HM (1963) Analysis of 460 deaths from venomous animals in the United States. Am J Med Sci 245: 129–141
*Patton WS, Evans AM (1929) Insects, ticks, mites and venomous animals of medical and veterinary importance. Part I Medical. HR Grubb, Croydon
Perlman E (1955) Near fatal allergic reactions to bee and wasp stings. A review and report of seven cases. J Mount Sinai Hosp 22: 336–348
Reed H (1946) Asthma and urticaria following a bee sting. East Afr Med J 23: 245–246
Reisman RE, Wypych JI, Yeagle N, Arbesman CE (1974) Stinging insect hypersensitivity. III Detection and clinical significance of IgE antibodies to insect venom in man. J Allergy Clin Immunol 53: 110–111
Rhoades RB, Schafer WL, Schmid WH, Wubbena PF, Dozier RM, Townes AW, Leifer KN, Cohan RM, Wittig HJ (1974) Hypersensitivity to the imported fire ant. J Allergy Clin Immunol 53: 112
Richards OW (1980) Scolioidea, Vespoidea and Sphecoidea; Handbook for the identification of British insects. vol VI, pt 3(b). Royal Entomological Society of London, London
Richards OW, Davies RG (1977) Imms general textbook of entomology, 10th edn. Chapman and Hall, London
Rubenstein HS (1980a) Allergists who alarm the public; a problem in medical ethics. JAMA 243: 793–794
Rubenstein HS (1980b) Bee venom immunotherapy. JAMA 244: 1672
Rubenstein HS (1982) Bee sting diseases: Who is at risk? What is the treatment? Lancet I: 496–499
San Martin PR (1971) The venomous ants of the genus *Solenopsis*. In: Bücherl W, Buckley EE (eds) Venomous animals and their venoms. Vol III Venomous invertebrates. Academic, New York, pp 95–121
Schenken JB, Tamiesia J, Winter FD (1953) Hypersensitivity to bee sting. Am J Clin Pathol 23: 1216–1221
Schmid WH (1977) Medical implications; imported fire ants, *Solenopsis invicta*. Cutis 19: 794–797
Settipane GA, Boyd GK (1970) Prevalence of bee sting allergy in 4,992 boy scouts. Acta Allergol (Kbh) 25: 286–291
Settipane GA, Hopson CJ (1971) Hymenopteran allergy; precipitation and passive cutaneous anaphylaxis tests in human and rabbit sera. Acta Allergol (Kbh) 26: 121–130
Settipane GA, Newstead GJ, Boyd GK (1972) Frequency of hymenoptera allergy in an atopic and normal population. J Allergy Clin Immunol 50: 146–150
Shilkin KB, Chen BTH, Khoo OT (1972) Rhabdomyolysis caused by hornet venom. Br Med J I: 156–157
Smith JD, Smith EB (1971) Multiple fire ant stings; a complication of alcoholism. Arch Dermatol 103: 438–441
Snodgrass RE (1935) Principles of insect morphology. McGraw-Hill, New York, p. 619
Sobotka AK, Valentine MD, Lichtenstein LM (1974a) Lack of cross-reactivity to vespid venom in sensitive patients. J Allergy Clin Immunol 53: 111
Sobotka AK, Valentine MD, Benton AW, Lichtenstein LM (1974b) Allergy to insect stings. I Diagnosis of IgE mediated hymenoptera sensitivity by venom induced histamine release. J Allergy Clin Immunol 53: 170–184
Sobotka AK, Adkinson NF, Valentine MD, Lichtenstein LM (1976a) IgE studies of patients with insect hypersensitivity. Fed Proc 35: 673
Sobotka AK, Franklin RM, Adkinson NF, Valentin M, Baer H, Lichtenstein LM (1976b) Allergy to insect stings. II Phospholipase A: The major allergen in honeybee venom. J Allergy Clin Immunol 57: 29–40
Sobotka AK, Lessoff MH, Lichtenstein LM (1976c) Absolute blocking antibody levels in passively and actively treated honeybee sensitive patients. J Allergy Clin Immunol 57: 247
Spencer JT (1968) Treatment of yellow jacket stings. JAMA 206: 649
Spruce R (1908) Notes of a botanist on the Amazon on Andes, Vol I. Macmillan, London, pp 362–365
Tauphaichitr VS, Tuchinda M (1982) Severe thrombocytopenic purpura following a bee sting. Ann Allergy 49: 229–231
Thomas JW (1958) The treatment of severe allergic reactions to insect stings and bites. Va Med Monthly 85: 415–422
Torsney PJ (1973) Treatment failure: insect desensitisation. J Allergy Clin Immunol 52: 303–306
Urbanek R, Karitsky D, Forster J (1978) Die Hyposensibilisierungbehandlung mit reinem Bienengrift. Dtsch Med Wochenschr 103: 1656–1660
Urbanek R, Zuipa J, Forster J, Kuhn W (1982) Bee stings Lancet I: 798–799
Valentine MD, Hunt KJ, Sobotka AK, Lichtenstein LM (1976) Venom immunotherapy for Hymenoptera sensitivity: Results in whole body extract (WBE) treatment failures and newly diagnosed patients. J Allergy Clin Immunol 57: 247
Weber NA (1939) The sting of the ant, *Paraponera clavata*. Science 89: 127–128
Wilson EO (1971) the insect societies. Belknap-Harvard Press, Cambridge, Mass
Winer LH (1957) In discussion of Caro et al. (1957). Arch. Dermatol 75: 486
Zahradnik J (1977) A field guide in colour to insects. English version translated by Kuthanova O. Octopus, London.

11 Flea Bites and Other Diseases Caused by Fleas

Fleas have been associated with man and animals from time immemorial. There must be few people who have never been bitten by a flea. They cause local reactions to their bite and are the vectors of some serious infectious diseases (Table 11.1). The latter fact is important because their biology requires that they partake of a meal of blood from some warm-blooded animal (bird or mammal) in order to reach maturity or to lay fertile eggs. This makes them voracious feeders and therefore biters. Their distribution is geographically and socially cosmopolitan, but they are most commonly encountered in conditions of overcrowding or primitive dwelling. They appear to be present in California in astronomical numbers and are prominently recorded in the history of that state (Anonymous 1936; Lunsford 1949). A significant note was made by the anonymous author in 1936 that a French traveller, La Perouse, had observed that "the indigenous Indians live in huts . . . which they can conveniently set fire to . . . when the fleas become troublesome and they can build another in less than two hours." Many other interesting tales of the effects of fleas on immigrants are told in these two papers, which also serve to emphasise the importance of immunological reactions following bites.

Morphology of Fleas

Fleas are wingless, laterally compressed insects with a hard, shiny integument. They have a common basic structure (Figs. 11.1, 11.2) and are ectoparasitic on warm-blooded animals. The body

Table 11.1. Infections and other diseases transmitted by fleas. The figures in parentheses indicate the degree of certainty of the fleas being the vector. (Compiled from James and Harwood 1969; Maegraith 1971; Smit 1971; White 1982)

Disease	Casual organism	Flea vectors
Bubonic plague	*Yersinia pestis*	*Xenopsylla cheopis* (1) *X. braziliensis* (1) *Pulex irritans* (2)
Pseudotuberculosis	*Y. pseudotuberculosis*	"Fleas"; very rare in man (2)
Tularaemia	*Francisella tularensis*	"Fleas"; possible vector (2)
Murine typhus	*Rickettsia mooseri* (*typhi*)	*X. cheopis* (1) *X. braziliensis* (1)
Haemorrhagic nephrosonephritis	*R. prowazekii*	Fleas; rodent reservoir (3) (USSR; eastern Asia)
Boutonneuse fever	*R. conori*	*R. conori* found in rabbit flea (3)
Q fever	*Coxiella burnetti*	Rodent flea vector in Asiatic Russia (3)
Lymphocytic choriomeningitis	An arenavirus	Virus found in three species of flea in USSR (3)
Tick-borne encephalitis	An arbovirus	Virus found in several species of flea in Poland and USSR (3)
Intestinal tapeworm	*Hymenlepis diminuta* *Dipylidium caninum*	Cysticercal stage passed in rat and dog fleas, repectively. Human infestation by accidental swallowing of the flea, with intestinal helminthiasis. Rare (1)
Vesicular and tonsillar forms of plague		Occurs in Indians in Ecuador after ingestion of fleas (1–2)

1. Fleas are definite vectors; 2, fleas are possible transmitters of the disease concerned; 3, these diseases are usually vectored by ticks but the causal organism has been found in fleas in the regions concerned.

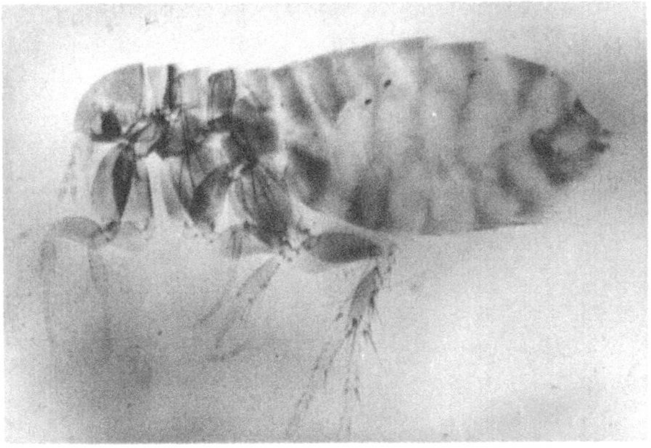

Fig. 11.1. Female poultry flea (*Ceratophyllus gallinae*) showing the general structure of a flea. This picture should be studied along with Fig. 11.2 for annotated details.

has three regions: head, thorax and abdomen. The head (Fig. 11.3) is rounded or angulated anteriorly with inconspicuous antennae. A lateral eye may be present or absent, as may a conspicuous genal comb with strongly chitinised tines. The mouthparts, consisting of paired maxillary palps, maxilla and mandibles, together with a central hypopharynx and labial palps, are adapted for piercing and sucking (Fig. 11.4). The head is applied directly to the three-segmented thorax. There is no neck. A well-marked comb may be present or absent at the posterior margin of the first segment. A pair of legs is attached to each thoracic segment. Each leg has five distinct parts: the coxa, trochanter, femur, tibia and tarsus, the last bearing two strong claws at its tip. The legs are strongly developed for jumping. The abdomen has at least

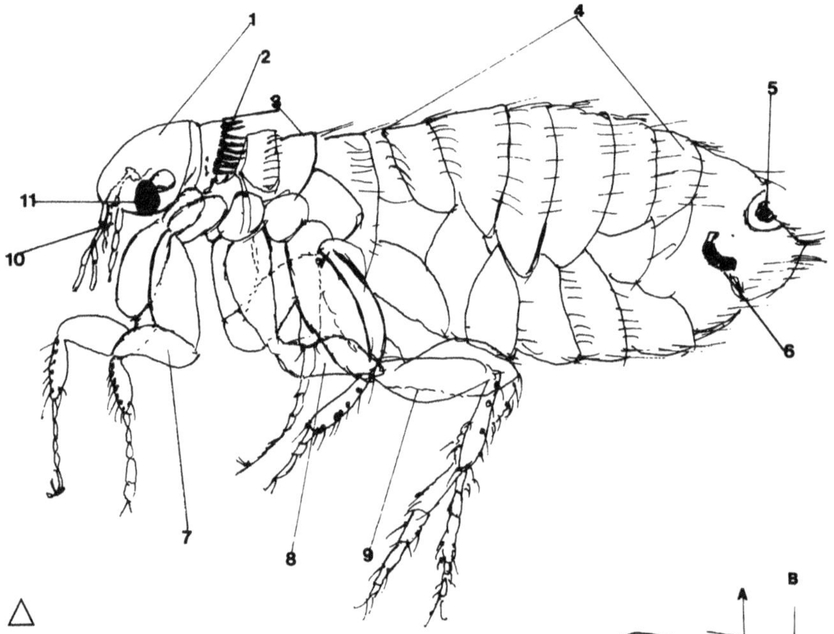

△

Fig. 11.2. Outline drawing of Fig. 11.1 to show some of the basic details, as commonly seen by ordinary microscopic examination. *1*, head; *2*, pronotal comb; *3*, thoracic segments; *4*, abdominal segments; *5*, pygidium; *6*, spermatheca; *7*, leg I; *8*, leg II; *9*, leg III; *10*, mouthparts; *11*, eye.

Fig. 11.3. Head and thorax of a flea (*Ctenocephalides canis*). *A*, metathorax; *B*, mesothorax; *C*, pronotal comb; *D*, prothorax; *E*, head; *F*, antennal fossa; *G*, antenna; *H*, eye; *I*, genal comb; *J*, maxillary palps; *K*, hypopharynx; *L*, mandibles; *M*, labial palps; *N*, maxilla; *O*, gena; *P*, the three sternal plates of thoracic segment. [After Ewing HE (1929) A manual of external parasites. Thomas, Springfield, Ill, by kind permission of the publishers] ▷

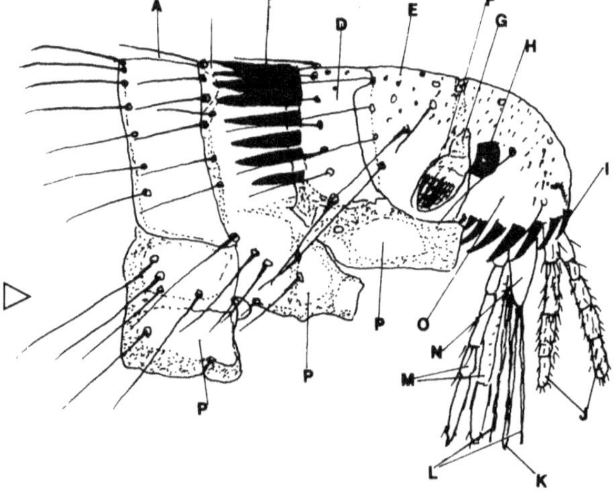

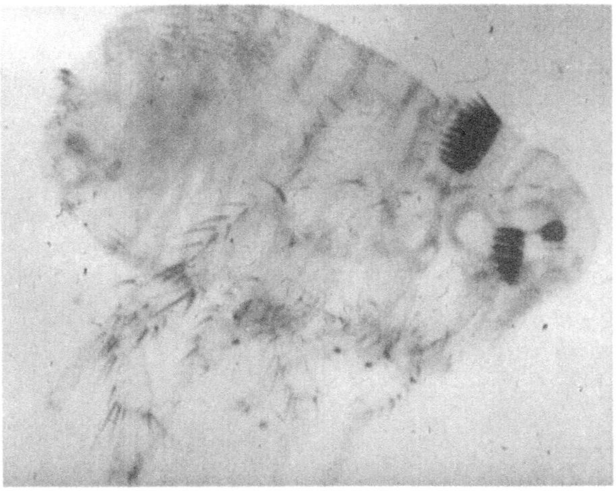

Fig. 11.4. *Ctenocephalides canis*, female. Note the presence of both genal and pronotal combs and the position and shape of the spermatheca.

nine segments, usually 10 or 11. The ninth segment bears the pygidium, the function of which is unclear but probably sensory. The male aedigus and the female spermatheca (Fig. 11.5) are easily visible near the posterior end of the abdomen and have shapes which are characteristic for each species or genus.

Classification of Fleas

White (1982) has noted some guidelines to distinguish the genera which attack man most frequently. These are set out in Table 11.2. The species of fleas which attack man and are associated directly with diseases or cause prominent lesions are shown in Table 11.3. Other fleas may bite man but the reactions they produce do not differ from those of the species shown.

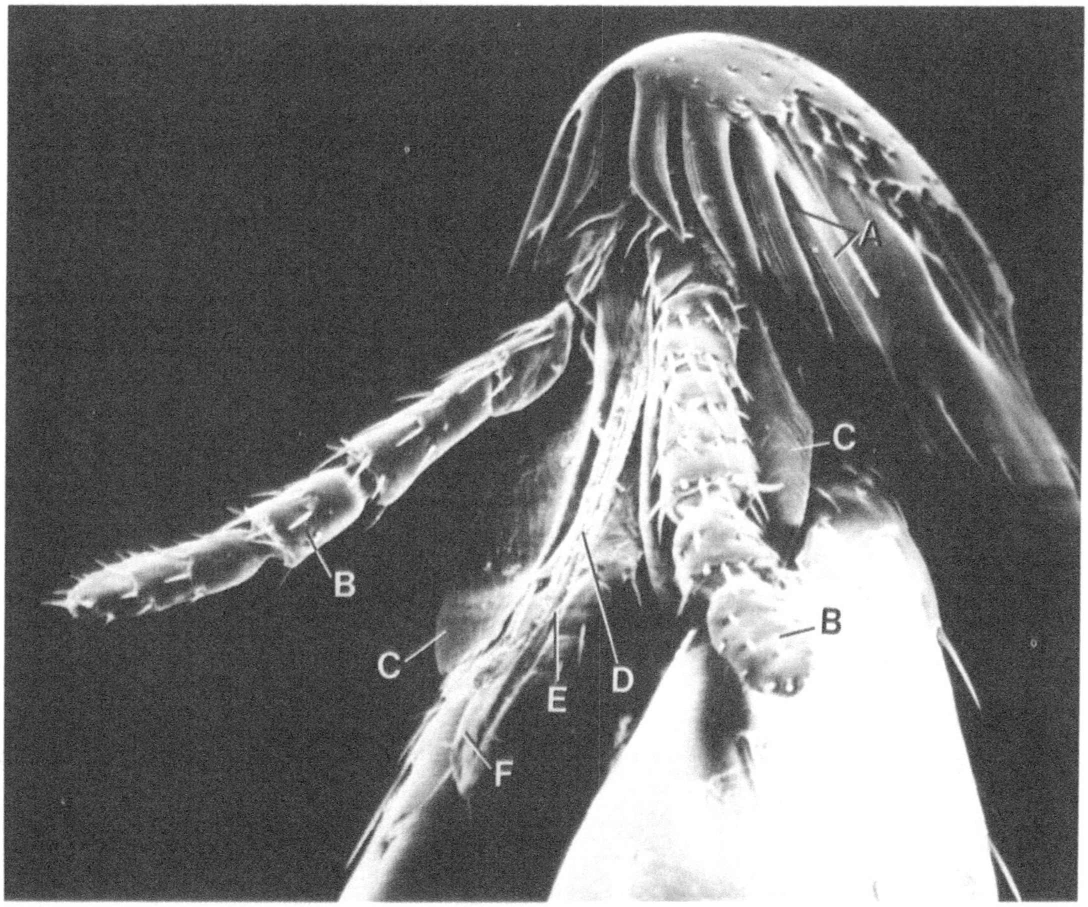

Fig. 11.5. Scanning electron micrograph of mouthparts of cat flea (*Ctenocephalides felis*). A, genal comb; *B*, maxillary palps; *C*, maxillae; *D*, hypopharynx; *E*, mandibles; *F*, labial palps. (Courtesy of Dr. H. V. Smith, Bacteriology Department, Stobhill Hospital Glasgow, and Dr. R. N. Titchener, Zoology Department, West of Scotland Agricultural College, Auchincruive, Ayrshire) × 250

Table 11.2. Features which can be used to distinguish the different genera of fleas which attack man most frequently. (Compiled from White 1982)

Features	Genus
1. Head rounded: combs absent	*Pulex*; *Xenopsylla*
a) Mesopleural rod present; cephalic bar above eyes absent	*Pulex*
b) Mesopleural rod absent; cephalic bar above eyes present	*Xenopsylla*
2. Head biangular anteriorly; combs absent	*Echidnophaga*
3. Head sharply pointed anteriorly; combs absent; large postabdominal spiracles	*Tunga*
4. Head and prothorax with combs	*Ctenocephalides*
5. Head without comb; prothorax with comb	*Nosopsyllus*
6. Head without comb; with 2 anterior spines; eyes absent	*Leptopsylla*

Table 11.3. Various flea species which bite man, some of which are vectors and all of which, apart from *Tunga penetrans* and *Leptopsyllus*, cause local reactions with hypersensitivity

Species	Region	Remarks
Pulicidae		
Pulex irritans	Cosmopolitan	Human flea; causes PU
P. similans	North and South America	
Xenopsylla cheopis	Cosmotropical	Bite reaction; plague and murine typhus vector
X. braziliensis	Africa; India; South America	Bite reaction; plague and murine typhus vector
Ctenocephalides (9 species)	Africa and Europe	Mostly on carnivores
C. canis	Widespread	Interchangeable hosts; commonly attacks man and causes PU in children
C. felis	Widespread	Interchangeable hosts; commonly attacks man and causes PU in children
Leptopsyllidae		
Leptopsyllus musculi		Rodent flea, known to harbour *Rickettsia prowazekii*; doubtful vector as it never attacks man (Mooser and Castenada 1938)
Ceratophyllidae		
Ceratophyllus gallinae	Europe	A large poultry flea; bite very painful
C. colombae	Europe	Pigeon flea; common biter of man in Finland (Reunala et al. 1979)
C. farreni	Europe	House martin flea; bites man (Bolam and Burtt 1956)
C. hirundis	Finland	Bites man (Reunala et al. 1979)
Monopsyllus sciurorum	Finland	Squirrel flea; bites man (Reunala et al. 1979)
Nosopsyllus fasciatus	Ne- and palaearctic Australia; South Africa	Brown rat flea; often bites man
Tungidae		
Tunga penetrans	Central and South America; tropical Africa; Madagascar; India	Causes tungiasis

Biology and Habits of Fleas

The biology and habits of fleas have been comprehensively described by Rothschild and Clay (1952). The most important biological requirement is a blood meal, which may be necessary to ensure the fertility, copulation or egg laying of the adult female. For example, *Ceratophyllus gallinae* (see Fig. 11.1) can copulate with fertilisation of the egg without such a meal but the female must take a blood meal for the eggs to mature (Rothschild 1965). In some species the blood meal must be from the preferred host, but in others any suitable host will suffice. Eggs are usually deposited within 24 h on the ground, in the nest of the host or on the host's fur. However, being non-adherent, they fall to the ground, where they have the appearance of a fine sprinkling of caster sugar. Some species (e.g. the rabbit flea, *Spilopsyllus cuniculi*) will only breed during the breeding season of the host, the circulating hormones in the blood of the latter being essential for egg maturation. The corticosteroid hormones appear to be the most important in this respect (Rothschild 1965).

In some species the host, such as man, is only visited for the purpose of feeding; in others, the host, such as furry mammals, provides both food and shelter; and in yet others the host provides the food and its nest the sheltered accommodation. The abandoned nests of such hosts are often teeming with fleas. The larvae (Fig. 11.6) do not suck blood but live on detritus and vegetable matter in dust. Blood is necessary for pupation, however, and this is obtained from the maternal excreta. The female flea is a voracious feeder and, according to Rothschild and Clay (1952) may feed continuously for up to 4 h if undisturbed. The majority of the ingested blood passes straight through the gut more or less unchanged, is excreted and falls to the ground for the larva to feed on.

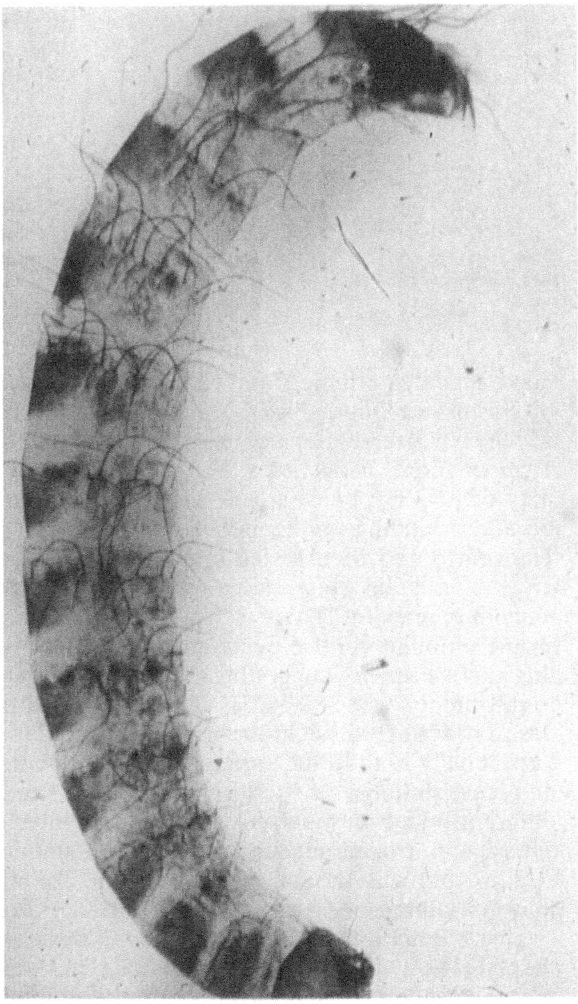

Fig. 11.6. Larva of *Ceratophyllus gallinae.* (Courtesy of Dr. R. N. Titchener, Zoology Department, West of Scotland Agricultural College, Auchincruive, Ayrshire)

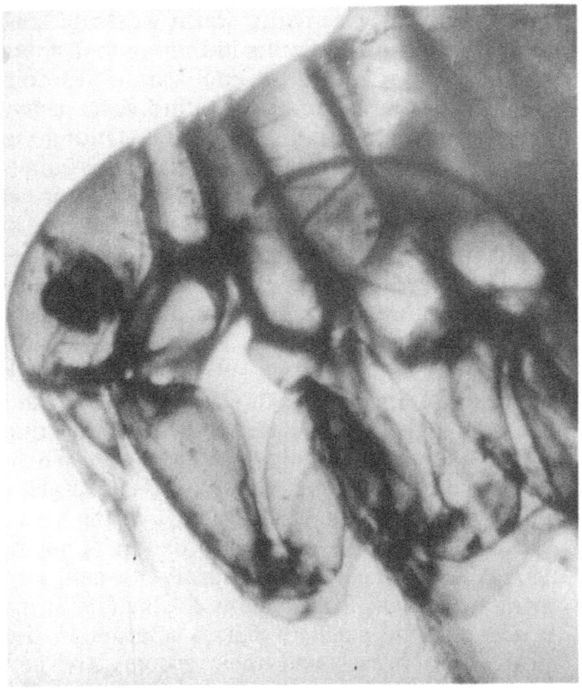

Fig. 11.7. Head and thorax of the human flea (*Pulex irritans*). Note the absence of combs but the presence of eyes.

The life cycle of fleas varies considerably not only between species—for example, it is 4–6 weeks for *Pulex irritans* (Imms 1938; Fig. 11.7) and 17 days for *Tunga penetrans* (Maegraith 1971)—but also amongst the same species, because of differing environmental temperature (Cotton 1970) or humidity and ready availability of a suitable food supply. For example, in India *Xenopsylla cheopis* has a life cycle of 3 weeks, but on the far eastern Pacific coast line it has one of 9–11 weeks (Imms 1938). The individual stages can each be modified by the circumstances mentioned so that the average larval stage of 9–15 days may be extended by adverse conditions to over 200 days. Similarly the pupal stage may be as brief as 7 days or as long as 1 year (James and Harwood 1969). James and his colleague gave the average life span as 30–75 days, taking all these factors into account. All stages can withstand starvation for long periods. This ability, plus the fact that the vibration of footsteps is the type of stimulus necessary to provoke the emergence of the adult flea from the pupa, explains why persons entering unoccupied but flea-ridden premises are liable to be severely attacked by hungry fleas.

Fleas are most active in warm weather; hence their liability to bite occurs in the summer in temperate climates and in the cool season in tropical climates. Extremes of temperature deter activity and very low temperatures are fatal. During their active phase they are on the lookout for suitable hosts. In this respect their jumping ability is very helpful. The average jump is about 20 cm, but White quotes Rothschild as noting that in search of food or to escape enemies they can reach a height of 2 m or more. This phenomenal performance is achieved by the storage of energy in the pad of resilin (a rubbery protein) at the junction of leg with thorax. In the case of *Ceratophyllus gallinae*, the waiting flea is stimulated to jump at the critical moment by a change in incident light: When a passing host casts its shadow on the flea (Humphries 1968) the thigh is turned, and the tension released throws the insect into the air (Chapman 1971). The host is found by the aid of smell, which attracts the flea. Rothschild and Clay (1952) have noted that the smell of horses appears to repel fleas, since horses and their grooms are never bitten.

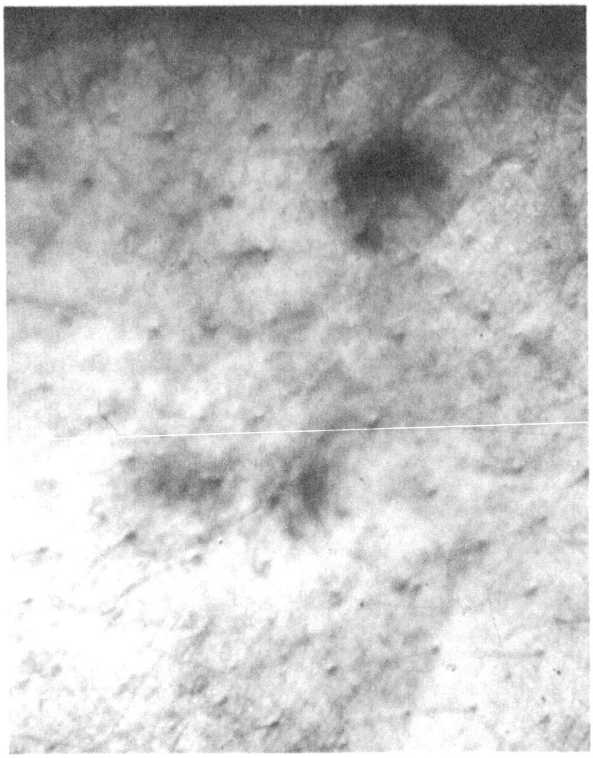

Fig. 11.8. Papular lesions of flea bites. Note clustering of three close together and the central papules with diffuse,.ill-defined surrounding erythema.

Clinical Features of Skin Lesions

The lesions produced by fleas vary in appearance according to the immunological stage reached by the victim in relation to flea antigen (see under Immunology, p. 170). The flea *Tunga penetrans* causes quite a different lesion, which will be considered separately.

Flea Bites

Probably the commonest skin lesion caused by an arthropod in man is a flea bite. The flea may begin to feed as soon as it reaches the skin. It may, however, be disturbed by movement of either the host or his clothing and therefore search for a more sheltered feeding place, or it may hide for a variable period in the clothing. Bites at the point of access usually appear around the ankle or wrist, but it is evident that the first meal can be taken almost anywhere on the body, although the scalp and face are seldom if ever attacked.

Infestation by a single flea usually results in one or perhaps two or three bites grouped irregularly over a small area of a few square centimetres (Fig. 11.8). The first bite may be unsuccessful in finding blood, or the flea may be disturbed so that two or three attempts may be necessary to feed. (Rothschild and Clay 1952 noted that most fleas make repeated attempts to feed, an opinion shared by Basex and Dupré 1965). The lesion produced is usually an irregular, very itchy, red weal, up to 1 cm or more in diameter (Fig. 11.9). Its margin may or may not be clearly defined and there may be a surrounding erythematous halo (Fig. 11.10). The centre may be elevated into a papule, vesicle or even a bulla (Fig. 11.11), depending on the individual reaction. There is usually a red haemorrhagic pinpoint central punctum (Fig. 11.12), but this may be absent, suggesting that the flea has not found a blood vessel. There is an almost irresistible desire to scratch these lesions and such action may occasionally abrade the surface causing exudation and encrustation of the lesion. Some persons react differently and may present with only papules or even haemorrhagic macules (see under Immunology, p. 169) with the same arrangements. The itch may be minimal or absent in such instances.

These lesions subside within 2 or 3 days and fade, leaving only an evanescent pale red stain within a week, and do not recur. However, rubbing or scratching may prolong this involution or may reactivate the oedematous weal. Additionally, in a proportion of cases the flea is unable to leave the

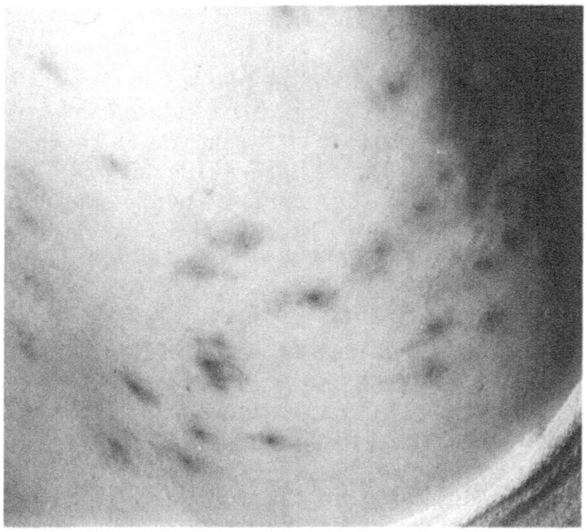

Fig. 11.9. Weals of flea bites.

host immediately after feeding and hides in seams in the clothing. It may remain hidden for 24 h or longer and then emerge to feed again in an entirely different area. If its feeding is constantly interrupted by scratching this process may be repeated over several days and result in crops of fresh lesions with a haphazard, bizarre distribution, which to the experienced eye are instantly recognisable as flea bites.

A similar appearance may be produced over a single 24 h period if several fleas attack simultaneously, the eruption then appearing at once and not in crops but with the same haphazard distribution (Fig. 11.13). With very heavy infestation the eruption is widespread, excoriation severe and itch almost intolerable.

Persons who become immune to flea bites show only an evanescent erythema with a central haemorrhagic punctum. The erythema fades very quickly, almost within minutes, but the central punctum may develop a purpuric halo from 0.5 to 1 cm in diameter, which persists for 3–4 days. These lesions do not itch. The present writer, who has been subject to occupational sporadic urticarial flea bites all his adult life, suddenly, at about the age of 63, changed to this type of purpuric macular eruption (see under Immunology, p. 169).

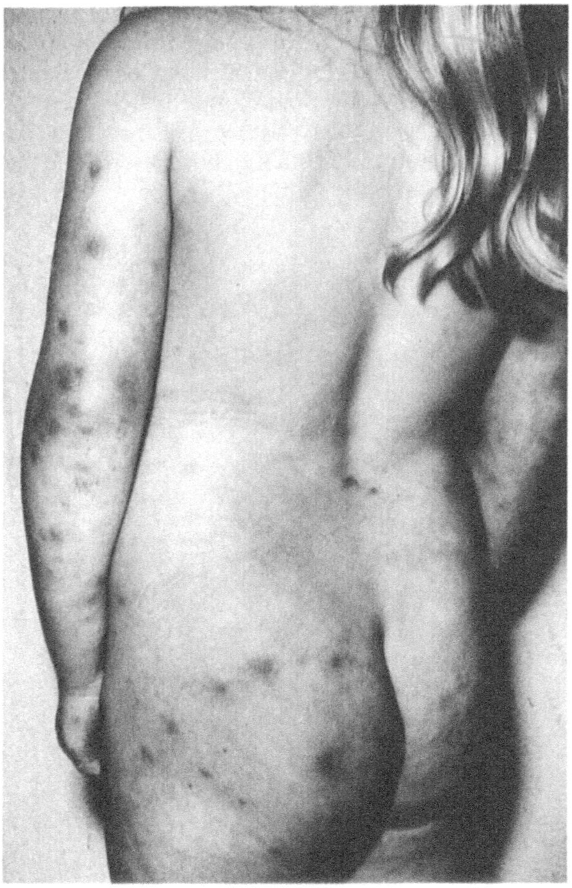

Fig. 11.10. Multiple flea bites. Note irregular distribution, tendency of clustering and the central papule with ill-defined surrounding erythema. (Courtesy of Dr. Alan Lyell, Glasgow)

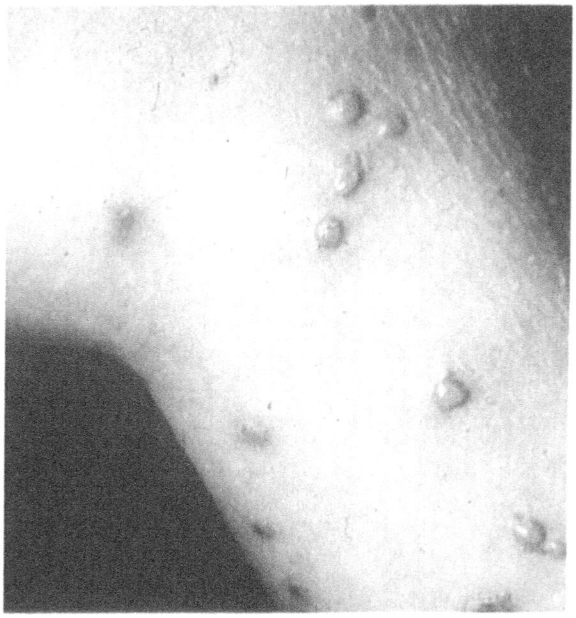

Fig. 11.11. Bullous flea bites on lower legs. Note tendency to grouping. Note also the papular lesion at the *left* of the picture.

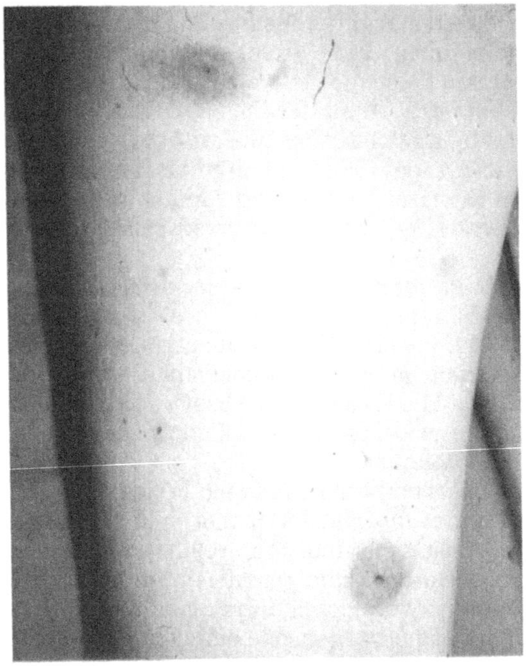

Fig. 11.12. Flea bites on thigh. Note the marked haemorrhagic central punctum and the dark erythematous maculopapule around, with vague halo of erythema at the periphery.

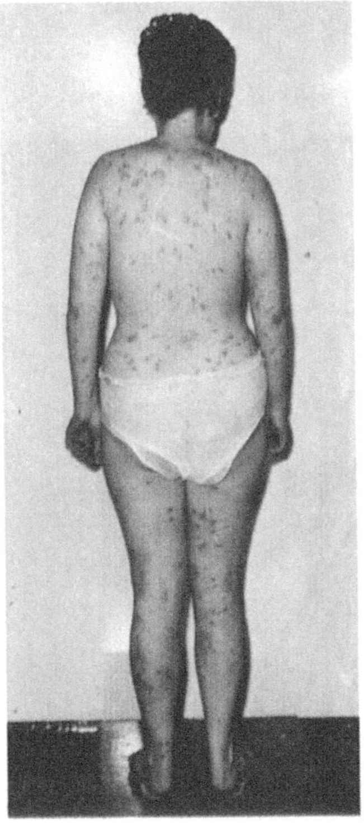

Fig. 11.13. Multiple flea bites showing all stages present at once. Note large irregular weals with erythematous flare, many with central haemorrhagic punctum, and tendency to grouping.

Papular Urticaria

Chronic re-infestation in persons constantly exposed to fleas produces the condition known as papular urticaria (PU), commonly known as "hives", "heat spots", lichen urticatus or strophulus. Clinically this is manifested by the appearance of recurrent lesions exactly similar to those described above. The lesions appear irregularly in crops (first noted by Barber 1914) and are chiefly seen on the limbs (Fig. 11.14) and around the waist (Fig. 11.15), but may also occur elsewhere on the trunk, the buttocks, neck, hands and feet (including the palms and soles in babies) (Fig. 11.16). Since the lesions recur in crops, all stages can be seen simultaneously, so that a patient may present with fresh weals with central puncta, accompanied by more persistent papules, vesicles, scratch marks (Fig. 11.17), exudation, encrustation and frequently secondary impetigo or ecthyma. The distribution remains characteristically bizarre, but two features are noticeable in the majority of cases: Firstly, new lesions still appear in small groups, all at the same stage, and, secondly, there is a marked tendency to clustering of lesions around the waistline, where tight clothing forms a barrier to the flea's progress (first emphasised by Rook and Frain-Bell 1953). This feature is also seen in many other infestations, notably those associated with various mites (see Chaps. 17, 18, 19 and 22).

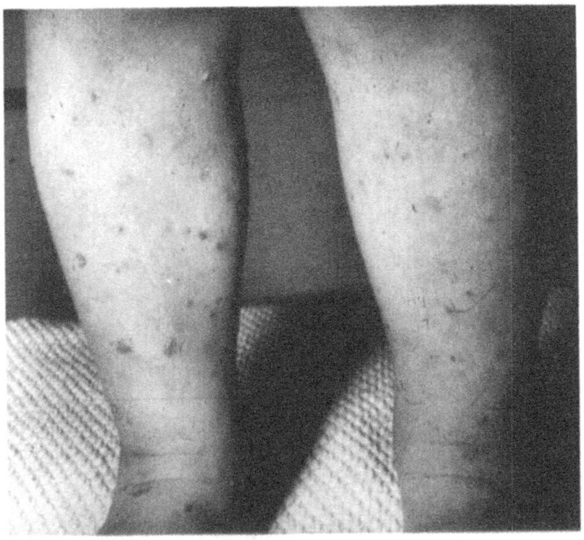

Fig. 11.14. Papular urticaria in a young child. Scattered irregular lesions consisting of papules, stain and small pinpoint crusts on many of the papules.

Residual staining or pigmentation of healed lesions is not uncommon, and, where scratching has been severe, there may be small scars. The patients are commonly young children between the ages of 2 and 7, but older children and rarely teenagers and adults may be affected. Delaimy (1978) has reported that PU in Iraq is commonly bullous, although papular and urticarial lesions are also seen. It may sometimes be extensive and rather like other bullous diseases.

Epidemiology

Patients of any age and either sex are liable to be bitten by fleas. Children who are developing immunity show more severe reactions than do adults and are consequently seen by physicians and dermatologists relatively more often in this context. There may be a familial incidence of flea bites because everyone in an infested dwelling is at risk.

No social class is exempt, but in overcrowded houses, whose owners keep one or more pet dogs or cats, bites are more likely, if only because of greater proximity to the animals' bed or sleeping place. Fox (1873) and Massie (1974) both considered PU to be commonest in the lower socioeconomic classes. Furniture or bedding on which

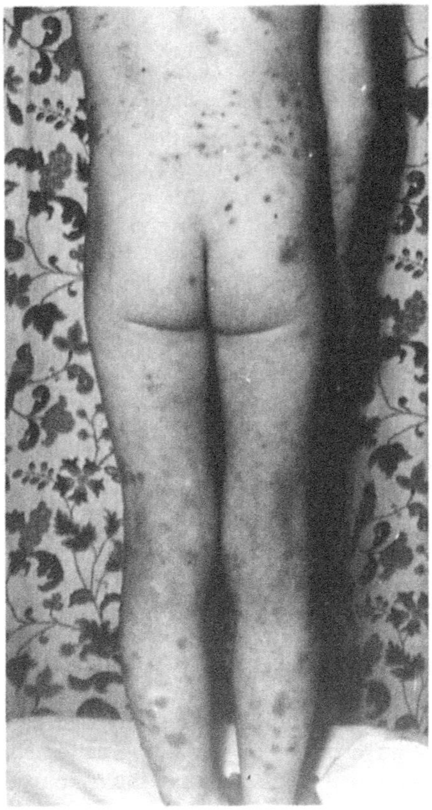

Fig. 11.16. General distribution of papular urticaria.

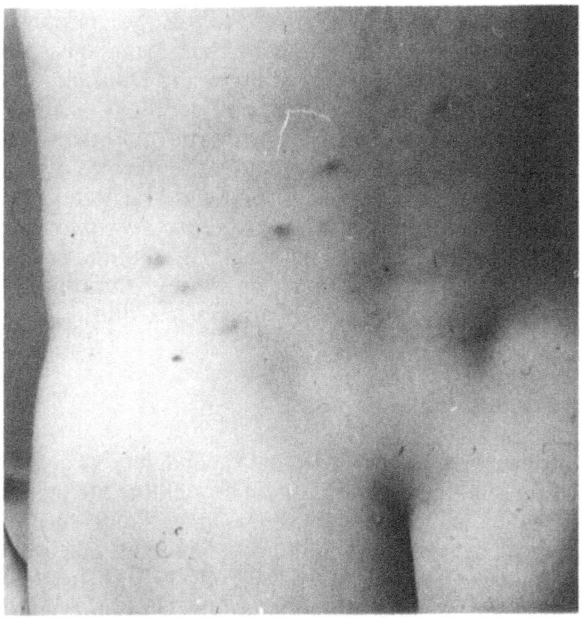

Fig. 11.15. Papular urticaria showing scattered lesions around the waist with a few on the buttocks.

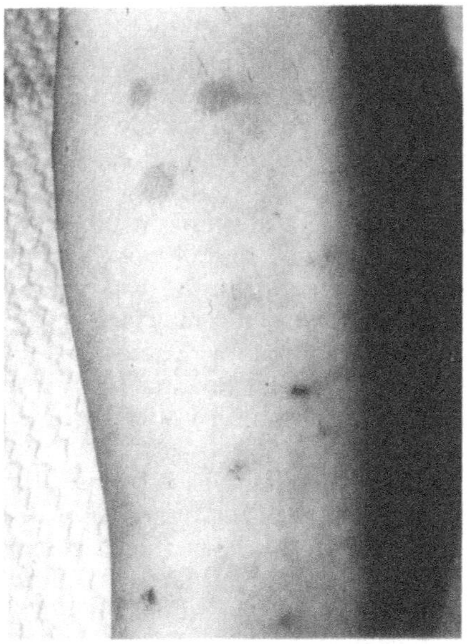

Fig. 11.17. Papular urticaria on forearm of child. Note the grouping of the lesions. The three at the *top* of the picture are recent weals. Two faint stains representing healed lesions are seen below these and on the *lower half* of the picture are four papules, two of which have tiny crusts of blood.

such pets lie are sources of fleas. The care with which these pets are groomed and housed is an important factor. Control of fleas will eliminate bites. On the other hand, some owners lavish the wrong kind of care on their pets allowing them the free run of the furniture and bedding and often keeping them on their lap, but not doing the necessary grooming or controlling of fleas. The present writer remembers such a patient, whose irritating "neurodermatitis" was only cured when it was realised that, clean and respectable as she was, her cat was flea-ridden. Suitable measures against the fleas cured both patient and cat.

Outbreaks of flea bites sometimes occur in the absence of pets. Dickey (1967) recorded an invasion of a living room by a horde of fleas 3 months after the death of a pet dog. The child in the house had been severely bitten and only recovered when the fleas were controlled. Parsons (cited by Dickey 1967), discussing this incident, noted that such sudden increases in numbers of fleas is not uncommon after the departure of a flea-ridden pet. Rothenburg (1975) cited another outbreak of flea bites caused by a swarm of fleas in a central heating tunnel beneath a children's day nursery. Three of the children were bitten by the fleas, which suddenly increased in number after the departure of a family of foxes from the tunnel. When the natural host of these fleas (*Ctenocephalides canis* or *C. felis* as a rule) disappears they quickly look for another host, which may well be man.

Whilst fleas may bite at any time of year they are more active during warm weather, when they breed. For example, *Ceratophyllus gallinae* overwinters in the host's nest in the pupal stage, the adults emerging in the spring. Coincident with this event there is an increase of clinical cases of flea bites (Wolff 1975). Flea bites are less frequent in winter; when the temperatures fall drastically fleas die, which is the probable reason why flea-borne epidemics tend to die down in the winter (Rothschild and Clay 1952). Flea bites may be an occupational hazard, as recorded by Titchener (1979) amongst laboratory workers investigating an outbreak of *C. gallinae* infestation in broiler breeder houses.

PU was suspected of being caused by insect bites by Bateman (1813) on clinical grounds. Fox (1873) attributed some cases to bedbugs, which Hamburger and Dietrich (1937) considered a common cause. Hutchinson (1879) pointed out that 75% of 109 children developed their eruption in the summer months. This finding was confirmed by Adamson (1907). It should be emphasised that the summer is the breeding season for cat and dog fleas. Fox (1873) had also noted that the eruption cleared when the children were admitted to hospital and relapsed on return home. He attributed this to good hygiene in hospital and poor hygiene at home. Porter (1910) had said that PU in children would clear up if they were confined to bed and protected from flea bites and would remain clear as long as these conditions were maintained. This statement was amplified and confirmed by Hallam (1927), who demonstrated that the lesions were associated with the home environment. They cleared on admission to hospital, or even if only kept overnight for several consecutive nights, but relapsed on full return home. Similarly Kinnear (1933) observed that the eruption cleared in children who had emigrated to the United States from Dundee but relapsed when they returned home. Lancashire (1928) also confirmed Hallam's findings. Tate (1935), whilst denying that vermin were the cause, nevertheless stated that "the exciting agent is something connected with the patient's home". Gordon (1933) noted a familial incidence.

Rook and Frain-Bell (1953) and later Rook (1961) were convinced of the arthropod origin of PU, a view which was shared by Hamburger and Dietrich (1937) and also by Wulf and Holtschmidt (1952). The circumstantial evidence cited above could equally apply to insect bites in every particular. The immunological development of the lesions of PU and of flea bites appear to be identical (see below). Further evidence was provided by Bolam and Burtt (1956), who demonstrated the presence of cat fleas in the furnishings (upholstery, rugs, bedding, pets' beds, etc.) of the houses where children with PU lived. Add to this the undoubted benefit derived by these patients from measures against arthropods (Hamburger and Dietrich 1937) and the case for an arthropod aetiology is almost overwhelming. Fleas are the principal arthropods responsible, but others at times induce a similar picture. Rook has listed bedbugs, rat mites, dog lice, mosquitoes and *Scleroderma domesticum* as other causes. The evidence is summarised in Table 11.4. PU in most instances, therefore, is equivalent to chronic recurring flea bites.

Immunology

It has long been known that the indigenous population of a flea-infested region are seldom affected by flea bites, whilst newcomers may suffer severely until they acquire immunity. This may take years or never occur (Cherney et al. 1939). Reactions may be of the immediate or delayed type on testing. Cherney and his colleagues noted a delayed reaction in eight of nine susceptible persons

Table 11.4. Summary of evidence in favour of flea bites (or other insect bites) being the cause of papular urticaria

Common features	References
General clinical appearance	Bateman (1813)
Seasonal variation (summer)	Hutchinson (1879); Adamson (1907)
Clears in hospital	Fox (1873); Hallam (1927)
Clears if protected from fleas	Porter (1910)
Familial incidence	Gordon (1933)
Clustering of lesions around clothing constrictions	Rook and Frain-Bell (1953)
Presence of fleas in houses of PU patients	Bolam and Burtt (1956)
Clears with antiarthropod measures	Hamburger and Dietrich (1937); Rook (1961)
Identical immunological features	Rook (1961)

and an immediate reaction in the ninth, whereas only three of 18 "immune" individuals showed even a mild response. They noted improvement in the sensitised persons following immunisation with whole body extract (WBE) of fleas. This prompted them to conclude that immunisation could prevent flea bites and could be used as a measure to combat the spread of flea-borne disease. This was a mistaken idea. Sensitive and immunised individuals are equally susceptible to being bitten, but the immunisation modifies or prevents the *reaction*, a point emphasised by Feingold and Benjamini (1961). Lunsford (1949) confirmed the reactivity of sensitised persons and noted that people not regularly exposed to flea bites are sensitive and that infants who have never been bitten show no reaction to their first flea bite. Shaffer et al. (1948) found that the majority of patients with PU reacted on testing with antigen, whilst controls had uniformly negative reactions. Shaffer et al. (1952) indicated that patients with PU showed similar immediate or delayed reaction to insect allergen and postulated that the clinical appearance of papular lesions in PU is due to a prolonged phase of delayed reaction, which may be so severe as to dominate the picture, whereas in those without PU this phase is transient and mild.

Benjamini et al. (1960) sensitised guinea pigs either by controlled exposure to flea bites or by the intradermal injection of WBE. Subsequent testing of both groups showed similar direct and cross reactions with the original sensitising stimuli. At first these reactions were delayed and then delayed and immediate. The same workers (1961) confirmed Mellanby's (1946) observed sequence of reactions to insect bites, viz. (1) delayed, (2) delayed and immediate, (3) immediate and (4) no reaction. The final non-reactive stage lasted at least 5 months. Without repeated exposures (in these tests the exposures were twice a week) the hypersensitive stage 2 could persist for at least 18 months. Feingold and Benjamini (1961), contrary to the experience of other workers, failed to desensitise patients by immunisation over periods varying from 5 to 25 months. They attributed this difference to the fact that they judged their results by objective challenge, whereas others had relied upon patients' subjective reaction as criteria. They also found inconsistent correlation between the clinical appearances and skin test reactions and attributed this partly to the fact that some of their patients were atopic with abnormal reactions. This finding was especially applicable to immediate reactions.

Feingold and his colleague concluded from their tests that the sensitizing agent in flea saliva was probably a hapten and that it acted as a complete antigen only when conjugated with Freund's adjuvant. Benjamini et al. (1963) collected flea antigen and demonstrated that this was correct, whilst Michaeli et al. (1965) showed that the substance conjugated with hapten was collagen or a collagen derivative.

It has been remarked on in the past (Kaposi, cited by Chipman 1910; Smith 1949) that a generalised urticaria may sometimes occur in association with flea bites. Feingold and Benjamini (1961) noted in their experiments that weals never appeared outside the special biting chambers and suggested that the generalised eruptions referred to were in reality an exacerbation of previously healed lesions in skin which had become sensitised.

Histopathology

Shaffer et al. (1952) showed that histological appearances were similar in skin test reactions and in lesions of PU, provided that they were at the same stage of development. Shaffer et al. (1954)

Table 11.5. Relationship between immunological stages, clinical appearance and histological changes in flea bite reactions and papular urticaria. (Compiled from Feingold and Benjamini 1961; Larrivée et al. 1964)

Immunological stage	Clinical lesions	Histological picture
1. Induction stage	Nil	No abnormal changes
2. Delayed reaction only	Indurated papules after 12–24 h	Intense mononuclear infiltrate at bite site after 24 h
3. Immediate and delayed reactions	Weal without erythema after 5–30 min; indurated papule after 12–24 h	Eosinophilic infiltrate with immediate reaction. Delayed reaction characterised by mononuclear infiltrate after 24 h
4. Immediate reaction only	Weal after 20 min	Eosinophilic infiltrate at bite site
5. Non-reactive	Nil	No abnormal changes

described these changes in more detail. In the immediate type of reaction and in the urticaria of PU there was oedema and dense perivascular and periappendicular infiltrate of lymphocytes and eosinophils in the middle and lower thirds of the corium. There were two types of reaction in the late papular stages of PU: The first was an "inflammatory" type, equating with a delayed tuberculin-type of reaction, with a dense cellular infiltrate, mainly of lymphocytes and eosinophils similarly distributed. There was no oedema, but at times some focal necrobiosis was seen. The second type of reaction had subsiding "non-inflammatory" papular lesions with a scanty lymphocytic infiltrate in the same region. The epidermis in the late stages was hyperkeratotic with moderate acanthosis. Occasional ulceration and crusting suggested scratching. Larrivée et al. (1964) correlated the clinical and histological appearances of flea bites at the various immunological stages. Their findings, in conjunction with the clinical description of Feingold and Benjamini, are summarised in Table 11.5.

Differential Diagnosis

The history and the clinical appearance of the lesions, which occur mainly in young children in the warm months of the year with a tendency to recur (Blank et al. 1950), are almost diagnostic. Careful and persistent questioning may be necessary to establish the possibility of flea contacts (Bolam 1958) and may cause parental resentment at supposed aspersions being cast on housekeeping ability. It should be stressed in cases of PU, which are often wrongly blamed on diet, that the problem is "not what the patient has been eating but rather what has been eating the patient" (Lunsford 1949). Conditions which have to be distinguished from flea bites, including PU, are:

1. *Ordinary urticaria*, which is acute and non-persistent and often affects the face
2. *Scabies*, which has its own specific lesions and distribution and may affect others in the household. (This may cause difficulty if more than one member of a family has PU.)
3. *Pediculosis corporis*, in which pediculi will be found in the clothing
4. *Pyogenic infection*, such as impetigo and ecthyma without underlying PU
5. *Chickenpox*, which is associated with malaise, fever, headache and often mucous lesions. This condition may cause diagnostic difficulties for inexperienced doctors unfamiliar with its appearance.

Treatment

Topical application of Vioform with hydrocortisone cream is usually adequate, but heavy secondary infection may require topical or even oral antibiotics. Topical insecticides for human patients, although recommended by Shaffer et al. (1948) and by Blank and his colleagues (1950) are unnecessary. Insect repellent powders, creams or lotions may help but must be used continuously over the season of flea activity to be effective. Burrows (1967) found a month's application of Flypel (12.5% each of diethyltoluamide and dimethylphthallate) insufficient as complete protection. Kochman (1956) found a solution of oil of citronella and dimethylphthallate to be satisfactory. Fleas will not feed through petrolatum (Lunsford 1949), and smearing the body lightly with this at night should be effective in avoiding flea bites.

According to Anderson (1949), Shannon had suggested in 1933 that oral vitamin B_1, possibly by its effect on body odour, repelled fleas. Eder (1945) reported complete success using 40 mg t.i.d. for 3 days followed by 40 mg daily for at least 1 month (10 mg for infants; 20 mg for children). Relapses did not occur for several months and responded to further dosage. Lunsford (1949) stated that opinion as to the value of this treatment varied from complete faith to total disbelief. He noted that 100 mg given intramuscularly was effective. Some further research on vitamin B_1 seems indicated.

Treatment of all suspected pets is essential. Destruction of pets is quite unnecessary; they can be disinfested satisfactorily by weekly application of pyrethrum dust or other suitable insecticide, providing it is not toxic to them. Regular grooming, using insecticides when required, is an effective means of controlling infestation (Canadian Ministry of Supply and Services 1980). It is equally important to disinfest the pet's bedding and the floor and skirting boards nearby, and all carpets, mats, cushions, upholstery, furniture and bedding where infestation has been possible. Pyrethrum dust, 3% malathion or 0.5% carbaryl are effective for this purpose and should be used once a month, for at least two or three applications. Regular vacuum cleaning is an essential part of this treatment (Bolam and Burtt 1956). It is advisable to keep children away whilst disinfestation is being carried out and subsequently to keep them away from possible sources of fleas as much as is reasonably possible. Drastic measures are seldom advisable for mild cases (Basex and Dupré 1965). Pets should be actively discouraged from sleeping on beds or other furniture. This is especially applicable to cats.

It is doubtful whether hyposensitisation is of much value at present.

For those bitten casually it is valuable to find and destroy the flea. Bedding should be carefully searched in the morning. For the person bitten during the day, it is advisable, if the opportunity arises, to remove all clothing in the bathroom, while standing on a white sheet or towel, and to inspect each garment meticulously, inside and out, while holding it over a basin or bath. The sheet or towel should be inspected on both sides last of all. More than one flea may be found. If the flea is spotted it can be captured by quickly placing a piece of wet soap upon it. A repeat search the next day may be necessary.

Tungiasis

The disorder known as tungiasis is caused in man by the flea *Tunga penetrans*, the common names for which are listed in Table 11.6 (Nuñez-Andrade 1952). A native of Central and South America, this flea infested Columbus' sailors in 1492; it played a not unimportant role in the subsequent history of those countries and spread to Africa, where it was recorded on the west coast in 1634. A second invasion from Brazil, caused by infested sailors and sand, introduced it to Angola in 1872 and it has since spread to Central and East Africa, to Madagascar and the west coast of Pakistan and India (Hoeppli 1963).

Morphology and Biology of *T. penetrans*

T. penetrans has a structure similar to that of other fleas. It is the smallest known flea (1 mm long). It is reddish-maroon in colour with a pointed head to assist its penetration of the host's skin (Giron 1981). There are two larval instars, described in detail by Hicks (1931). The life cycle, influenced to some extent by environment, is about 3 weeks (Smit 1973).

The larvae, adult males and virgin females live for preference in dry sandy soil around pigsties, poultry runs, stables etc. and feed on vegetable material and other detritus (Jelliffe 1953; Smit 1973; Giron 1981). They also require blood meals to complete the life cycle. The male dies after

Table 11.6. List of common names for *Tunga penetrans* in various countries. (Compiled from Nuñez-Andrade 1952)

Common name	Country
Nigua	Mexico; Peru; Paraguay
Chica	Colombia
Pico	Peru
Pique	Northern Argentina; Lower Bolivia; Uruguay
Suthi	Bolivia
Ton; *tomsico*; *tunga*; *catecuba mijor*; *bicho dos pes*; *bicho do porco*	Brazil
Moukardam	Sudan
Pulga de la arena; *pulga penetrante*; *pulga se encaja*; *puce de sable*	France (?)
Sandfloh	Germany
Chigoe; jigger; burrowing flea; sand flea	USA

copulation, but the gravid female is very active, jumping up and down, reaching a height of about 35 cm, until she dies or finds a host and burrows into its skin (Connor 1976). It "claws violently to get below the surface" (Connor) and insinuates its pointed head between the cells of the stratum corneum, working its way inwards until only the posterior aspect of the terminal abdominal segments are visible, flush with the surface (Fig. 11.18). It breathes through the posterior spiracles. The head is in the papillary dermis and here the flea can feed, at first on exudate, then on exudate containing inflammatory cells and finally on a pool of blood. Lavoipierre et al. (1979a) studied the gut contents of fleas removed at varying periods after embedding; their findings would seem to reflect the progress of the host's inflammatory reaction. In a second paper (1979b) they noted that different hosts may react somewhat differently, the preferred host producing the favourite cellular elements earlier than the other hosts.

The flea's abdomen enlarges to the size of a pea over a period of 7–14 days and is spherical in shape as a result of the maturation of the contained eggs (Smit 1973; Connor 1976; Fig. 11.18). Giron (1981) held that it then burst and presumably discharged its contents all at once; however, according to Connor (1976), the eggs are extruded over a period of 2 weeks by a muscular process, whilst Zalar and Walther (1980) noted that they were discharged singly over 7–10 days. Smit (1973) numbered the eggs in thousands, but most other authors put the figure at between 150 and 300. The flea then collapses and dies, either being extruded or remaining in situ.

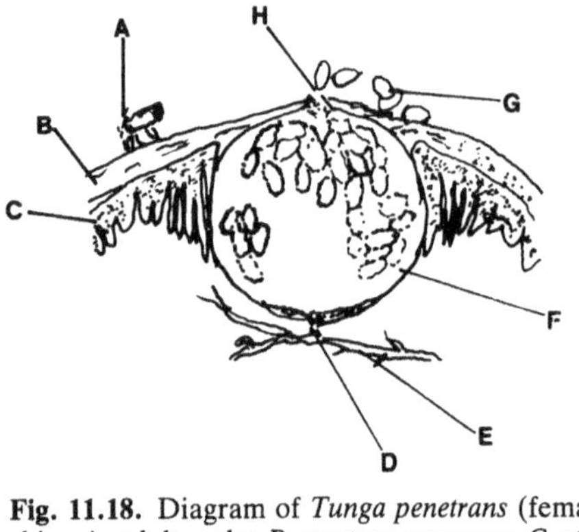

Fig. 11.18. Diagram of *Tunga penetrans* (female) in situ in the skin. *A*, adult male; *B*, stratum corneum; *C*, stratum malpighii; *D*, head and mouthparts of gravid female; *E*, superficial dermal blood vessel; *F*, gravid female abdomen containing eggs; *G*, eggs liberated on the skin surface; *H*, genital opening of female. (After Zalar and Walther 1980, by kind permission of the authors and the publisher, the American Medical Association. Copyright 1980, American Medical Association)

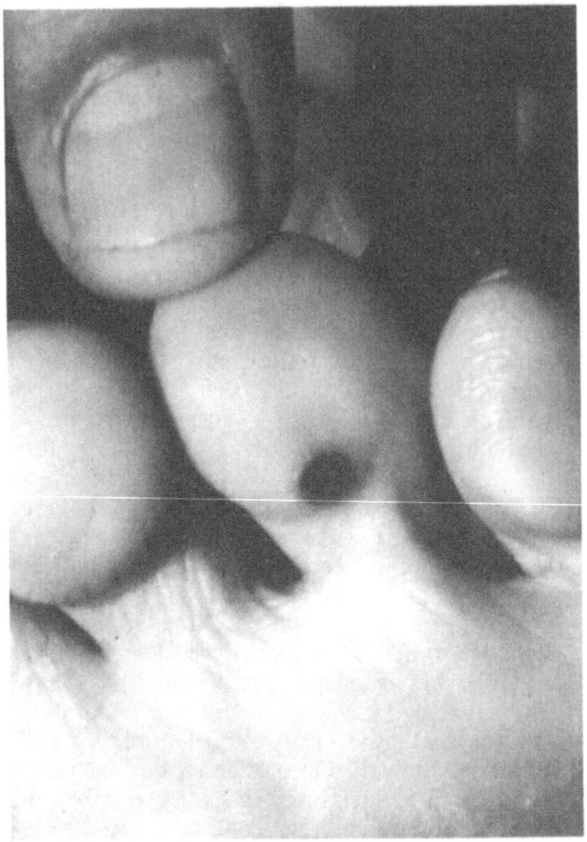

Fig. 11.19. Lesion of *Tunga penetrans* on the plantar aspect of right fourth toe. Note the large black blood crust on the surface and the slightly elevated peripheral margin. (Courtesy of Dr. Ney Romiti, Santos, Sao Paulo, Brazil)

Clinical Features

Lesions can occur almost anywhere on the body (Connor 1976) but much the commonest sites are on the feet and—in native children—on the thighs, perineum and genitalia (Maegraith 1971). Connor said that the weightbearing areas tended to be avoided, whilst Nuñez-Andrade (1952) maintained that the fleas preferred calloused skin. On the feet the commonest area is around the nail folds and especially just below the free edge of the nail (Fig. 11.19). The interdigital web is also commonly affected. Lesions may be single but are often multiple and may be very numerous. Giron (1981) has seen as many as 300 on a single patient.

During burrowing by the flea there is mild itch and slight pain. The itch persists and the pain increases as the flea enlarges, so that the lesions become very tender; if there are several lesions on the feet, standing or walking may be impossible.

The individual lesion consists of a firm, somewhat hard, slightly tender nodule with a flat surface of whitish-yellow keratin having a minute black spot in the centre, which is the posterior end of the flea abdomen (Jelliffe 1953). The lesion may be from 1–2 cm across. There is often a central black crust of blood on the surface. Basex et al. (1968) noted slight surrounding oedema in a lesion formed in an interdigital fissure, and in the subungual type they pointed out that although the lesions have a keratotic surface the base is inflammatory. Goldman (1976) observed that by transillumination such a lesion shows a dark central mass.

Secondary infection with pyogenic organisms is not uncommon in these lesions and is indicated by increased tenderness and by the formation of a pustule around the lesion accompanied by lymphangitis and enlargement and tenderness of regional lymph nodes. When this happens with multiple lesions they may coalesce to give an appearance like a honeycomb (Nuñez-Andrade 1952; Giron 1981). Severe cellulitis or erysipelas may occur (Reiss 1966). Thrombophlebitis was noted by White (1982), and bone necrosis was mentioned by Giron (1981). These complications may result in autoamputation of a toe or be severe enough to merit amputation of part or all of a foot or even a leg (Guyon 1870).

Faust and Maxwell (1930) recorded a very unusual instance of multiple infestation by *Tunga penetrans* in the inguinal, pubic and right lower abdominal regions, which was acquired by the patient by sitting on a cargo of infested sisal hemp from Yucatan. Scrapings from the surrounding excoriated skin surface revealed hundreds of *Tunga* larvae in various stages of development. These authors cited Newstead, who, in 1907, reported having found larvae easily in skin scrapings around tungiasis lesions rather than on the ground.

Tetanus has often complicated tungiasis in the past (Guyon 1870), probably following the extraction of fleas by natives using dirty implements. Vincent alleged that the administration of quinine for malaria in the Congo and in Madagascar precipitated or aggravated this complication, and this opinion was endorsed by Brumpt in South Africa and by Queiro in Costa Rica, where he also saw two patients who developed gas gangrene in their lesions. (All these instances were cited by Nuñez-Andrade 1952). *T. penetrans* is not infrequent in persons with anaesthetic leprosy lesions of the feet, and severe multiple lesions may occur (Fig. 11.20.)

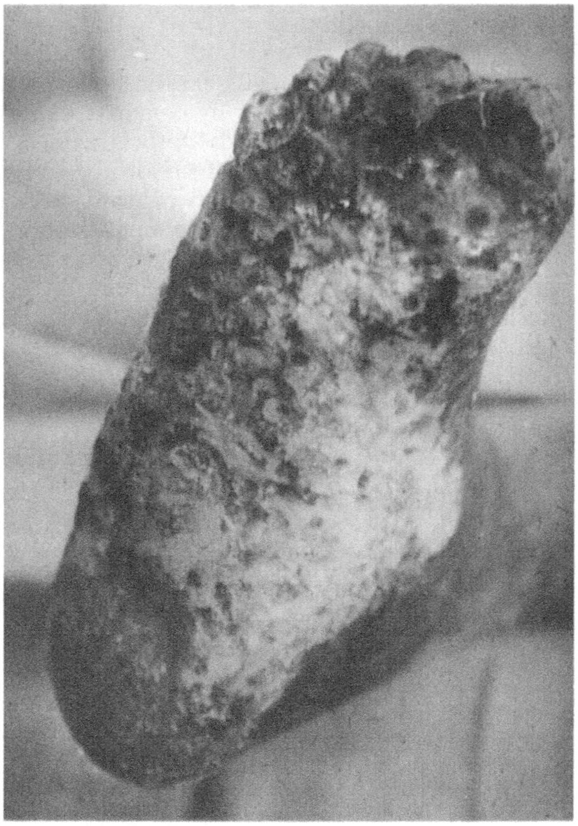

Fig. 11.20. Tungiasis on the foot of a leper. Note the multiple rounded black lesions scattered over the plantar aspect of the whole foot, causing gross disfigurement and disability. Patient is a Kenyan. (Courtesy of Dr. W. S. Douglas, Monklands Hospital, Airdrie)

Histopathology

The most detailed description is that given by Giron (1981), whose findings were as follows:

A punch biopsy of skin close to the drainage opening of the nodule revealed an irregular epidermis with moderate acanthosis, an increase in the granular layer and marked hyperkeratosis with parakeratotic zones. At the extremity of the horny covering an amorphous mass could be seen, which was eosinophilic, with a dentate border, enclosed between layers of horn cells. Amongst the material it was possible to discern some corresponding to chitinous remains and fragments of exoskeleton. In the upper dermis there were foci of haemorrhage, oedema, dilatation of blood vessels with a granulomatous infiltrate of lymphocytes, plasma cells and eosinophils, areas of mirco-abscesses formed by polymorphonuclear cells, foci of epithelioid cells and scaly crusts at the margins. The diagnosis was of an inflammatory granuloma due to a living agent.

Reiss (1966) and also Zalar and Walther (1980) had noted some of these features. Several authors have recorded finding pieces of exoskeleton and numbers of eggs in the material extruded from the lesions. Goldman (1976) noted that cross sections of completely excised lesions showed the arthropod in the centre, mainly in the epidermis.

Differential Diagnosis

The diagnosis of tungiasis is easy in endemic regions but may be difficult if a patient exhibits symptoms in a place remote from such regions, as has occurred in the past and is increasingly likely in these days of air travel. A history of having been in such an area, especially of going about barefoot or wearing sandals, and the clinical development and appearance of the lesion(s) are sufficient for diagnosis. Nevertheless, alternative diagnoses may have to be considered and these are summarised in Table 11.7.

Epidemiology

Persons of either sex or any ethnic group are liable to be attacked. The flea commonly lies in the dry dusty soil around farm buildings such as pigsties and stables, and persons working in these areas, especially with pigs, are the most exposed to attack. Those who go barefoot or wear open-toed sandals are especially susceptible. Since the feet and buttocks are the most commonly affected parts, those who walk, sit or camp on infested soil are potential victims (Jelliffe 1953). Tungiasis is endemic in infested areas, but the native inhabitants, being well aware of the risk, can remove the parasites early. Unsuspecting immigrants or travellers, however, can easily fall prey to attack, and in the past this has had serious consequences for explorers or even whole armies, e.g. the French army in Mexico (cited by Guyon 1870). Short-term visitors do not usually present with symptoms until they return home (see Table 11.8). Tungid fleas are not disease vectors but their invasion of human skin may be complicated by various secondary infections (see under Clinical Features, p. 173).

Table 11.7. Conditions to be considered in the differential diagnosis of tungiasis

Alternative diagnosis	Features
1. Plantar wart, especially subungual	Slow growing; tender; central black spots when involuting; seldom inflamed or infected
2. Subungual exostosis	Bony hard; non-tender; hyperkeratotic surface may displace nail; shown on radiograph
3. Malignant melanoma	Usually chronic but may be subacute; granulomatous; bleeds easily; may be pigmented; history of naevus
4. Acute paronychia	Solitary; acute; painful; tender; inflamed; swelling around nail; may suppurate; regional lymphadenopathy with lymphangitis
5. Mycotic granuloma	Slow growing; soft; very vascular granuloma bleeds easily; mycelium on microscopy (see Fuga et al. 1977)
6. Verruga peruana	History of being recently in the Andes. Granulomatous bartonellosis. Associated anaemia; lesion bright red; bleeds easily; not on toenail or interdigital area (see Basex et al. 1968)

Table 11.8. Sporadic cases of tungiasis contracted in endemic areas but recorded in the countries where the affected travellers lived

Origin of infestation	Where symptoms presented	Reference
Mexico	Paris	Guyon (1870)
Mexico	New Orleans	Faust and Maxwell (1930)
Gabon (West Africa)	New York	Reiss (1966)
Peru	Paris	Basex et al. (1968)
Cameroon (West Africa) Surinam (South America)	Holland	Tan-Lim et al. (1971)
Dahomey (West Africa)	France	Leques et al. (1973)
East and West Africa	Denmark	Fogh (1973) cited by Fuga et al. (1977)
East Africa	Germany	Laugier et al. (1975); Bäurle et al. (1981)
Africa	USA	Goldman (1976)
Angola	Italy	Fuga et al. (1977)
East Africa	USA	Zalar and Walther (1980)

Treatment

The infesting parasite should be removed, preferably intact, as early as possible (Jelliffe 1953). In the first 48 h a sterile needle may achieve this; during maturation of the eggs, curettage of the contained flea and cautery of the hollow are sufficient, whereas the mature flea must be totally excised under local anaesthesia. Whatever is removed should always be examined microscopically to confirm the diagnosis. For secondary infection topical and systemic antibiotics may be required. Complications should be treated as and when they arise.

Prevention

Persons visiting endemic areas are advised to be inoculated against tetanus. They should wear stout shoes or boots and never sit or camp on infested ground (Jelliffe 1953). The feet should be inspected daily for unsuspected lesions. An ointment containing a little cresol was recommended by Jelliffe. Infested ground and buildings should be disinfested regularly with insecticides such as lindane, dimethylphthallate or dimethyl carbamate. A high level of prophylaxis can be provided by good regular general hygiene measures for domestic and farm buildings (Nuñez-Andrade 1952). This author also advocated the use of adhesive paper (flypaper) for collecting fleas, as recommended by South Africans.

References

Adamson HG (1907) Skin affections in childhood. Oxford University Press and Hodder and Stoughton, London, pp 255–263

Anderson NP (1949) In discussion of Lunsford (1949). Arch Dermatol Syphilol 60: 1200

Anonymous (1936) The flea in Californian history and literature. Cal Hist Soc Q 15: 329–337

Barber HW (1914) Urticaria papulosa. Practitioner 2: 820–826

Basex A, Dupré A (1965) Le prurigo strophulus, syndrome parasitaire par piqûres d'insectes. Modalities, étiologiques, cliniques et évolutives. Ann Dermatol Sylphiligr (Paris) 92: 371–382

Basex A, Salvador R, Dupré A, Vites P, Balas D (1968) Sarcopsyllose (Tungiase) ou puce chique d'origine peruvienne. Bull Soc Fr Dermatol Syphiligr 75: 143–146

Bäurle G, Stroothenke M (1981) Tungiasis—eine "Urlaubsdermatose". Hautarzt 32: 372–373

Bateman T (1813) A practical synopsis of cutaneous diseases. Longman, Hurst, Rees, Orme and Brown, London, pp 13–14

Benjamini E, Feingold BF, Kartman L (1960) Allergy to flea bites III: The experimental induction of flea bite sensitivity in guinea pigs by exposure to flea bites and by antigen prepared from whole flea extracts of *Ctenocephalides felis felis*. Exp Parasitol 10: 214–222

Benjamini E, Feingold BF, Kartman L (1961) Skin reactivity in guinea pigs sensitized to flea bites. The sequence reaction. Proc Soc Exp Biol Med 108: 700–702

Benjamini E, Feingold BF, Young JD, Kartman L, Shimizu M (1963) Allergy to flea bites IV: In vitro collection and antigenic properties of the oral secretion of the cat flea *Ctenocephalides felis*. Exp Parasitol 13: 143–154

Blank H, Shaffer V, Spencer MC, Marsh WC (1950) Papular urticaria. Pediatrics 5: 408–413

Bolam RM (1958) L'Urticaire papuleuse. Enquête sur les causes de cette malade. Bull Soc Fr Dermatol Syphiligr 65: 388–391

*Bolam RM, Burtt ET (1956) Flea infestation as a cause of papular urticaria; a preliminary investigation. Br Med J 1: 1130–1133

Burrows D (1967) Papular urticaria, insect repellent and seasonal variation. Br J Dermatol 79: 497–499

Canadian Ministry of Supply and Services (1980) Control of fleas. Publ No 1187. Information Services for Agriculture. Acland, Ottawa

Chapman RF (1971) The insects; structure and function, 2nd edn. The English Universities Press, London, p 153.

Cherney LS, Wheeler CA, Reed AC (1939) Flea antigen in prevention of flea bites. Am J Trop Med 19: 327–332

Chipman ED (1910) Urticaria—with special reference to the cause in the papular form of children. Cal State J Med 8: 207–209

*Connor DH (1976) Tungiasis. In: Binfield CH and Connor DH (eds) Pathology of tropical and extraordinary diseases, vol 2. Armed Forces Institute of Pathology, Washington DC, pp 610–614

Cotton MJ (1970) The life history of the hen flea *Ceratophyllus gallinae* (Schrank) (Siphonaptera: Ceratophyllidae). Entomologist 103: 45–48

Dickey RF (1967) Papular urticaria—hordes of fleas in the living room. Cutis 3: 345–348

Dilaimy M (1978) Bullous papular urticaria. Cutis 21: 666–668

Eder HL (1945) Flea bites. Preventive treatment with thiamine hydrochloride. Arch Paediatr 62: 300–301

Faust CE, Maxwell TA (1930) The finding of the larva of the chigoe *Tunga penetrans* in scrapings from human skin. Arch Dermatol Syphilol 22: 94

*Feingold BF, Benjamini E (1961) Allergy to flea bites. Clinical and experimental observations. Ann Allergy 19: 1275–1289

*Fox T (1873) Diseases of the skin, 3rd edn. Henry Renshaw, London, pp 124–127

Fuga GL, Fabbro G dal, Provini M, Ribuffo A (1977) Osservazzioni su tre casi di Tungiasi. Minerva Med 68: 4115–4120

*Giron GP (1981) Tungiasis (nodulo solitario) Dermatol Venez 19: 49–56

Goldman L (1976) Tungiasis in travellers from Tropical Africa. JAMA 236: 1386

Gordon H (1933) Observations on lichen urticatus. Lancet II: 126–128

Guyon M (1870) Histoire naturelle et medicale de la chique *Rhinchoprion penetrans* (Oken). CR Acad Sci (Paris) 70: 785–792

*Hallam R (1927) Papular urticaria. Br J Dermatol 39: 95–111

Hamburger, Dietrich (1937) Lichen urticatus exogenes. Acta Paediatr 22: 420–421

Hicks EP (1931) The early stages of jigger *Tunga penetrans*. Ann Trop Med Parasitol 24: 575–586

Hoeppli R (1963) Early references to the occurrence of *Tunga penetrans* in tropical Africa. Acta Trop (Basel) 20: 143–153

Humphries DA (1968) The host finding behaviour of the hen

flea *Ceratophyllus gallinae* (Schrank) (Siphonaptera) Parasitology 58: 403–414

Hutchinson J (1879) Lectures on clinical surgery, vol I. Churchill, London, pp 79–87, 98–99

Imms AD (1938) A general text book of entomology, 4th edn. Methuen, London, pp 688–693

James MT, Harwood RF (1969) Herms's medical entomology, 6th edn. Macmillan, London, pp 299–319

*Jelliffe DB (1953) Tungiasis. In: Simons RDG Ph (ed) Handbook of tropical dermatology and medical mycology. Elsevier, Amsterdam, pp 895–900

Kinnear J (1933) Urticaria papulosa: with notes of fourteen cases with unusual history. Br J Dermatol 45: 65–68

Kochmann R (1856) Strophulus par piqûres de puces. Dapim Refuiim 15: VII

Lancashire GH (1928) Papular urticaria. Br Med J II: 1196

*Larrivée DH, Benjamini E, Feingold BF, Shimizu M (1964) Histologic studies of guinea pig skin: different stages of allergic reactivity to flea bites. Exp Parasitol 15: 491–502

Laugier P, Hunziker N, Orusco M, Brun R, Reiffers J, Posternak F (1975) Tungiose africaine. Dermatologica 150: 221–222

Lavoipierre MMJ, Radovsky FJ, Budwiser PD (1979) The feeding process of a tunga flea, *Tunga monositus* (Siphonaptera: Tungidae) and its relationship to the host inflammatory and repair response. J Med Entomol 15: 187–217

Lavoipierre MMJ, Radovsky FJ, Budwiser PD (1979) The host-parasite interaction of *Peromyscus mamiculatus* and the embedded female of *Tunga monositus* (Siphonaptera: Tungidae). J Med Entomol 16: 85–94

Leques B, Comby F, Sevrat P, Bullier R, Jasserna R (1973) Presentation de photos cliniques et parasitologiques d'un cas bordelais importé de Tungose. Bull Soc Fr Dermatol Syphiligr 80: 152

*Lunsford CJ (1949) Flea problem in California. Arch Dermatol Syphilol 60: 1184–1202

Maegraith BG (1971) In: Adams and Maegraith: Clinical tropical diseases, 5th edn. Blackwell, Oxford, pp 297, 383–384

Massie FS (1974) Papular urticaria; etiology, diagnosis and management. Cutis 13: 980–986

*Mellanby K (1946) Man's reactions to mosquito bites. Nature 158: 554

Michaeli D, Benjamini E, Buren FP de, Larrivée DH, Feingold BF (1965) The role of collagen in the induction of flea bite sensitivity. J Immunol 95: 162–170

Mooser H, Castenada MR (1938) The multiplication of the virus of Mexican typhus fever in fleas. J Exp Med 55: 307–323

Nuñez-Andrade R (1952) Tungiasis. Gac Med Mex 82: 11–15

*Patton WS (1931) Insects, ticks, mites and venomous animals of medical and veterinary importance. Part II Public Health. HR Grubb, Croydon, pp 232–271, 650–659

Porter L (1910) In discussion of Chipman (1910). Cal State J Med 8: 209

Reiss F (1966) Tungiasis in New York City. Arch Dermatol 93: 404–407

Reunala T, Ulmanen I, Siltanen I (1979) Animal fleas attacking man (in Finnish). Duodecim 95: 119–123

*Rook A (1961) Papular urticaria. Pediatr Clin North Am 8: 817–833

Rook A, Frain-Bell W (1953) Papular urticaria. Arch Dis Child 28: 304–310

Rothenburg HW (1975) Of fleas and foxes. Arch Dermatol 111: 1215

Rothschild M (1965) The rabbit flea and hormones. Endeavour 24: 162–168

Rothschild M, Clay T (1952) Fleas, flukes and cuckoos. Collins, London, pp 61–117

Shaffer B, Spencer MC, Blank H (1948) Papular urticaria. Its response to treatment with DDT and the role of insect bites in its etiology. J Invest Dermatol 11: 293–298

Shaffer B, Jacobsen C, Pori PP (1952) Papular urticaria. Its relationship to insect allergy. Ann Allergy 10: 411–421

*Shaffer B, Jacobsen C, Beerman H (1954) Papular urticaria; Histopathologic correlation of lesions of papular urticaria and positive skin test reactions to insect antigens. Arch Dermatol Syphilol 70: 437–422

Smit FGAM (1973) Siphonaptera. In: Smith KGV (ed) Insects and other arthropods of medical importance. The Trustees of the British Museum (Natural History), London, pp 325–371

Smith LM (1949) In discussion of Lunsford (1949). Arch Dermatol Syphilol 60: 1199

Tan-Lim KM, Pluis AHG (1971) Tungiasis. Dermatologica 143: 245–246

Tate BC (1935) Papular urticaria (lichen urticarus). Arch Dis Child 10: 27–48

Titchener RW (1979) Infestation of broiler breeder houses with hen fleas. Parasitology 79: xiii

White GB (1982) Fleas. In: Manson-Bahr PEC, Apted FIC (eds) Manson's tropical diseases, 18th edn. Baillière Tindall, London, pp 734–823

Wolff K (1975) Vogelflohe als fakultative Aktoparasiten des Menschen. Schweiz Rundischau Med (Praxis) 64: 1173–1175

Wulf K, Holtschmid J (1952) Zur Ätiologie und Therapie des Strophulus. Hautarzt 3: 267–270

Zalar GL, Walther RR (1980) Infestation by *Tunga penetrans*. Arch Dermatol 116: 80–81

12 Reactions to Lepidoptera

Lepidoptera comprise butterflies and moths, which are characterised by two pairs of wings covered by easily detachable scales, often vividly coloured in striking patterns. The developmental stages of egg, larva, pupa and adult correspond to similar stages in other endopterygote insects. Although there is no clear-cut distinction between moths and butterflies, it can be stated that in general butterflies have clubbed antennae and almost without exception rest with the wings pressed closely together over the back, whilst most moths have thread-like or feathery antennae and rest with the wings folded close to the sides of the body (Hyde 1974; M. R. Shaw 1982, personal communication).

There are many species of Lepidoptera, estimates varying between 120 000 and 165 000, and some 150 or so of these are recorded as causing damage to human skin. A classified list of the latter with their principal geographical distribution and appropriate references is given in Table 12.1.

Mechanism of Damage to Human Skin

Damage to human skin and mucosa, which has been known since Roman times (Phisalix 1922), arises from contact with and penetration of the skin or mucosa by the poison hairs or spines of larvae (caterpillars) or, sometimes, by the poison hairs of adults. (These are described in more detail below.) There may be direct contact between the caterpillar and the skin, either as the result of deliberate handling (by children, entomologists or other collectors) or accidentally, by the caterpillar falling from a tree onto a person below. Contact may also be indirect, by windborne hairs and spines or by the deliberate or accidental handling of cocoons or caterpillar webs into which the spines or hairs have been incorporated by the larvae, or of dead larvae, moulted skins or the bodies of adult Lepidoptera which have been contaminated during emergence from cocoons etc. or themselves bear irritant hairs. Entomological specimens, especially those kept in closed boxes, also give rise to irritating dust which can retain its potency for months or years. Dust from imagines of certain Lymantridae, from all *Hylesia* species, from *Dirpha* species and *Tryporyza innotatus* can similarly cause skin and eye lesions.

General Structure of Caterpillar Hairs and Spines

Many workers have described the irritating hairs and spines of caterpillars. The illustrations in Figs. 12.1 to 12.5 have been kindly loaned by Dr. R. V. Southcott of Adelaide and the descriptions to follow are based on his findings (Southcott 1978) and the paper by Maschwitz and Kloft (1971). The interested reader is advised to consult these two papers for full details.

Poisonous hairs and spines appear to be derived from ordinary covering hairs or setae. The latter develop from trichogen cells of the epidermis, the details of which are shown in Fig. 12.1. Such setae may be modified into sensory receptors of mechanical or chemical stimuli (Chapman 1971) or may develop poisonous properties if their cavity communicates with a poison-secreting gland. The structure of the various types of poisonous hairs and spines are illustrated in Figs. 12.2–12.5. Different species have different types and these with their principal structures are set out in Table 12.2. De Jong et al. (1976) confirmed by scanning electron microscopy that the shaft of these hairs is hollow (a fact already known for over 50 years), communicating with the outside by means of circular holes placed laterally near the tip and at the points of the barbs. The tiny Spiegelhaare (type 3a of Table 12.2) or dart hairs or flechets occur in enormous numbers. Maschwitz and Kloft (1971) estimated that there were about 630 000 on a single caterpillar of the Thaumetopoeidae family, whilst De Long (1981) calculated that a single larva of *Euproctis similis* had up to 2 000 000.

Table 12.1. Various species of Lepidoptera which have been reported as affecting human skin. (The superscript letters in the third column indicate references in the footnotes)

Species	Region	References
Superfamily ZYGAENOIDEA		
Family Limacodidae		
(= Eucleidae=Cochlididae)		
Sibine stimulea	Neotropical; nearctic	[b,c,e,f] Foot 1922; Allard and Allard (1958)
Natada nasoni		[a] Foot (1922)
Parasa hilarata	Ne- and palaearctic	[a,e,f] Mills (1925)
P. chloris	Ne- and palaearctic	[a,b,c,f]
P. latistigra	Ne- and palaearctic	[a,b,c,f]
P. indetermina	Nearctic	[f]
Sisyrosea textula	Nearctic; Australia	[b,e,f]
Doratifera vulnerans	Southeastern Australia	[e]
D. oxleyi	Southeastern Australia	[e]
D. quadriguttata	Southeastern Australia, New South Wales	[e]
Phobetron hipparchus	Australia; Brazil	[e,f]
P. pithecum	North America	[f]
Euryda variolans	Brazil	[d]
Scopelodes nitens	Australia	[e]
S. dinaria	Australia	[e]
Hydroclada kenrickii	New Guinea	[e]
Pymaomorpha modesta	New Guinea	[e]
Androneta spinuloides	Nearctic	[b,e,f]
Euclea delphinii	USA	Allard and Allard (1958)
Family Megalopydidae		
Megalopyge opercularis	Southern USA; Central and South America	[a,f] Foot (1922); Bishopp (1923); Micks (1952); McGovern et al. (1961)
M. crispata	USA	Jones and Mills (1959)
M. pyxiafera	USA	Jones and Mills (1959)
M. urens	Uruguay	[f] Mazella and Patetta (1948); Piaggio-Blanco and Paseyro (1946)
M. lanata	Brazil; Panama	[d,e,f] Foot (1922); Smith (1982)
M. albicollis	Brazil	Foot (1922)
M. krugii	Puerto Rico	[f]
M. superba	Brazil	[d,f]
M. radiata	Brazil	[d,f] Foot (1922)
M. undulata	Brazil	[d,f]
Carama cretata	USA; Brazil	[a,f] Foot (1922)
Podalia radiata	Brazil	[d,f]
P. chrysocoma	Brazil	[d,f]
P. albescens	Brazil	[d,f]
P. orsilochus	Brazil	[d,f]
Lagoa crispata	Nearctic	[a,b,c,f] Foot (1922); Allard and Allard (1958); Gordon and Lavoipierre (1962)
L. pyxidifera	Eastern USA	[f]
Norape spp.	Nearctic	[b,f]
Aidos amanda	Brazil	[d,f]
Trosia fallax	Brazil	[d,f]
Superfamily PAPILIONOIDEA		
Family Nymphalidae		
Inachis (=*vanessa*) *io*	Ne- and palaearctic	[a,b,c,f]
Mymphalis (=*Euvanessa*) *antiopa*		[a,b,f]
Euptoreta spp.	Nearctic	[c]
Family Morphidae		
Morpho hercules	Brazil	[d,f]
M. achillaena achillaena	Brazil	[d,f]
M. anaxibia	Brazil	[d,f]
M. menelaus	Brazil	[d,f]
M. rhetenor	Brazil	[d,f]
M. laertes	Brazil	[d,f]
M. cypis	Brazil	[d,f]

Table 12.1. *(continued)*

Species	Region	References
Superfamily BOMBYCOIDEA		
Family Lasiocampidae		
Macrothylacia spp.	Mostly tropical	[a]
M. rubi	Europe	Carter (1979)
Arctacea cribaria	Europe and Brazil	[d,f]
Cosmotriche spp.	Mostly tropical	[a,f]
Macromphala lignosa	Brazil; tropical	[a,d,f]
Gastropacha quercifolia		[f]
Dendrolimus pini	South Japanese islands	[a] Geserick (1952);
Titya proxima	Brazil	[d,f]
Lasiocampa quercus	Ne- and palaearctic	[a,b] Hellier and Warin (1967)
Euglyphus ornata	Brazil	[d,f]
Malacosoma americana	Nearctic	[b,f]
M. nuestria		South (1885); Thresh (1906); Tyzzer (1907)
Taragama igniflua	Philippines	[a,c] Tyzzer (1907); Foot (1922)
Suana concolor	Malaya	[e] Keegan (1963)
Philadoria potatoria	UK	Shaw (1982, personal commun.)
Eriogaster lanestris	UK	Hellier and Warin (1967)
Family Saturniidae		
Automeris io	Nearctic	[a,f] Tyzzer (1907); Allard and Allard (1958); Jones and Miller (1959)
A. corisus	Uruguay	Dallas (1928); Piaggio-Blanco and Paseyro (1946)
A. viridescens	Brazil; Argentine	[d] Foot (1922); Dallas (1928)
A. cinctistriga	Colombia	Foot (1922)
A. melanops	Brazil	[d,f]
A. ilustris	Brazil	[d,f]
A. aurantiaca	Brazil	[d,f]
A. acuminata	Brazil	[d]
A. incisa	Brazil	[d,f]
A. complicata	Brazil	[d,f]
Rotschildia spp.	Neotropical	[b]
Cricula spp.	Neotropical; Afrotropical	[a]
Coloradia spp.	Nearctic	[b]
Dirphia sabina	Tropical South America	[a,d,f]
D. multicolor	Colombia; Brazil	[d,f]
Hemileuca oliviae	New Mexico; tropical South America; nearctic	[a] Caffrey (1918)
H. lucina		[f]
H. nevadensis	Mid-western USA	Menwood and McDonald (1983)
H. maia	North America	[c,f] Allard and Allard (1958)
Hylesia urticans	French Guiana	[a,b]
H. linda	Mexico	[a,b]
H. canitia	Guianas	Boyé (1932)
H. continua	Guianas	Boyé (1932)
H. nigricans	Argentina	Dallas (1928)
H. nanas	Argentina	Dallas (1933)
H. metapyrrha	Argentina	Dallas (1933)
H. sorana	Argentina	Dallas (1933)
H. minasia	Argentina	Dallas (1933)
H. falcifera	Argentina	Dallas (1933)
H. remax	Argentina	Dallas (1933)
H. fulviventris	Argentina	Dallas (1933)
H. tapaber	Venezuela	Hill et al. (1948)
H. volvex	Peru	Pesce and Delgado (1966)
Lonomia achelosis	Venezuela	Smith (1982)
Ludia spp.	Afrotropical	[a]
Samia spp.	Neo- and Afrotropical	[a,f]
Eacles spp.	Neotropical	[b]
Eudyana venata	Argentina	Dallas (1928)
Pseudohazis eglantina	Nearctic	[b,f]
P. hera		[f]

Table 12.1. *(continued)*

Species	Region	References
Family Anthelidae		
Anthela spp.	Australia	Musgrave (1924, 1941)
Cheleptyrex collesi	Australia	
Family Eupterotidae		
Panacela lewinae	Australia	Froggatt (1911); Musgrave (1924)
Superfamily SPHINGOIDEA		
Family Sphingidae		
Sphinx spp.	Nearctic	[b] (European species said to be hairless; Shaw 1982, personal commun)
Superfamily NOTODONTOIDEA		
Family Thaumetopoeidae		
Thaumetopoea wilkinsonii	Palaearctic, Afrotropical	Numerous
T. pityocampa	Palaearctic, Afrotropical	Numerous
T. pinivora	Palaearctic, Afrotropical	Numerous
T. processionea	Palaearctic, Afrotropical	Numerous
Ochrogaster (= *Teara*) *contraria*	Australia	[e] Frogatt (1911); Flecker and McSweeney (1944)
O. linifer	North Australia; Papua New Guinea	Smith (1982)
Anapha venata	Africa	Smith (1982)
A. infracta		
Superfamily NOCTUOIDEA		
Family Lymantriidae		
Euproctis (= *Porthesia*) *chrysorrhoea*	Ne- and palaearctic	Numerous
E. similis	Palaearctic	Numerous
E. edwardsii	Australia	[e]
E. flava	Oriental	[e] Saito (1930); Keegan (1963)
E. flavociliata	Malaysia	[e] Keegan (1963)
E. funeralis	Malaysia	[e] Keegan (1963)
E. stenomorpha	North Australia	[e]
E. xutha	Papua New Guinea	[e]
E. phaeorrhoea	USA	[f] Tyzzer (1907); Jones and Miller (1959)
E. pseudoconspersa	Far East	Kawamoto et al. (1978)
Lymantria dispar	Australia	[a,f] Froggat (1911); Musgrave (1941)
L. monachis		[f]
Orgyia antiqua	Europe	Carter (1979)
O. pseudotsugato	Northwestern America	Perlman et al. (1976)
O. anartoides	Australia	[a,e,f]
Leptocneria reducta	Australia	[e]
Acryphas leucomelas	Australia	[e]
Dasychira pudibunda	UK	[a,f] Thresh (1906); Tyzzer (1907)
Hemerocampa leucostigma	Nearctic	[a,f] Knight (1922); Gilmer (1923)
Leucoma (= *Stilpnotia*) *salicis*	Ne- and palaearctic	[b,f]
Ocneria spp.		[a]
O. monacha		Henwood and McDonald (1983)
Family Arctiidae		
Arctia caja	Ne- and palaearctic	[a,f] Thresh (1906); Tyzzer (1907)
A. villica	Ne- and palaearctic	[a,f] Thresh (1906); Tyzzer (1907)
Spilosoma virginica	Europe (not UK)	Henwood and McDonald (1983)
S. lubricepeda	UK	Hellier and Warin (1967)
S. glatignyi	Nearctic; Australia	[b,f]
S. luteum	UK	Henwood and MacDonald (1983)
Utethesia ornatrix	Brazil	[d,f]
U. pulchella	Brazil	[d,f]
Antarctica fusca	Brazil	[d,f]
Ecpantheria orsa	Brazil	[d,f]
Eupseudosoma aberrans	Brazil	[d,f]

Table 12.1. (*continued*)

Species	Region	References
E. involutum	Brazil	d,f
Eutans terminalis	Australia	e
Adolia spp.	Neotropical; Oriental	a,f
Lithosia caniola		a,b,f
L. griseola		f
Parasemia spp.		a,b,f
Euchaetia egle	Nearctic	b,c,f
Halisodota caryae	Nearctic	b,f
Callimorpha spp.		a
Family Nolidae		
Uraba lugens	Australia	e
Family Noctuidae		
Acronicta (= *Apatele*) *americana*	Nearctic	a,b,c,f
Catocala spp.	Nearctic	a,b,c,f
Family Phycitidae		
Plodia interpunctella[a]*	India	Grosdanov (1959)

* Non-hairy.
[a] Maschwitz and Kloft (1971); [b] Pesce and Delgado (1971); [c] Picarelli and Valle (1971); [d] Rotberg (1971); [e] Southcott (1978); [f] Delgado Quiroz (1978)

Table 12.2. Types of poisonous hairs and spines found in different species of Lepidoptera, together with some of their characteristic features. (Compiled from Maschwitz and Kloft 1971; Southcott 1978)

Type of hair/spine	Features	Group
1. Normal	Usually long; may have outward directed barbs; stiff tips may penetrate human skin	Arctiidae; Nymphalidae; Noctuidae
2. Urticating hairs with modified tips (see Fig. 12.4)	Sharp free end; barbed hooks directed toward the base at sharp end (visible by phase contrast)	Lasiocampidae
3. Urticating hairs with pointed bases	Sharp pointed bases; barbed hooks directed against free end; easily detachable	
a) Spiegelhaare	Very short thin hairs (70–100 μm by 4–5 μm); hollow	Lymantriidae
b) Spiegelhaare of Thaumetopoeidae (see Fig. 12.3b)	Like a, but arise from a base which is invaginated and concealed at rest; appears in third instar and increases in size up to sixth instar from 106 μm to 213 μm; released in a cloud when disturbed; woven into cocoons	Thaumetopoeidae
c) Brush hairs (Fig. 12.3a)	Long urticating hairs in thick bundles	Lymantriidae; Noctuidae
d) Hairs of anal tufts of imagines	More numerous in females; two types (1) long and tapered at each end; (2) short with barbs directed against the base	
4. Poison spines (see Figs. 12.4, 12.5)	Usually associated with tubercles on caterpillars; tip may be broken off on contact but rest of the spine penetrates the human skin; pressure of touch and penetration together with internal pressure from caterpillar body enables poison to be injected into victim's skin	Megalopygidae; Limacodidae; Saturniidae; tropical Noctuidae

The various kinds of poison hairs are found in circumscribed discs or cups or tubercles arranged in parallel rows on the dorsal and lateral surfaces of the caterpillars on one or more of the abdominal segments, depending on the species. They are often vividly coloured and some can be erected by the caterpillar if disturbed. The poison in the stouter spines may actually be injected into the human skin as a combined result of the pressure of contact and internal compression by the caterpillar. In other instances the poisonous toxins may ooze out onto the surface of the skin (e.g. with *Auto-*

meris io; Maschwitz and Kloft 1971) and cause a contact reaction on the abraded surface. Apart from acting as a defence mechanism for the living caterpillar, these poisonous hairs are often woven into the cocoon or web by the silk-spinning caterpillars. Non-poisonous hairs may also cause irritation of a mechanical nature.

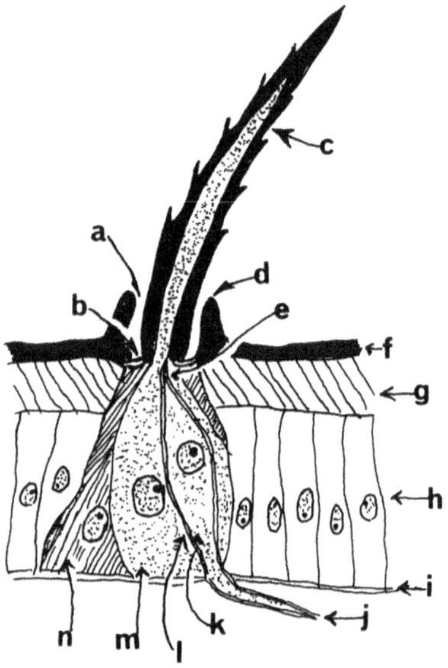

Fig. 12.1. Seta (macrotrichia) of an insect. *a*, alveolus; *b*, setal membrane; *c*, seta; *d*, annulus; *e*, dendrite of sensory neurone with stretch receptor; *f*, exocuticle; *g*, endocuticle; *h*, epidermis; *i*, basement membrane; *j*, proximal process of neurone; *k*, sensory neurone; *l*, neurilemma; *m*, trichogen cell; *n*, tormogen cell. (After Southcott 1978, by kind permission of the author and the Editor of *Records of the Adelaide Children's Hospital*)

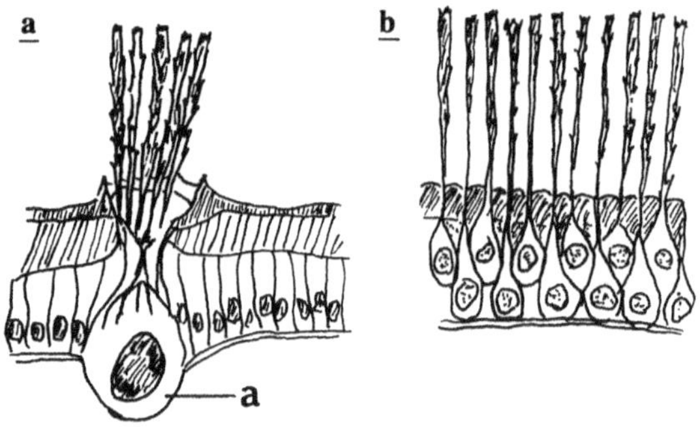

Fig. 12.3a, b. The origin of small dart hairs or flechets. **a** Multiple darts from single "cup" arising from simple cell, as in *Euproctis chrysorrhoea*. **b** Dart hairs each arising from a separate cell in a stratified layer of trichogen cells, as in *Thaumetopoea pityocampa*. *a*, Poison gland cell. (After Southcott 1978, by kind permission of the author and the Editor of *Records of the Adelaide Children's Hospital*)

Nature of Venom

The nature of the venoms in the poisonous spines and hairs of caterpillars has not yet been fully elucidated. According to Picarelli and Valle (1971), some undoubtedly contain histamine and also hitherto unidentified adenyl compounds. They could find no histamine, acetylcholine or 5-hydroxytryptamine in the setae of *Megalopyge* species but did find agents with spreading properties and also doubtful proteolytic and haemolytic activities. De Jong and Bleumink (1977a) identified histamine in the hairs of *Euproctis chrysorrhoea* but not apparently in sufficient concentration to account for skin reactions, except those of a sensi-

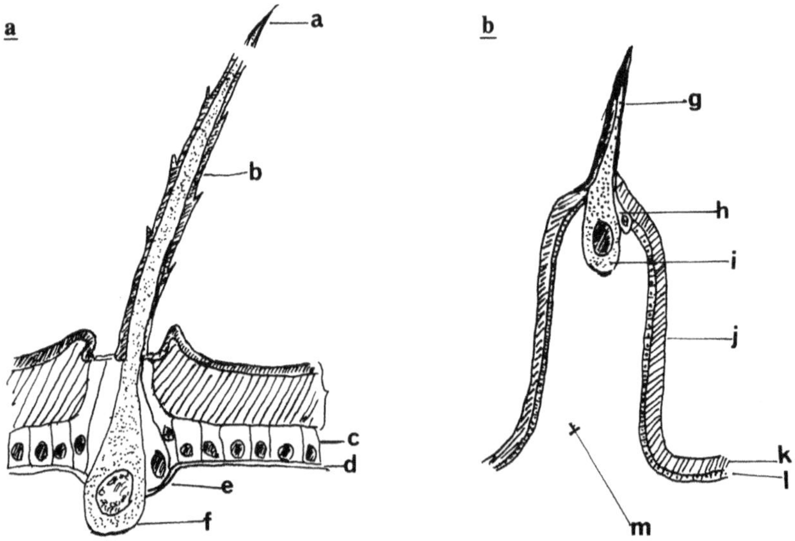

Fig. 12.2a, b. Showing conversion of a seta to a poison-bearing organ. **a** Seta communicates with poison cell. Its cavity contains poison released by setal fracture. **b** Seta elevated on a projection of insect cuticle enhancing its mechanical effectiveness. *a*, broken seta; *b* and *g*, seta; *k*, cuticle; *c* and *l*, epidermis; *d*, basement membrane; *e* and *h*, trichogen cell; *f* and *i*, gland cells; *j*, spine; *m*, body cavity of insect. (After Southcott 1978, by kind permission of the author and the Editor of *Records of the Adelaide Children's Hospital*)

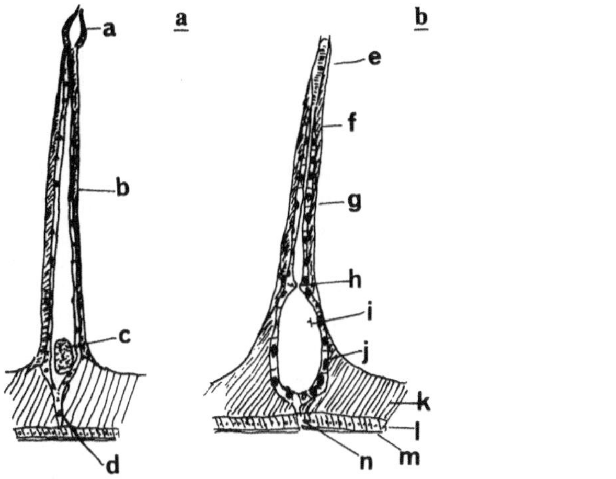

Fig. 12.4a, b Structure of a stinging spine. **a** Capped by a terminal detachable piece. Poison is liberated by rupture of thin membrane between this piece and the spine. (Seen in *Doratifera larvae.)* **b** Stinging spine with plugged terminal orifice. Mechanical pressure at tip releases the plug and venom is extruded. *a*, Terminal piece; *b* and *g*, epidermal lining of spine space; *c*, poison cell; *n*, pore canal; *e*, pigmented plug; *f*, shaft; *h*, diaphragm; *i*, cavity; *j*, epidermal cells of bulb sac; *k*, cuticle; *l*, epidermis; *m*, basement membrane. (After Southcott 1978, by kind permission of the author and the Editor of *Records of the Adelaide Children's Hospital*)

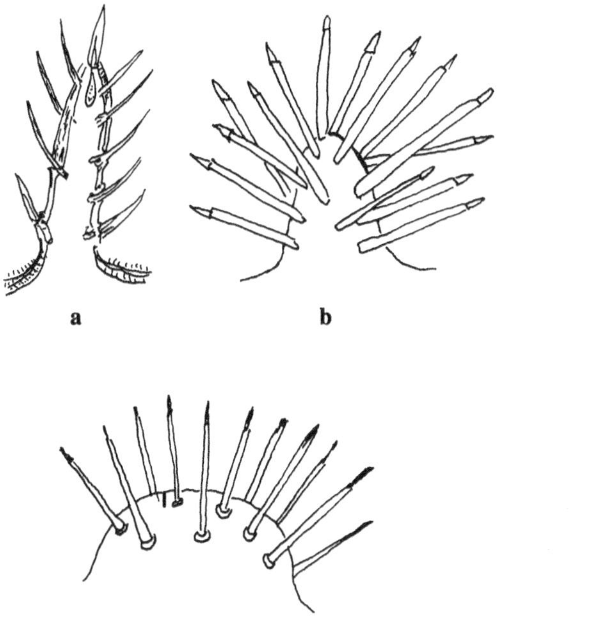

Fig. 12.5a–c. Three types of grouping of venomous spines. **a** short conical spines with tiers of stinging setae; **b** multiple long, strong spines arising from a conical eminence; **c** multiple spines with terminal plugs. (After Southcott 1978, by kind permission of the author and the Editor of *Records of the Adelaide Children's Hospital*)

tivity nature. However, Hall-Smith and Graham (1980) found serotonin and histamine (1 μg/g and 30 μg/g, respectively on caterpillar skin including hairs. Moreover, they also found that when minced caterpillar skin was incubated with histidine it proved to be a powerful histamine producer—20 times more than human skin in this respect. Valette and Huidorro (1954) had already indicated that the venom of the poison hairs of *Thaumetopoea pityocampa* larvae contained a histamine liberator. Goldman et al. (1960) indicated by chromatographic and electrophoretic techniques that the toxin of caterpillar hair was a polypeptide rather than a protein. De Jong and Bleumink (1977a) also isolated substances with trypsin-like and chymotrypsin-like activity, which they considered were probably due to peptidases. Proteolytic and phospholipase A^2 activity were also observed and regarded by De Jong as equivalent to the non-haemolytic "sphering" action on erythrocytes of the venom of many snakes and insects (see pp. 5, 139, 195, 220). De Jong and his colleague (1977b) also indicated that components giving rise to IgG antibodies in rabbits were present in the hair extracts and that the peptidases referred to might also be responsible for both complement and plasminogen activation. Bleumink et al. (1982) confirmed these findings and stated that the assumption was warranted that such proteases, especially kallikreinase, are major factors in the elicitation of the clinical symptoms seen after contact with caterpillar spines.

The venom of *Hylesia* is water soluble, which prompted Zaias et al. (1969) to suggest that sweating, by dissolving the venom, could spread the effect of a single contact. Pesce and Delgado (1971) noted its histamine-like action but held the view that the rarity of sensitisation phenomena associated with this species denoted the probable absence of a protein moiety. Arocha-Pinango and Layrisse (1969) reported five patients who developed a long-standing fibrinolytic bleeding disorder after contact with caterpillars of the Saturniidae family restricted to a defined region in Venezuela. The syndrome, apart from initial burning irritation, occipital headache and generalised aching, showed the appearance of extensive ecchymoses some 8–72 h after contact, with bleeding from all orifices. The patients recovered after treatment with epsilon amino caproic acid. The caterpillar hairs were shown to have a fibrinolytic activity. Mills (1925) reported the occurrence of marked "gooseflesh" around sites of penetration by caterpillar hairs of *Parasa hilarata* in patients in North China, which suggests a possible liberation of acetylcholine.

Clinical Picture

Skin Reactions

South (1885) quoted a traveller in South America, T.P. Bigg-Wither, as follows:

Varieties of caterpillar are legion. Bodies are protected by triple coats of mail, i.e. covered with hairy substance which in some resembled moss and in others stag antlers. To attempt to touch the creatures with the naked hand was a scarcely less hazardous undertaking than plunging one's hand into a live hornet's nest. Each hair or point has the power of inflicting a sting as painful as that of certain venomous species of red ant very common in parts of the forest, so that, if by chance, as not infrequently befell us when working on the picada, one of these caterpillars happens to drop off a tree on to the hand or worse still on to the nape of the neck, the pain is almost unbearable, the spot on which the creature falls immediately becoming inflamed and afterwards swelling up to a great size.

The clinical reaction of the skin to the poisonous hairs of caterpillars has a certain basic uniformity whatever the species, with the exception of the Megalopygidae, and therefore a general description will be given, with variations where relevant.

Visible lesions are almost always preceded by itch, often of a burning character, sometimes amounting to pain, which at first increases rapidly in intensity. With *Hylesia* moth the peak of intensity is reached in about 2 h and persists for 2–3 days. The onset in these cases can be delayed by up to 1 week (Hill et al. 1948). With Thaumetopoeidae larvae (processionary and "bag-shelter" caterpillars) the onset is always delayed for about 3 h and occasionally for up to 1 week (Touraine et al. 1947b). With *Euproctis* and related species the onset may be immediately after contact (Balding 1884; Thresh 1906; Cleland 1920; Knight 1922; Musgrave 1941; De Long 1981), or may be delayed for 8–12 h (Blair 1979; Shama et al. 1982) or even for 2–3 days (Hellier and Warin 1967). Itch is usually continuous but may exhibit intermittent exacerbations (Musgrave 1941; Touraine et al. 1974b; Blair 1979). It is aggravated by warmth (Musgrave 1941; Blair 1979) or by repeated exposure to the caterpillars (Hellier and Warin 1967), The burning character with *Hylesia* was also prominent in the epidemic caused by *Euproctis flava* (Randel and Doan 1956), whereas De Long (1981) noted that pain was completely absent in the lesions associated with *E. similis*. Succumbing to the urge to scratch increases the itch (Touraine et al. 1974b).

The itch is followed very quickly in many instances by the appearance of tiny, rose-red, maculopapules or papules from 2 to 5 mm across. A central vesicle may often be seen, which rarely may become pustular. The larger lesions seem to be the result of more intimate contact with the caterpillar (Blair 1979). Lesions caused by the larva of *Lymantria dispar* are rather smaller (1–3 mm) and when excoriated reveal a necrotic centre (Beaucher and Farnham 1982). A linear or streaky appearance may be seen where the larvae have crawled over the skin (White 1901; Torchi 1952–1953; Hall-Smith and Graham 1980; Beaucher and Farnham 1982), but this feature can equally well be absent in the same circumstances (Meek 1901; Hellier and Warin 1967; Fig. 12.6). Touraine and his colleagues (1974b) pointed out that with *Thaumeto-*

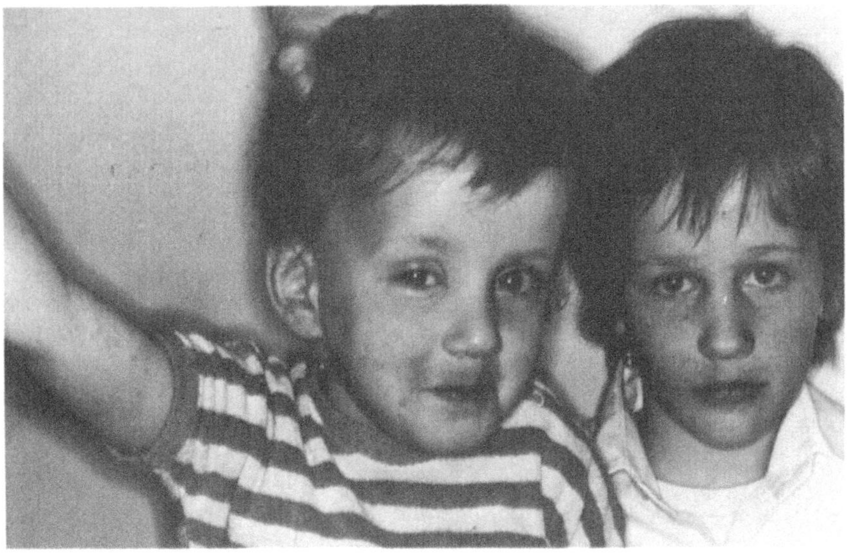

Fig. 12.6. Slightly urticated papular lesions on the arms and face of twin children caused by racing caterpillars of *Euproctis chrysorrhoea* on their arms. (Courtesy of Dr. S. Alexander, Barking, Essex)

poea species the papules, which were slightly oedematous with an erythematous base, itched most markedly at their acuminate tip, scratching of which produced tiny serous crusts. These fell off in about 3 days with relief of the itch. The papules, which could number hundreds, subsided in 3–4 days leaving faint brown macules which disappeared in a further 5–8 days. Blair (1979) noted similar pigmentation after involution of *Euproctis* lesions. With *Hylesia* contamination, itch was quickly followed by erythema which could become generalised, but the papular lesions did not appear until about 4 h after the onset of itching. They, too, were very numerous and could remain discrete or coalesce into plaques. Not infrequently they assumed a morbilliform appearance. Scratching also resulted in crust formation and, if secondary infection supervened, pustules appeared (Boyé 1932; Zaias et al. 1969). Tiny petechial lesions were sometimes scattered throughout the papular lesions (Hill et al. 1948; Allard and Allard 1958; Pesce and Delgado 1966).

Shama et al. (1982), in addition to the above lesions, noted the presence of weals on many patients. These have sometimes not been recorded and this could be because, as Blair (1979) observed, dermatologists often do not see patients in the earliest stages. She noticed that the lesions in her patients urticated when rubbed. The papules in *Hylesia* eruptions have an urticated appearance (Boyé 1932) and were reported as slightly oedematous in *Thaumetopoea* lesions (Touraine et al. 1974a, b). Urticaria as such has been a prominent feature of many outbreaks (Anderson 1884; Balding 1884, 1885; South 1885; White 1901; Meek 1901; Thresh 1906; Tyzzer 1907; Potter 1909; Cleland 1920; Knight 1922; Musgrave 1924; Hellier and Warin 1967; Southcott 1978; Hall-Smith and Graham 1980; Shama et al. 1982); (Fig. 12.7). Generalised urticaria with eyelid oedema was recorded by both South (1885) and Thresh (1906). In some of the latter's patients the eyelid oedema seemed to be a local reaction to conjunctivitis, but in South's patients it was apparently unrelated to areas of contact, a feature noted by Hellier and Warin (1967) and emphasized by Hall-Smith and Graham 1980; (Fig. 12.8). This suggests the development of hypersensitivity, a state which would

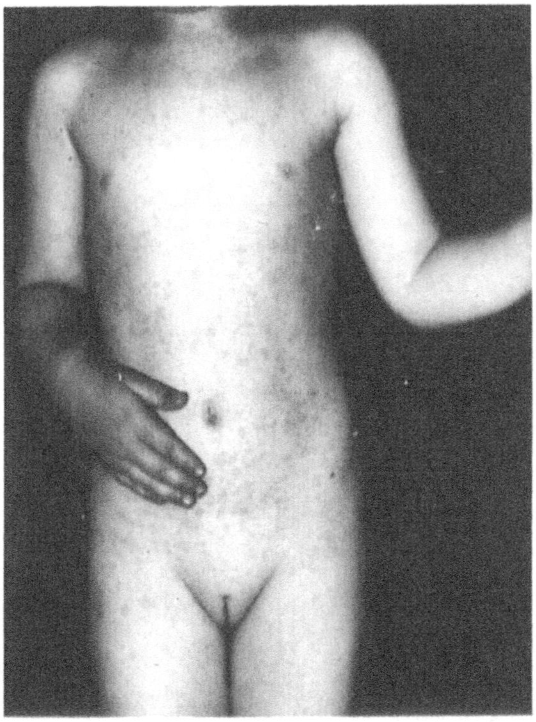

Fig. 12.7. Widespread eruption caused by yellow-tail moth caterpillar. (From Hellier and Warin 1967, by kind permission of Prof. F. F. Hellier and the Editor of the *British Medical Journal*)

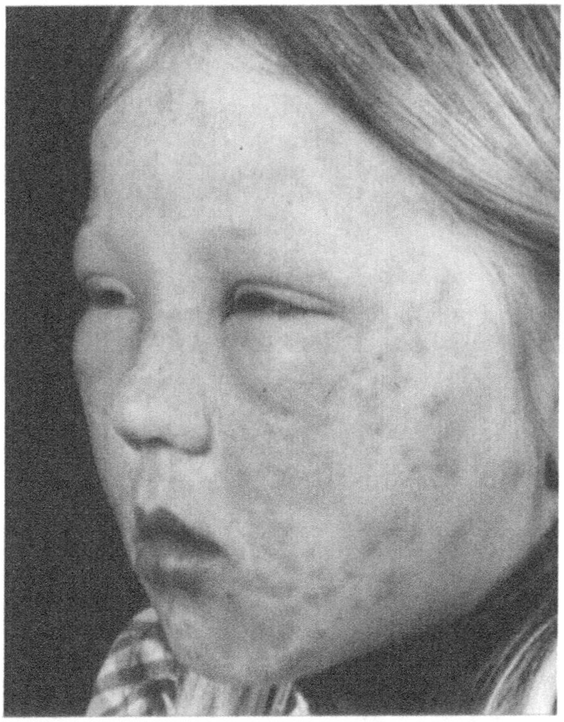

Fig. 12.8. Urticated lesions and eyelid oedema caused by contact with "hairy caterpillars." (Courtesy of Dr. Patrick Hall-Smith)

also account for the increase of itch with repeated exposure. Delbos (1948) regarded lesions caused by *T. pityocampa* as hypersensitive and noted that natural immunity could occur. Localised oedema was reported in association with lesions of the neck, eyelids and forearms by Touraine et al. (1974b) and observed in many patients contaminated by *Hylesia* (Leger and Mouzels 1918; Dallas 1928; Allard and Allard 1958). Dallas (1928) also recorded generalised oedema in this context.

Chronicity with the development of lichenification or secondary eczema was noted as a result of repeated, more or less continuous re-exposure for weeks to *Hylesia* (Boyé 1932; Pesce and Delgado (1966) and to *Euproctis chrysorrhoea* (Potter 1909; Blair 1979). Hellier and Warin (1967) pointed out that many lesions associated with contact with *Eriogaster lanestris* and *Lasiocampa quercus* showed a tiny central black dot, visible only with a lens, which they thought represented the penetrating caterpillar hair. Local numbness, lymphangitis and lymphadenopathy have been recorded in some patients with *Euproctis flava* stings (Saito 1936; Randel and Doan 1956). Malaise may occur in severe eruptions, and mild fever is not uncommon in children (Knight 1922; Hellier and Warin 1967).

The distribution of eruption is very similar, whatever species of caterpillar or moth is responsible: The most common sites are on the exposed areas—back of the hand, wrist, forearm (Fig. 12.9), cubital fossa, upper arm and neck, and, less commonly, the upper trunk and anterior abdomen (Blair 1979). Torchi (1952–1953) found the popliteal fossae and thighs, as well as the retroauricular folds, conchae and sides of the neck, were not uncommonly affected. For some reason

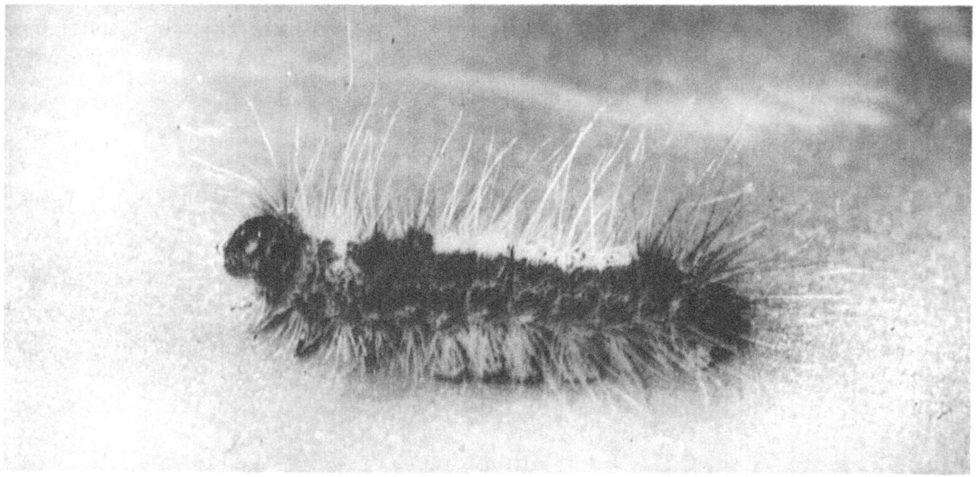

a

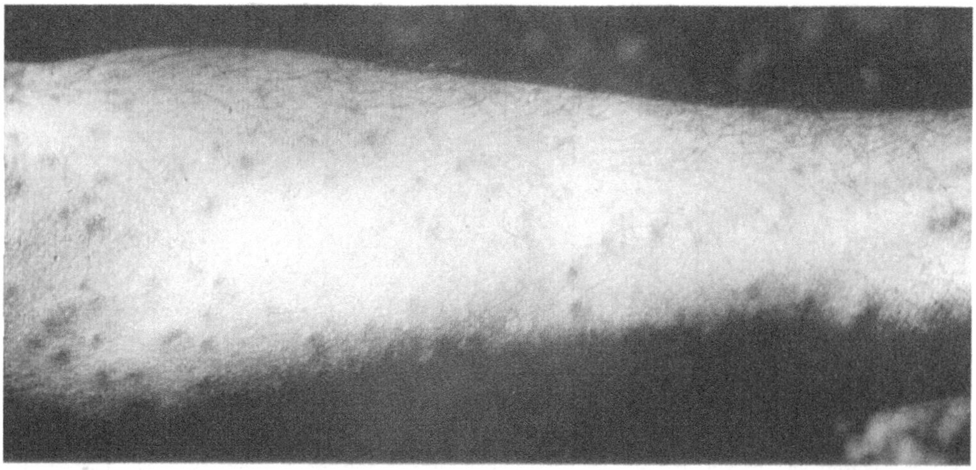

b

Fig. 12.9. a Caterpillar of *Euproctis edwardsii*; **b** papular eruption caused by this caterpillar. (From Southcott 1978, by kind permission of the author and the Editor of *Records of the Adelaide Children's Hospital*) the face is usually spared (Musgrave 1941; Hellier and Warin 1967; Blair 1979; Hall-Smith and Graham 1980; Beaucher and Farnham 1982), except for urticarial reaction; however, in Thresh's (1906) series of 20 children only the face and hands were involved (see Fig. 12.6). Rendall (1884) noted that children had a habit of collecting caterpillars in their handkerchiefs and pinafores, which were then often used to wipe their faces after the caterpillars had been emptied out. Touraine and his colleagues (1974a, b) laid stress on the tiny pearly vesicular lesions on the interdigital areas of the hand; these are similar to some lesions of scabies in the same area but disappear after 2 or 3 days. South (1885) had also noted itching between the fingers. The palms and palmar surface of the fingers are said to be seldom involved; however, Katzenellenbogen (1955) noted that they were not infrequently affected in children who play with caterpillars. Indeed the present writer has seen erythematous macular lesions 2–3 mm across on a child's palm several days after collecting caterpillars. Areas covered by clothing but where the skin is thin are sometimes affected, e.g. axillae, clavicular and pectoral regions, the waistline and genital areas (Katzenellenbogen 1955). Castle (1924) records lesions on the buttocks of a patient who was alleged to have sat on a caterpillar.

Areas contaminated by *Hylesia* are much the same as regards exposed sites and those where the skin is thin, but the eruption quickly becomes widespread (Pesce and Delgado 1966). Rotberg (1971) concluded that no area was exempt, but most authors have regarded the face, palms and soles as seldom if ever involved. Any area except these can be quite severely affected by indirect contact because of the all-pervasive nature of the irritating dust released from the hundreds of thousands of fluttering moths. This dust lands on clothing, bedding, laundry and upholstery unless special precautions are taken and can affect any part of the body coming into contact with these contaminated articles. Leger and Mouzels (1918) noted that the pulp of the fingers used for rubbing and scratching lesions induced by *Hylesia* became numb and later developed tiny vesicles.

Any of the above lesions usually clear in about 7 days, but the petechial lesions of *Hylesia* rash take 2 weeks (Pesce and Delgado 1966) and residual pigmentation about 3 weeks (Zaias et al. 1969).

Reactions to "Stings" from Megalopyge Larvae

Two *Megalopyge* spp. commonly cause sting reactions: *M. opercularis* Smith and Abbot in Texas, New Mexico and Central and South America (Foot 1922; Bishopp 1923; Micks 1952; McGovern et al. 1961) and *M. urens* in Uruguay and elsewhere in South America (Piaggio-Blanco and Paseyro 1946; Mazzella and Patetta 1948). They produce similar reactions but different from those caused by other lepidopterous larvae (Micks 1952). All victims react, but some are more susceptible than others. Multiple contact does not necessarily increase symptoms significantly, according to McGovern and his team (1961), although experimentally Foot (1922) had noted that reaction increased in severity with repeated exposure. There is no increased incidence at any particular age and both sexes are equally affected. Foot held that the severity of reaction could vary with the location of the sting, but this was not so in Micks' (1952) series of patients. Areas of thicker skin (e.g. palms) seem to react less severely than areas where it is thinner.

The usual areas involved are (1) the hand or arm, (2) the foot or leg and (3) the neck or face, in that order of frequency (Micks 1952). After contact with the caterpillar there is immediate, increasingly intense local burning pain, which often radiates proximally to the root of the affected limb and may have a shooting character. Erythema develops almost simultaneously around the site punctured by poison spines and spreads peripherally to produce a halo, often several centimeters in diameter, around a small central papule. In some instances the central lesion may be haemorrhagic and sometimes after about 2–3 h may become vesicular and remain so for several hours (Bishopp 1923). The affected area frequently swells rapidly, at times even involving the whole limb, which may double in volume. Radiating lymphangitis is common and regional lymphadenopathy often develops, sometimes within 45 min (McGovern et al. 1961). Areas not contaminated by the larvae and not contiguous with affected areas are not as a rule involved, although one of McGovern's patients developed a widespread maculopapular rash. Local lesions and erythema may persist for days and sometimes there is residual pigmentation (Bishopp 1923). The rapidity of development of the reaction was a feature stressed by Micks (1952), who also pointed out that symptoms could persist for up to 48 h in the absence of treatment.

In addition to the lesions described and the pain, children may be feverish and restless and complain of nausea and vomiting. Headache is a common early symptom and may be severe and persist for 24 h. Foot (1922) noted that severe swelling may be accompanied by general numbness and pseudoparalysis, rendering the victim incapable of work. Of McGovern's (1961) patients 5% showed evidence of mild to severe shock with hypotension, bradycardia and respiratory embarrassment. Some even became comatose. Convulsions were seen in five patients. Although death was not recorded, the authors considered it to be a possibility which could not be excluded. Table 12.3 shows the frequency of occurrence of the principal features.

Table 12.3. Frequency of features in reactions to contact with larvae of *Megalopyge opercularis*. (Based on McGovern et al. 1961)

Feature	Number of patients	Percentage
Severe local pain	2093	98.3
Local swelling	1964	92.0
Regional lymphadenopathy	679	31.9
Headache	626	29.4
Shock-like syndrome	104	4.96
Convulsions	5	0.24

Foot (1922) induced similar reactions by rubbing caterpillars or their hairs onto the skin of volunteers. Repeated tests evoked painful oedema rather than simple erythema. Mazzella and Patetta (1948) produced the same effects in dogs by local injection of toxin from poison spines. Regional lymphadenopathy was a marked feature in their experiments.

Grosdanov (1959) noted that *Plodia interpunctella* (Phycitidae) caterpillars caused an itching contact dermatitis in workers cleaning and removing the kernels from infested nuts. These caterpillars had neither hairs nor spines, but extracts of the caterpillars or their excrement gave positive confirmatory epicutaneous tests.

Eye Lesions

Mucosal lesions may accompany the skin lesions from contact with any of the damaging species of caterpillar. Rhinitis and tracheitis may occur on rare occasions (Pesce and Delgado 1971), whilst smarting of the lips and nostrils has been recorded amongst entomologists dissecting *Hylesia* moths (Boyé 1932; Dallas 1927). Phisalix (1922) noted nodular conjunctivitis as a not uncommon reaction. Although eye lesions are less common than skin lesions, under some circumstances they may be much more serious. The following account has been compiled from six papers concerned only with ocular lesions viz. Gunderson et al. (1950) Geserick (1952), Dreyer (1953), Corkey (1955), Watson and Sevel (1966) and Bishop and Morton (1968).

Dreyer (1953) recognised two groups of eye lesion: (1) resulting from contact with airborne poison hairs, not infrequently bilateral; and (2) resulting from the forcible striking of the eye by a whole caterpillar, usually unilateral and causing the disorder called ophthalmia nodosa. The first group is relatively benign but may still cause considerable inconvenience. It can be caused by any species of caterpillar which damages the skin, some more than others (Gunderson et al. 1950). Geserick (1952) described 22 instances in 18 persons where single pointed hairs were observed on the palpebral conjunctiva causing painful inflammatory conjunctivitis. The pain and inflammation disappeared quickly and without sequel when the offending hair was removed. Not all patients in this group seek help at once. Bishop and Morton (1968) recorded a series of 132 patients injured in the eye of whom only 19 sought advice within 24 h; at least 30 waited a week or longer before asking for help. Examination does not easily reveal the cause, especially if an adequate history is lacking, e.g. with children. Conjunctivitis and corneal haziness may be evident on naked eye inspection. No obvious foreign bodies will be seen. Even with fluorescein a foreign body will only be visible with suitable magnification. Many patients are therefore treated initially as examples of simple conjunctivitis or keratoconjunctivitis, usually without success. Slit lamp examination is essential. Minute scarification may then be seen on the cornea and minute barbed hairs will be seen embedded in the conjunctiva and especially in the cornea. Scratch marks will be found on the upper half of the cornea when the upper eyelid is affected and on the lower half when the lower eyelid is involved. When the contact is by airborne hairs they are not usually deeply embedded and can be removed with the aid of a fine needle or very fine epilating forceps. If they are more deeply embedded, removal may be impossible. In the case of a single hair, excision may be effective, but this is quite impracticable with multiple hairs.

The much more serious condition of ophthalmia nodosa is caused by the eye being struck suddenly and usually forcibly by a caterpillar, which may be thrown by a child (Dreyer 1953), may be accidently wiped onto the eye by a towel (Gunderson et al. 1953), may fall onto the eye from a tree (Corkey 1955; Watson and Sevel, 1966), or may be suddenly and sharply blown into the eye by a gust of wind (Watson and Sevel 1966). There is immediate severe smarting or burning pain. Opening the eye becomes almost impossible. There is much lacrimation, and the conjunctiva becomes severely reddened, swollen and raised by as much as 5–6 mm above the sclera. Focal haemorrhages may be seen, and the cornea becomes oedematous and lustreless. Slit lamp examination at this stage will show many hairs embedded in the conjunctiva, sclera and cornea. Those with projecting free ends may be removed, as above, with forceps, but those with no projecting portion cannot be removed. There may be some alleviation of symptoms at this stage as the result of the removal of projecting hairs. Irrigation seems to be quite useless (Gunderson et al. 1953). Within a few days pain will return and inflammation continue. This pattern of remission and exacerbation is characteristic. Iritis and iridocyclitis may develop with posterior synechiae. The aqueous humor may become turbid and corneal opacities develop. Repeated slit lamp examination will show that the caterpillar hairs wander through the ocular tissues; this penetration is due to a combination of eye movement and the barbs on the hairs themselves, which encourage such movement in one direction only. The penetration becomes deeper and deeper. In the solid tissues the irritant hairs induce surrounding inflammatory reaction, and tiny foreign body granulomata form with the hair in the centre (Geserick 1952). These are visible as nodules in the conjunctiva, sclera and iris. Some of these granulomata may persist after the hair has passed through the layer of tissue. Vision becomes progressively impaired and may be totally lost. If pain is not relieved, enucleation of the eye becomes necessary. Full details of the clinical and pathological findings in such a case are described by Gunderson et al. (1953)

Histopathology

The microscopic changes in human skin caused by penetration of poison-containing hairs and liberation of the poison are basically similar for all species of caterpillar or adult moth, with minor species variations. The following description has been taken from papers by Tyzzer (1907) Foot (1922), Hill et al. (1948) Zaias et al. (1969), Rotberg (1971), Blair (1979) and De Jong et al. (1976).

In all cases there are focal epidermal changes related to the presence of poison hair fragments. Around these fragments there is cell necrosis which may very quickly result in a superficial bulla formation. This is followed by a rapidly developing localised spongiosis of the malpighian layer. With *Hylesia* hairs bulla formation and cell necrosis are less evident, but ballooning or hydropic degeneration of the epidermal cells is seen. In all cases there is a moderate cellular exocytosis into the epidermis. With *Euproctis* and *Hylesia* stings the migrating cells are mainly neutrophils with ocasional lymphocytes and eosinophils, but with *Megalopyge* stings the predominant cell is the lymphocyte, and much fibrin is also present.

The superficial dermis shows dilatation of otherwise normal blood vessels, which are often engorged, especially in *Hylesia* and *Megalopyge* reactions. In all instances there is a perivascular infiltrate. In *Hylesia* reactions the infiltrate is mainly neutrophil with a few lymphocytes and pyknotic histiocytes. A mild circulatory eosinophilia may sometimes also be present. *Megalopyge* induces a perivascular infiltrate of lymphocytes, eosinophils, neutrophils and mast cells in that order of frequency, the vessels themselves containing lymphocytes and eosinophils. Experimentally Piaggio-Blanco and Paseyro (1946) and Mazzella and Paketta (1948) confirmed the dominance of eosinophil cells in *Megalopyge* reactions, noting also an eosinophilia of the peripheral blood and regional lymph nodes. With *Euproctis* the infiltrate begins like that of *Hylesia* but within 24–48 h becomes predominantly lymphocytic. Blair (1979) and De Jong et al. (1976) noted particularly the non-involvement of the cutaneous appendages, which would seem to indicate that the earlier theories (Gilmer 1923) that penetrating hairs only entered the skin through hair follicles was incorrect. Hall-Smith and Graham (1980) noted the presence of increased histamine in the victim's skin, which they attributed to an increased histamine forming capacity (see p. 183). Jones and Miller (1959) noted rapid oedema of the corium with neutrophil perivascular infiltrate, which they attributed to histamine effect, with *Automeris io*. With *Hylesia* hairs, if penetration was deep, a foreign body giant-cell reaction around the fragments could be seen. Repair of the immediate reaction described began after 72 h. It had been suggested by early workers (Rossiter 1924) that the changes could be regarded as similar to those induced physically by fibreglass fragments. Kemper (1955) indicated that penetrating hairs do not induce a simple mechanical reaction but one like the toxic reaction of an insect bite. Cuypers et al. (1975) have shown that fibreglass induced only microtraumatic changes in the epidermis together with eczematous spongiosis and a dermal perivascular lymphocytic infiltrate. There was no cell necrosis in the epidermis. Zaias et al. (1969) suggested that the cell necrosis represented the reaction to the lepidopterous toxin, with the underlying dermal changes being an inflammatory reaction, an opinion originally expressed in 1918 by Leger and Mouzels.

Epidemiology

A knowledge of the epidemiology is important and frequently necessary for diagnosis.

Hylesia

The skin eruption caused by the various species of the *Hylesia* genus of Saturniidae (see Fig. 12.10) is well known in South America. The moths are found from Mexico to Argentina, their prevalence being determined by the prevailing climatic conditions. Recognised in Cayenne, French Guiana since 1912 (Boyé 1932), the first full description of skin eruption caused by *Hylesia* species was published by Leger and Mouzels (1918). Outbreaks of skin reaction have also been recorded by Dallas (1926, 1927, 1928, 1933) and Jorg (1933) in Argentina, by Hill et al. (1948), D'Avanzo (1952) and Zaias et al. (1969) from Venezuela, by Allard and Allard (1958) and Pesce and Delgado (1966) from Peru and by Rotberg (1971) from Brazil.

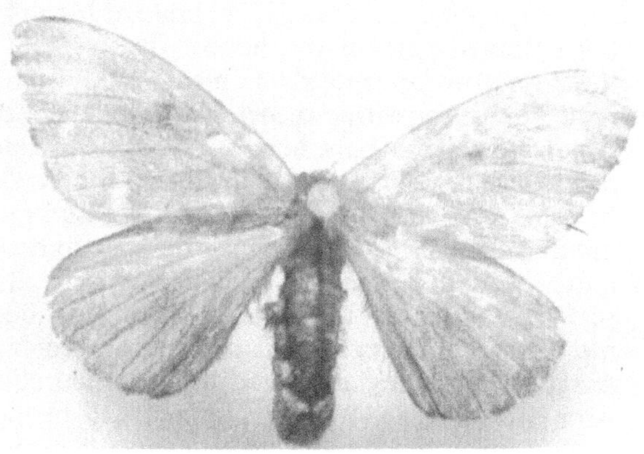

Fig. 12.10. *Hylesia nigricans*. (Courtesy of the Curator, Scottish Natural History Museum)

The age and sex incidence of those exposed and reacting is the same as for the general population concerned. The onset of the eruption is invariably preceded by a sudden invasion of an area at dusk by vast numbers of moths attracted by the lights of a village, town or ship at anchor. The swarm of insects fluttering and banging against the lights and other fittings releases a cloud of dust, grey, brown or yellowish in colour (depending on the local species), which covers the unclothed body of persons below as well as their clothes, furniture, bedding, floor etc., even gaining entry to drawers and cupboards injudiciously left open (D'Avanzo 1952). The number of outbreaks per year is dependent on the number of moth generations per year. In equatorial climates such as in Venezuela or French Guiana there are four generations annually; outbreaks occur in January, April, July and October, but are often more irregular (Boyé 1932). In Peru moths generally appear from the end of April to early June, the end of the rainy season (Allard and Allard (1958); Pesce and Delgado 1966); however, every 4 or 5 years, more than one generation may appear annually, and outbreaks may then also occur in August–September and December–January (Pesce and Delgado 1971). In Argentina cases occur in the summer months between January and March (Dallas 1928).

The occurrence of an outbreak in a particular inhabited area also depends on the direction of the prevailing wind. Where outbreaks have been a regular occurrence it has been the custom of villagers to extinguish their fires just before dusk for an hour or two until the wind has died down (Boyé 1932).

The crews of oil tankers calling at ports in Venezuela (Caripito in particular) are especially liable to attack, being obliged to anchor in enclosed areas for one or two nights with their lights on and fully exposed to swarming (Hill et al. 1948; D'Avanzo 1952; Zaias et al. 1969). In addition to the immediate occurrence of many cases of eruption there are also several instances of the eruption appearing for the first time a week or more after the ship has left the area. This is due to contamination of clean clothing and bed linen, which, when these are issued later, produces new cases. Hill and his colleagues (1948) noted that in 9 of 31 cases arising in a tanker crew of 45 the victims had their first attack on the seventh day after exposure and 24 h after the issue of fresh but contaminated bed linen. This finding raised the possibility of a infectious exanthema at the time. In village outbreaks up to 80% of the population may be affected (Allard and Allard 1958). Rotberg (1971) observed that affected persons had a diminished capacity for work.

Other Species

Larvae and some adult moths of the family Lymantridae, notably several species of *Euproctis* (see Figs. 12.9, 12.11) and *Lymantria dispar* (Fig. 12.12), have caused outbreaks of varying severity in many parts of the world. In the United Kingdom relatively small numbers have been involved (though most cases have gone unrecorded): e.g. Thresh (1906), 20 patients; Blair (1979) 36; and Hellier and Warin (1967) 45. Larger numbers have been reported in Europe, where the disorder

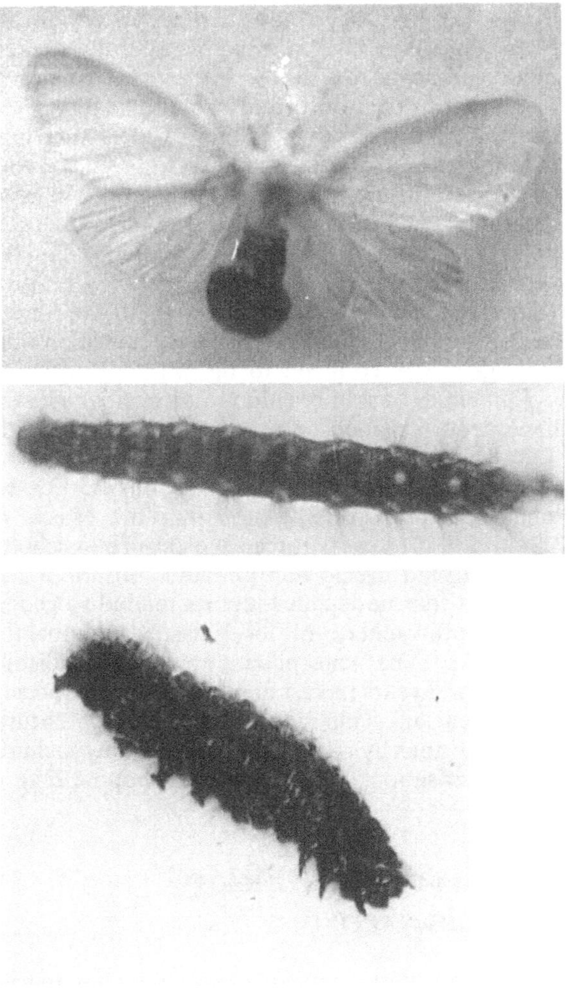

a b c

Fig. 12.11a–c. *Euproctis chrysorrhoea*. **a** adult moth; **b** larva; **c** larva showing walking legs. (**a** and **b** Courtesy of the Curator, Scottish Natural History Museum; **c** courtesy of Dr. S. Alexander, Barking, Essex)

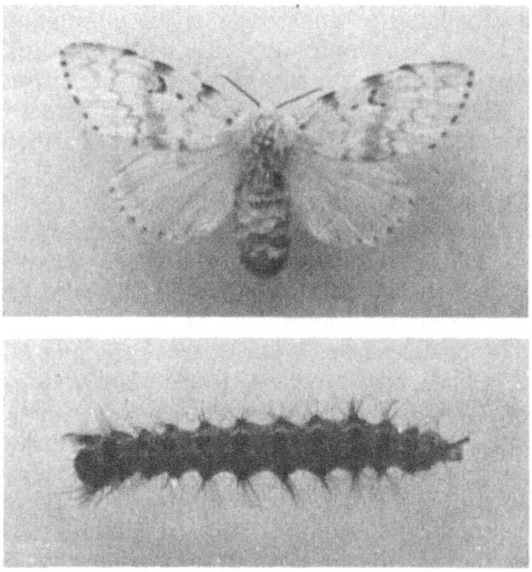

a b

Fig. 12.12a, b. *Lymantria dispar*. **a** adult moth; **b** caterpillar. (Courtesy of the Curator, Scottish Natural History Museum)

has been familiar for at least 250 years (De Jong et al. 1975). Polano (1935) noted an outbreak in the Friesian islands amongst workers and bathers. In the United States, where *Euproctis chrysorrhoea* had been introduced in 1892 (Potter 1909), Fernald and Kirkland (1897) first recorded severe defoliation damage to fruit trees by the caterpillars, and epidemics involving large numbers of persons were subsequently reported by White (1901), Meek (1901), Potter (1909) and by Kephart (1915). More recently Beaucher and Farnham (1982) and Shama et al. (1982) have recorded thousands of people affected by the larvae of *Lymantria dispar*, which have caused severe economic damage to trees in the northeastern states of the United States. Cleland (1920) and Musgrave (1924) reported numbers of cases in Australia which were caused by *Euproctis edwardsii*. These outbreaks pale into insignificance beside those in Japan, where up to 300 000 patients were affected by hairs from *E. flava* caterpillars and adults (cited by Keegan 1963 and by Smith 1982), and in Shanghai where De Long (1981) described an epidemic of over half a million cases due to *E. similis*. Outbreaks of dermatitis caused by different species of *Thaumetopoea* have been recorded: in Cyprus by Cheverton (1936), caused by *T. wilkinsonii*; in France by Touraine et al. (1974a, b) and in Italy by Torchi (1952–1953), caused by *T. processionea* (Fig. 12.13); and in Israel by Katzenellenbogen (1955) and Ziprowski et al. (1959), caused by *T. pinivora*. From Australia came reports by Froggatt (1911) and Flecker and McSweeney (1944) of numerous cases caused by the bag-shelter moth larva of *Ochrogaster* (= *Teara*) *contraria*. Caterpillars of many other species have also been recorded as causing cutaneous reactions (see Table 12.1).

With all these epidemics there is a certain similarity in the circumstances of exposure. The larvae, some of which have a processionary habit of looking for food, live gregariously in webs in trees or shrubs, which vary according to species and also to the geographical location: e.g. fruit and hedgerow trees and shrubs in the British Isles; pines and forest trees in Europe and the Middle East—parts of the Bois de Boulogne were closed to the public in 1866 because of a great epidemic of caterpillars (Phisalix 1922); fruit trees in northeastern America; and eucalyptus, acacia and mistletoe in Australia. Sudden increases in the number of cases are correlated with increases in the population of the larvae, which probably result from favourable climatic conditions in sucessive years. For example, De Long (1981) observed a 23-fold increase in larval numbers of *Euproctis similis* the year before the great Shanghai epidemic.

Persons who venture into the vicinity of these swarms of caterpillars or moths will probably suffer from falling caterpillars or windborne dust. The victims include children playing with, and especially collecting, caterpillars (Hellier and Warin 1967), picnic parties beneath trees (Shama et al. 1982), bathers, whose towels are often contaminated (Polano 1935), soldiers bivouacking beneath trees (Flecker and McSweeney 1944; Ziprowski et al. 1959), men collecting domestic firewood (Torchi 1952–1953) or merely people walking in the countryside (many authors, from Balding 1884 onwards). In some instances caterpillar rash may be an occupational hazard, e.g. workers engaged in removing nests (Froggatt 1911; Katzenellengoben 1955), forestry workers (Touraine et al. 1974a, b), hop pickers irritated by larvae of *Dasychira pudibunda* (Thresh 1906; Whitwell 1943) and especially entomologists (Cockerell 1885; Knight 1922) and to a lesser extent pharmacologists. Collecting boxes and specimen jars are bound to be contaminated and careless opening of these will release a cloud of irritating dust (Balding 1884). In this context De Jong (1980) has devised a vacuum technique for collecting poisonous hairs for pharmacological testing which avoids any handling by the research worker.

Other materials contaminated include children's handkerchiefs and pinafores used for collected caterpillars (Rendall 1884; Thresh 1906; Hellier and Warin 1967), infested firewood (Cleland 1920), laundry hung out to dry beneath infested trees (De Long 1981), as well as the clothing of those already affected (Cleland 1920). Blair (1979) has pointed out that some caterpillars may enter buildings to pupate and thus be a source of contamination. In the great epidemic of the village of Somerville near Boston, Massachusetts in 1897 the walls and piazzas of the houses had to be washed down daily to prevent such human contamination (Meek 1901).

De Long (1981), in his epidemiological appreciation of the Shanghai outbreak, noted several important features. There was a sudden increase in larvae and dispersal of their poison hairs from many foci simultaneously. These hairs came into contact with a large number of people at the same time and the potential victims were in a position to be contaminated. Considered from the point of view of incriminating the larvae as the source of the trouble he noted that (1) there were infested trees in the areas where the dermatitis occcurred; (2) where there was no dermatitis there were few or no larvae on the trees; (3) in areas of prevalence more cases occurred in houses which were near infested trees than in those which were not; (4) the rise in the number of cases correlated with an increase in the number of larvae; (5) when the caterpillars were eradicated the number of cases quickly fell; and (6) poison hairs were found on the skin of patients. He also noted that in a hospital with infested trees in the grounds there were more cases amongst patients allowed outside than amongst those confined to the ward.

Epidemics of skin reaction to *Megalopyge* larvae have been recorded on at least three occasions in Texas (Foot 1922; Micks 1952; McGovern et al. 1961). McGovern et al. reported on 2130 cases, whilst Bishopp (1923) noted that the effects of "thousands" of cases forced the closure of schools until infested trees were treated. Bishopp also observed that newspaper reports tended to generate an atmosphere of local hysteria about the outbreaks. The caterpillars appear periodically every 4 or 5 years in vast numbers and do not occur every year in such numbers because of natural control, either by bacterial infection or by tachinid fly parasitisation of the larvae (Bishopp 1923).

Morphology and Biology of Lepidoptera

It is obviously impracticable to consider any species in great detail here. For fuller information readers are advised to consult the appropriate reference cited in Table 12.1 or special works on Lepidoptera. Nevertheless, some indication of the general morphology of one or two selected species should help to a basic understanding of the defence mechanisms of these insects which can cause reactions in man.

Hylesia spp.

Hylesia moths have a wing span of 3–5 cm and a body length of 1.5–3 cm. The northern species are a golden colour, whilst those from Peru and Argentina have dark brown or black stripes on the body. The wings and body are heavily coated with scales and long hairs (see Fig. 12.10); on the dorsal surface of the body there are clusters of shorter hollow spines about 150 μm × 2–3 μm situated on a narrow median band and intermingled with longer hairs. The latter are brightly coloured but the spines are a dull yellow, which changes to brown shortly after being shed (Boyé 1932). Leger and Mouzels (1918) and Boyé (1932) gave detailed biological descriptions of the hairs and spines. The males have no poison spines except those acquired from the female during mating. Any hairs found on eggs, larvae or exuviae come from the same source.

The life cycle is about 3 months (Boyé 1932), the eggs being laid in clusters adhering to the branches of forest trees and other plants (Dallas 1933) and coated with urticating spines by the female. They hatch in 2–3 weeks; the larvae moult four times and emerge about 1 month later as imagines.

Euproctis chrysorrhoea

Euproctis chrysorrhoea is a smaller whitish moth which has a wing-span of 2.5–4 cm and a prominent anal tuft of long brown hairs at the posterior end of the abdomen, forming a sort of tail (hence the name, "brown-tail" moth; see Fig. 12.11). These hairs are more prominent on the female and are easily detached.

Some 300–400 small round eggs, which are thickly covered with hairs from the female anal tuft, are laid, especially on the undersurface of the twigs and leaves of fruit trees, forming small masses about 2 × 1 cm. The young caterpillars hatch after about 1 month and weave a communal web of silk in which they spend the winter. Emerging in the spring they feed voraciously on the leaves of the host tree, undergoing four moults inside the web before pupating there. The web thus becomes liberally coated with larval hairs and may cause skin irritation if handled. The larvae disperse before pupation and spin cocoons amongst the foliage. The caterpillar hairs break off during and after cocoon construction and become incorporated in it. (This may also occur with some Lasiocampidae species.) It has been suggested by Potter (1909) and others that the anal tuft of the emerging female imago is contaminated by these hairs in the cocoon. This is unlikely in natural conditions. Moreover, the irritating properties of the anal tuft are due to the hairs of the latter being themselves noxious (M. R. Shaw 1982, personal communication). Goossens (1881) thought that the caterpillar tubercles oozed a sticky poisonous secretion when disturbed. This, he said, dried almost instantaneously to an irritating dust. It seems more likely, however, that Cleland's (1920) view that the rash was due to poison spines was correct. This appears to have been confirmed by several workers (see Maschwitz and Kloft 1971; Southcott 1978).

Thaumetopoea spp.

Thaumetopoea pityocampa (see Fig. 12.13) and related species appear as adults in mid-summer, as does *Euproctis*, at the end of July and early August. Its eggs are laid in the lower branches of pine trees because it is a poor flyer. Larvae hatch about 1 month later and begin to feed at once. Between meals they rest on temporary platforms of silk. About November the colony, which has by this time developed the processionary habit, enabling them to go as far afield as possible and retrace their steps, like Ariadne, along the silken thread which they have left in their trail, begin to construct a stout winter home, usually near to the top of the tree. This is made of silk threads and bands woven around the supporting framework of needles, twigs and branches and containing caterpillar hairs amongst its meshes. The mature larvae emerge in March, descend to the ground and bury themselves to pupate, the imagines emerging about 4 months later in July.

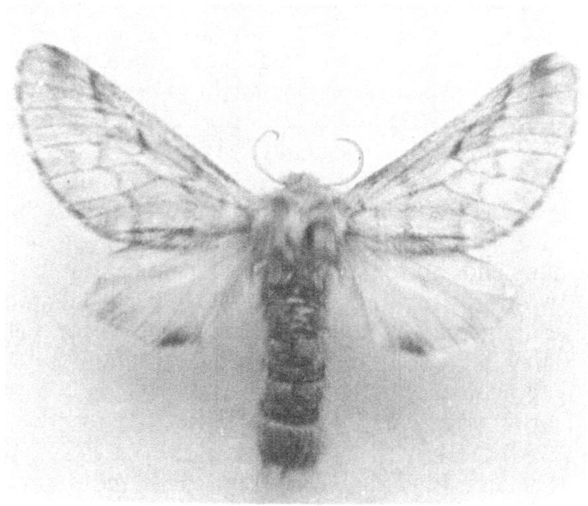

Fig. 12.13. *Thaumetopoea processionea*, adult moth. Note long hairs on body and wings. (Courtesy of the Curator, Scottish Natural History Museum)

Ochrogaster (= *Teara*) *contraria*

The bag-shelter moths, *Ochrogaster* (= *Teara*) *contraria*, behave in a similar fashion. Their webs are large irregular bag-shaped structures built in shrubs and trees such as acacia and eucalyptus. Much dust is released from them when the bushes are disturbed, for example by men sleeping below them (Flecker and McSweeney 1944). Horses may suffer even more severely than men. Froggatt (1911) described how they developed severe swelling of the lips, tongue and oral mucosa, making feeding impossible and thus having a fatal outcome at times. Cattle and sheep are not affected, apparently because their oral mucosa is more resistant (Froggatt 1911).

Megalopyge opecularis

The morphology and biology of *Megalopyge opercularis* are fully described by Bishopp (1923). The adult moths are yellowish-brown with a scattering of long white hairs, which imparts a silvery sheen to them. The female is slightly larger than the male and has a wing span of about 4 cm. The eggs are usually laid (300–400 per female) on the leaves of trees and hatch in 4–8 days. The larvae undergo five to six moults before reaching maturity in 30–60 days. After pupation the imago emerges and lives for about 9 days. Two generations are produced annually: The adults emerging from overwintered cocoons appear in April–June and the second generation appear in September to October (in Texas). The larvae are variously known as "puss caterpillars", "possum bugs" and "Italian asps" in the United States, as *perrito* (little dog) in Mexico (Bishopp 1923) and as *Bicho peludo negro* (black hairy bug) in Uruguay (Piaggio-Blanco and Paseyro 1946). The mature larva is about 2.5 cm long, tapers somewhat posteriorly and has three rows of warts on each side from which arise long hairs and shorter spines. The hairs are about half to two-thirds as long as the larval body. The spines contain the toxin secreted by basal poison cells. They increase in number with each moult and are yellowish with a black tip. The larva as a whole varies from dark brown to tawny red to grey.

All the larval stages can sting (Foot 1922), but the later (and larger) instars cause more severe reactions (Bishopp 1923), probably because of the greater number and size of the poison spines and greater amount of toxin injected (Micks 1952). Freshly moulted skin and recently dead larvae can also cause a lesser degree of reaction. Gilmer (1923) thought that this toxin was probably not a protein but capable of conjugating with one.

Doratifera spp. and *Uraba lugens*

Southcott (1978) has described in detail the rash caused by different species of *Doratifera* (Limacodidae) and by *Uraba lugens* (Nolidae). The latter group especially cause a very persistent irritating skin reaction, which may be evident for up to 6 weeks. The life cycle of this caterpillar includes no less than 11 instars. Southcott's work should be read for full details.

Diagnosis

In the case of *Hylesia*, where the swarms of moths cannot avoid being noticed and their association with the onset of the eruption is easily recognised, diagnosis is fairly obvious. However, when the onset is delayed and the victims have left the area, an accurate history is very important. Similarly, obvious epidemics of caterpillars soon come to the public attention in the relevant area (as will be evident from the epidemiological notes), but smaller outbreaks, where the cases are almost sporadic, are more difficult to diagnose. The lesions described are very like those resulting from attacks by several kinds of mite, bugs, fleas etc., but the distribution may be somewhat different. Predatory mites frequently attack covered areas of the body. Pyemotid, cheyletiellid or trombiculid mites often attack exposed areas, but at times the eruption they induce may be widespread and indiscriminate. Flea bites tend to have a bizarre asymmetrical distribution. Whatever distribution is dominant with these parasites, there is generally a noticeable tendency for the lesions to concentrate in the vicinity of constricting garments such as belts, garters etc. This is not a feature of lepidopterism. The history and circumstances in which the eruption develops are also points of diagnostic importance. Other diseases such as scabies, lichen planus, pityriasis rosea and sensitisation eczema have their own special characteristics, physical features, distribution, mode of onset and response to treatment.

Confirmatory tests for the reactions to larvae or imagines of many species have been carried out. Those for *Megalopyge* have been noted on pp. 187 and 188. Tests for other species—applying patch tests of extracts from living or dead caterpillars, their skin or hairs of various types, their cocoons or the dust from caterpillars or moths, or by rubbing the material directly onto the skin of patients or volunteers—have all been recorded. The results are usually a replica of the clinical picture but sometimes are demonstrated as a weal and flare reaction. They are mostly immediate but some may persist for several weeks (Southcott 1978). Positive reactions have been obtained to *Hemerocampa leucostigma* (Knight 1922), to *Euproctis edwardsii* (Musgrave 1924) and to *E. chrysorrhoea* (Kemper 1955), to *Eriogaster lanestris* and *Spilosoma lubricipeda*—a species not otherwise recorded as causing skin reaction (Hellier and Warin 1967), to *E. similis* (De Long 1981), to *Lymantria dispar* (Shama et al. 1982; Beaucher and Farnham 1982) and to many other species, including *Doratifera* spp., *Uraba lugens* and species of Eupterotidae and Lymantriidae (Southcott 1978), by various tests. De Jong et al. (1975) obtained a positive reaction to *E. chrysorrhoea* by the intradermal injection of a saline extract of poison hairs and with his colleagues in 1976 he confirmed a finding of Tyzzer (1907) that the spines of *E. chrysorrhoea* caused spherocytosis of human erythrocytes in vitro. In South America confirmation of the pathogenic role of the dust shed by *Hylesia* was obtained by Leger and Mouzels (1918) by Allard and Allard (in 1952 but reported in 1958), by Pesce and Delgado (1966) and by Zaias et al. (1969).

Treatment

Early treatment of lesions caused by *Hylesia* with a 50% solution of sodium hyposulphite was claimed by Pesce and Delgado (1966) to alleviate the symptoms quickly and to suppress lesions, provided it was used within an hour of contact, and the earlier the better. Similarly, Fabré (1916), confirmed by Knight (1922) on several patients, found that a pulp of the leaves of purslane (*Portulaca oleracea*) was surprisingly beneficial when applied to the lesions. It would seem that this would be worth investigating pharmacologically. Other topical treatment is purely symptomatic, and calamine lotion, as recommended by D'Avanzo (1952), is probably as effective as anything. An oily preparation is best as it does not cake and spreads easily. Topical corticosteroids, benzocaine etc. are not helpful. The pain often experienced in severe cases is alleviated by oral codeine but may even require morphine (Keegan 1963). That encountered from *Megalopyge* hairs is promptly relieved by 10 ml of 10% calcium gluconate intravenously (Micks 1952). Oral antihistamines are of little help except in the eruption caused by *Thaumetopoea wilkinsonii*, where Ziproski et al. (1959) found they helped greatly. For the shock syndrome associated with *Megalopyge* lesions Micks (1952) recommended subcutaneous 1 in 1000 adrenaline solution twice daily if necessary. *Megalopyge* eruptions were helped greatly by the removal of excess hairs and spines by Sellotape stripping (McGovern et al. 1961). This remedy might also apply to other reactions to Lepidoptera.

Precautions

Contamination can be avoided to a large extent by refraining from handling with the naked hands any stage of Lepidoptera known to be harmful. Walking, picnicking or sleeping beneath infested trees should be avoided. Where *Hylesia* is prevalent, people should keep indoors when they are swarming. Lights of any kind should be extinguished at dusk and kept out for 1–3 h, unless they are inside adequately screened buildings. Personal clothing and bed linen should be kept in closed drawers or cupboards in these regions. Control measures depend on local conditions (Keegan 1963). Infested trees and shrubs should be sprayed with appropriate insecticides. Buildings should have adequate screens on the windows and doors. Schools and other places of communal gathering should be temporarily shut if infestation is likely to be spread by their remaining open. Caterpillars' webs should be removed only by properly protected personnel.

References

Allard HF, Allard HA (1958) Venomous moths and butterflies. J Wash Acad Sci 48: 18–21

Anderson J (1884) The urticating properties of the hairs of some lepidoptera. Entomologist 17: 275–276

Arocha-Pinango CL, Layrisse M (1969) Fibrinolysis produced by contact with a caterpillar. Lancet I: 810–812

Balding G (1884) Of the irritating properties of the hairs of *Liparis chrysorrhoea*. Entomologist 17: 256–257

Balding G (1885) Concerning the irritating properties of caterpillars. Entomologist 18: 41–43

Beaucher WN, Farnham JE (1982) Gypsy moth caterpillar dermatitis N Eng J Med 306: 1301–1302

Bishop FC (1923) The puss caterpillar and the effects of its sting on man. US Dept of Agriculture Circular No 288. US Govt Printing Office, Washington DC, pp 1–14

Bishop JW, Morton MR (1968) Caterpillar hair keratoconjunctivitis. Med J Aust 2: 995–997

Blair CP (1979) The browntail moth, its caterpillar and their rash. Clin Exp Dermatol 4: 215–222

Bleumink E, De Jong MCJM Kawamoto F, Meyer GT, Kloostermuis AJ, Slijper-Pal IJ (1982) Protease activities in the spicule venom of *Euproctis* caterpillars. Toxicon 20: 607–613

*Boyé R (1932) La papillonite Guyanaise. Bull Soc Pathol Exot 25: 1099–1107

Caffrey DJ (1918) Notes on the poisonous urticating spines of *Hemileuca oliviae* larvae. J Econ Entomol 11: 363–367

Carter DJ (1979) The observer's book of caterpillars. Warne, London

Castle WF (1924) Dermatitis due to caterpillars. Br Med J 2: 218

Chapman RF (1971) The insects. Structure and function. English Universities Press, London

Cheverton RL (1936) Irritation caused by contact with the processionary caterpillar (larva of *Thaumetopoea wilkinsonii* Tams) and its nest. Trans R Soc Trop Med Hyg 29: 555–558

Cleland JB (1920) Papulo-urticarial rashes caused by the hairlets of caterpillars of the moth (*Euproctis edwardsii* Newman). Med J Aust 1: 169–170

Cockerell TDA (1885) On *Porthesia similis* (*chrysorrhoea*) irritation. Entomologist 18: 74–75

Corkey JA (1955) Ophthalmia nodosa due to caterpillar hairs. Br J Ophthalmol 39: 301–306

Cuypers JMC, Hoedemaeker PhJ, Natel JP, and De Jong MCJM (1975) The histopathology of fibreglass dermatitis in relation to von Hebra's concept of eczema. Contact Dermatitis 1: 88–95

Dallas ED (1926) Eritema generalizado producida por un lepidoptero. Rev Soc Entomol Argent 2: 63–64

Dallas ED (1927) Nota sobre dermitis por "Hylesia". Sem Med 14: 896

Dallas ED (1928) Nota sobra Lepidopterismo en la Republica Argentina. Cuarta Reunion Soc Argent Patol Reg Norte 4: 691–694

Dallas ED (1933) Otro caso de dermitis extendida producida por un lepidoptero y notas sobre *Hylesia nigricans* Berg (Lip. Bombycidae). Reunion Soc Argent Patol Reg 2: 469–470

*D'Avanzo G (1952) La dermatite da contatto provocata da farfalle del Genere *Hylesia* ('Yellowtail moth dermatitis' o 'Caripito itch'). Med Lav 43: 439–452

De Jong MCJM (1980) A safe and rapid method of collecting the urticating hairs from *Euproctis* caterpillars (Lepidoptera; Lymantriidae). Clin Exp Dermatol 5: 357–359

*De Jong MCJM, Bleumink E (1977a) Investigative studies of the dermatitis caused by the larva of the browntail moth *Euproctis chrysorrhoea* L. (Lepidoptera: Lymantriidae). III Chemical analysis of skin reactive substance. Arch Dermatol Res 259: 247–262

*De Jong MCJM, Bleumink E (1977b) Investigative studies of the dermatitis caused by the larva of the browntail moth *Euproctis chrysorrhoea* L. (Lepidoptera: Lymantriidae) IV. Further characterisation of skin reactive substances. Arch Dermatol Res 259: 263–281

*De Jong MCJM, Bleumink E, Nater JP (1975) Investigative studies of the dermatitis caused by the larva of the browntail moth (*Euproctis chrysorrhoea* Linn.) I. Clinical and experimental findings. Arch Dermatol Res 253: 287–300

*De Jong MCJM, Hoedemaeker PHJ, Jongebloed WL and Nater JP (1976) Investigative studies of the dermatitis caused by the larva of the browntail moth (*Euproctis chrysorrhoea* Linn.) II. Histopathology of skin lesions and scanning electronmicroscopy of their causative state. Arch Dermatol Res 255: 177–191

Delbos J (1948) A propos de la dermatite des chenilles (Cnetocampa pityocampa). Bull Soc Fr Dermatol Syphiligr 55: 321

Delgado Quiroz A (1978) Venoms of Lepidoptera. In: Bettini S (ed) Arthropod venoms. Springer, Berlin Heidelberg New York, pp 555–611 (Handbook of experimental pharmacology, vol. 48)

*De Long S (1981) Mulberry tussock moth dermatitis. A study of an epidemic of unknown origin. J Epidemiol Community Health 35: 1–4

Dreyer V (1953) Ophthalmia nodosa. Acta Ophthalmol 31: 429–436

*Fabré JH (1916) The life of the caterpillar. Translated by Teixeria de Mattos A. Dodd, Mead, New York

Fernald CH, Kirkland AH (1897) The brown tail moth (*Euproctis chrysorrhoea* L). Spec Bull Hatch Exp Station Mass Agric Coll, pp 3–15

Flecker H, McSweeney A (1944) Irritation produced by the procession caterpillar (*Ochrogaster contraria*). Med J Aust 2: 137–138

Foot NC (1922) Pathology of the dermatitis caused by *Megalopyge opercularis*, a Texan caterpillar. J Exp Med 35: 737–753

Froggatt WW (1911) Bagshelter caterpillars of the family Liperidae that are reported to kill stock. Agric Gaz N S Wales May 3, 443–447

Geserick H (1952) Beobachten bei Raupenhaarerkrankungen der augen. Uber Konjunktivitis durch Raupenhaare, über das Eindringen und über die Wanderung von Raupenhaaren. Klin Monatsbl Augenheitk 120: 373–393

Gilmer PM (1923) The poison and poison apparatus of the white marked tussock moth *Hemerocampa leucostigma* Smith and Abbot. J Parasitol 10: 80–86

Goldman L, Sawyer F, Levine A, Goldman J, Goldman S, Spinanger J (1960) Investigative studies of skin irritations from caterpillars. J Invest Dermatol 34: 67–78

Goossens Th (1881) Des chenilles urticantes. Ann Soc Entomol Fr 1: 230–236

Gordon RM, Lavoipierre MMJ (1962) Entomology for students of medicine. Blackwell, Oxford, p 286

Grosdanov A (1959) Berufsbedingte Ekzeme und Hautentzundungen durch Raupen der *Plodia interpunctella*. Berufsdermatosen 7: 30–35. Cited by Henwood and MacDonald (1983)

Gunderson T, Heath P, Garron LK (1950) Ophthalmia nodosa. Trans Am Ophthalmol Soc 48: 151–169

Hall-Smith PJ, Graham P (1980) Beware the furry caterpillar. Clin Exp Dermatol 5: 261–263

Hellier FF, Warin RP (1967) Caterpillar dermatitis. Br Med J II: 346–348

*Henwood BP, MacDonald DM (1983) Caterpillar dermatitis. Clin Exp Dermatol 8: 77–93

Hill WR, Rubinstein AD, Kovacs J (1948) Dermatitis resulting from contact with moths (genus *Hylesia*). JAMA 138: 737–740

Hyde GE (1974) British moth book I. Jarrold nature series books. Jarrold, Norwich

Jones DL, Miller JH (1959) Pathology of the dermatitis produced by the urticating caterpillar, *Automeris io*. Arch Dermatol 79: 81–85

Jorg ME (1933) Nota previa sobre el principo activo urticante de *Hylesia nigricans* (Lepidoptera: Hemileucidae) y las dermitis provocadas por el mismo. Reunion Soc Argent Patol Reg 2: 482–495

Katzenellenbogen I (1955) Caterpillar dermatitis as an occupational disease. Dermatologica 111: 99–106

Kawamoto F, Suto C, Kumada N (1978) Studies in the venomous spicules and spines of moth caterpillars I. Fine structure and development of the venomous spines of the *Euproctis* caterpillars. Jpn J Med Sci Bio 31: 291–299

Keegan HL (1963) Caterpillars and moths as public Health problems. In: Keegan HL and MacFarlane WV (eds) Venomous and poisonous animals and noxious plants of the pacific region. Oxford, Pergamon, pp 165–170

Kemper H (1955) Experimentelle Untersuchungen über die durch Aftervolle von *Euproctis chrysorrhoea* (Lepidoptera) erzeugte Dermatitis vergleichen mit der Wirkung von Arthropodensticken. Z Angew Zool 4: 37–59

Kephart CF (1915) The poison glands of the larva of the browntail moth (*Euproctis chrysorrhoea* Linn). J Parasitol 1: 95–103

Knight HH (1922) Observations on the poisonous nature of the white-marked tussock moth (*Hemerocampa leucostigma* Smith and Abbot). J Parasitol 8: 133–135

*Leger M, Mouzels P (1918) Dermatite prurigineuse determiné par des papillons saturnides du genre *Hylesia*. Bull Soc Pathol Exot 11: 104–107

McGovern JP, Barkin GY, McElhenney TR, Wende R (1961) *Megalopyge opercularis*. Observations of its life history, natu-

ral history of its sting in man and report of an epidemic. JAMA 175: 1155–1158
*Maschwitz UWJ, Kloft W (1971) Morphology and function of the venom apparatus of insects—bees, wasps, ants and caterpillars. In: Bücherl W, Buckley EE (eds) Venomous animals and their venoms, vol III Venomous invertebrates. Academic, New York, pp 1–60
Mazzella H, Patetta MA (1948) Estudio experimental de la accion local de la toxina del *Megalopyge urens* Berg. Arch Soc Biol Montevideo 13: 131–136
Meek RR (1901) Further observations on the browntail moth. Boston Med Surg J 144: 651
Micks DW (1952) Clinical effects of the sting of the "puss caterpillar" (*Megalopyge opercularis* S. and A.) on man. Tex Rep Biol Med 10: 399–405
Mills RG (1925) Some observations and experiments on the urticating properties of the larva of *Parasa hilarata* Standiger. Am J Hyg 5: 342–363
Musgrave A (1924) Some caterpillars injurious to man. Aust Museum Mag 2: 34–36
Musgrave A (1941) Harmful moth caterpillars. Aust Museum Mag 7: 391–396
Perlman F, Press E, Googins JA, Malley A, Poarea H (1976) Tussockosis: reaction to Douglas fir tussock moth. Ann Allergy 36: 302–307
Pesce H, Delgado A (1966) Lepidopterismo y erucismo. Epidemilogia y aspectos clinico en el Pais. Mem Inst Butantan. Simposio internacional sobre venanos animais 3, Suppl comemorativo: 829–834
*Pesce H, Delgado A (1971) Poisoning from adult moths and caterpillars. In: Bücherl W, Buckley EE (eds) Venomous animals and their venoms, vol III Venomous invertebrates. Academic, New York, pp 119–156
Phisalix M (1922) Lépidoptères. In: Animaux venimeux et venins. Masson et Cie, Paris, pp 343–357
Piaggio Blanco RA, Paseyro P (1946) Lesiones cutaneas provocados por las crugas del "*Megalopyge urens*" (Bicho peludo negro) y del "*Automeris coresus*" (Bicho peludo verde). Arq Urug Med Cirug Spec 29: 30–39
Picarelli ZP, Valle JR (1971) Pharmacological studies in caterpillar venoms. In: Bücherl W, Buckley EE (eds) Venomous animals and their venoms, vol III Venomous invertebrates. Academic, New York, pp 103–118
Polano MK (1935) Rupsendermatitis (in Dutch). Ned Tijdschr Geneeskd 79: 2400–2401 (English translation by Polano MK)
Potter RA (1909) Browntail moth dermatitis. JAMA 53: 1463–1464
Randel HW, Doan GB (1956) Caterpillar urticaria in the Panama Zone. Report of five cases in venom. Publ No 44 AAAS, Washington DC. Cited by Keegan (1963)
Rendall P (1884) Urticating by *Liparis chrysorrhoea*. Entomologist 17: 275
Rossiter CB (1924) Dermatitis due to caterpillars. Br Med J II: 348
*Rotberg A (1971) Lepidopterism in Brazil. In: Bücherl W and Buckley EE (eds) Venomous animals and their venoms, vol III Venomous invertebrates. Academic, New York, pp 157–168
Saito J (1936) Über hautreizenden Giftstoff eines japanischer Giftschmelterlings *Euproctis flava* Bremer. Jpn Dermatol 30: 230–243
Shama SK, Etkind PH, Odell TM, Canada AT, Finn AM, Soter NA (1982) Gypsy moth caterpillar dermatitis. N Engl J Med 306: 1300–1301
Smith KGV (1982) Arthropod dermatoses, stings, bites, allergies and neuroses. In: Manson-Bahr PEC and Apted FIC (eds) Manson's tropical disease, 18th edn. Baillière Tindall, London, pp 739–741
South R (1885) On the urticating hairs of some lepidoptera. Entomologist 18: 3–6
*Southcott RV (1978) Lepidopterism in the Australian region. Rec Adelaide Children's Hosp 2: 87–173
Thresh JC (1906) Caterpillar rash. Lancet II: 291–292
Torchi M (1952–1953) Dermatiti da processionarie. Arch Ital Dermatol Sifil 25: 272–274
Touraine A, Thomas J, Caldera R (1947a) La dermatite des chenilles. Presse Med 55: 654–655
Touraine A, Thomas J, Caldera R (1947b) Dermatites par chenilles processionaires du cheine. Bull Soc Fr Dermatol Syphiligr 7: 202
*Tyzzer EE (1907) The pathology of the browntail moth dermatitis. J Med Res 16: 43–64
Valette G, Huidorro H (1954) Pouvoir histaminoliberation du venin de la chenille processionaire du Pin (Thaumetopoea pityocampa Schift). C R Soc Biol (Paris) 158: 1605–607
Watson PG, Sevel D (1966) Ophthalmia nodosa. Br J Ophthalmol 50: 209–217
White CJ (1901) Dermatitis produced by a caterpillar. Boston Med Surg J 144: 599
Whitwell GM (1943) Hop dermatitis. Lancet II: 305
Zaias N, Ionnides G, Taplin D (1969) Dermatitis from contact with moths (genus *Hylesia*). JAMA 207: 525–527
Ziprowski L, Hopshi E, Tahori AS (1959) Caterpillar dermatitis. Isr Med J 18: 26–31

13 Scorpion Stings

Scorpions, like spiders, have been regarded with justifiable fear in certain parts of the world since the times of the ancient Greeks and Romans. Their poisonous stings have caused innumerable deaths. The statistics for Mexico speak for themselves (Mazzotti and Bravo-Becherelle 1963: The records for the period 1940–1949 combined with those for 1957–1958 show that there were 20 352 deaths caused by scorpions, 2068 by snake bites, 274 by spider bites and a further 1933 unspecified but most likely caused by scorpion stings). In spite of these figures, and rather similar ones for other regions, Mazzotti and his colleague pointed out that scorpion sting was not listed as a specific cause of death in the International Classification of Diseases in 1963.

Morphology of Scorpions

Scorpions are easily recognisable. They are large arthropods and can reach a length of up to 18 cm. Fig. 13.1 shows the basic structure of a scorpion—a body and five obvious pairs of appendages. The body consists of a trunk and a tail. The trunk comprises the unsegmented cephalothorax (prosoma) and the seven-segmented preabdomen (mesosoma). The tail or postabdomen (metosoma) has six segments. The cephalothorax is covered dorsally by a hardened shield, the carapace, which carries a pair of median eyes (simple or ocelli) and from two to five pairs of eyes on its lateral edges (also ocelli), arranged in one or two groups. The cephalothorax bears six pairs of appendages. Anteriorly, just each side of the midline are relatively small chelicerae, which have three segments. Each terminal segment has a fixed and a movable finger forming a pincer. The second pair of appendages are the pedipalps, arising lateral to the chelicerae. They are massive, leg-like structures. The coxae together act as crushing maxillae for gripping prey. The trochanter is short and ringed, the femur long and cylindrical, the tibia toothed and the tarsus enlarged and conspicuous. It comprises a large pincer (the hand) which has a fixed section and mobile finger. The shape of the pincer varies from species to species. In Buthinae the distinguishing feature between many of the different species is the row of denticles on the cutting edge of the movable finger (Shulov and Levy 1978).

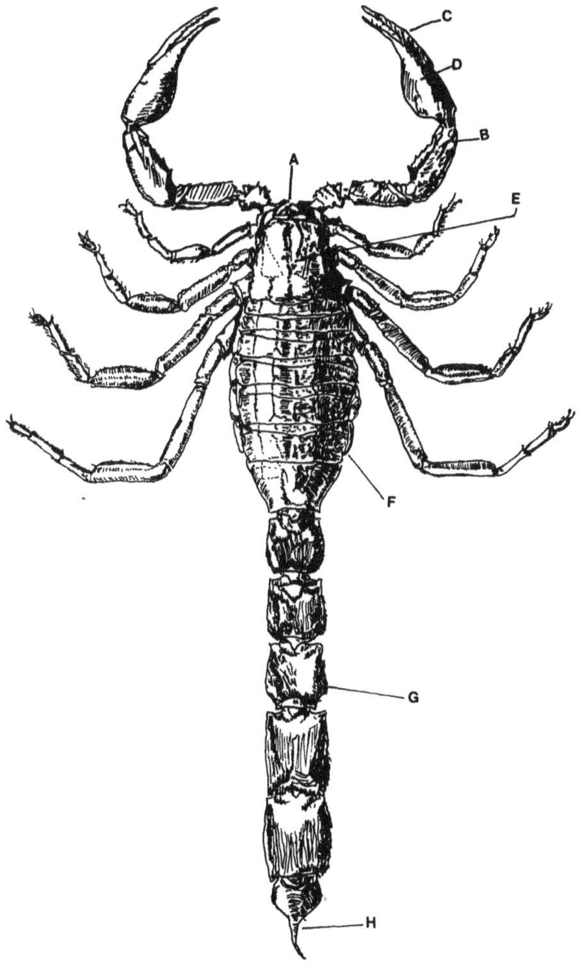

Fig. 13.1. Scorpion, showing the general morphology. *A*, chelicerae; *B*, palp; *C*, movable digit of palpal claw; *D*, fixed digit of palpal claw; *E*, carapace of cephalothorax; *F*, abdomen with seven segments; *G*, tail with six segments, including the sting; *H*, sting. [After Sheals (1973), by kind permission of the Trustees of the British Museum (Natural History)]

There are four pairs of seven-jointed walking legs articulating with chitinised plates on the ventral surface of the prosoma. The coxae of legs I and II have maxillary plates and house salivary glands. They exercise a masticatory function. Only the terminal tarsal segment carries claws.

The mesosoma has a ventral genital opening, immediately behind which are the comb-like pectines; these are unique to scorpions, but their function is imperfectly understood. There are paired respiratory openings on the ventral surface of segments III and IV leading to book lungs.

The tail, of more or less uniform thickness, terminates in the telson, which has a bulbous base tapering to a curved sting. The bulbous portion contains two poison glands with independent ducts opening onto the surface of the sting. The latter can be directed in any direction except downwards, hence the necessity for erecting the tail to sting forwards or laterally. At rest the sting is curved laterally (Stahnke 1978). In walking, the tail is stretched out behind—unless the sting is about to be used, when it is curved upwards and forwards. (These morphological details are taken from Cloudsley-Thompson 1958; Bücherl 1971; Sheals 1973, in addition to personal observation.)

Classification of Scorpions

There are six families (see Tables 13.1 and 13.2), of which Buthidae contains almost all the dangerous species (Bücherl 1971). Other species which are said to have caused trouble are also shown in the tables. See Sheals (1973) for identification data of each family.

Scorpions are ovoviviparous or oviparous, producing between 12 and 36 young which begin independent life on their mother's back. After six or seven moults spread over 3 years they reach the adult stage (Bücherl 1971). They are nocturnal predators feeding on other arthropods and even small vertebrates (Minton 1974). Their mating

Table 13.1. Scorpions of the family Buthidae which have been reported as attacking man. (Based on data in Bücherl 1971)

Species	Regions	References
Subfamily Buthinae		
Androctonus australis[a]	North Africa	Balozet (1964); Minton (1974)
A. amoreuxis[a]	North Africa; Mauretania	Balozet (1964)
A. aeneas[a]	North Africa	Balozet (1964)
A. crassicauda[a]	Turkey; Libya; Egypt	Balozet (1964)
A. hoggarensis[a]	Sahara Mountains	Balozet (1964)
A. maroccanus[a]	Morocco	Bücherl (1971)
Buthacus arenicola[a]	North Africa; eastern Mediterranean	Balozet (1964)
Buthus occitanus[a]	North Africa	Bouisset and Larrouy (1962); Balozet (1964, 1971); Minton (1974)
B. tamalus	Southern India	Devi et al. (1970); Balozet (1971); Minton (1974)
B. martensi	Manchuria; Korea	Balozet (1971)
Buthotus judaicus[a]	Israel	Balozet (1971)
Parabuthus transvaalius	South Africa; Abyssinia	Grasset et al. (1946); Balozet (1971)
P. triradulatus	South Africa	Grasset et al. (1946); Balozet (1971)
P. granulatus	South Africa	Bücherl (1971)
Leiurus quinquestriatus[a]	Southeastern Sahara; Egypt; Israel; Iran; Pacific area	Goldstein (1956); Whittemore et al. (1963); Balozet (1964); Gueron and Yaron (1970); Minton 1974
Subfamily Rhopalurinae		
Centruroides sculpturatus[a]	Arizona	Stahnke (1950, 1966, 1972); Ebeling (1975); Minton (1974)
C. gertschi[a]	Arizona; Texas	Stahnke (1950)
C. suffusus[a]	Mexico (Durango)	Baerg (1924); Whittemore et al. (1963); Minton (1974)
C. irritans	USA	Minton (1974)
C. margaritatus	Panama	Baerg (1925)
C. panthenensis		Minton (1974); Ebeling (1975)
C. chisosarium		Ebeling (1975)
C. vittatus[a]	Northwestern Arkansas	Baerg (1924); McGregor and Flanagan (1962); Ebeling (1975)

Table 13.1. *(continued)*

Species	Regions	References
C. limpidus[a]	Mexico	Whittemore et al. (1963); Minton (1974)
C. noxius	Mexico	Whittemore et al. (1963); Minton (1974)
Subfamily Tityinae		
Tityus bahiensis[a]	Brazil; Argentina (north east)	Abalos (1963); (Da Silva 1952)
T. trinitatus[a]	Brazil; Argentina (north east); Trinidad	Ridgeway et al. (1962); Poon-King (1963); Abalos (1963); Bartholomew (1970); Minton (1974)
T. sectus	Argentina	Abalos (1963);
T. serrulatus[a]	Brazil	Da Silva (1952); Corrado et al. (1966); Minton (1974)
T. trivittatus[a]		
Subfamily Isometrinae		
Isometrus maculatus	Cosmopolitan in Australia	Southcott (1978)

[a] Dangerous species which may cause death.

Table 13.2. Scorpions of families other than Buthidae which have been reported as attacking man. (Based on data in Bücherl 1971)

Species	Regions	References
Family SCORPIONIDAE		
Subfamily Scorpioninae		
Scorpio maurus	Algeria	Bouisset and Larrouy (1962)
Opisthophthalmus wahlbergi[a]	South Africa	Grasset et al. (1946); Balozet (1971)
O. glabriformis[a]	South Africa	Grasset et al. (1946); Balozet (1971)
Heterometrus spp.	India	Balozet (1971)
Subfamily Ischurinae		
Hadogenes troglodytis dentatus[a]	South Africa; Madagascar; Mozambique; Congo	Grasset et al. (1946); Balozet (1971)
Opisthacanthus lepturus	Panama	Baerg (1925)
Subfamily Urodacinae		
Urodacus excellens	Northern and central Australia	Southcott (1978)
U. yashenkoi	Central Australia	Southcott (1978)
Family VEJOVIDAE		
Subfamily Vejovinae		
Vejovis spinigeris	New Mexico	Baerg (1924)
V. flavus	Arizona	Stahnke (1950)
Family DIPLOCENTRIDAE		
Diplocentria whitei	Southern USA	Sheals (1973)
Family BOTHRIURIDAE		
Bothriurus bonaviensis	Brazil	Da Silva (1952)
B. marghalaensis	Brazil	Da Silva (1952)
Cercophonius spp.	Tasmania; Victoria; Western Australia	Southcott (1978)
Family CHACTIDAE		
Subfamily Euscorpioninae		
Euscorpius italicus	Southern Europe; North Africa	Balozet (1971)

[a] Dangerous species which may cause death.

dance, very like a human square dance, involves the male and female grasping each other's pedipalpal claws and moving to and fro over a limited area about 15 cm in diameter, which is swept clean by the pectine combs before the spermatophore is deposited by the male on the ground and cemented there. When the male succeeds in dragging the female over it so that the genital aperture touches it, the spermatophore explodes depositing seminal fluid in the genital tract (Shulov and Levy 1978).

There seem to be two principal groups of scorpion, according to Stahnke (1950). Bank scorpions (Bücherl's forest scorpions) live on the surface beneath bark, logs, stones and crevices, whilst ground scorpions (Bücherl's field, desert and semi-desert scorpions) are intrinsically burrowing scorpions. In warm humid climates these may live in canefields, banana plantations etc., at the roots of bushes, beneath old palm fronds and in other damp spots. In drier areas they actively burrow to seek moisture and in arid regions have been found as much as 2.4 m (8 ft) below ground level (Stahnke 1966). On the surface in these areas they shelter in the daytime beneath stones etc. Their colour tends to match their surroundings, but not always. (The present writer has seen very dark brown as well as sand-coloured specimens in the sandy desert of Iraq). Like many other arthropods they adapt to human dwellings and are often found in the vicinity of these beneath piles of wood, stones or bricks, below boxes or in outhouses. Inside dwelling houses they frequent dark sheltered spots and show special preference for clothing discarded at night and the inside of footwear and gloves. They also favour warm.damp areas such as beneath or behind kitchen furniture. In most instances people are stung in houses when they are dressing without first examining their clothing. As Maegraith (1971) remarked, scorpions sting the careless and unwary.

Scorpions are commonest in dry arid regions, although they do not tolerate excessive heat (Southcott 1978). They are also moisture dependent, for which reason they burrow into the ground in search of water (and coolness). They can resist starvation for 4–5 months (Ebeling 1975). A well-fed specimen can even survive being corked up in a dry test tube for 30 days (Stahnke 1966). Some species of Vejovidae and Chactidae can survive freezing and it is not therefore surprising that they can be encountered at altitudes of up to 2130 m (7000 ft, Cloudsley-Thompson 1958; Stahnke 1966). Nevertheless, scorpions as a whole prefer warmer climates and in the Americas are confined between latitudes 40°N and 45°–50°S. They are most liable to sting when active and hungry. According to Balozet (1971), stings are more frequent at night than in the daytime, and in hot stormy weather.

The clinical effects can be classed as local and systemic. Most of the species which cause marked local effects may produce relatively minor systemic effects, whilst those which cause severe systemic effects may cause some local reaction but frequently do not. Species which are deadly in some regions appear to be less so in others. Children always react more severely than adults, and the younger the child the worse the reaction. Most fatalities occur in children.

Clinical Features

Local Effects

Baerg (1924, 1925) described most of the local effects noted by subsequent observers. Initially an instant sharp burning pain is felt by most of the victims, lasting from a few minutes to several hours. There may be a feeling of numbness or a dull ache which may extend beyond the sting site. Commonly the sting is on the limbs, head or neck (Balozet 1971). Da Silva (1952) found that of 1331 stings seen in a 7-year period in Brazil, 55% were on the hands, 20% on the feet, 7% on the legs, 4.5% on the head and neck and 8.5% were not specified. Burning pain was the only symptom in some stings from *Tityus* species (Abalos 1963; Bartholomew 1970). Other local sensations recorded include prickling associated with "gooseflesh" ("horripilatus" of Balozet 1971) and tenderness or hypersensitivity (Stahnke 1950; Ebeling 1975). Cloudsley-Thompson (1958) observed that this hypersensitivity could persist at the sting site after all other evidence had disappeared, whilst Stahnke (1972) noted persistent hyperaesthesia at the sting site for up to 10 days after sting by *Centruroides sculpturatus*. A sting by *C. vitattus* produced a white halo around the site (Baerg 1924), but whether this indicated ischaemia or oedema is uncertain. A local weal may occur (Bücherl 1971; Maegraith 1971), which may be evanescent but can extend well beyond the sting area and be accompanied by transient systemic symptoms. Redness of the sting site has been described (Baerg 1924, 1925; Mundle 1961), but Reid (1982) regarded it as unusual. Discolouration by punctate oozing of blood or by marked ecchymosis has been noted (Minton 1974; Ebeling 1975). Most authors agree that local swelling often extending well beyond the sting site is quite common, although Minton thought it was rare. On the other hand, its absence was regarded by Rook (1979) as a sign of impending severe systemic effects. In stings by *Vejovis* species Stahnke (1950) noted that marked, often widespread swelling of an allergic nature, even to the extent of general anaphylaxis, could occur. Ebeling (1975) also declared that vesicles could appear at the bite site. Ansari (1948) reported gangrene of a fingertip after a scorpion sting in which a small blister appeared very soon after the sting, whilst Marsh (1948), confirming this observation, noted that sometimes a young adult putting on a shirt with an unsuspected scorpion in its folds could be bitten several times. Interestingly he noted that the first bite caused a black disc of dead skin with surrounding inflammation, the second an inflamed plaque with a small 5 mm central necrotic zone, the third a vesicular erythematous disc with no necrosis and the fourth a faintly reddened area only, suggesting that the potency of the venom diminished with successive stings.

Systemic Effects

The following description of systemic symptoms and signs is based on Balozet (1971). The patient is agitated and restless and may have a feeling of impending death. Small children may try to climb their cot wall (Stahnke 1950). Waterman (1938) observed that infants gave a sudden cry before becoming ill, which could be important in diagnosis if the scorpion was not suspected. Muscle tone is greatly increased, perhaps causing spontaneous twitching (Barsoum et al. 1954; Cloudsley-Thompson 1958), and characteristically leads to muscle spasm of limbs, abdomen and pharyngeal muscles. The tongue feels thickened (Stahnke 1966) and there may be difficulty in swallowing (Ebeling 1975). Similarly, there may be tightness of the chest and difficulty with speech (Cloudsley-Thompson 1958; Minton 1974; Ebeling 1975). In severe cases opisthotonos may be seen. In small children chaotic convulsions are common and may be a herald of early death. Priapism is not uncommon. Balozet (1971) found the tendon reflexes to be lost and the plantar and corneal reflexes diminished or absent, but Minton (1974) asserted that they were typically exaggerated, which would be in conformity with increased muscle tone. There is a marked increase in salivary, sweat and tear gland secretion. The pupils are widely dilated and there is clouding of vision. Exophthalmos may be noted.

Tachycardia has been observed by some, bradycardia by others (e.g. Mundle 1961), but Minton (1974) has pointed out that bradycardia is followed by tachycardia. There may be associated palpitation, and arrhythmia is not uncommon. It was first recorded by Waterman (1938) in stings by *Tityus trinitatus* and confirmed by Poon-King (1963) with ECG changes suggestive of myocardial infarction. Gueron and Yaron (1970) and Minton (1974) agreed, adding that urinary catecholamine excretion was greatly increased. The prominence of these findings lead Mundle (1961), Bartholomew (1970) and Maegraith (1971) all to conclude that death was primarily cardiac, but Balozet (1971) and others felt that respiratory failure was the primary cause of death. Respirations are irregular, pulmonary oedema is frequent (Mundle 1961) and it has been shown that the venom acts directly on the respiratory centre. It is likely, because of the variation in venom composition in different species and different parts of the world, that the conclusions of each group were correct for their own region.

The temperature is variable. Hypothermia is said to have a bad prognosis (Mundle 1961). Vomiting occurs in a number of patients, and sometimes the vomit is tinged with blood. Balozet (1971) believed this was an early indication of involvement of nerve centres. An increase in peristalsis is noticeable and may be associated with diarrhoea or meloena. There is usually oliguria, but polyuria and incontinence also occur. Haematuria and occasionally glycosuria may be observed. Waterman (1938) noted the latter in his patients and pointed out that there was also hyperglycaemia, which has been a consistent finding by others since his observation. He also recorded acute pancreatitis and the occurrence of pancreatic cysts. This seems to be a fairly regular finding in patients stung by *T. trinitatus* and was confirmed by Bartholomew (1970), who found raised SGPT enzymes but normal bilirubin. The plasma potassium is usually elevated and sodium depressed. Balozet (1971) emphasised that exacerbation after apparent improvement is a very bad sign and often presages death.

Pathology

Post-mortem examinations (Devi et al. 1970; Gueron and Yaron 1970) have shown general congestion of many organs with haemorrhages in occasional instances (subendocardial, adrenal or cerebral). Devi and his colleagues found thrombosis in some vessel walls of the heart and, on histological examination, occlusion and thrombosis of small vessels in many organs, indicating toxic fibrinolysis. Reid (1982) reported that intravascular coagulation occurred with stings by *Buthus* species in India. Gueron and Yaron (1970) noted myocardial changes, e.g. muscle fibre degeneration, focal necrosis and interstitial oedema, with maximal involvement of papillary muscle and subendothelial tissues equivalent to that seen as a result of catecholamine overdosage.

Venom of Scorpions

According to Minton (1974), scorpion venom is an apocrine secretion. The first drop is clear but subsequently it becomes increasingly turbid (Balozet 1971). Up to eight different proteins have been isolated, the number and amount depending on the species. They are of low molecular weight and low antigenicity (Balozet 1964). Venom yield varies widely, ranging from 0.075 mg (*Centruroides noxius*) to 4.8 mg. (*Parabuthus* spp.; Minton 1974). For a given species the toxic effects are proportional to the amount injected, and with repeated stings the potency appears to fall (Marsh 1948). The weight for weight toxicity of venom varies greatly from species to species, some being much more virulent than others.

The principal component is a neurotoxin with adrenergic and cholinergic effects (Barsoum et al. 1954; Corrado et al. 1966; Gueron and Yaron 1970; Balozet 1971). This activity explains most of the effects seen clinically. 5-Hydroxytryptamine is present in some venoms, especially that of *Leiurus*, and is said to account for the severe pain (Minton 1974). Some venoms, especially *Tityus* have trypsin activity, held by Bartholomew (1970) to account for the pancreatitis which not infrequently follows their sting. In experimental work Grasset et al. (1946) also noted a haemorrhagin toxin, most noticeable in *Opisthophthalmus* and *Hadogenes* species, which may account for local bruising and the occasional necrotic lesions recorded (Ansari 1948; Marsh 1948). The venom also inhibits the respiratory centre. There is no histamine or lipoprotein present (Balozet 1971).

Antivenin serum is difficult to produce because of the low antigenicity of the venom. The first and most potent antivenin was produced in Turkey against *Androctonus crassicauda*, but since then numerous specific antivenins have been produced in different regions. Some are of help for stings from heterogenous species but most have only homologous specificity. Shulov and Levy (1978) noted that scorpion haemolymph neutralises scorpion venom and cited the instance of a child being saved in Israel by treatment with this when antivenin was unavailable.

Waterman (1938) made the important observation that scorpion venom is excreted in breast milk and can be fatal to a neonate by this route.

Epidemiology

As has already been stated, the danger of scorpion stings has been known for centuries. In Mexico it was well known in the pre-Colombian era (Mazzotti and Bravo-Becherelle 1963). Consistent tabulation of incidence and death rates is not possible because of the diverse manner of previous reports. However, all writers are agreed that the younger the victim the more deadly the effects of the venom. The sexes are equally vulnerable, but males are probably more often affected because of their outdoor occupations. Season affects the incidence only in so far as temperature affects the activity of the scorpions, which are more lively in warm weather. They only sting by accident or in self-defence.

The incidence in Mexico has been very high for a very long time. Baerg (cited by Mazzotti and Bravo-Becherelle 1963) quoted the average number of deaths in the city of Durango alone over the period 1890–1926 as 45 per annum. This gave a death rate of about one for every thousand inhabitants. The figures are known with some accuracy because the city has had a health service since Spanish colonial times. A later compilation given by the same authors for the whole of Mexico from 1940 to 1949 indicated an annual death rate per 100 000 population of 7.4–8.9. (Total deaths from this cause in this period ranged from 1588 to 1944.) As indicated at the beginning of this chapter, scorpions account for about ten times the number of deaths in Mexico that result from all other venomous animals together. Children aged between 1 and 4 years were the most vulnerable, followed by those under 1 year.

In neighbouring Arizona state Ebeling (1975) noted 75 deaths caused by scorpions in the period 1926–1965, again a considerably higher number than all other poisonous animals combined. *Centruroides sculpturatus* caused most of the trouble. Stahnke (1972) pointed out that whilst the population of the state had trebled between 1940 and 1970, the deaths from scorpion stings in the same period had fallen threefold as a result of improved scorpion control and better means of treatment (antivenin).

In Trinidad Waterman (1938) described 698 cases of scorpion stings (mostly caused by *Tityus* species) between 1929 and 1933. Table 13.3 shows the incidence and mortality in relation to age

Table 13.3. Incidence and mortality of scorpion stings in Trinidad 1929–1933. (Based on Waterman 1938)

Age group	Number of cases	Mortality
1–5 years	88	25%
6–10 years	96	5.2%
11–20 years	190	2.6%
over 20 years	324	0.25%

groups. The fewest cases but highest mortality were in infancy. The majority of patients were over 13 years of age.

In Brazil 1331 scorpion stings were registered in Ribeirao Preto (population 77 500) (Da Silva 1952). The majority occurred in daylight, with only a small number at night (103), and at the beginning of the rainy season, when the scorpions are most active; seven of the eight deaths occurred at this period, which prompted Da Silva to speculate on a possible seasonal variation in the virulence of the venom.

In the Old World many scorpions are dangerous (see Table 13.1). Balozet (1964), discussing scorpions in southern Algeria, noted that 20 164 stings had been recorded in a 17-year period, with 386 deaths. The incidence and mortality relative to age groups are shown in Table 13.4. Once again infants are the most vulnerable to the effects, although adults and children are more liable to be stung. *Androctonus australis* was responsible for 80% of the stings and 95% of the deaths.

Table 13.4. Incidence and mortality of scorpion stings in southern Algeria in a 17-year period. (Based on Balozet 1964)

Age group	Number of cases	Number of deaths	Mortality
Infants	411	32	7.78%
Children	5 211	191	3.66%
Adults	13 130	145	1.10%
Elderly	1 412	18	1.27%

Diagnosis

With an obvious history of being stung there is no difficulty in making a diagnosis. However, with infants and children it is not so easy. Waterman (1938) emphasised that the diagnosis is unlikely to be made if not suspected and that therefore a high index of suspicion is helpful. He stated that a patient who showed excessive salivation, vomiting, glycosuria and a low pulse and respiration rate should be strongly suspected of having been stung by a scorpion. Poon-King (1963), working in the same region (Trinidad), added to these signs epigastric pain, abdominal tenderness and profuse sweating. In severe cases shock, muscular twitching and carpopedal spasms are also important evidence. Minton (1974) considered excessive salivation and sweating to be very suggestive, and of course pain at the sting site increases suspicion. He also pointed out that scorpion stings are single and bleed little, whereas snake bites show more than one puncture and often bleed profusely.

Waterman (1938) included infectious fevers and malignant malaria in the differential diagnosis and stated that in pregnant patients with convulsions the distinction from eclampsia could be difficult. An ECG in which the RTS segment may be significantly deviated, the presence of increased catecholamines in the urine and an increase in serum SGPT are aids in making the diagnosis.

Treatment

The treatment of scorpion stings consists of antivenin serum, measures to combat the pharmacological effects of venom and symptomatic remedies. First aid measures include ice-packs applied to the sting area, which give some relief of pain and reduce local circulation. Stahnke (1972) stated that such treatment should be started within 5 min to have the best effect. Local anaesthetic injections around the sting site provide the best means of relieving pain (Waterman 1938; Reid 1982). A tourniquet applied proximal to the sting site has been advocated. Ebeling (1975) thought it should only be used if there was evidence of developing anaphylaxis. Early hospitalisation is essential.

Antivenin serum must be given early. It is effective if given within 2 h after the sting (Bücherl 1971). Precautions against hypersensitivity to horse or goat serum should be taken (Stahnke 1972). It is generally accepted that specific antivenin serum raised against the species which has stung the patient should be used. If this is unavailable, serum against *Androctonus crassicauda* should be used for stings from Old World scorpions and against *Centruroides sculpturatus* for New World scorpion stings (Bouisset and Larrouy 1962). Practitioners and hospitals in scorpion-infested regions should know of and have access to the nearest poison centre (Ebeling 1975). Maegraith (1971) advised that, where possible, the offending scorpion should be killed and retained for identification. The dosage of antivenin recommended by Bücherl (1971) should be large enough to neutralise at least 2 mg of dried venom, which is usually the equivalent of five to ten ampoules of serum. It should be given at one time, half intravenously and the other half by intravenous drip or intramuscularly.

The venom, especially of the Old World species, causes acute sympathetic and parasympathetic stimulation. Barsoum et al. (1954) reinforced by Gueron and Yaron (1970) recommended an α-adrenergic blocking agent, phentolamine (Rogitine), given intravenously in a dose of 1.0 mg/kg as very effective. Labetalol (Trandate) which is a combined α- and β-blocker could be used instead but is liable to cause bradycardia and thus accentuate the bradycardia present in the early stages of venom intoxication. It should be given with the patient in the supine position, intravenously, 50 mg over a period of 1 minute, repeated if necessary after a 5-min interval. A dose of 200 mg should not be exceeded (manufacturer's advice). Efrati (1978) reported that a blood pressure of 260/190 induced by scorpion stings returned to normal in a few minutes after the intravenous injection of Rogitine. Following this, 4 mg propanalol, also given intravenously, cleared all the remaining symptoms in 30 min. Efrati was dubious of the value of antivenin, probably because the amount given is usually far too small, and stated that adrenergic blocking agents should always be used as well.

The cholinergic effect of venoms are counteracted by atropine (Marsh 1948; Barsoum et al. 1954), which Reid (1982) advised in a dose of 2 mg for adults, 0.5 mg–1.0 mg for children aged 6–12 years, 0.25–0.5 mg for children aged 1–5 years and 0.25 mg for infants under 1 year. This drug complements phentolamine or labetalol.

Central nervous system excitability and convulsions, which are more prominent with *Centruroides* scorpions, are best counteracted by barbiturates; Stahnke advocated a dose of 240 mg for a young child, adding 60 mg per year up to a maximum of 1200 mg for an adult. Barbiturates induce relaxation, avoid stress and allow time for evaluation and administration of antivenin serum. Tranquillizers are also helpful, being adrenolytic (Balozet 1971). Stahnke (1972), whilst agreeing with the benefit of barbiturate-induced relaxation, stated that some tranquillisers, such as diazepam, were contraindicated. Calcium gluconate (10 ml of 10% solution intravenously) has also been said to help (Biery 1977; Reid 1982), but according to Balozet it is ineffective.

Morphia and morphine derivatives and pethidine are contraindicated (Stahnke 1972; Minton 1974), although Reid (1982) had advocated pethidine. Adrenaline and corticosteroids are also contraindicated because of hypertension and glycosuria.

Barsoum et al. (1954) recommended that facilities for assisted respiration and oxygen should be available. Intravenous fluids, except as a vehicle for drugs, are best avoided because of pulmonary oedema.

Prevention

There are several ways in which prevention can be helped. Public education concerning the appearance, biology and habits of the local scorpions should be undertaken (Da Silva 1952), and should include advice about inspecting and shaking clothing before dressing in the morning, the wearing of footwear at night and always using a light when walking about at night indoors (Biery 1977). Ebeling's aphorism (1975), "never put your hand or foot where you cannot see", is very apt.

Measures should be taken to prevent scorpions entering houses. These include installing wire screens on doors and windows, fixing a continuous horizontal strip of glazed tiles or rustproof metal sheeting on outside walls to prevent insects climbing (Mazzotti and Bravo-Becherelle 1963), raising the floor and tiling it, and using smooth concrete tiles on the roof. Cracks on the outside walls of dwellings, store houses etc., should be filled, and lumber and firewood should be stored off the ground (Ebeling 1975).

Hiding and breeding places should be removed or destroyed. This involves the removal of domestic and farmyard debris, wearing suitable protective gloves. Such areas can also be treated with suitable scorpionicides. The most rapidly effective is lindane (gamma-benzene hexachloride; Whittemore and Keagan 1963). Ridgeway et al. (1962) found a concentration of 2.24 mg per square foot to be rapidly lethal to scorpions within 24 h. If inadequate concentrations are used the scorpions recover after a period of coma. Moreover, they are initially rendered very excitable and more liable to sting. Chlordane (5%) is less effective but more persistent (Ebeling 1975) and valuable against any scorpions not killed by lindane. Malathion is also effective but much less so than lindane. It induces cannibalism amongst scorpions in inadequate doses (McGregor and Flannigan 1962).

Indoor spraying of places likely to harbour scorpions is valuable, providing it is remembered that in very hot weather with temperatures about 38°C (100°F) scorpions are liable to migrate to the coolest places in the house, namely the bathroom and around the waste outlet in the kitchen (Ebeling 1975). It is also important to remember that lindane should not be used in occupied rooms; the room should be evacuated first and when it is re-entered the windows should be opened.

Head-hunting competitions and bounty schemes have also been used as a means of reducing the scorpion population (Da Silva 1952). Mazzotti and Bravo-Becherelle (1963) noted that one health inspector along with his aides caught half a million scorpions in a few days.

References

Abalos JW (1963) Scorpions of Argentina. In: Keegan HL and MacFarlane WV (eds) Venomous and poisonous animals and noxious plants of the Pacific region. Pergamon, Oxford, pp 111–117

Ansari MY (1948) Gangrene after scorpion sting. Br Med J II: 388

Baerg WJ (1924) The effect of the venom of some supposedly poisonous arthropods. Ann Entomol Soc Am 17: 343–352

Baerg WJ (1925) The effect of the venom of some supposedly poisonous arthropods of the Canal Zone. Ann Entomol Soc Am 18: 471–478

Balozet L (1964) Le scorpionisme en Afrique du Nord. Bull Soc Pathol Exot 57: 33–38

*Balozet L (1971) Scorpions in the Old World. In: Bücherl W and Buckley EE (eds) Venomous animals and their venom, vol III Venomous invertebrates. Academic, New York, pp 349–371

*Barsoum GS, Nabawy M, Salama S (1954) Scorpion poisoning. Its signs, symptoms and treatment. J Egypt Med Assoc 37: 857–894

Bartholomew C (1970) Acute scorpion pancreatitis in Trinidad. Br Med J I: 666–668

Biery TL (1977) Venomous arthropod handbook. Disease Surveillance Branch, Epidemiology Division, USAF School of Aerospace Medicine. US Gov Printing Office, Washington DC

Bouisset L, Larrouy G (1962) Envenimations par *Scorpio maurus* et *Buthus occitanus* dans le department de Tlemcen. Bull Soc Pathol Exot 55: 139–146

* Bücherl W (1971) Classification, biology and venom extraction of scorpions. In: Bücherl W and Buckley EE (eds) Venomous animals and their venoms, vol III Venomous invertebrates. Academic, New York, pp 371–394

*Cloudsley-Thompson JL (1958) Spiders, scorpions, centipedes and mites. Pergamon, London

Corrado AP, Antonio A, Diniz CR (1966) Recent advances on the mechanism of action of Brazilian scorpion venom, *T. serrulatus*. Mem Inst Butantan. Simposio internacionale sobre venenos animais 33, Suppl comemorativo: 957–960

Da Silva TL (1952) The scorpion problem in Ribeirao Preto, Sao Paulo, Brazil. Notes on epidemiology and prophylaxis. Am J Trop Med Hyg 1: 508–513

Devi CS, Reddy CN, Devi SL, Bhatt HV, Suvarnakuma NG, Murthy DG, Reddy CRRM (1970) Defibrination syndrome due to scorpion venom poisoning. Br Med J 1: 345–347

Ebeling W (1975) Urban entomology. University of California, Division of Agricultural Science, Los Angeles, Cal, pp 343–345

Efrati P (1978) Epidemiology, symptomatology and treatment of Buthinae stings. In: Bettini S (ed) Arthropod venoms. Springer, Berlin Heidelberg New York, pp 312–317 (Handbook of experimental pharmacology, vol 48)

Goldstein R (1956) Les piqûres des scorpions. Dapim Refuiim 15: VI

Grasset E, Schaafsma A and Hodgson JA (1946) Studies on the venom of South African scorpions (*Parabuthus*, *Hadogenes*, *Opisthophthalmus*) and the preparation of a specific antiscorpion serum. Trans R Soc Trop Med Hyg 39: 397

Gueron M, Yaron R (1970) Cardiovascular manifestations of severe scorpion sting; clinicopathologic correlation. Chest 57: 156–162

McGregor T, Flanigan JF (1962) Effects of insecticides in the scorpion *Centruroides vittatus*. J Econ Entomol 55: 661–662

Maegraith BG (1971) In: Adams ARD and Maegraith BG (eds). Clinical tropical diseases, 5th edn. Blackwell, Oxford, pp 400–410

Marsh F (1948) Gangrene after scorpion sting. Br Med J II: 498

Mazzotti L, Bravo-Becherelle MA (1963) Scorpionism in the Mexican Republic. In: Keegan HL and MacFarlane WV (eds) Venomous and poisonous animals and noxious plants in the Pacific region. Pergamon, Oxford, pp 119–131

*Minton SA (1974) Venom diseases. Thomas, Springfield, Ill, pp 27–37

Mundle PM (1961) Scorpion stings. Br Med J I: 1042

Poon-King T (1963) Myocarditis from scorpion stings. Br Med J I:374–377

Reid HA (1982) Animal poisons—scorpion stings. In: Manson-Bahr PEC and Apted FIC (eds) Manson's tropical diseases, 18th edn. London, Baillière Tindall, pp 563–564

Ridgway RL McGregor T, Flanigan JF (1962) The effect of residual deposits of insecticides in the scorpion, *Centruroides vittatus*. J Econ Entomol 55: 1012–1013

Rook A (1979) Scorpions. In: Rook A, Wilkinson DS and Ebeling FJG (eds) Textbook of dermatology, 3rd edn. Blackwell, Oxford, p 935

Sheals JG (1973) Scorpions. In: Smith KGV (ed) Insects and other arthropods of medical importance. Trustees of the British Museum (Natural History), London, pp 417–424

Shulov A, Levy G (1978) Venoms of Buthinae. In: Bettini S (ed) Arthropod venoms. Springer, Berlin Heidelberg New York, pp 309–369 (Handbook of experimental pharmacology, vol 48)

Southcott RV (1978) Australian harmful arachnids and their allies. Southcott, Mitcham, South Australia

Stahnke HL (1950) The Arizona scorpion problem. Ariz Med 7: 23–29

*Stahnke HL (1966) Some aspects of scorpion behaviour. Bull South Cal Acad Sci 65: 65–80

Stahnke HL (1972) Arizona's lethal scorpion. Ariz Med 29: 490–493

Stahnke HL (1978) The genus *Centruroides* (Buthinae) and its venom. In: Bettini S (ed) Arthropod venoms. Springer, Berlin Heidelberg New York, pp 277–307 (Handbook of experimental pharmacology, vol 48)

*Waterman JA (1938) Some notes on scorpion poisoning in Trinidad. Trans R Soc Trop Med Hyg 31: 607–624

Whittemore FW Keegan HL (1963) Medically important scorpions in the Pacific area. In: Keegan HL and MacFarlane WV (eds) Venomous and poisonous animals and noxious plants of the Pacific region. Pergamon, Oxford pp 107–110

Whittemore FW, Keegan HL, Borowitz JL (1961) Studies of scorpion antivenins. Bull WHO 25: 185–188

14 Spider Bites

For centuries spiders have been the subject of superstitious fear by man. In many parts of the world there has been good reason for this fear, because several species have caused human death by their bite. For example, the black widow spider (*Latrodectus mactans*) in its various forms has caused death in many countries. The notorious Australian funnel-web spiders (*Atrax robustus* and *A. formidabilis*), the *Phoneutra* and *Loxosceles* spiders in South America and *Harpactirella* in South Africa have all killed many people in their respective regions. This is to say nothing of the suffering induced in the far larger number of victims who did not succumb to bites. With the exception of *Loxosceles* spiders and, to a very secondary extent, of *Latrodectus*, none of the dangerous arachnids affect the skin, except in so far as the venom is injected through the skin. Bite marks, often practically invisible, are inevitable, and very occasionally evanescent bruising or even an urtiçarial reaction may be seen.

Spiders produce three types of venomous toxin. Some species, e.g. *Latrodectus*, *Atrax*, *Phoneutra* or *Harpactirella*, secrete a potent neurotoxin with central nervous system effects. *Loxosceles*, *Lycosa*, *Chiracanthium* and some other genera inject a venom containing a cytotoxic factor, the effect of which is to produce changes resulting in necrosis of skin and surrounding tissues. *Loxosceles* also produces a haemolytic toxin which can cause severe fatal effects on the victim. Bücherl (1971) said that no male of any species was capable of injecting a deadly dose of venom into human beings, but this does not seem to apply to *Atrax* species (see p. 223; Sutherland 1972). According to Bücherl, over 1000 papers had been published up to 1971 on the medical importance of dangerous spiders, and many more have appeared since. Only those instances of spider bites involving damage to or lesions of the skin are discussed in this chapter. The species concerned are enumerated in a classified manner in Tables 14.1, 14.2 and 14.3.

General Morphology of Spiders

Spiders show two distinct body regions, the cephalothorax and the abdomen (see Fig. 14.1). Both are unsegmented and joined by a narrow stalk. A pair of chelicerae, a pair of pedipalps and four pairs of walking legs are appendages of the cephalothorax.

The head, the anterior portion of the cephalothorax, carries the eyes and mouthparts. Spiders have from two to eight simple eyes, usually eight. There are two types: pearly, white lustreless nocturnal eyes and black, shiny diurnal eyes. In many species they are arranged in two rows, which are curved forwards (procurved) or backwards (recurved). The curvature, which is not always in the same plane, may give the impression of three or even four rows. The clypeus is the space between the eyes and the chelicerae. The face is that part of the head which can be seen from in front. The chelicerae are the first pair of appendages lying in front of and above the mouth. They consist of a basal segment and a terminal claw or fang and are homologous to the second antennae of crustaceae. The poison glands discharge through an opening near the tip of the fangs, on the convex surface so that it avoids getting blocked during biting. The chelicerae of the Orthognatha (trap-door spiders) are horizontal and when the fang is erected it points downwards (as with snakes), whereas in the Labidognatha (or true spiders) the chelicerae are vertical and the erected fang points inwards. Thus the Orthognatha fangs strike downwards in a vertical plane whilst the Labidognatha bite with a lateral pincer movement. Russell and Waldron (1967) cited a personal communication from Gertsch to the effect that all spiders except two groups were venomous, but that the fangs for most species were too short or too fragile to penetrate human skin.

The second pair of appendages on the head are the six-segmented pedipalps lying on each side of the mouth. These are sensory organs resembling

Table 14.1. List of various species of spiders (excluding *Latrodectus*, *Lycosa* and *Loxosceles* species) whose bite causes skin lesions in man. Most are relatively minor (see text). (Based on Bücherl 1971)

Species	Region	References
Superfamily MYGALOMORPHAE (ORTHOGNATHA)		
Family Ctenizidae		
Aganippe raphiduca	Western Australia	Southcott (1978)
Missulena spp.	Australia	Main (1976)
Family Banychelidae		
Idiomma blackwalli (Cambridge)	Australia	Southcott (1978); Main (1976)
Family Theraphosidae:		
Grammostolinae		
Eurypelma californica	Panama	Horen (1963)
Aphonopelma spp.	California	Russell and Waldron (1967)
Lampropelma violaceopedes	Malaysia	Lim and Davie (1970)
Brachypelma smithi[a]	USA	Cooke et al. (1973)
Theraphosinae		
Sericopelma communis F. Cambridge	Panama	Baerg (1925)
Pamphobetus spp.	California	Horen (1963)
Selenocosmia crassipes[b]	Australia	Southcott (1978)
S. sterlingi[b]	Australia	Southcott (1978)
Family Dipluridae		
Dekana spp.	Australia	Main (1976)
Superfamily ARANEOMORPHAE (LABIDOGNATHA)		
Family Argiopidae (=Araneidae)		
Argiope argentata	Argentina	Gorham (1968a)
A. aurantia	USA etc.	Gorham (1968a)
Glyptocranium gasteroacanthoides (Simon)	Peru	Phisalix (1922); Vellard (1954); Pirosky et al. (1962)
Family Clubionidae:		
Clubioninae		
Chiracanthium inclusum (Hentz)	USA	Gorham (1968a)
C. mordax (=*C. diversum*) L. Koch	USA; Hawaii; Australia; Central and southwestern Pacific area	Groham (1968a); Main (1976)
C. punctorium (Villiers)	Europe (Germany)	Habermehl and Habermehl (1979)
C. japonicum (Bosenberg and Strand)	Japan	Ori (1975)
C. mildei	USA (Boston area)	Spielman and Levi (1970)
C. brevicalcaratum	Australia	Southcott (1978)
Family Salticidae		
Phidippus formosus	USA	Russell (1970)
Mopsus mormon Karsch	Australia (Queensland)	Southcott (1978)
Thiodina sylvana (Hentz)	California	Waldron (1968)
Family Gnaphosidae		
Herpyllus ecclesiasticus Hentz	USA (South Carolina)	Majeski and Durst (1975)
Family Theridiidae		
Achaearanea tepidariorum	Australia	Main (1976)
Family Sparassidae		
Otios calligasta	Australia	Main (1976)
Family Dysderidae		
Dysderca crocata	Australia (introduced)	Main (1976)
Family Dictynidae		
Ixeuticus robustus	Australia	Main (1976)

[a] These spiders have urticating hairs.
[b] Not stated whether this species causes skin lesions.

Table 14.2. List of various species of *Loxosceles* and *Lycosa* species which cause necrotic arachnidism. (Based on cited references and Bücherl 1971)

Species	Region	References
Superfamily ARANAE (LABIDOGNATHA)		
Family Scytodidae: Loxoscelinae		
Loxosceles laeta (Nicolet)	South America	Very numerous
(= *L. rufipes* Lucas)	Australia	Vellard (1954)
L. rufescens (Dufour)	Israel (USA: Australia)	Efrati (1969)
L. spadicea Simon		Bücherl (1971)
L. reclusa Gertsch and Malik	Southwestern USA	Numerous
L. decemdentata Franganillo		Bücherl (1971)
L. distincta (Lucas)		Bücherl (1971)
L. unicolor von Keyserling	Southwestern USA	Gorham (1968b)
L. arizonica	Southwestern USA	Gorham (1968b)
L. devia	Southwestern USA	Gorham (1968b)
L. caribbaea	Puerto Rico	Gorham (1968b)
L. spinulosus	South Africa	Newlands (1975)
Family Lycosidae: Lycosinae		
Lycosa raptoria Walck (= *L. erythrognatha* Lucas)	Brazil	Vellard (1954); Horen (1963); Bücherl (1971)
L. tarentula (Rossi)	Europe	Phisalix (1922); Bücherl (1971)
L. miami Wallace		Grothaus and Teller (1968)
L. antelucana	USA (Tennessee and southwest)	Redman (1974)
L. minima	Chile	Horen (1963)

Table 14.3. *Latodectus* species (Based on Levi 1959, also cited by Bücherl 1971)

Species	Region	References
Superfamily ARANAE		
Family Theridiiade: Latrodectinae		
Latrodectus mactans mactans Fabr. (= *L. variolus*)	Cosmopolitan	Numerous
L. m. tredecimguttatus (Rossi) (= *L. revivensis*=*L. malmignathus)*	Southern Europe; Israel; Corsica	Bettini (1964); Efrati (1969); Maretic (1971); Minton (1974)
L. m. cinctus Blackwall (= *L. indistinctus*)	South Africa	Finlayson (1955); Minton (1974)
L. m. menovadi Vinson		
L. m. hasselti	Australia; southeast Asia	Ingram and Musgrave (1933); Wiener (1961); Keegan (1963); Southcott (1978)
L. geometricus C.L. Koch	South Africa	Finlayson (1955); Pirosky and Abalos (1963); Minton (1974)
L. pallidus Cambridge		
L. curacoviensis (Muller) (= *L. m. bishopi*)	USA; Mexico; Argentina	Pirosky and Abalos (1963); Minton (1974)
L. hystrix Simon		
L. dahli Levi		

legs. In male spiders the terminal segment is expanded into a complex storage organ for sperm and is characteristically different for each species or genus. Sperm is transferred from the abdominal reproductive organ prior to courtship and during mating is introduced into the female genital opening.

From the ventral surface of the thoracic portion of the cephalothorax four pairs of seven-segmented legs arise, supported by the sternum and chitinised epimera. The tarsi are armed with a pair of claws and sometimes a third claw or pulvillus. They are also supplied with bundles of sticky hairs which enable them to walk on smooth surfaces. Those spiders with spinning organs have one or two rows of spines on the upper surface of the metatarsus, which are used to comb silk into bands.

On the abdomen the genital opening lies anteriorly in a midline ventral furrow leading to the reproductive organs. There are also three spiracu-

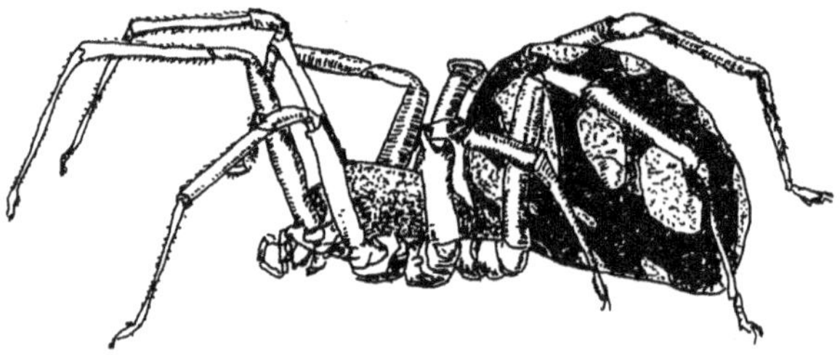

Fig. 14.1. *Latrodectus mactans*, illustrating the general structure of a spider. (After Sheals 1973, by courtesy of the Trustees of the British Museum)

lar openings on the ventral surface. They are of two kinds, namely lung slits leading to one or two pairs of lung-like organs (lung books) and tracheal spiracles. The spinning organ is near the caudal end of the abdomen ventrally. As a rule there are three pairs of finger-like spinnerets.

The above description owes much to Comstock (1948) and Main (1976). For full details of mouthparts, male palpal organs, spinning organs and other internal organs the reader is advised to read these two books.

Individual Reactions not Commonly Recorded

Several Mygalomorph spider bites cause skin reaction. The venom of *Eurypelma californica* is cytotoxic but is neutralised by serum if deeply injected. It causes only superficial reaction, therefore, and this also applies to *Pamphobetus* species (Horen 1963). One of the very large "tarantulas", the bird-eating Malaysian species, *Lampropelma violaceopedes*, has been reported as causing an instant painful reaction to its bite, quickly followed by an intermittent sensation of thoracic compression. Swelling of the bitten finger with oedematous erythema followed in minutes. All this reaction had gone within 72 h (Lim and Davie 1970). A Panamanian species, *Sericopelma communis*, produced similar effects, which lasted only 6 h (Baerg 1925). Several Australian species are also said to cause severe effects. According to Main, *Idiomma blackwalli* and some species of *Dekana* can cause local swelling and redness. Southcott (1978) has cited other trap-door spiders, *Aganippe raphiduca* and *Selenocosmia crassipes* and *S. stirlingi* (the latter two the so-called barking spiders) as causing severe but unspecified effects on man in Australia.

Theraphosid spiders are large and hairy. In species of *Grammostola* and *Brachypelma* (Grammostolinae) and *Lasiodora* and *Acanthascurria* (Theraphosinae) some hairs have urticating properties, which are set out in Table 14.4 (Cooke et al. 1973). They are used defensively, being "flicked off" in clouds in the face of an aggressor, leaving the spider with a "motheaten" appearance. They are renewed by moulting every 12–18 months over a life span of up to 30 years. Type III hairs seem to be those which cause urticaria in man. Cooke and his colleagues described how a 36-year-old male arachnologist (who handled *Brachypelma smithi* daily) developed punctate, itching urticarial lesions 20–30 min after contact. The individual lesions were related to penetration of the skin by the barbed hairs, which were shown histologically to be present from the stratum corneum to a depth of 2 mm. The effect subsided after 1–2 h but tended to recur for the next 2–3 weeks. It could be reproduced experimentally by the hairs concerned. These lesions are an occupational hazard which could also occur in those who keep these "tarantulas" as pets.

Bites by Argiopidae have been recorded. *Argiope aurantia* has caused trivial lesions (Gorham 1968a). *Glyptocranium gasteroacanthoides*

Table 14.4. Details of urticating hairs found on many Theraphosidae. (Based on Cooke et al. 1973)

Type	Size (mm)	Barb details on hairs	Spiders with this type	Region	Clinical effect
I	0.2–0.6	Reversed at base; two rows helically arranged large barbs	Only spiders in the USA		Cannot penetrate skin
II	0.5–1.5	Very small barbs	Avicularinae only; mostly *Avicularia*		Incorporated into webs; cause pricking but not urticaria
III	0.3–1.2	Sturdy barbs along half length	Many species	Mexico; Caribbean; Central and South America	Cause inflammation on touch; can penetrate at least 2 mm into skin
IV	0.06–0.2	Dart-like; few barbs at base only	Mainly *Grammostola*		? Respiratory effects on small animals

was incriminated by Escomel (1918, cited in detail by Phisalix 1922) as the cause of necrotic arachnidism in the Arequipa region of Peru. It is an easily identified spider on account of its unusually large abdomen, in both absolute and relative terms. It is well known to the local vineyard workers as *pododora* and is much feared by them. It lives amongst the vines and bites the hands of the workers or falls to the ground and bites their exposed feet. The effects are remarkably similar to those of loxescelism, even to the extent of occasional fatal haemolytic reactions, and will therefore not be described separately. Phisalix and some others (e.g. Pirosky and Abalos 1963) accepted Escomel's opinion as to the cause, but Vellard (1954), who carried out research in the area, was sceptical. He never encountered any effects in experiments with this species and considered that there had been confusion in identifying the cause, which he felt was a species of *Loxosceles*. Bücherl (1971) classed *Glyptocranium* as a "non-proven dangerous species", whilst Keegan (1963) grouped it amongst species with potent venom which seldom bit man.

Bites from two species of jumping spider, *Thiodina sylvana* and *Phidippus formosus*, have been reported from the United States (Waldron 1968; Russell 1970). The former caused sharp, brief local pain followed by an itching ecchymotic swelling, whilst the latter evoked local pain, swelling of the whole hand and a tiny 2-mm wide ulcer. Both had quite recovered within 2 weeks. The Australian jumping spiders *Mopsus mormon* and *Dysderca crocata* have been listed by Main (1976), along with the huntsman spider *Otios calligasta*, as causing swelling, redness, burning or itching at the site of the bite. The theridiid spider *Achaearanea tepidariorum* and the dictynid species *Ixeuticus robustus* are both recorded by Main as causing painful weeping erosions in the bitten area; those caused by the latter species persisted for weeks. In a personal experience Main also noted that the former species caused itching and burning at the bite site. The gnaphosid spider *Herpyllus ecclesiasticus* caused trivial erythema and induration around the site of its bite, associated with malaise, nausea and joint pains for 2 days. All evidence of bites had disappeared within 9 days (Majeski and Durst 1975).

Chiracanthium Bites

Various species of *Chiracanthium* can bite man (see Table 14.1). The toxicity of their venom varies from species to species, probably from one part of the year to another and apparently in the same species from one country to another (Horen 1963). Simon (cited by Phisalix 1922) regarded *Chiracanthium punctorium* as a dangerous spider, and Maretic (1975) ranked it next to *Latrodectus tredecimguttatus* in Europe. Bücherl (1971) even considered that some species of *Chiracanthium* might cause death. These spiders are both urban and rural and many invade houses. Their epidemiology resembles that of *Loxosceles* (Minton 1974). They are nocturnal, and therefore most bites occur at night. Exposed parts of the body are commonly bitten, usually a finger or hand. In the 19 patients recorded by Ori (1975) the majority of the bites occurred in summer months, almost all in June. Curiously nearly all the spiders and their victims in the series were male. In Australia *C. mordax* caused similar lesions (Main 1976).

Clinical Effects

Clinical effects included pain, occasional itch, erythema, oedematous swelling, petechiae, pigmentation, lymphangitis, lymphadenopathy and sometimes necrosis and gangrene. Symptoms, usually not severe, included chills, fever, malaise, headache, dizziness, nausea, vomiting, anorexia and even shock. The mild cases usually suffered pain and showed erythema, oedema, often extending beyong the bite site, and sometimes lymphangitis and enlargement of lymph glands for 2 to 3 days (Phisalix 1922). The pain in some patients radiated from the hand to the axilla and even in one instance caused a sense of constriction of the chest (Gorham 1968a). In a case cited by Phisalix (1922), a second bite reactivated pains and itch at the site of the first bite, where it persisted for 2 weeks. The oedematous swelling may involve a whole hand and wrist and persist for several weeks (Habermehl and Habermehl 1979). More severe reaction with early necrosis progressing to small dry gangrenous spots with a surrounding erythematous halo have been recorded by Spielman and Levi (1970) (with no other symptoms of any kind), by Maretic (1975) and by Southcott (1978). Some of Spielman's patients took up to 8 weeks to recover.

Histology

Spielman and Levi (1970) demonstrated early dermal oedema with intra- and perivascular collections of neutrophils progressing to epidermal and fat necrosis within 24 h. Some of the blood vessels became blocked and degenerate, whilst after 3 days some muscle degeneration was also seen.

Treatment

Treatment was symptomatic and included pethidine for pain, and systemic antibiotics.

Lycosa Bites

Spiders of the genus *Lycosa* (see Table 14.2) were thought for centuries to be the cause of frenzied or epidemic dancing (tarantism). The Italian species *L. tarentula* was blamed. It occurs not only in Italy but also in Greece, Spain, Southern France and Germany. According to Phisalix (1922) various Italian physicians in the seventeenth century disproved the role of this species in tarantism by experimental bites in man and animals. The effects were entirely local. Phisalix suggested that perhaps *Lycosa* bites had stimulated neurotic behaviour in psychologically predisposed persons. Nevertheless, *L. tarentula* causes swelling and itching of affected limbs, and a related species *L. infernalis* was said to have caused the death of 70 000 cattle in Russia in 1838–1839 (Moutschoulsky, cited by Phisalix 1922).

Clinical Effects

Brazil and Vellard (1925) in Sao Paulo noted that *L. erythrognatha* (= *L. raptoria*) was the principal cause of necrotic arachnidism in that region of Brazil. They reproduced identical lesions by the injection of the venom into the skin of animals. This venom resists cold but is heat labile and considerably inactivated by potassium permanganate. Horen (1963) noted that it is a cytolytic toxin with a particular affinity for the skin and has a weak proteolytic action. He pointed out that its effect is inhibited by human serum, which would account for most of its effects being superficial and for the absence of any systemic effect, since it would be neutralised if absorbed into the circulation. Moreover, it is known to have no haemolytic effects (Horen 1963; Bücherl 1971). Thus in man necrotic skin lesions are produced with little or no systemic reaction (Vellard 1954).

Horen (1963) noted that bites by *L. erythrognatha* (in Brazil) and *L. minima* (in Chile) both cause erythema, local oedema and some vesiculation. After 3–4 days early necrosis occurred in the centre of the lesion, with eschar separation and ulceration after 2–3 weeks. Pain was minimal but the scars became keloidal and tender. Grothaus and Teller (1968) reported a bite on the finger by *L. miami* which caused dizziness and nausea for about half an hour. Pain lasting for 2 h began 1 h after the bite and was quickly followed by swelling of the hand and forearm, which subsided on the second day.

Evanescent ischaemia was seen at the bite site but no other ill effect. Redman (1974) was bitten on the index finger by *L. antelucana*, which caused intense pain within 10 min. There was a small laceration with a drop of liquid (? venom) on the surface. There was early hyperaemia for about 1 cm around with swelling, giving the appearance of perionychia. The actual bite was depressed. By the third day the finger was twice its normal size with a 2-cm dark violaceous centre and lymphangitis of the hand and forearm. The lymphangitis settled in 24 h, but the swelling required a further 2 days to clear. On the sixth day the dark area sloughed off as an eschar and a further small area around the nail bed 3 days later. Healing then proceeded.

These examples indicate the superficial nature of the lycosid lesion, although it does leave a scar. Bites from this genus are not uncommon in Brazil, and probably also in many other countries, but have been much less frequently reported than the more dramatic *Loxosceles* lesions.

Treatment

In Sao Paulo, Brazil and Vellard (1925) produced a species-specific anti-*Lycosa* serum which proved effective in preventing necrosis. It will not protect against bites by other species, nor are *Lycosa* bites prevented by antisera for other species, such as anti-*Latrodectus* serum or anti-*Loxosceles* serum. Other treatment is symptomatic and includes antibiotics, preventive antitetanus injections and analgesics. Corticosteroids are unlikely to help.

Loxoscelism

Vellard (1954), in his detailed account of arachnidism in South America, cited Puga Borne [1892–1896] and Guzman [1894] as the first to describe necrotic lesions and occasionally associated severe systemic manifestations and to ascribe them to spider bites. Macchiavello (1937) gave Prada [1873–1894] priority. In none of these reports was the spider identified. Escomel [1918, 1919, 1940] attributed the lesions to *Glyptocranium gasteroacanthoides* (see pp. 212–213) according to Vellard (and Phisalix 1922); however, he considered that Escomel was mistaken. Macchiavello (1934) was the first to associate *Loxosceles laeta* with the disorder, which had been familiar to the inhabitants of the coastal regions of Chile and Peru long before the first medical reports appeared (Costa 1949). Macchiavello (1947b) was later to demonstrate that identical necrotic skin lesions could be produced by injecting the venom of *L. laeta* intradermally into rabbits' ears. Many reports have now been published involving hundreds of cases in South America. In recent years several instances have been reported in the United States, Israel (Efrati 1969), in South Africa (Newlands 1975), and *Loxosceles* species have recently been identified in Australia (Main 1976). Table 14.2 lists the various species said to have caused lesions, the signs and symptoms being more or less identical for all species. Vellard (1954) successfully produced an anti-*Loxosceles* serum at Lima, which afforded protection against most of the effects of *L. laeta* (see p. 219), but whether it protects against other species of *Loxosceles* is not yet known as it is unavailable elsewhere.

There are two distinct clinical forms of loxoscelism: Necrotic cutaneous arachnidism (NA), with occasionally mild systemic symptoms (*mancha gangrenosa* of Chile), is at least ten times as common as the viscerocutaneous form (VCA), in which similar skin lesions are overshadowed by severe, sometimes fatal haemolytic effects. The following descriptions of the two types, unless otherwise stated, are based on the account of Gajardo-Tobar (1966), itself the distillation of 200 personal cases of *L. laeta* bites.

Anyone living in a "*Loxosceles* area" is liable to attack, although most bites in South America occur in the patient's own home (Mackinnon and Witkind 1953). Most victims are bitten when in bed or getting dressed, but in the United States, where *L. reclusa* is the cause of most cases, an appreciable number of bites occur in children playing in infested premises (Lessenden and Zimmer 1960; James et al. 1961; Nance 1961; Nicholson and Nicholson 1962; Minton and Olson 1964), or in adults working in infested outhouses or elsewhere out of doors (Pitts 1962; Micks 1963). The sex incidence is equal, but women were said by some authors to predominate (Macchiavello 1937; Schenone 1959; Schenone and Prats 1961). Any part of the body can be bitten, but the limbs are involved in almost 70% of cases. Other areas in order of frequency are face, neck, thorax, abdomen and genitalia. It is noteworthy that only 3% of Gajardo-Tobar's 200 cases were bitten on the genitalia, whereas in *Latrodectus* bites between 60% and 70% of the bites are in this area in domestic cases, thus contrasting the habits and habitat of the different spiders. Majeski and Durst (1976) noted in the case of *L. reclusa* that over 50% of their patients were bitten on the thighs, feet or buttocks. The age range can be anything from 1 month to 70 years, over two-thirds being between 15 and 50 years.

Necrotic Cutaneous Arachnidism

Clinical Features

About 75% of Gajardo-Tobar's patients felt the bite as a sharp prick, although Anderson (1971) said it was generally painless. In those who felt the bite there was a brief asymptomatic period of 5–10 min, extended rarely to 24 h. There was then an explosion of increasing, burning, local pain, followed shortly by itching in a few patients, usually evanescent (Fardon et al. 1967) and rarely generalised (Berger 1973b). Many patients bitten by *L. reclusa* or other North American species experienced a delay of up to 8 h before the onset of pain (Pitts 1962; Micks 1963; Dillaha et al. 1963; Russell et al. 1969). The pain, which is almost invariably present, may be exceptionally severe and not even completely controlled by pethidine (meperidine) or morphine (Pitts 1962). Once established, its intensity increases continuously or intermittently up to an unbearable peak where suicide may be contemplated and amputation of an affected limb fervently desired. It tends to diminish as the necrotic lesion ages but usually persists until separation of the eschar (see below), although in many cases the most severe pain ends after 24 h (Macchiavello 1947a). Movement and function of the affected limb may be impeded or inhibited by the pain. Insomnia is the rule and anxiety frequent.

The bite is marked initially by hyperaemia and the development of a tiny red papule or papules (Vellard 1954). Very shortly after (within 2 or 3 h), however, a clear-cut central zone of ischaemic pallor appears, which may be up to 30 cm across and is surrounded by an erythematous halo. At the same time the whole area becomes oedematous, giving the central ischaemic zone a pale indurated appearance, with a peripheral, erythematous oedematous margin. This central pallor persists after the initial erythema has faded (Dillaha et al. 1963). The peripheral oedema, which is not well demarcated, may spread extensively, especially to dependent parts, and can involve a whole limb or more than half of the trunk. The central zone loses its sensitivity, but the reddened oedematous halo around is often exquisitely tender. Discolouration of the central ischaemic zone begins after the first 48 h (Fardon et al. 1967), as the result of ecchymotic extravasation (Mackinnon and Witkind 1953) and small haemorrhages. It also becomes red, then violaceous, the whole producing a marbled or mottled effect. On the third day one or more small sterile, serous or serosanguineous vesicles may appear in the centre of this central zone in the region of the bite site. The mottled area darkens steadily. By the fifth or sixth day the oedema begins to subside, except for the immediate periphery of the lesions, and the by now blackened central area has the appearance of a dry, clear-cut, parchment-like eschar (Fig. 14.2). The exact size of the eschar is not evident until the sixth or seventh day (Fardon et al. 1967). It is always bacteriologically sterile (Mackinnon and Witkind 1953; Anderson 1971). It begins to separate at the edges and is shed painlessly in the third week after the bite (Figs. 14.3, 14.4), although this event may not occur until several weeks later in some cases. The burning pain which may have persisted in the oedematous areas around now begins to abate.

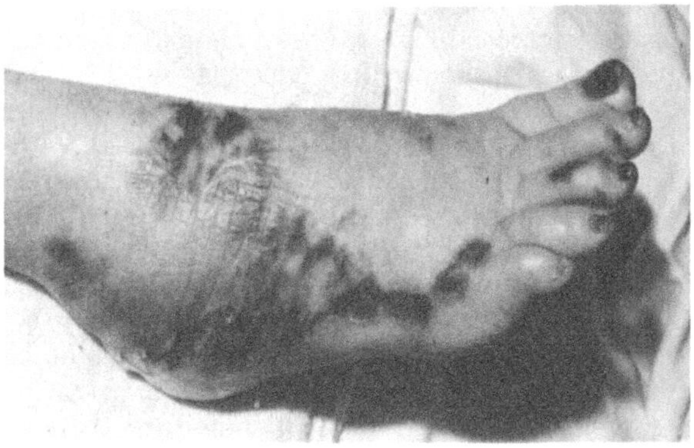

Fig. 14.2. Gangrenous bite of *Loxosceles reclusa* showing the extent of the affected area, clear-cut edge beginning to develop and early ulceration in one area after separation of the slough. Black eschar can be seen in other areas. (Courtesy of Dr. A. L. Schroeter, the Mayo Clinic, Rochester, Minnesota)

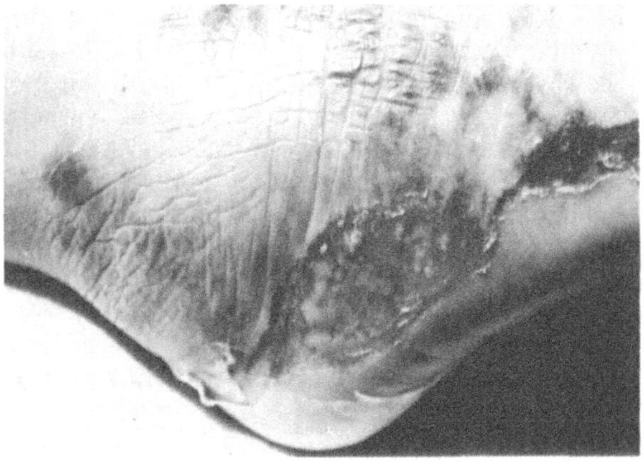

Fig. 14.3. Closer view of the ulcerated portion of Fig. 14.2. Note that only skin and subcutaneous fat are involved. (Courtesy of Dr. A. L. Schroeter, The Mayo Clinic, Rochester, Minnesota)

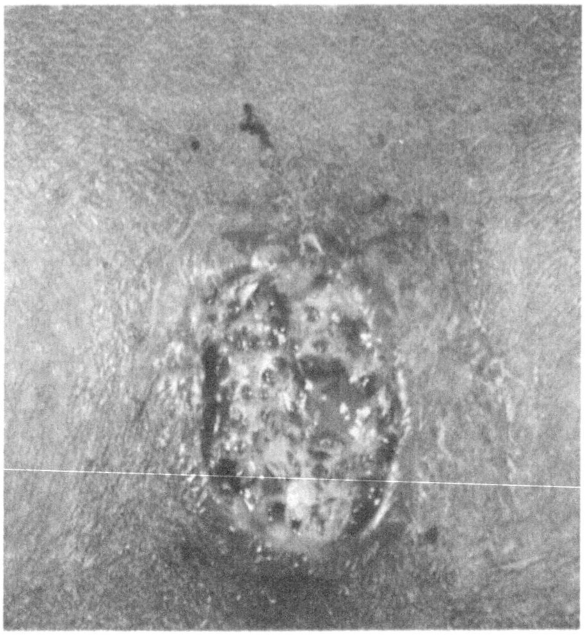

Fig. 14.4. Ulcerated, relatively small lesion caused by the bite of *Loxosceles reclusa*. Note the sharply demarcated edge and the superficial nature of the ulceration. (Courtesy of Dr. A. L. Schroeter, The Mayo Clinic, Rochester, Minnesota)

Lymphadenopathy is not a feature of this condition. It occurred in 13.5% of Gajardo-Tobar's patients and was reported in ten of Micks' 80 patients. Dillaha et al. (1972) noted it as a feature, whilst it was present in one of seven patients seen by Russell et al. (1969). It is probable, as Gajardo-Tobar (1966) indicated, that the lymphadenitis was associated with secondary infection rather than with the necrotic process as such. The same applies to the very occasional lymphangitis seen by all these groups. Repair of the pale, usually shallow ulcer left after separation of the eschar is very slow and if unaided may take up to 6 months (Macchiavello 1947a). A stellate, disfiguring scar is left. The depth of the ulcer depends on the situation. For example, Anderson noted that an ulcer resulting from a bite on an obese thigh measured 40 cm by 15–20 cm and was 4 cm deep because of the thick layer of fat. The ulcers never penetrate below the subcutaneous fascia. The scars show a bluish or brownish pigmentation and not infrequently develop painful keloids.

Systemic Symptoms

Gajardo-Tobar reported general symptoms in NA in 39% of his patients, which is in keeping with the findings of others. Dillaha et al. (1972) estimated the incidence as some 25%. Such symptoms include headache, mild fever, vertigo, nausea, vomiting, diarrhoea, sweating and nervousness. Some patients develop a widespread skin eruption after some 24–36 h which lasts about 3 days (Schmaus 1929; Atkins et al. 1957; Lessenden and Zimmer 1960; Pitts 1962; Micks 1963; Dillaha et al. 1963; Fardon et al. 1967). Lessenden and his colleague noted that fever and arthralgia developed when the rash appeared. The rash has been scarlatiniform (Mackinnon and Witkind 1953; Pitts 1962; Russell et al. 1969), erythematous and purpuric (Costa and Salveraglio 1949), maculoerythematous (Fardon et al. 1967), morbilliform (Lessenden and Zimmer 1960; Dillaha et al. 1963; Berger 1973b) or urticarial with itch (Micks 1963). Majeski and Durst (1976) claimed that such skin eruptions only occurred in the more severe cases, but this view is not supported by the case descriptions in which they appear.

Laboratory Data

Laboratory findings in NA are scanty in the literature. Atkins et al. (1958) and Schenone (1959) noted a moderate leucocytosis, whilst Lessenden and Zimmer (1960) pointed out that laboratory evidence of haemolysis could be detected frequently, although there was no clinical evidence of such.

Diagnosis

The diagnosis is made on the grounds of known or suspected history of spider bite and would be greatly enhanced if the offending spider could be produced and identified. The lesion is solitary and the increasing pain with central ischaemia is very suggestive. When necrosis has already started, the appearance and history, including details of where the incident occurred, are very indicative of NA.

The differential diagnosis includes carbuncle, furunculosis and other insect bites (Gajardo-Tobar 1966); injury, firearms burns, erysipelas, caustic chemical burns and cutaneous anthrax (Macchiavello 1947a); thermal burns (Vellard 1954); acute Chagas' disease, especially of the oculopalpebral type, angio-oedema, ophthalmic zoster, cutaneous diphtheria and other types of cutaneous gangrene (Schenone and Prats 1961); and cellulitis and ecthyma (Dillaha et al. 1963).

Viscerocutaneous Arachnidism

Clinical Features

VCA begins in exactly the same manner as the local form just described. For the first 24 h it is impossible to forecast the onset of serious symptoms, and if patients should die quickly the necrotic lesion scarcely progresses beyond the cyanotic, marbled indurated phase. The severe generalised burning pain does not materialise. The onset of systemic involvement is indicated by severe malaise, restlessness, headache and fever, one or more of which always occurs. In small children convulsions may occur early (James et al. 1961). Of Gajardo-Tobar's 22 patients with visceral effects 13 exhibited vertigo, tachycardia and hypotension and some experienced nausea and vomiting, even of blood. The most alarming symptoms occur between 12 and 24 h after the onset of general symptoms and consist of ecchymoses, jaundice, haematuria and haemoglobinuria. In the next few hours headache increases, chills may occur, together with general weakness, cessation of sweating and rise of temperature and pulse rate. The skin sometimes takes on an earthy colour. As the condition deteriorates dyspnoea may develop, cyanosis increases, jaundice deepens and anaemia becomes apparent. Signs of pulmonary congestion and oedema may cause stertorous breathing with the production of much frothy blood-stained mucus. The pulse becomes thready, hypotension is accentuated, urine is suppressed and extreme restlessness is followed by coma and death. Not all patients reach this severity, but even with energetic treatment Izu in Lima recorded five deaths in 31 patients (cited by Vellard 1954) and Gajardo-Tobar (1966) had seven deaths in his 22 patients (32%). Examination will confirm the above features and often, especially in children, reveals that the liver and spleen are palpable. Careful examination may also be necessary to reveal the local lesion produced by the bite, although it may be obvious.

Laboratory Data

There is a massive and rapid haemolysis, the effects of which could account for all the general symptoms. The erythrocyte count in the peripheral blood may fall below 1.0 million per mm^3, with corresponding reduction in haemoglobin. James et al. (1961) recorded a fall of the latter from 12.0 g/100 ml to 6.0 g/100 ml in 24 h, and Weiner et al. (1960) a drop from 12.0 g/100 ml to 4.0 g/100 ml in 6 h. At the same time there is a fall in the platelet count, often by as much as 50%. There is a marked polymorphonuclear leucocytosis with many immature cells. The count may reach 55 000/mm^3 (Minton and Olson 1964). Many counts recorded have been over 30 000/mm^3. In favourable cases there is a return to normal in about 10 days. Meneghello and Emparanza (1952) recorded a fall to leucopenic levels (3500) 3 weeks after the onset, whilst in a patient mentioned by the Nicholsons (1962) the leucocyte count 24 h after being bitten was 3400. Eosinophils are conspicuous by their absence, although Vellard (1954) noted that a discrete eosinophila appearing during treatment heralded the onset of convalescence. The serum is markedly tinged with haemoglobin to the extent of being black on occasion.

The urine, usually scanty, shows some haematuria and massive haemoglobinuria and it too may be black. Occasionally methaemoglobin may be detected in both urine and blood. Blood, haemoglobin and haemosiderin casts may be noted as well as albuminuria. The blood urea nitrogen may be raised above 200 mg/100 ml (James et al. 1961). Serum potassium may be raised to toxic levels (James et al. 1961; Vorse et al. 1972). The blood coagulation time is normal but the bleeding time is prolonged. The erythrocyte sedimentation rate is raised in VCA, but normal in NA.

Histopathology of the Gangrenous Lesions

The progress of events has been described in part in material from excision and post-mortem specimens and various stages recorded by Lessenden and Zimmer 1960, Gajardo-Tobar (1966), Taylor and Denny (1966), Dillaha et al. (1972) and Vorse et al. (1972). The process appears to be as follows. Capillary dilation (probably that following initial ischaemia) is accompanied by developing dermal oedema, which extends deeply as far as the fascia–muscle boundary. There is early dermoepidermal separation with a neutrophil polymorphonuclear (PMN) infiltrate in this area, but tending to accumulate around the small superficial arterioles and venules as the venom diffuses. After about 18 h there is early oedema of the endothelial cells of these small vessels, which, with the formation of microthrombi, ultimately leads to their occlusion. At this time a few scattered discrete eosinophil cells may be seen in the corium. This vascular thrombosis extends to deeper vessels. Erythrocytes escape through the damaged vessel walls forming small subdermal haemorrhages. The ultimate result of the vascular occlusion is necrosis of the area supplied by the damaged vessels with subepidermal sloughing. Eventually a necrotic demarcation zone caused by microthrombi delineates the whole area of the future eschar, which includes skin, subcutaneous fat and superficial fascia but not muscle. Foamy macrophages can be seen in the necrotic fat, and the dying or dead dermal material shows fibrocollagen, swelling, disintegrated or dissolved. Granulation tissue forms beneath the eschar, healing by fibrosis.

These changes have been produced experimentally with spider venom injected into animals, either by the experimenter or by controlled spiders. The sequence of events has been described in papers by Pizzi et al. (1957), Smith and Micks (1970), Butz et al. (1971) and by Berger et al. (1973). Pizzi and his colleagues and Berger et al. have remarked on the resemblance of the lesions to the Arthus phenomenon. However, the latter consists of changes induced by the influence of antigen–antibody reaction and complement activation, whereas there is no indication of antibodies to spider bites being formed in NA or VCA. This has been explained by Berger and his collaborators, who noted that in the Arthus reaction the immunological process induced aggregation of PMN leucocytes, which in turn damage the vascular endothelium as they migrate through the wall in large numbers. Thrombus formation ensues. In NA the venom toxin initially damages the vascular endothelium lining of the vessel wall. This leads to fibrin formation, platelet aggregation and thrombus formation. This is *followed* by PMN leucocyte infiltration. These early changes are seldom if ever seen in the *clinical* specimens presented for histological examination, because the PMN infiltrate has already arrived in them. The sequence of events, however, would seem to be as described above, since the clinical and experimental lesions appear to be identical. Smith and Micks (1970) stated that their experiments indicated that PMN leucocytic infiltration was essential for the development of the lesions caused by *L. reclusa* and that this infiltration was complement dependent.

The pathological changes in VCA were fully described by Gajardo-Tobar (1966) and confirmed by Taylor and Denny (1966) and by Vorse et al. (1972). They are due to intravascular haemolysis and haemoglobin liberation and complicated by intravascular coagulation (Vorse et al. 1972). All organs show, in some degree, hyperaemia, oedema and focal haemorrhages. Liver cells show cloudy swelling, fatty degeneration or even focal necrosis, with marked haemosiderosis (especially in the Kupfer cells) and iron deposition in the intertrabecular spaces. Renal changes are concentrated in the epithelial cells of the proximal convoluted tubules, which also reveal swelling, fatty degeneration and necrosis. The tubules and Bowman's capsule are filled with blood and haemosiderin casts and necrotic debris. There is acute pulmonary oedema and possibly haemothorax or haemopericardium. There is cloudy swelling and fatty degeneration of cardiac muscle. The bone marrow is filled with primitive cells. Multiple gastric ulcers were found by Taylor and Denny (1966).

Treatment

Treatment may be specific or non-specific. Specific treatment involves administering anti-*Loxosceles* serum, as prepared by Vellard (1954). It is only available at present in South America and only against *L. laeta*. Its action is delayed for 2–3 h; even if given immediately after the bite some minimal skin changes will occur before its effects begin. If given within 4 h all systemic reactions can be inhibited. However, once the necrotic process has started it cannot be reversed by the serum but may be limited to a smaller area than it might otherwise have involved. In severe cases, even if given after the onset of haemolysis, the latter can be stopped when the serum's effect begins. Vellard (1954) recommended 5 ml subcutaneously as being sufficient to inhibit systemic effects if given within 4 h. If given later, 10 ml is required and this may have to be repeated after 12 h if necessary. Results depend on how early the serum is given.

There are various forms of non-specific treatment. Surgery, until quite recently, was used to excise granulating ulcers or disfiguring scars preparatory to skin grafting. For this purpose it is best undertaken after separation of the eschar (Butz 1971). However, surgery can also be curative, if the bite area and the surrounding tissues down to and including subcutaneous fascia are excised early, within 2–4 h of the bite, and providing there is no secondary infection. The whole reactive process can be aborted and spontaneous healing brought about. (Butz 1971; Auer and Hershey 1974; Minton 1974). Such treatment is not always possible and then other measures are required.

Analgesics are needed to control the pain. Pethidine (meperidine) is often used in doses of up to 100 mg, but even morphine may fail to relieve the pain. The curative measures mentioned above abolish pain.

There is some diversity of opinion about the value of corticosteroids. If given early enough in doses equivalent to 80–100 mg of prednisolone daily they may prevent the area of necrosis from increasing (Dillaha et al. 1963; Minton 1974); however, they can delay healing if not given early. Others have found them of no value (Atkins et al. 1958; Anderson 1971; Berger 1973a) and similarly if given intralesionally (Jansen et al. 1971; Berger 1973a). On the other hand, systemic symptoms can be limited if large doses are given, the earlier the better (Weiner et al. 1960; James et al. 1961; Chu et al. 1978).

Some authors have claimed benefit from the use of antihistamines (Vellard 1954; Prats and Schenone 1957; Schenone 1959; Lessenden and Zimmer 1960), but the consensus now is that their value is doubtful. Antibiotics are of no help except in controlling secondary infection. Heparin has been advocated on the grounds that it may help to prevent or diminish intravascular coagulation, especially if given early (Anderson 1971; Berger 1973a; Auer and Hershey 1974; Minton 1974). In Anderson's patient heparin produced prompt improvement, and he advised that it should not be withheld to await gross evidence of fibrinogen or platelet depletion. It seems that it could be a particularly valuable drug for severe systemic loxoscelisem.

Blood transfusion can be life saving in this disease. Many cases do not reach hospital early, and precipitate haemolysis may result in a dramatic fall in erythrocyte count and haemoglobin level, which can very rapidly have fatal consequences in small children. Exchange transfusion, the earlier the better, has brought about remarkable recoveries, not only by replacing lysed erythrocytes but by diluting and removing the toxin (Gotten and McGowan 1940; Meneghello and Amparanza 1952; Nance 1961; Nicholson and Nicholson 1962).

Topical treatment does not help the local necrotic process, but until skin grafting is carried out in those cases which reach the ulcerating stage the local application of lead subacetate lotion (1%) or an antibiotic tulle could relieve discomfort.

Oliguria and anuria in the haemolytic phase may be alleviated by diuretics and kidney function helped by dialysis.

Loxosceles Spiders: Morphology and Biology

The species differences amongst *Loxoceles* (family Scytodidae) are a matter for experts. These spiders are all small, averaging 8–12 mm in length, depending on species. Their six eyes are arranged in a recurved row. They have simple external reproductive organs. The cephalothorax is low and the body coloured various shades of brown, light brown or yellow. All have a characteristic dark violin-shaped pattern on the dorsum of the carapace (Fig. 14.5).

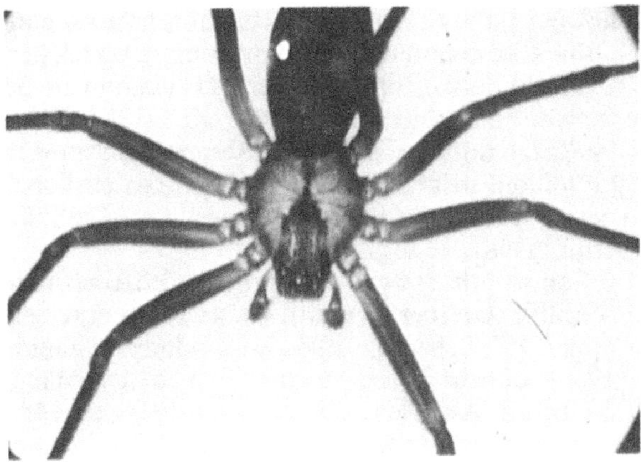

Fig. 14.5. *Loxosceles reclusa.* Note the violin-shaped marking on the dorsal surface of the cephalothorax. (Courtesy of Dr. A. L. Schroeter, The Mayo Clinic, Rochester, Minnesota)

Their bodies are covered with short, macroscopically invisible hairs (Dillaha et al. 1963; Lewis and Regan 1966; Arnold 1976).

According to Gorham (1968b), *L. reclusa* mates once and lays several batches of eggs. This activity occurs principally in the warm weather months and never in midwinter, whether in North or South America (Mackinnon and Witkind 1953). The eggs hatch in 33 days, the developmental period is between 266 and 444 days and adult life ranges from 356–894 days for females and 301–796 days for males. Only 25% live more than 350 days as adults.

The natural habitat is in dark places under bark, logs, stones, lumps of peat or in the crevices of ruins of bygone towns (Prats and Schenone 1957; Dillaha et al. 1963; Delgado 1966). Dry conditions are essential for *L. laeta* (Delgado 1966), but *L. reclusa* tolerates a humid environment (Anderson 1971). Most species, especially *L. laeta* and *L. reclusa*, have become adapted to living in buildings, in cracks in walls and ceilings, in the roof space, behind furniture and pictures, in cellars and outhouses, where they are often found beneath boxes or crates, and particularly amongst clothing hung on walls or in cupboards. Waldron et al. (1975) found signs of infestation by *L. laeta* in 127 out of 700 contiguous commercial buildings in California and concluded that this infestation was of long standing. With the advent of central heating, houses are more frequently invaded and the spiders are spreading to areas usually too cold for them (Gorham 1968b). Waldron and Russell (1967) have pointed out that they can be imported in furniture, packing cases etc. They tend to avoid areas inhabited by other spiders.

They are actively mobile nocturnal and crepuscular predators, stimulated by the slightest movement. Their web is small and irregular. They are not aggressive towards man and only bite if disturbed or in self-defence. *L. laeta* specimens in the United States (imported) may owe the absence of aggression to lower environmental temperatures (Levi and Speilman 1964).

Loxosceles Venom

The venom of *Loxosceles* contains at least eight fractions (Elgert et al. 1973). All workers agree that hyaluronidase, levarteranol, protease and esterase are present. Elgert et al. isolated a fraction with dermonecrotic properties. Geren et al. (1973) separated two fractions, which could each cause lesions and death in experimental animals. Geren et al. (1976) noted that these fractions acted independently of hyaluronidase, alkaline phosphatase or 5-nucleotide phosphohydrolase. Antisera against the whole venom extract protected against their effects. Morgan et al. (1978) demonstrated a haemolytic factor (which many workers had hitherto failed to do), which damaged red cells so that they lysed in the presence of normal blood group-compatible human serum. The degree of haemolysis appeared to vary with the serum, which might explain why some victims of bites experience severe haemolytic reactions and many others do not.

Majeski and Durst (1976) regarded the neutrophil leucocyte response to the venom as very important. They attributed much of the damage to lysosomes from these cells. Incidentally, this theory suggests that it might be worthwhile trying the therapeutic effect of dapsone, which is effective in several conditions associated with neutrophil aggregations (e.g. dermatitis herptiformis and Sneddon and Wilkinson syndrome). It may act by inhibiting lysosome activity. Smith and Micks (1968) showed that the components which they separated from venoms by immunoelectrophoresis were identical for *L. rufescens* and *L. reclusa*.

Machiavello (1947b) has summarised other important points about *Loxosceles* venom. In some species its activity varies from spider to spider; darker specimens are alleged to have the more potent venom. Potency tends to diminish with age and shows seasonal variation, being highest in warm weather, although the amount is greatest at periods of climatic stability (Morgan 1969). Imprisonment and starvation reduce the potency. On the rare occasion of a second bite, the repeat bite always has less severe effects. Only venom injected intradermally can cause lesions. It is destroyed by heat. It has no relation to arachnolysin, an extract of whole crushed spider, which is intensely haemolytic. In Macchiavello's day only necrotising and coagulant activity could be demonstrated in the laboratory.

Control

Control means, in practice, control of spiders indoors. The indoor increase of *Loxosceles* varies in different areas. There is a direct relationship between habitat and environmental temperature (Gorham 1968b). These spiders are very susceptible to contact insecticides, e.g. gamma-benzene hexachloride, malathion or dichlorvos; however, according to Gorham, good housekeeping is the best means of avoiding contact between man and spider. Regular dusting of furniture and pictures, and airing and shaking of stored clothing should be carried out. Always clean behind furniture. Storage bags and boxes should be airtight, and those not required suitably disposed of. Individuals in *Loxosceles* areas would be well advised to shake their clothing prior to dressing. Prophylaxis of this kind is particularly important because of the difficulty in preparing effective antisera (Vellard 1954). It follows that education of the general public in these areas is important.

Prognosis

Several writers have expressed the view that many persons are probably bitten and experience trivial reactions which are never reported or pass unnoticed (Pesce and Lumbreras 1954; Vellard 1954; Denny et al. 1964). Because of this Anderson (1978) has suggested that some householders may develop immunity, although it has never been shown that antibodies to *Loxosceles* are present.

The prognosis in NA is always good as regards survival, but untreated cases may leave grossly disfiguring scars. Severe haemolysis is unlikely if it is not evident in the first 48 h. Pesce and Lumbreras (1954) assessed the mortality in children as between 15% and 20%.

Latrodectism

Latrodectus bites are principally notable for their effects on the central nervous system, but skin lesions, though evanescent, do occur; since there has been confusion in the past between latrodectism and loxoscelism they must be described in some detail, especially since either can be fatal.

Latrodectus Spiders: Morphology and Biology

Table 14.3 shows the modern classification of the genus, based on information gleaned from Bücherl (1971). This should make for easier understanding of the literature on the bites. *L. mactans* in all its varieties is cosmopolitan between latitudes 55°N and 50°S (Newlands 1975), although different conditions in various regions have resulted in taxonomic variations, which cause difficulties even for experts (Levi 1959). For example, the United States variety is jet black viewed dorsally, in Brazil it shows many light markings, whilst in Australia *L. mactans hasselti* has a characteristic red diagonal stripe across its back. Other species of *Latrodectus* may be found in colder areas such as Canada and the USSR and parts of the United States.

L. mactans is a fairly small spider (see Figs. 14.1, 14.6), the adult female body being 8–15 mm long

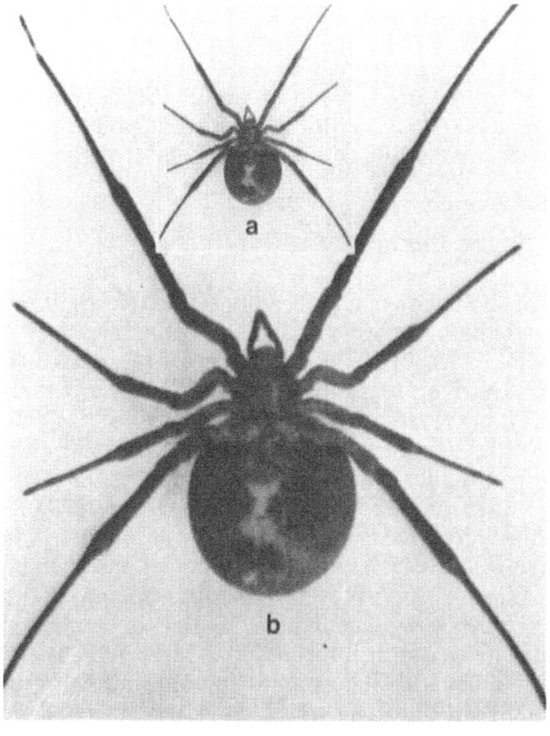

Fig. 14.6a, b. *Latrodectus mactans* (the black widow spider), ventral aspect. **a** male; **b** female. (Photograph taken by Wayne Book and supplied by courtesy of the Wellcome Museum of Medical Science, Director Dr. A. J. Duggan)

and the male much smaller (3 mm). It has eight eyes arranged in two rows, the front of which is procurved and the other recurved. The fangs operate on a lateral plane. The globose abdomen has an orange-red hour-glass marking on the ventral surface. There are combs on tarsi IV, which enable it to cast a band of sticky silk around its prey (D'Amour et al. 1936). In spite of its very small size the male has legs almost as long as those of the female.

The habitat of *Latrodectus* spiders under natural circumstances is in ready-made holes, abandoned nests and burrows of small mammals, beneath banks, tufts of grass, cacti, stones, pieces of wood or tree stumps. They can be found below heaps of rubble, old tins, flower pots, inside dry watering cans, in outbuildings, beneath the eaves and especially below the lavatory seat in outside toilets (Ingram and Musgrave 1933; D'Amour et al. 1936; Wolcatt 1948; Finlayson 1955; Levi 1959; Pirosky and Abalos 1963). In New Zealand and Jamaica it is found on beaches (Levi 1959). *L. mactans* is not aggressive but will bite in self-defence or if disturbed. Where *Latrodectus* is more domesticated, as in the United States, attacks tend to be indiscriminate, whereas in South America and Italy it is essentially rural, and epidemics occur during harvest time (Bettini 1964). Pirosky and Abalos (1963) reported hundreds of cases annually during flax harvesting in Argentina, and similarly Finlayson (1955) reported cases in South Africa amongst grape pickers. The incidence is seasonal in temperate climates but continual in tropical areas.

Clinical Picture

The cutaneous manifestations are overshadowed by general neurotoxic effects. The bite may be painless (Reid 1971), a sharp prick (Gertsch 1949) or a burning sensation (Wiener 1961). Fang marks may be revealed by two puncta (Phisalix 1922). Within 10 min increasingly severe pain develops, appearing first in the regional lymph nodes (Maretic 1971), spreads centrifugally (Greer 1949) and especially affects the limbs and abdomen. It has been variously described as being "intense, violent, agonising, exquisite, excruciating, griping, cramping, shocking, lancinating, aching or numbing", and incessant or intermittent (Gertsch 1949). It is not relieved by morphine (Ingram and Musgrave 1933). In the early stages the bite site is oedematous with a red halo, but this does not appear to persist (Gertsch 1949; Wiener 1961; Reid 1971). According to Phisalix (1922), Escomel stated that this local change always occurred and resembled cellulitis. Sweating, tenderness and numbness appear at the bite site within a few hours. General symptoms include headache, backache, faintness, dizziness, pronounced restlessness, dyspnoea, urinary retention and hysterical fear. There are often flexor muscular spasms of the limbs so that the victim involuntarily assumes a curled-up position. The outstanding feature in many patients is the cramp-like or colicky abdominal pain, which, together with rigidity, nausea and less commonly vomiting, simulates an abdominal emergency. Neuromuscular involvement causes weakness, tremors, loss of muscle tone, incoordination, interference with speech or paralysis. Convulsions may occur in young children. There may be collapse or shock. Sweating is pronounced, and excessive salivation and lacrimation may also occur. There is considerable thirst (Phisalix 1922; Ingram and Musgrave 1933; Gertsch 1949; Greer 1949; Wiener 1961; Reid 1971). Ingram and Musgrave pointed out that pains in the small joints of the hands and feet can occur, whilst Greer regarded a complaint of burning of the soles of the feet as almost pathognomonic of latrodectism; Maretic (1971) also regarded this as an important symptom. Phisalix noted general cutaneous hypersensitivity. Oedema of the eyelids accompanied by a scarlatiniform eruption may occur on rare occasions (Wiener 1961; Maretic 1971; Minton 1974). Reid (1982) said an itching eruption may occur around the bite site in severe attacks.

Physical examination confirms the local oedema and erythema, the abdominal rigidity and skin hypersensitivity. Maretic (1971) has described the typical "facies latrodectisma" as a reddened, sweat-covered face, with oedema of the eyelids, marked blepharoconjunctivitis, painful grimace and latterly trismus of the masseter muscles (Fig. 14.7). The calf muscles may be tender.

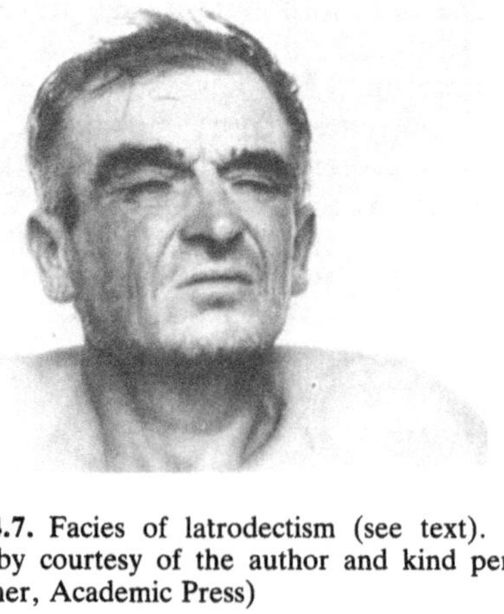

Fig. 14.7. Facies of latrodectism (see text). (From Maretic 1971, by courtesy of the author and kind permission of the publisher, Academic Press)

Limb movement is hindered by spasm. There will be profound shock and hypotension, although the blood pressure may be normal or even raised (Greer 1949). The temperature is variable. The pulse is full and bounding and may be rapid, but Phisalix (1922) stressed its normality, a useful sign in differentiating from an acute abdominal catastrophe, as is the absence of abdominal tenderness (Minton 1974). Wiener (1961) noted that regional lymphadenopathy with lymphangitis occurred, often within 30 min of the bite. Moderate leucocytosis and albuminuria may be found (Greer 1949; Maretic 1971).

The pain begins to diminish within 24 h, and the other symptoms also subside, seldom persisting for longer than 2–3 days. Rarely there may be pain for a little longer, but not enough to prevent the patient from returning to work (Phisalix 1922). Weakness and lethargy may last for 3–4 weeks (Wiener 1961).

It should be emphasized that *L. mactans* often bites with little or no symptoms. This is because it has the power to bite without injecting much or any venom and can in fact control the amount it injects. The toxicity of the venom also shows seasonal variations (Keegan et al. 1960). Bites are therefore probably commoner than has been recorded.

The diagnosis of acute symptoms presents little difficulty if a spider bite is suspected, and such symptoms occurring in an area where *Latrodectus* spiders are known to exist should always raise this possibility. Acute abdominal incidents are excluded by the absence of tenderness, more or less normal pulse and no developing distension.

Prognosis

The death rate seems to vary between 4% and 6% in the reported outbreaks where specific treatment is unavailable, although Phisalix (1922) maintained that the bite was never fatal. Specific antivenom serum prevents all fatalities. In the absence of such therapy, death may supervene in a few hours in very young children, or not until over 4 weeks later in previously healthy adults (Ingram and Musgrave 1933).

Treatment

Specific antivenin serum (horse serum) is available in most if not all countries where the spider exists. It should be given as early as possible in a dose of 5 ml subcutaneously or intravenously and the patient kept quiet. If there is no improvement 5–10 ml intravenously should be given an hour later. Precautions against possible anaphylactic reactions to horse serum should be at hand for immediate use (adrenaline solution and soluble corticosteroids ready in a syringe; Newlands 1975). This serum should only be used where symptoms are severe, but always in children (Horen 1963); it is unnecessary for milder cases. Symptomatic treatment is aimed at relieving muscle spasm. Calcium gluconate in doses of 10–20 ml intravenously gives relief, although its action is brief. Muscle relaxants give better results (Minton 1974). Russell (1962) found methocarbamol (Robaxin) intravenously or mephenesin (Myanesin) gave excellent results. However, these drugs have no effect whatever on skin eruptions, oedema or itch. As a first aid measure before development of severe symptoms an ice pack applied to the bite and a tourniquet applied between the bite site and the heart and released briefly at intervals may help.

Control

To eradicate the spider from buildings Pirosky and Abalos (1963) recommended 0.5% gamma-benzene hexachloride spray, which kills spiders in 60–90 min.

Bites Caused by *Atrax* Species

Dangerous spiders which produce very mild or no apparent skin lesions are the funnel-web spiders of Australia, *Atrax* species (Dipluridae). The most venomous is *A. robustus*, which caused five deaths in the Sydney region between 1927 and 1949. All the deaths were caused by bites from the male, although bites from the female have been recorded (Musgrave 1949). The venom contains a neurotoxin, hyaluronidase and other ingredients. This spider gains entrance to dwellings through doors, windows, ventilators etc. and hides beneath bathroom furniture, in clothing, cupboards and in shoes (Sutherland 1978). According to Musgrave (1949) considerable force is required to remove these spiders during the process of biting. Not all bites are envenomated.

The only treatment is a tourniquet, which should not be released en route to hospital. Atropine, diazepam and frusemide are all said to help. The patient may require to be in intensive care for a period (Sutherland 1978).

Bites Caused by *Phoneutria* Species

The largest spiders in South America are the *Phoneutria* species (Ctenidae), which are nocturnal in habit. They are aggressive and their venom causes severe local pain. The bite may be invisible or be seen as a small erosion or red macule. The pain radiates over the whole affected limb and to the trunk. The symptoms in man suggest histamine and adrenaline overdosage, with hypothermia, sweating, tachycardia and hypertension amongst other symptoms. Sedation against the pain also suppresses all other symptoms. Death is very rare and only occurs in the weakly and in young children.

Treatment, apart from analgesics (including local anaesthesia), includes vascular dilatation, intravenous antihistamines and one to five ampoules of specific antivenin intramuscularly, followed by the same amount intravenously. A watch should be kept for signs of anaphylaxis. A polyvalent vaccine is now available from the Butantan Institute, Sao Paulo (Schenberg and Pereira-Lima 1978).

Solifugae (Solpugida)

These arachnids should be considered briefly here. Solifugae (false spiders, camel spiders or Galeodes) superficially resemble spiders and are easily mistaken for them. They are commonest in Africa but occur in every continent except Australia and New Zealand (Cloudsley-Thompson 1958). The present writer encountered large specimens in the southern Iraqi desert during World War II. They were taken by the soldiers serving there as spiders, possibly poisonous and feared as such. However, they were not recorded as biting men in that area.

Morphology

They have the general structure of an arachnid, with a prosoma (cephalothorax) and opisthosoma (abdomen) united by a much stouter waist than is the case with true spiders. They have four pairs of legs but the first pair are used as tactile organs. The pedipalps have six segments, the terminal one having a suctorial function. The chelicerae are relatively very large, being sometimes as long as the prosoma. Proportionately they are said to be the most formidable jaws in the animal kingdom (Cloudsley-Thompson 1958). There are no poison fangs or glands. Most species are from 1 to 5 cm overall but larger specimens (e.g. *Galeodes* spp.) may have a span of up to 12.5 cm (5 in.). They are hairy and yellow or brown in colour. Those seen in Iraq were a pale sandy colour, apparently hairless, but close inspection revealed a considerable number of discrete hairs, reddish in colour on the body and limbs.

Biology

Solifugae are nocturnal carnivores, a vivid account of whose hunting prowess has been given by Hutton (1843). They have a voracious appetite for insects of all kinds and sizes and fight viciously with one another over disputed prey, although once beaten they tamely allow themselves to be eaten by the victor. They live in burrows excavated by the chelicerae. Their eggs hatch after 2 weeks and the young are assiduously protected by their ferocious mother during the 3 weeks until the first moult. They are very rapid runners and with the aid of their suctorial pedipalps can walk up glass. They can capture and consume small lizards and even mice but as a rule do not eat warm-blooded animals. The prey is killed by the powerful chelicerae and not by any toxin.

Clinical

On the rare occasions on which they have been recorded as biting man it is the result of their getting into his clothing or bedding. The present writer can vouch for their ability to do this as they have a penchant for entering tents. Cloudsley-Thompson (1977) noted that many of the alleged attacks on man were uncertain or mythical but there are authentic records of such bites (Phisalix 1922). The effect is said to be severe but descriptions of the actual bites are not available. It seems certain that they are entirely the result of trauma, although secondary infection may be superimposed. Toxic and sensitivity reactions do not occur.

References

Anderson PC (1971) Treatment of severe loxoscelism. Mo Med 68: 609–612, 618

Anderson PC (1978) Brown recluse spider bites; an update. J Ky Med Assoc 76: 172–173

Arnold RE (1976) Brown recluse spider bites; five cases with a review of the literature. J Am Coll Emergency Physicians 5: 262–264

Atkins JA, Wingo CW, Sodeman WA (1957) Probable cause of necrotic spider bite in the Mid-West. Science 162: 73

Atkins JA, Wingo CW, Sodeman WA, Flynn JC (1958) Necrotic arachnidism. Am J Trop Med 7: 165–185
Auer AI, Hershey FB (1974) Surgery for necrotic bites of the brown spider. Arch Surg 108: 612–618
Baerg WJ (1925) The effect of the venom of some supposedly poisonous arthropods of the Canal Zone. Ann Entomol Soc Am 18: 471–478
Berger RS (1973a) A critical look at therapy for the brown recluse spider bite. Arch Dermatol 107: 298
Berger RS (1973b) The unremarkable brown recluse spider bite. JAMA 225: 1109–1111
Berger RS, Adelstein EH, Anderson PC (1973) Intravascular coagulation; the cause of necrotic arachnidism. J Invest Dermatol 61: 142–150
Bettini S (1964) Epidemiology of latrodectism. Toxicon 2: 93–102
*Brazil V, Vellard J (1925) Contribuicao ao estudio do veneno das aranhas. Mem Inst Butantan 2: 5–77
Bücherl W (1971) Spiders. In: Bücherl W and Buckley EE (eds) Venomous animals and their venom, vol III Venomous invertebrates. Academic, New York, pp 197–277
Butz WC (1971) Evenomation by the brown recluse spider (Aranae: Scytodidae) and related species. A public health problem in the United States. Clin Toxicol 4: 515–525
Butz WC, Stacy LD, Heryford NN (1971) Arachnidism in rabbits. Necrotic lesions due to the brown recluse spider. Arch Pathol 91: 97–100
Chu JY, Rush CT, O'Connor DM (1978) Haemolytic anaemia following brown spider (*Loxosceles reclusa*) bite. Clin Toxicol 12: 531–534
*Cloudsley-Thompson JL (1958) Spiders, scorpions, centipedes and mites. Pergamon, London
*Cloudsley-Thompson JL (1977) Adaptational biology of Solifugae (Solpugida). Bull Br Arachnol Soc 4: 61–71
Comstock JH (1948) The spider book. Cornell University Press, Ithaca, NY, pp 95–136
Cooke JAL, Miller FH, Grover RW, Duffy JL (1973) Urticaria caused by tarantula hairs. Am J Trop Med Hyg 22: 130–133
Costa RS (1949) Araneismo en nuestro pais. An Inst Hig Montevideo 3: 57–66
Costa RS, Salveraglio F (1949) Accidentes por picardores de Aranas. An Inst Hig Montevideo 3: 51–56
D'Amour FE, Becker FE, van Riper W (1936) The black widow spider. Q Rev Biol 11: 123–160
Delgado A (1966) Investigacion ecologica sobre *Loxosceles rufipes* (Lucas) 1834, en la region costera del Peru. Mem Inst Butantan. Simposio internationale sobre venenos animais. 33, Suppl comemorativo: 683–687
Denny WF, Dillaha CJ, Morgan PN (1964) Hemotoxic effect of *Loxosceles reclusus* venom—*in vivo* and *in vitro* studies. J Lab Clin Med 64: 291–297
Dillaha CJ, Jansen GT, Honeycutt WM, Hayden CR (1963) The gangrenous bite of the brown recluse spider in Arkansas. J Arkansas Med Soc 60: 91–94
Dillaha CJ, Jansen GT, Honeycutt WM (1972) North American loxoscelism. In: Demis DJ, Crounse RG, Dobson RL, McGuire J (eds) Clinical dermatology, vol 4. Harper and Row, Philadelphia, pp 1–8
Efrati P (1969) Bites of *Loxosceles* spiders in Israel. Toxicon 6: 239–241
Elgert K, Wright RP, Camber BJ, Barrett JT (1973) Radiolabelling of the polypeptide components of Missouri brown spider venom. Fed Proc 32: 223
Fardon DW, Wingo CW, Robinson DW, Masters FW (1967) The treatment of brown spider bite. Plast Reconstr Surg 40: 482–488
Finlayson MH (1955) Spider-bite in South Africa. S Afr Med J 29: 509–510
*Gajardo-Tobar R (1966) Mi experiencia sobre loxoscelismo. Mem Inst Butantan. Simposio internationale sobre venenos animais 33, Suppl comemorativo: 689–698
Geren CR, Chan TK, Ward BC, Howell DE, Pinkston K, Odell GV (1973) Composition and properties of extract of fiddleback (*Loxosceles reclusa*) spider venom apparatus. Toxicon 11: 471–479
Geren CR, Chan TK, Howell DE, Odell GV (1976) Isolation and characterisation of toxins from brown recluse spider venom (*Loxosceles reclusa*). Arch Biochem Biophys 174: 90–99
Gertsch WJ (1949) American spiders. D. van Noskrand, New York
Gorham JR (1968a) Envenomation by the spiders *Chiracanthium inclusum* and *Argiope aurantia*. JAMA 206: 1958–1962
Gorham JR (1968b) The brown recluse spider, *Loxosceles reclusa*, and necrotic spider bite. J Environ Health 31: 138–145
Gotten HB, MacGowan JJ (1940) Blackwater fever (haemoglobinuria) caused by spider bite. JAMA 114: 1547
Greer WER (1949) Arachnidism; effect of calcium gluconate in six cases. N Engl J Med 240: 5–8
Grothaus RH, Teller LW (1968) Envenomation by the spider *Lycosa miami* Wallace. J Med Entomol 5: 500
Habermehl GG, Habermehl IA (1979) Araneism in Western Germany; two case reports. Toxicon 17: 183–184
Horen WP (1963) Arachnidism in the United States. JAMA 185: 839–843
Hutton T (1843) Observatins on the habits of a large species of Galeodes. Ann Mag Nat Hist 13: 81–85
Ingram WW, Musgrave A (1933) Spider bite (arachnidism): a survey of its occurrence in Australia and case history. Med J Aust 2: 10–15
James JA, Sellars WA, Austin ON, Terrill BS (1961) Reactions following suspected spider bite a form of loxoscelism? Am J Dis Child 102: 395–398
Jansen GT, Morgan PN, McQueen JW, Bennett WE (1971) The brown recluse spider bite. Controlled evaluation of treatment using the white rabbit as an animal model. South Med J 64: 1194–1202
Keegan HL (1963) Venomous spiders of the Pacific. In: Keegan HL, MacFarlane WV (eds) Venomous and poisonous animals and noxious plants of the Pacific region. Pergamon, Oxford, pp 133–136
Keegan HL, Hedeen RA, Whittemore FW (1960) Seasonal variations in venom of black widow spiders. Am J Trop Med Hyg 9: 477–479
Lessenden CM, Zimmer LK (1960) Brown spider bites. J Kans Med Soc 61: 379–385
*Levi HW (1959) The spider genus *Latrodectus* (Aranae: Theridiidae). Trans Am Microsc Soc 78: 7–43
Levi HW, Spielman A (1964) The biology and control of the South American brown spider *Loxosceles laeta* (Nicolet) in a North American focus. Am J Trop Med Hyg 13: 132–136
Lewis MI, Regan JF (1966) Necrotic arachnidism. Cal Med 105: 457–462
Lim BL, Davie CE (1970) The bite of a bird eating spider *Lampropelma violaceopedes*. Med J Malaysia 24: 311–313
Macchiavello A (1934) Nota preliminaria sobre el aracnoidismo cutaneo gangrenosa de la provincia Antofagasta. Comunicacion al Prima Congreso Medico Sanitario, Santiago de Chile, 1934. Cited by Macchiavello (1937)
Macchiavello A (1937) La *Loxosceles laeta* causa del aracnoidismo cutaneo o mancha gangrenosa de Chile. Rev Chil Hist Nat 41: 11–19
*Macchiavello A (1947a) Cutaneous arachnoidism or gangrenous spot of Chile. Puerto Rico J Public Health Trop Med 22: 425–466

Macchiavello A (1947b) Cutaneous arachnoidism experimentally produced with the glandular poison of *Loxosceles laeta*. Puerto Rico J Public Health Trop Med 23: 266–279
*MacKinnon JE, Witkind J (1953) Aracnoidismo necrotico. An Fac Med Montevideo 38: 75–100
*Main BY (1976) Spiders. Sydney, Collins
Majeski JA, Durst GG Sr (1975) Bite by the spider *Herpyllus ecclesiasticum* in South Carolina. Toxicon 13: 377
Majeski JA, Durst GG Sr (1976) Necrotic arachnidism. South Med J 69: 887–891
*Maretic Z (1971) Latrodectism in Mediterranean countries, including South Russia, Israel and North Africa In: Bücherl W, Buckley EE (eds) Venomous animals and their venom, vol III Venomous invertebrates. Academic, New York, pp 299–309
Maretic Z (1975) The medical importance of the bite of *Chiracanthium punctorium* Villers. In: Proceedings of sixth international arachnological congress, Amsterdam, 22 April 1974, pp 183–186. Cited by Southcott (1978)
Meneghello J, Emparanza E (1952) Loxoscelismo cutaneovisceral y cortisona. Bol Inform Parasit Chil 7: 11–12
Micks DW (1963) The current status of necrotic arachnidism in Texas. In: Keegan HL, MacFarlane WV (eds) Venomous and poisonous animals and noxious plants of the Pacific region. Pergamon, Oxford, pp 153–159
*Minton SA (1974) Venom diseases. Thomas, Springfield, Ill
Minton SA, Olson C (1964) A case of spider bite with severe haemolytic reaction. Paediatrics 33: 283–284
Morgan BB, Morgan PN, Bowling RE (1978) Lysis of human erythrocytes by venom from the brown recluse spider, *Loxosceles reclusa*. Toxicon 16: 85–88
Morgan PN (1969) Preliminary studies on venom from the brown recluse spider *Loxosceles reclusa*. Toxicon 6: 161–165
Musgrave A (1949) Spiders harmful to man. Aust Museum Mag 9: 385–388, 411–419
Nance WE (1961) Hemolytic anemia of necrotic arachnidism. Am J Med 31: 801–807
Newlands SG (1975) Review of the medically important spiders of Southern Africa. S Afr Med J 49: 823–826
Nicholson JF, Nicholson BH (1962) Hemolytic anemia from spider bite; necrotic arachnidism. Okla State Med Assoc J 55: 234–236
Ori M (1975) Studies on the poisonous spider, *Chiracanthium japonicum*, as a pest of medical importance 1. Envenomation by the spider, *Chiracanthium japonicum*. Jpn J Sanit Zool 26: 225–229
*Pesce H, Lumbreras H (1954) Aracnidismo en Lima por "*Loxosceles laeta*". Rev Med Peruana No 301: 3–18
Phisalix M (1922) Animaux venimeux et venins. Masson et Cie, Paris, pp 256–314
Pirosky I, Abalos JW (1963) Spiders of the genus *Latrodectus* in Argentina. Latrodectism and *Latrodectus* antivenin. In: Keegan HL, MacFarlane WV (eds) Venomous and poisonous animals and noxious plants of the Pacific region. Pergamon, Oxford, pp 137–140
Pitts NC (1962) Necrotic arachnidism N Engl J Med 267: 400–401
Pizzi TP, Zacarias JS, Schenone HF (1957) Estudio histopatologico experimental en el envenenamienta por *Loxosceles laeta*. Biologica (Santiago) 23: 33–43
Prats F, Schenone H (1957) Mordedinas de aranas. Nueves consideraciones sobre Loxoscelismo. Bol Chil Parasitol 12: 7–9
Redman JF (1974) Human envenomation by a lycosid. Arch Dermatol 110: 111–112
Reid AH (1971) Spider bites. In: Maegraith BG (ed) Clinical Tropical medicine, 5th edn. Blackwell, Oxford, pp 401–402
Reid AH (1982) Animal poison; spider bites. In: Manson-Bahr PEC, Apted FIC (eds) Manson's tropical diseases, 18th edn. Baillière Tindall, pp 564–565
Russell FE (1962) Muscle relaxants in black widow spider (*Latrodectus mactans*) poisoning. Am J Med Sci 243: 159–161
Russell FE (1970) Bite by the spider *Phidippus formosa*; case history. Toxicon 8: 193–194
Russell FE, Waldron WG (1967) Letter concerning an article on necrotic arachnidism by Lewis MI and Regan JF. Cal Med 106: 248–249
*Russell FE, Waldron WG, Madon MB (1969) Bites by the brown spiders *Loxosceles unicolour* and *Loxosceles arizonica* in California and Arizona. Toxicon 7: 109–117
Schenberg S, Pereira–Lima FA (1978) Venoms of Ctenidae. In: Bettini S (ed) Arthropod venoms. Springer, Berlin Heidelberg New York, pp 217–245 (Handbook of experimental pharmacology, vol 48)
Schenone H (1959) Estudio de 27 casos de Loxoscelismo. Bol Chil Parasitol 14: 7–13
Schenone H, Prats F (1961) Arachnidism by *Loxosceles laeta*. Arch Dermatol 83: 139–142
Schmaus LF (1929) Case of arachnidism (Spider bite). JAMA 92: 1265–1266
Smith CW, Micks DW (1968) A comparative study of the venom and other components of three species of *Loxosceles*. Am J Trop Med Hyg 17: 651–656
Smith CW, Micks DW (1970) The role of polymorphonuclear leucocytes in the lesion caused by the venom of the brown recluse spider *Loxosceles reclusa*. Lab Invest 22: 90–93
Southcott RV (1978) Australian harmful arachnids and their allies. Southcott, Mitcham, South Australia
Spielman A, Levi HW (1970) Probable envenomation by *Chiracanthium mildei*, a spider found in houses. Am J Trop Med Hyg 19: 729–732
*Sutherland SK (1972) The Sydney funnel-web spider (*Atrax robustus*) 3. A review of some clinical records of human envenomation. Med J Aust 2: 643–647
*Sutherland SK (1978) Biology and venoms of Dipluridae. In: Bettini S (ed) Arthropod venoms. Springer, Berlin Heidelberg New York, pp 126–148 (Handbook of experimental pharmacology, vol 48)
Taylor EH, Denny WF (1966) Hemolysis, renal failure and death, presumed secondary to bite of brown recluse spider. South Med J 59: 1209–1211
*Vellard J (1954) L'araneisme au Perou et dans les region meridionale de l'Amerique du Sud. Preparation d'un serum specifique contre le venin de *Loxosceles laeta*. Trav Inst Fr Études Andines 4: 133–185
Vorse H, Seccareccio P, Woodroff K, Humphrey BG (1972) Disseminated intravascular coagulopathy following fatal brown spider bite (necrotic arachnidism) J Pediatr 80: 1035–1037
Waldron WG (1968) Bite by the spider *Thiodina sylvana* in Southern California. Toxicon 6: 71
Waldron WG, Russell FE (1967) *Loxosceles reclusa* in Southern California. Toxicon 5: 57
Waldron WG, Hadon MB, Suddarth T (1975) Observation on the occurrence and ecology of *Loxosceles laeta* (Araneae: Scytodidae) in Los Angeles County, California. Cal Vector Views 22: 29–36
Weiner RG, Stoffer RP, Chornock FW, Young RB (1960) Massive intravascular haemolysis. J Kans Med Soc 61: 206–207
*Wiener S (1961) Red back spider bite in Australia; an analysis of 167 cases. Med J Aust 2: 44–49
Wolcott GN (1948) The insects of Puerto Rico. J Agric Univ Puerto Rico 32: 1–973

15 Scabies

In discussing the history of scabies Pye-Smith (1893) wrote,

> Scabies is really one of the most important diseases from a scientific point of view; for it illustrates the whole progress of scientific medicine—the ancient method, which still survives, of inventing explanations instead of investigating circumstances, the fallacy of ascribing results to dyscrasias, of which the existence has never been proved, the survival of doctrines of pathology which have long since been exploded in physiology, the value of apparently useless knowledge, the bearing of pure science like zoology upon practical therapeutics, the nature of inflammation and the relation between an irritant and an irritable tissue, the radiation of sensations, the pathology of pruritus and the importance of a patient's nails in the production of cutaneous lesions. Finally scabies is the typical example of a disease which is now as fully known as we can, perhaps, know any disease, for we know its pathology and cause, we can explain its symptoms, we can diagnose it with certainty and, although the hypothetical "*vis medicatrix naturae*" is utterly powerless, we can cure it by definite and rational means, quickly, safely and completely.

The persistence of scabies as a major public health problem belies Pye-Smith's optimism. The difficulty in eradicating it from some communities remains as great as ever. Bearing in mind that probably the most important single factor in controlling scabies is an intelligent understanding of its behaviour in varying circumstances and of the limitations of individual treatment, a brief historical survey is both illuminating and valuable. Full historical accounts can be found in the writings of Hebra (1868), Beeson (1927), Heilesen (1946) and Friedman (1948). Table 15.1 gives a chronological sequence of steps in the knowledge of an understanding of scabies and speaks for itself.

Table 15.1. Tabulated history of scabies, outlining the stages in the understanding of the disease and development of its management

Dates	Authority	Remarks	Reference
c.1000 B.C.	Indian MSS	Clinical features known.	Nair B.K.H. (1973)
c.1000 B.C.	*Bible*	Contagious nature; public health measures	*Bible*; Hebra (1868)
4th cent. B.C.	Aristotle	"Lice-in-the-flesh"; removal of mites	Hebra 1868; Heilesen (1946)
7th cent. A.D.	Chinese lit.	Interdigital lesions	Hoeppli (1959)
10th cent. A.D.	At Tabari	Effects of warmth; extraction of mites	Heilesen (1946)
12th cent. A.D.	Abenzoar	Mites living in skin	Beeson (1927)
12th cent. A.D.	Hildegarde	Associated mites with scabies	Hebra (1868)
15th cent. A.D.	Guy de Chauliac	Contagious nature; distribution of lesions	Rayer (1835); Beeson (1927)
16th cent. A.D.	Rabelais	Interdigital lesions	Heilesen (1946); Beeson (1927)
16th cent. A.D.	Scaliger	Burrows described	Heilesen (1946); Beeson (1927)
16th cent. A.D.	Benedictus	Head never affected	Heilesen (1946); Beeson (1927)
16th cent. A.D.	De Vigo	Benefit of opening burrows in treatment	Heilesen (1946); Beeson (1927)
16th cent. A.D.	Ambrose Pafe	Mites live and feed in burrows and cause itch	Heilesen (1946); Beeson (1927)
16th cent. A.D.	Shakespeare	Burrows on fingers	Shakespeare
1623	Anonymous	Mites in burrows the cause of scabies	Vocabulario dell' Academia della crusta, cited by Hebra (1868); Heilesen (1946)

Table 15.1. (*continued*)

Dates	Authority	Remarks	Reference
1634	Thomas Mouffet	Nature of the mite; how and where to find it	Hebra (1868)
1689	Bonomo and Cestoni	First description of the morphology of the mite	Mead (1775); Lane (1928)
1726	Daniel Turner	Spread by contact in bed; topical therapy alone effective	Turner (1726)
1758	Linnaeus	Regarded the scabies mite and the flour mite as identical	Heilesen (1946)
1775	Richard Mead	Publicised the work of Bonomo and Cestoni	Mead (1775)
1778	C. DeGeer	First accurate description of *Sarcoptes scabiei*	DeGeer (1778); Heilesen (1946)
1786	J. E. Wichman	Detailed description of scabies and the mite	Beeson (1927)
1807	Joseph Adams	Experimental self-infestation; incubation period noted	Adams (1807)
1813–1829	Thomas Bateman	*Sarcoptes* a contaminant	Bateman (1813, 1819, 1829)
1834	Renucci	Public demonstration of *Sarcoptes scabiei*	Cumston (1924)
1835	Rayer	*Sarcoptes* still a contaminant	Rayer (1835)
1851	Boeck and Danielssen	First description of Norwegian scabies	Hebra (1868)
1868	F. von Hebra	Full and accurate account of clinical, therapeutic and zoological aspects of scabies	Hebra (1868)
1905	N. Hyde	Effects of mass migration on scabies	Hyde (1905)
1919	J. H. Munro	Biological study of *Sarcoptes*	Munro (1919)
1941–1945	K. Mellanby	Detailed study of parasitology, clinical behaviour and spread of scabies; prophylaxis tried	Mellanby (various)
1944	R. M. Gordon et al.	Prophylaxis with impregnated soap	Gordon et al. (1944)
1946	B. Heilesen	Exhaustive study of biology of *Sarcoptes*	Heilesen (1946)
1949	Prakken and van Vloten	Allergy studies	Prakken and van Vloten (1949)
1968	A. Fain	Detailed morphological study	Fain (1968)
1974	Barthelmes and Barthelmes	Allergy studies	Barthelmes and Barthelmes (1974)
1974	Hancock and Milford-Ward	Immunoglobulins in scabies	Hancock and Milford-Ward (1974)
1980	Falk et al.	Immunological aspects of scabies	Falk (1980); Falk et al (1980a, b)

General Clinical Appearances

Patients with scabies seek advice because they itch or have a widespread eruption in which itch is the dominant feature. The lesions associated with scabies may thus vary from almost none to very profuse. Since the diagnosis may be difficult it is essential to examine the patient thoroughly in a good light, preferably with the aid of a magnifying lens.

The itch, which may vary from mild to intolerably severe, is characteristically nocturnal and is scarcely noticeable in the daytime. It usually starts after the victim retires to bed and becomes warm. In some it may commence during undressing for bed (Epstein and Orkin 1977). Dubreuilh and Beille (1895) pointed out that persons on night duty developed itching about 4 a.m. which persisted for about 2 h but *did not recur* when they retired to bed in daytime. Mellanby (1943) maintained that the itch, which is generalised, was the result of sensitisation to the *Sarcoptes* and not to its burrowing. Dixon (1941), on the other hand, said that the itch only occurred when the mite was actively burrowing. The nocturnal character of the itch would seem to support this view, although the itch does not actually begin until after a latent period following initial infestation, which, Mellanby claimed, was necessary to the development of sensitisation. Perhaps this allergic phenomenon is only activated by burrowing and concomitant secretion of digestive juices by the mite. Some scabietics itch constantly and there are many variations.

There are two distinct types of itch in scabies. In addition to the generalised itch there is a localised reaction directly caused by the activity of the mite. This was noted by Hebra (1868), by Mellanby (1943) and by Heilesen (1946). It has a burning character, and those who have experienced it can easily distinguish it from the generalised itch (Mellanby 1943). On very rare occasions there is no itch (Mellanby 1943), but there are also patients who are scarcely bothered by the itch, even when it is present (Russell 1964), and others who declare that they do not itch, although the evidence of scratching belies their assertion. Gougerot (quoted by Beek and Mellanby 1953) said that sometimes the only symptom of scabies was the bedfellow's itch; however, this probably represents the asymptomatic stage prior to the development of sensitisation.

After scabies has been successfully treated the itch may persist for as long as a few weeks but eventually disappears without further treatment. Borda (1954) has noted that it may recur during menstruation. If a treated scabietic becomes reinfested, the itch returns promptly. The fact that there is no latent period is held by Mellanby to be supportive evidence that the itch is allergic in nature.

There are two principal components of the eruption of uncomplicated scabies. The burrows and the associated papules and vesicles are directly related to the presence of the *Sarcoptes*, whilst the generalised rash is related to the development of sensitisation.

The burrow or tunnel made by the adult female *Sarcoptes* lies in the horny layer of the epidermis and presents clinically as a greyish line resembling a pencil mark, about 5 mm long on average (Fig. 15.1) Hebra (1868) recorded one of 10 cm in length. These burrows may be more or less straight or serpentine. In clean persons of European origin they have a whitish colour with occasional dark specks (due to faecal scybala), but in those whose occupation renders their skin, especially of the hands, very dirty and who cannot or do not clean themselves adequately, the burrows appear darker because of extraneous particles becoming embedded in the burrow roof. When these burrows are thoroughly cleaned they appear even darker since the ingrained material cannot be removed (Hebra 1863). In contrast, burrows on the penis, buttocks, elbows and knees are much paler in all patients. In dark-skinned people such as Indians, burrows appear as distinctly white lines and are more easily seen. In a case of Norwegian scabies (see Fig. 15.28) there were multiple burrows on the anterior abdominal walls, each surmounted by a tiny linear blood-stained crust.

The point of entry of the mite into the burrow is marked by a tiny white scale. The blind end, where the mite lies, is scarcely visible to the naked eye but through a lens can be seen as a minute elevation with a tiny halo of erythema. Sometimes a vesicle is formed beneath the burrow. It is often oval and the burrow can be clearly seen on the roof. The blind end of the burrow is always beyond the edge of the vesicle (see p. 259). Occasionally, especially if the patients neglect to seek treatment, these vesicles may become purulent. In other instances the burrow may be seen lying on the surface of an elongated red papule. This occurs most frequently on

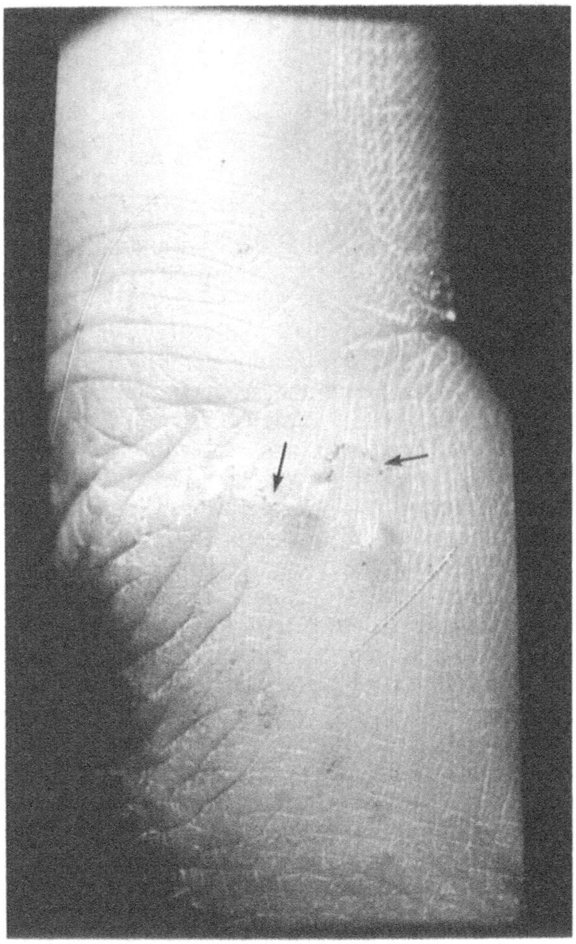

Fig. 15.1. Scabies burrows on the side of a finger. The darker areas represent the papule at the blind end of the burrows. (From Alexander 1969, by kind permission of the Editor of *Clinical Pediatrics*)

the penis and buttocks but may sometimes also be found on the axillary folds, the nipples, umbilicus and trunk. In babies and very young children such papules are often seen on the trunk and axillary folds (Alexander 1969).

Burrows are generally found in those areas where there are few or no hair follicles and usually where the stratum corneum is thin and soft. Johnson and Mellanby (1942) listed these in order of frequency, as shown in Table 15.2. In general terms this distribution conforms to what is seen in clinical practice but can vary considerably according to circumstances. For instance, Parlette (1976) found that in naval personnel the finger webs were the commonest site, followed by the genitalia, thighs, buttocks, sacral region, volar aspect of the wrists, the waistline, umbilicus, axillae, elbows, ankles and inframammary region, in that order.

Table 15.2. Distribution of burrows in scabies in men, according to Johnson and Mellanby (1942)

Hands and wrists	63%
Elbows	11%
Feet	9%
Genitalia	9%
Buttocks	4%
Axillae	2%
Elsewhere	2%

Sefton (1947) found that burrows in scabietics in a Japanese prisoner-of-war camp were usually limited to the penis. (Knowles 1918 had found a similar situation amongst soldiers in World War I.) He attributed this to acute awareness of the possibility of scabies amongst the inmates and the consequent desire for immediate treatment before there was time for lesions to appear elsewhere. In the absence of such treatment burrows appeared on the buttocks and ischial tuberosities and then the elbows, umbilicus, scrotal area and axillary folds. Lesions on the hands, wrists, feet and ankles were rare in these patients. Greenhough (1886) only found burrows on the hands, wrists and penis. In hospital practice in Glasgow, burrows are commonly found on the sides and, to a lesser extent, the dorsal surface of the fingers; on the interdigital webs (Fig. 15.2) (although usually concealed by eczematous scaling in this area); on the volar aspect of the wrist, the ulnar border and palm of the hand; and on the sole, instep and below the malleoli (Alexander 1968; Fig. 15.3). Penile lesions are less common than is the case in military establishments. Except in infants, burrows on the axillary folds, elbows and trunk are relatively uncommon.

Burrows occasionally occur in bizarre situations, for example behind the ears, under the nail or on the back (Beek and Mellanby 1953), in the cubital fossae (Dixon 1941) or on the little toe and on the back (personal observation).

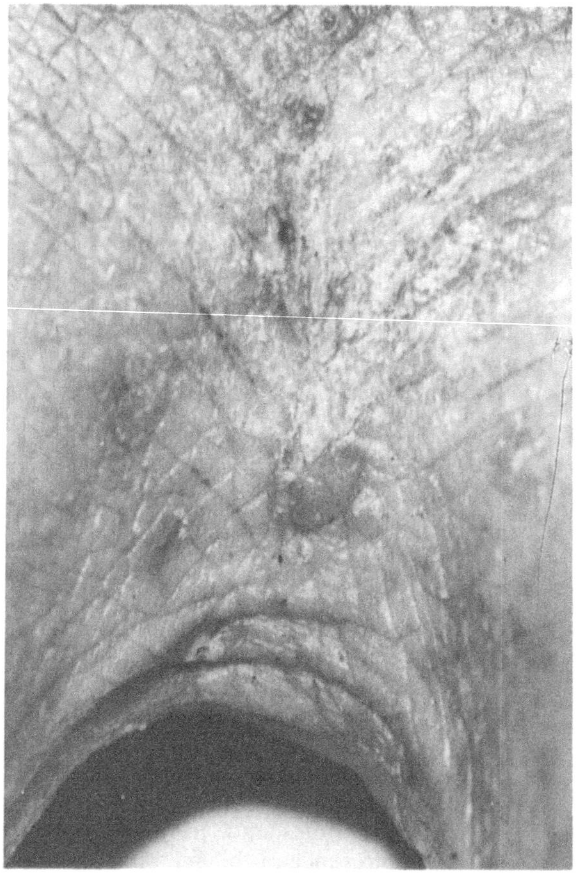

Fig. 15.2. Burrows and eczematised scaling and scratch marks on an interdigital web in scabies.

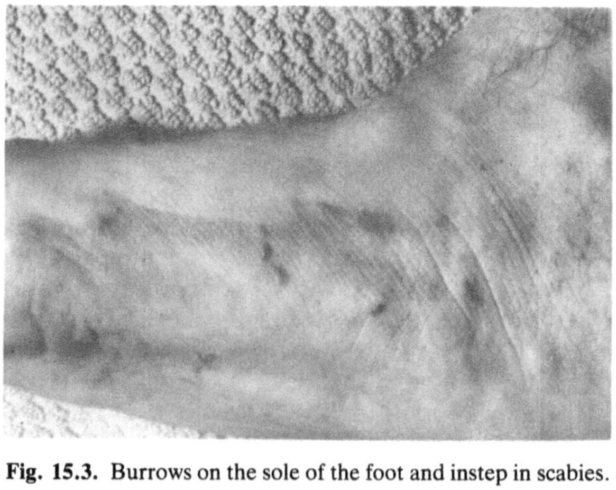

Fig. 15.3. Burrows on the sole of the foot and instep in scabies.

Burrows are often said to be absent. Sehgal et al. (1972) found burrows in only 7% of a large series of over 1000 cases, whilst Hurwitz (1977) said that the incidence varied between 7% and 13%, being less in infants. Greenhough (1886) said they were comparatively rare, even in well-developed scabies. It is true that there may be very few burrows present in an individual patient. Mellanby (1943) said that the average number of adult female mites (and therefore the number of burrows) per patient was approximately 11 and often fewer. Although it may be very difficult to find burrows, especially if there is marked secondary infection, a thorough search of the whole body in a good light, with a lens if necessary, is usually successful in finding at least one (Alexander 1968). This examination takes only a few minutes, but doubtless in an overcrowded clinic or in a refugee camp it may not be possible. Failure to make such an examination could well account for the low incidence reported in some series. The author has seen many patients in whom only single burrows could be found. The number of patients suspected of having scabies in the absence of burrows in a clinic where there was a high index of suspicion amongst the dermatologists was low, probably not much more than 10%. It is misleading to suggest that burrows are seldom found in scabies; their absence usually indicates an inadequate examination or inexperience on the part of the examiner. Moreover, such a suggestion encourages the diagnosis of scabies on inadequate grounds, which in turn tends to lead to the indiscriminate use of antiscabietics on every patient who itches.

Very often, especially on the sides of the fingers and wrists, tiny pinpoint papules (Fig. 15.4) or clear vesicles may be seen close to the burrows. They may be single or composed of small groups of discrete lesions. They have been somewhat inaccurately described by Shelley and Wood (1976) as "larval papules". They represent the reaction to the presence of larvae and other immature stages of the *Sarcoptes* in moulting pockets (see p. 258), which are invisible to all but the most acutely and usually short-sighted individuals (Heilesen 1946) and which, as a rule, can only be found with the aid of a strong lens and are about 0.5 mm long.

After a suitable incubation period a hypersensitivity eruption appears. This period varies from 4 to 6 weeks; however, according to Mellanby (1943), if the initial infestation is very heavy, it may be shorter. The eruption is usually quite profuse, composed of pinpoint papular erythematous lesions mainly on the anterior trunk, thighs, buttocks and sometimes on the forearms (Figs. 15.5, 15.6) and accompanied by severe pruritus. The involved area is frequently heavily scratched, adding excoriations to the clinical picture.

Certain areas are free of lesions in scabietics. In infants lesions may occur on any part of the body (Alexander 1969), but in all other persons scabietic

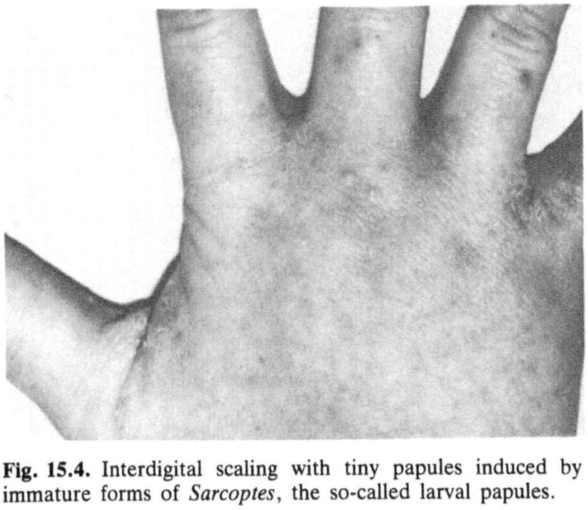

Fig. 15.4. Interdigital scaling with tiny papules induced by immature forms of *Sarcoptes*, the so-called larval papules.

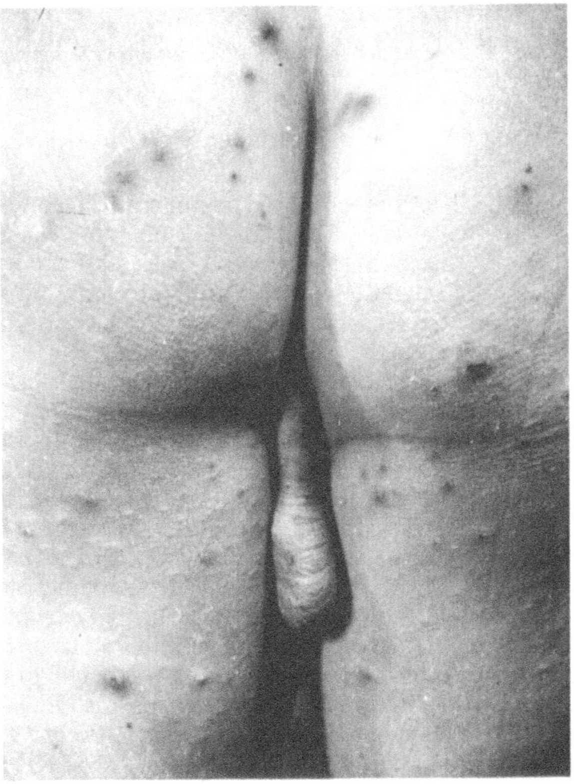

Fig. 15.5. Scabietic papules and pustules, some scratches, on the buttocks, thighs and scrotum in scabies. (From Alexander 1968, by kind permission of the Editor of *The Practitioner*)

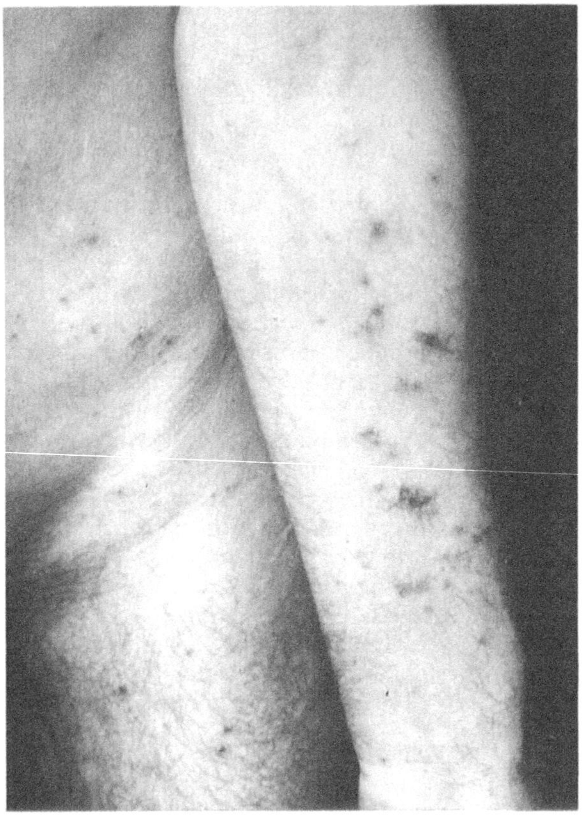

Fig. 15.6. Scratched papules of the sensitivity eruption of scabies.

lesions are not seen on the face or scalp (Dubreuilh and Beille 1885; Degos 1953) and rarely on the neck or back. Madsen (1970) suggested that on the scalp of young infants this ovigerous mite did not dig into the epidermis but rather into the crusts and "scale-crusts".

A fully developed case of uncomplicated scabies will thus present with a hypersensitivity eruption as above, together with a variable number of discrete, itching areas on the fingers, wrists, genitalia and perhaps the feet. However, the whole picture is considerably modified by age and sex because the distribution of burrows is influenced by these factors (Figs. 15.7, 15.8). Apart from being more profuse in the very young, the sensitivity eruption varies little. The distribution of the lesions associated with burrows in adult males and in children is shown in the accompanying diagrams, Fig. 15.9 and 15.10. Some authors (e.g. Hernandez-Perez 1971) go so far as to doubt the diagnosis of scabies in adult males if the penis is not involved. Bearing in mind the habits of the *Sarcoptes*, this is too extreme a view.

Because the itch in scabies is so marked, scratching is universal and unavoidable, except in the paralysed (see p. 249) and, as a rule, in Norwegian scabies. Complications such as secondary infection or eczematisation are therefore common. Secondary infection or pyoderma may take the form

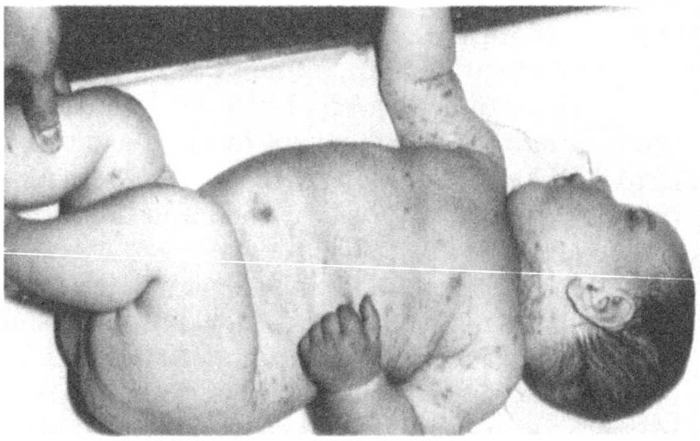

Fig. 15.7. Typical eruption of scabies in an infant. Note clustering of lesions around axillae and neck, which nevertheless retain their discrete nature.

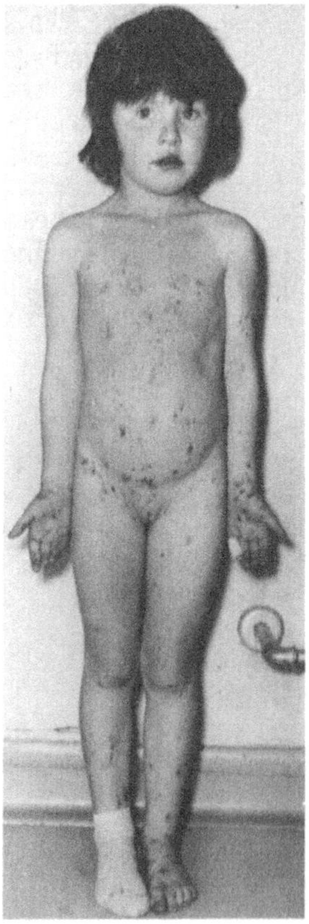

Fig. 15.8. Distribution of eruption of scabies in a child. Note pronounced lesions on hands and feet.

of staphylococcal or streptococcal impetigo (Figs. 15.11, 15.12), of the more deep-seated streptococcal ecthyma, of invasion of scabietic vesicles by organisms transforming them into pustules and of furuncles in the hairy areas (Figs. 15.13, 15.14). When secondary infection is severe or caused by organisms with additional specific properties, there may be complications of the infection. For example, staphylococcal infection may cause cellulitis or abscesses (even mammary abscesses; Borda 1954) associated with lymphangitis and lymphadenopathy, which may even suppurate, whilst streptococcal infections may give rise to acute glomerulonephritis.

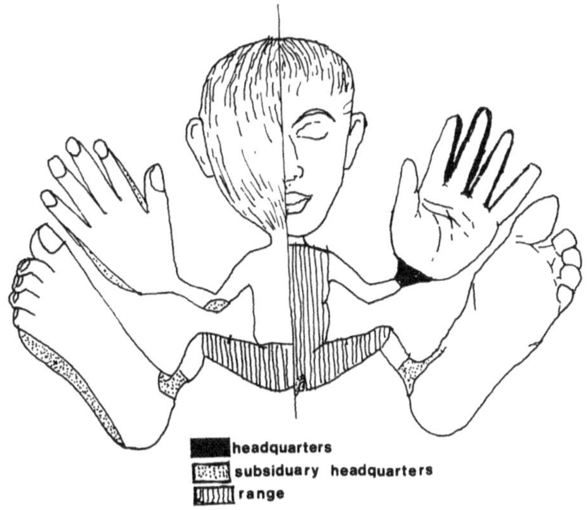

Fig. 15.9. The "headquarters" and "range" of *Sarcoptes scabiei* in adult male subjects. Constructed from figures in Johnson and Mellanby (1942). (From Marples 1965, by kind permission of the author and the publisher, C. C. Thomas)

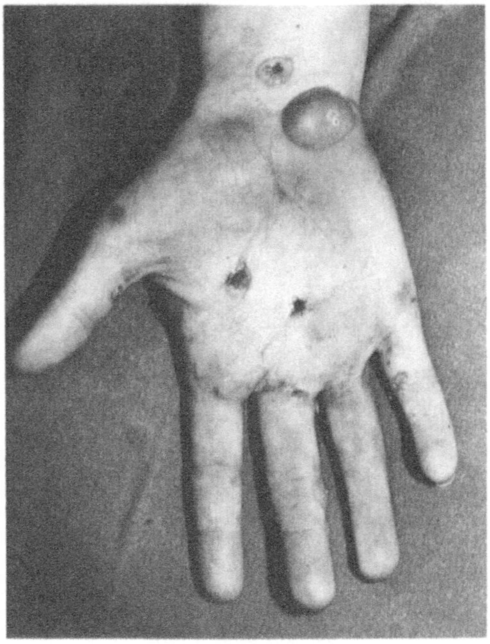

Fig. 15.11. Bullous lesions in scabies. This child was at first sight thought to have impetigo, but burrows were found at the periphery of the bullae, whether the latter were intact or not. The whole family were infested but unsuspected.

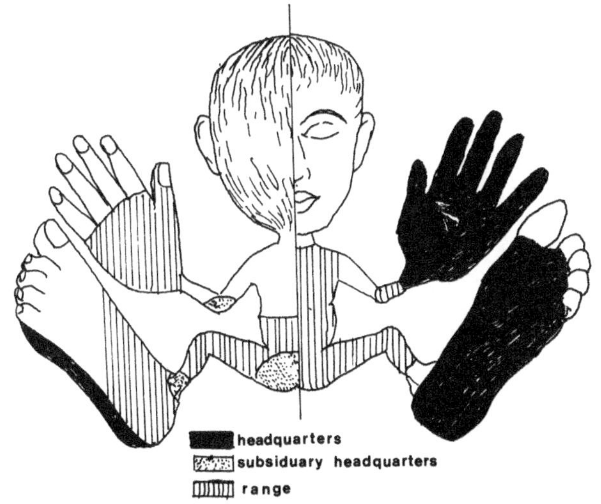

Fig. 15.10. The "headquarters" and "range" of *Sarcoptes scabiei* in adult male subjects. Constructed from figures in Bartley and Mellanby (1942) and in Marples (1950). (From Marples 1965, by kind permission of the author and the publisher, C. C. Thomas)

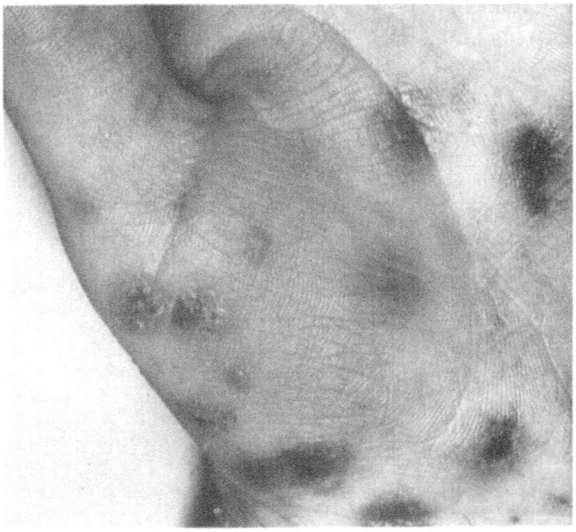

Fig. 15.12. Close view of hand of same patient as in Fig. 15.8 showing healing, impetiginised lesions on the palm and wrist together with new burrows and vesicles on the thenar eminence.

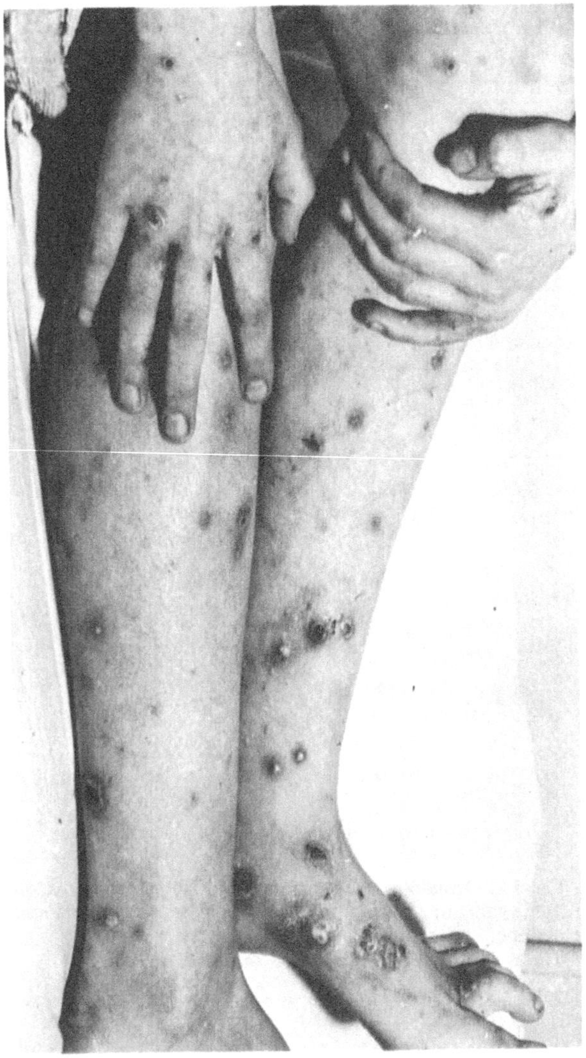

Fig. 15.13. Pustular and impetiginised lesions of pyoderma associated with scabies. Note the interdigital lesions on the hand and involvement of the instep of the foot. (From Alexander 1968, by kind permission of the Editor of *The Practitioner*)

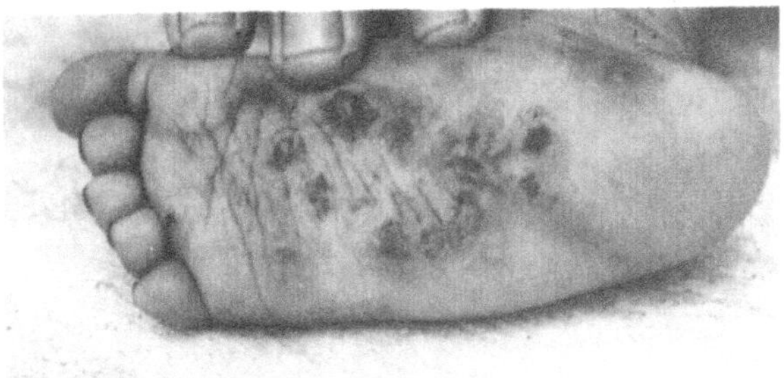

Fig. 15.14. Pustules and crusts of secondarily infected scabies in a Polynesian child. (Courtesy of Prof. Mary J. Marples)

Secondary eczema may be of the dry scaly type or exudative or lichenified. One special area where eczema is not infrequently seen is the areolar region of the breast in women. Scabies should always be kept in mind when such lesions are present (Fig. 15.15). Eczematous complications of scabies usually have the characteristic distribution of scabies. That is to say they occur mainly in those areas where the burrows or papules are most commonly found, such as the hands (Fig. 15.16) or feet (Fig. 15.17) and also over the area of hypersensitivity eruptions. Sometimes the lesions may

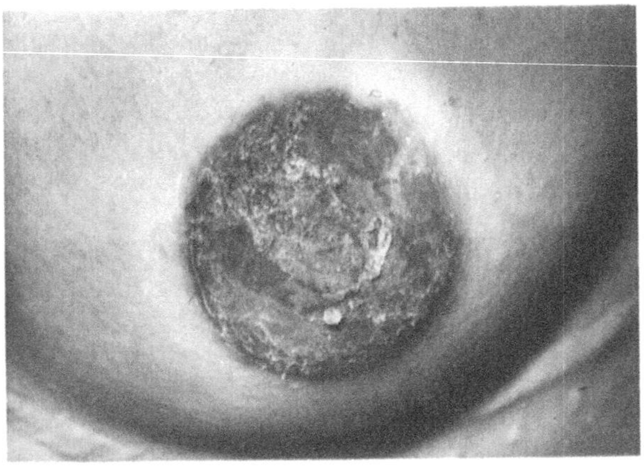

Fig. 15.15. Confluent eczema of the nipple and areolar areas in a woman with scabies.

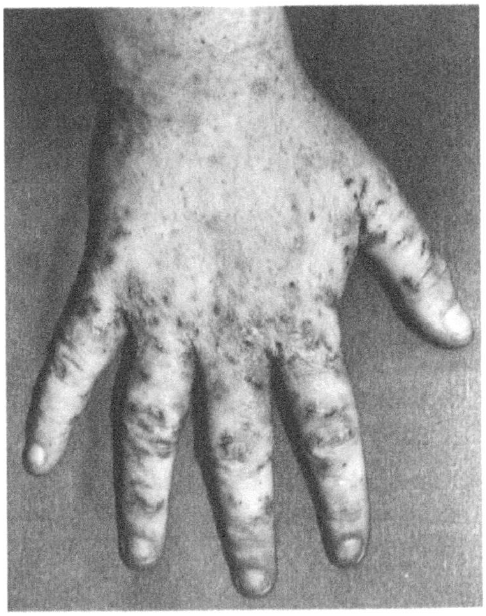

Fig. 15.16. Heavily excoriated and eczematised scabies of the hand. Note the pronounced involvement of the interdigital webs.

become very widespread (Fig. 15.18). Urticaria may also complicate scabies. The lesions will, as a rule, settle quickly after treatment of the underlying scabies, but at other times it may be many months before they recover.

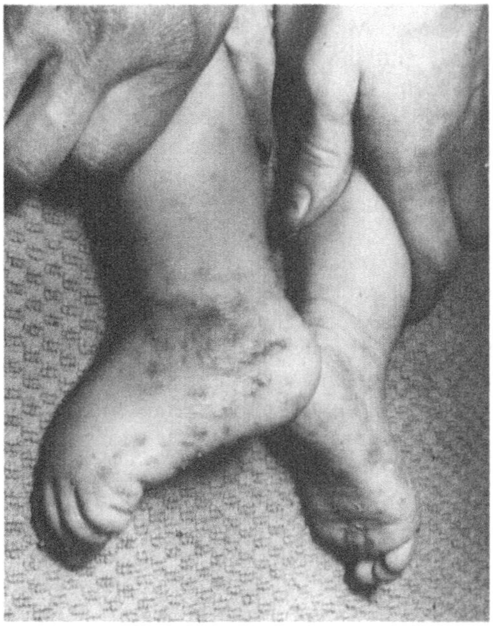

Fig. 15.17. Eczematisation of scabies in an infant. Unless burrows are deliberately sought (and they are not easy to see in such cases), the diagnosis will be overlooked. (From Alexander 1969, by kind permission of the Editor of *Clinical Pediatrics*)

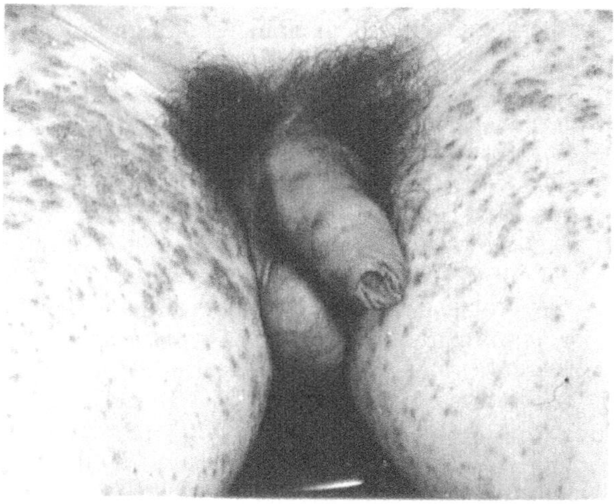

Fig. 15.18. Widespread eczematisation in scabies. This could easily be mistaken for a contact eczema hypersensitisation reaction unless burrows are noticed on the penis and elsewhere. (From Alexander 1968, by kind permission of the Editor of *The Practitioner*)

Intolerance of alcohol, with congestion of the skin, facial itch and an "asphyxial" sensation, has been noted to follow an attack of scabies (Borda 1954).

Complications which do not have the widespread distribution of scabies are pediculosis and toxic erythema. Pediculosis is associated with scabies in overcrowded living conditions of long standing, such as in bad city slums, refugee camps and amongst besieged or besieging armies. In sporadic instances these two diseases only occur together in persons of vagrant type. In fact, Greenhough (1886) said he had never encountered them in the same patient. Toxic erythema (what is called the dermal type of erythema multiforme by some dermatologists) may very occasionally occur as a complication of scabies (Fig. 15.19) It is acute and widespread and disappears quickly after treatment of the scabies. A feature of the complications mentioned is that they may present in their own right without a suspicion of scabies, the important point being that they did not respond in the expected manner to what is apparently correct treatment. Borda (1954) noted the curious tendency in some patients for lesions of other diseases such as papular urticaria or "psychological dermatitis" to recur in sites where scabies lesions had been present.

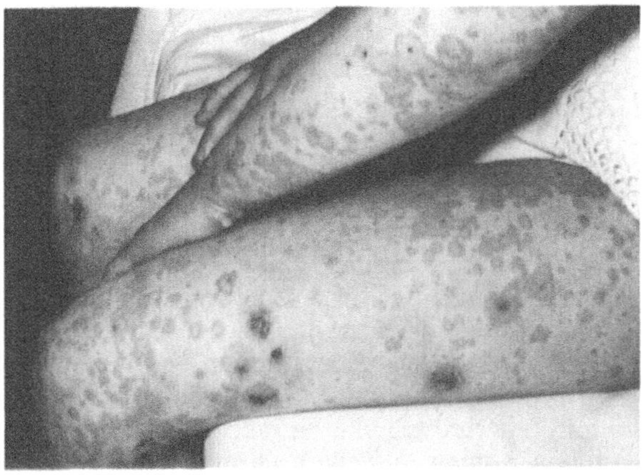

Fig. 15.19. Scabies complicated by toxic erythema.

In infants with scabies such complications are quite frequent, and when scabies has been contracted in the early weeks of life the result of perpetual itching prevents sleep. This results in weight loss and the appearance of marasmus. The present writer has seen 6-month-old twins weighing only 2.7 kg each entirely as the result of scabies.

After treatment for scabies the weight was regained in a few weeks without any additional measures being taken. It is of interest to note that Steigman (1967) attributed the severity of the eczematous eruption occurring in babies to passively acquired maternal antibodies from a scabietic mother.

Clinical Variants of Scabies

Scabies may sometimes mimic other skin diseases in its clinical manifestations. Dermatitis herpetiformis is frequently diagnosed as scabies in its early stages because of the widespread nature of the eruption and its persistent itch, especially if the distribution of the lesions is atypical. The reverse happening in less common, but Ackerman et al. (1975) have described such an instance.

Anolik and Rudolph (1976) described a patient with a scaly papular eruption resembling Darier's disease. Large numbers of *Sarcoptes* were found and it was then realised that this was the early stage of Norwegian scabies in a patient immunosuppressed because of a renal transplant. Aterman et al. (1976) reported a 13-month-old infant with a 2-month history of a diffuse erythematous papular eruption, the histology of which revealed epidermal thickening and a dense infiltrate mainly of histiocytes, which seriously raised the question of Letterer–Siwe disease. However, the child was in good general health; the discovery of many burrows on the palms revealed the true diagnosis. Hazelrigg and Jarrett (1975) reported a patient with exactly similar features.

A pre-existing disease may cause confusion if scabies develops. Pillsbury and Scully (1948) recorded a patient with discoid lupus erythematosus (DLE) on the forehead, nose, ears and neck of 18 months' duration. Lesions appearing on the right axillary fold were taken for the same condition until a diffuse scabietic eruption became apparent 10 days later. A. Lyell (1979, personal communication) reported a similar instance in Glasgow when a young woman, also with chronic DLE presented with curious papular telangiectatic lesions on the back. These were thought to be lesions of vasculitis until a biopsy revealed a *Sarcoptes* on the summit of a papule. Further search showed burrows on the feet. Saruta and Nakamizo (1978) reported involvement of a big toenail in scabies in a diabetic patient with gross thickening of the plate and large numbers of mites in various stages in the debris. This patient had evidence of other autoimmune phenomena and could well have been developing Norwegian scabies.

Treatment of scabies with topical corticosteroids may greatly alter the clinical appearance in a manner akin to the production of "tinea incognito" by these preparations applied to fungal infections (Ive and Marks 1968). Such preparations are used to relieve undiagnosed itch. The suppression of the latter and the scratching allows an increase in parasite numbers and in burrows, especially on the hands and feet. McMillan (1972) described a baby so treated, and the present writer has also seen more than one such case. Bean (1974) described a 22-month-old child in whom there were widespread excoriated papules and nodules on the trunk and the remains of numerous bullae on the hands, feet and thighs. A diagnosis of pemphigus or pemphigoid had been considered and topical and systemic corticosteroids prescribed. The correct diagnosis and treatment were only realised when several other members of the family were found to have scabies. An exactly similar situation occurred with a 10-year-old patient of the present writer. A similar state of affairs may frequently occur in hemiplegic patients, often without progressing to Norwegian scabies. The paralysed side may not itch and the normal side is not scratched. The result is the same—there is an increase in the number of burrows and parasites.

Patients with Brazilian pemphigus are peculiarly susceptible to scabies. Martins-Castro et al. (1974) reported an epidemic amongst a hospital population of such patients in whom 75% developed scabies. In such a generalised scaling eruption scabies could appear unnoticed until corticosteroid therapy had brought the pemphigus under control. The effect of this treatment on the scabies would be very unfavourable and the effect of antiscabietic treatment on the pemphigus would be equally poor.

Burrows et al. (1975) described a fine papular eruption on the trunk and limbs of a 13-year-old child with lymphatic leukaemia. This faded after each of two doses of methotrexate. The authors postulated that the reactivity of skin remote from the scabies lesions may have been altered and the patient developed unusual lesions but not Norwegian scabies. They felt that methotrexate could not have influenced the *Sarcoptes* because they had no evidence that it could do this. However, it is interesting in this connection to note that after Van Aerssen (1968) had treated demodicidosis in two rosaceous patients with oral methotrexate for about 6 weeks no mites could be found, whereas they had been abundant previously in follicular scrapings.

Nodular Scabies

Nodular lesions develop in about 7% of scabietic patients (Konstantinov and Stanoeva 1973; Orkin and Maibach 1978a). Han et al. (1983) found nodules in 11.2% of their 1061 patients. Although noted by Hebra (1868) they were first described in detail by Ayres and Anderson (1932). The lesions appear during active scabies and consist of itchy, round, smooth nodules about 5–8 mm in diameter (Fig. 15.20). H. L. Arnold Jr. (1981, personal communication) described a young man whose scabies (second attack in 5 years) showed diffuse, florid, nodular lesions up to 20 mm in diameter almost from the onset. Nodular lesions involve the whole skin thickness but move freely over the underlying tissues. They are firm, red or reddish-brown and characteristically persist after the rest of the eruption has cleared with treatment. A burrow may sometimes be seen on the surface of early lesions (Samman 1963; Grant and Keczkes 1964) but never in those of long standing (Konstantinov and Stanoeva 1973). They are commonest under the age of 15 years and especially below 5 years. They occur mainly on those areas where the skin is thinnest, such as the genitalia (Fig. 15.21) or axillary folds, but never on the hands or feet. It should be noted that non-persistent nodules are not uncommon on infants with scabies (Barale et al. 1971; Ramos y Silva 1977). Similarly, non-persistent haemorrhagic oedematous papules, which resembled chancres when they ulcerated, were described by Haber (1963) on the penis.

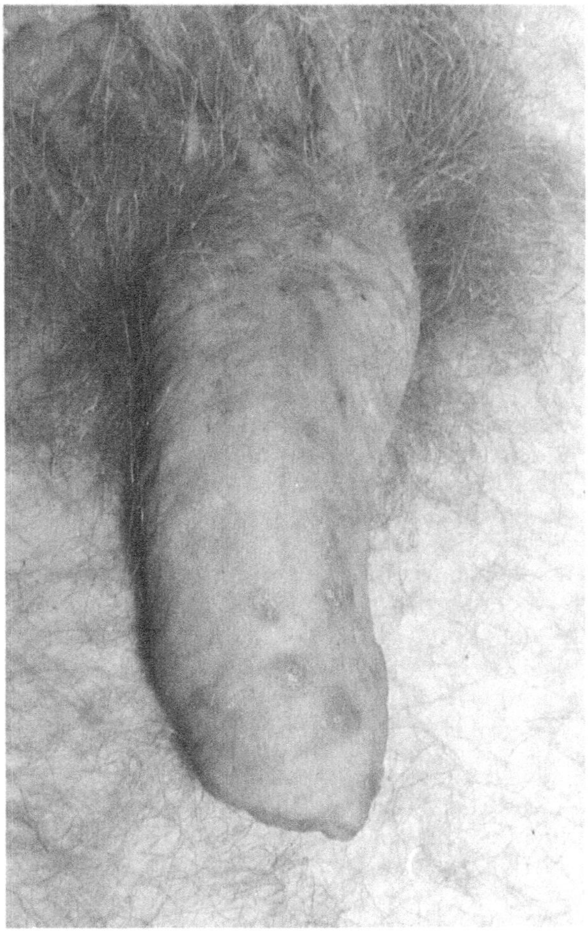

Fig. 15.21. Nodular penile lesions, which are not uncommon in scabies.

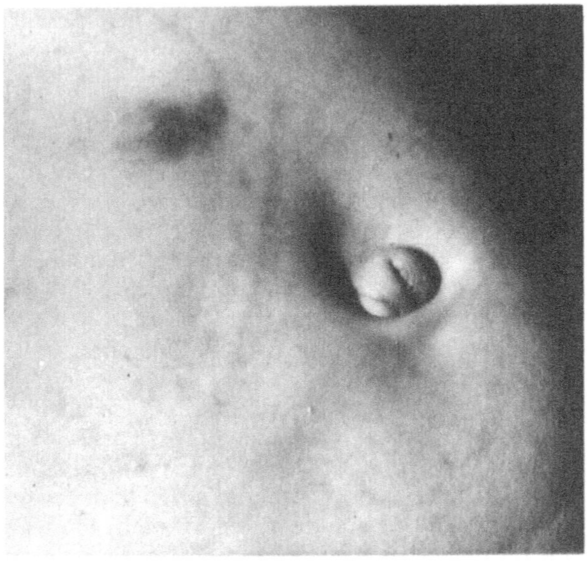

Fig. 15.20. Persistent nodular lesion of scabies on the anterior abdominal wall.

According to Konstantinov and Stanoeva (1973), the itch was inconstant, paroxysmal and nocturnal. Eighty per cent of cases resolve in 3 months, but the remainder may persist for up to 1 year. A persistent pigmented macule may remain after the nodule has disappeared, and both macule and nodule may urticate if rubbed.

The histology is described in the section on pathology (see p. 252). Histological diagnosis is not easy in the absence of evidence of scabietic infestation. Clinical diagnosis depends on the history and on the evidence of scabies.

Nodules have been regarded as a reaction of the reticuloendothelial system to mite antigen (Barthelmes and Barthelmes 1974), as a toxic reaction to sarcoptic material absorbed through lymphatics (Haber 1963), as a reaction to dissolved sarcoptic faeces similarly absorbed (Konstantinov and Stanoeva 1973) and as combined delayed and immediate hypersensitivity reaction (Garcovitch et al. 1978). The latter explanation possibly covers the suggestion by Arnold (1981) that perhaps second attacks of scabies are more apt to be nodular from the beginning. Topical therapy is usually ineffective, but Kocsard (1976), confirmed by Ely (1977) and by Arnold (1981), found that crude coal tar dabbed on the nodules was effective.

Scabies and Acute Glomerulonephritis

In certain tropical regions and places where the summer season is very hot, epidemics of scabies associated with acute glomerulonephritis (AGN) have been reported. Epidemic AGN associated with pyoderma was recorded by Symonds (1960), Blumberg and Feldman (1962), Poon-King et al. (1967) and by Anthony et al. (1967). New M-type nephritogenic strains of beta-haemolytic streptococci (BHS) were involved in the 1967 outbreak, and in many of the patients reported by Anthony et al. the pyoderma was found to be secondary to scabies. Further epidemics of AGN associated with infected scabies have been reported from South Africa (Hersch 1967), Israel (Lasch et al. 1971), Trinidad (Svartman et al. 1972; Poon-King et al. 1973), Nigeria (Whittle et al. 1973) and from Panama and Colombia (Potter et al. 1977).

The causal agent in most of these epidemics was an M-type strain of BHS. Not always the same strain was responsible; at least two were new strains. A feature of these organisms was their affinity for skin lesions. In the last two Trinidadian epidemics it was also noted that the outbreak of AGN was immediately preceded by a sudden increase in the incidence of scabies and that the BHS pyoderma was secondary to scabies in the great majority. Potter et al. (1971) found that amongst AGN patients five distinct dermopathic M-type strains of BHS had been successively prevalent, three of which had been associated with major epidemics of AGN over a 5-year period. The tendency for AGN to result from skin infections in these tropical regions contrasts with the respiratory origin of nephritogenic strains of BHS in the United Kingdom and in temperate regions in general. In this respect Borda (1954) should be credited with precedence in noting the association between AGN and infected scabies. In addition to two personal cases he indicated that Chilean workers had stressed that over 50% of their cases of AGN of infancy were related to skin infections, most of which were impetiginised scabies, whereas only 23% were related to pharyngitis and 4% to scarlatina (see p. 277 regarding race in this context). Sporadic instances of AGN related to infected scabies have been recorded by Allen (1972), by Moulin et al. (1977) and by Charmes et al. (1978).

Diagnosis of Scabies

Scabies can be one of the most difficult or one of the easiest diseases to diagnose (Stokes 1936). Much has been written about the inability of some physicians to diagnose scabies (Greenhough 1886; MacCormac 1918; Stokes 1936; Lunn 1944–1945; Hellier 1966, 1976; Hansen and Lynch 1976; Witkowski and Parrish 1978). This has been attributed to the inadequate experience (and possibly inadequate instruction) of medical students. The cyclical epidemic nature of the incidence of scabies, which will be discussed later (see pp. 265, 266, 276), results in a periodic scarcity of patients with the disease; those who have seen few or no patients with scabies during their study of Dermatology find if difficult to recognise the condition (Hansen and Lynch 1976).

The presenting symptom is usually itch. All patients with an unexplained itch should be suspected of having scabies until the contrary has been proved (Degos 1953; Alexander 1967a, b). A high index of suspicion is the physician's most important defence against overlooking scabies. The site, severity, duration and timing of the itch are all helpful diagnostic points. It may be localised initially and become generalised or it may be widespread from its inception with some areas itching more than others. For example, intractable interdigital itching, causing compulsive rubbing of the areas, was so well known in the sixteenth and seventeenth centuries as to carry the names of "Scotch fiddle" or "Welsh fiddle" (Boog-Watson 1971). Itching of the penis and scrotum has long been regarded as a valuable sign of scabies (Fox 1864; MacCormac 1918, Stokes 1936; Sefton 1947; Degos 1953), although Greenhough (1886) declared that penile lesions were rarely scratched. The nocturnal character of the itch is a feature of scabies (see p. 228), although it should be remembered that itch from other causes may be aggravated by the warmth of the bed.

A history of itching in other members of the family is an important feature of scabies and has been emphasised by most authors. It is particularly frequent in those who share the same bed, but other family contacts such as those between mother and child (especially with infants) and between brothers and sisters are also important. However, although such a history can be regarded as *prima facie* evidence of a patient having scabies (Hunter 1972), Dubreuilh and Beille (1895) pointed out that the conjugal partner of a scabietic may not be affected. The itching status of other members of the household such as lodgers, whether relatives or not, and of frequent visitors such as nearby relatives or baby-sitters should also be the subject of inquiry. When there is no family history of itch, inquiry about fellow inmates of institutions such as hospitals, schools, school dormitories, military accommodation, lodging houses, refugee camps etc. should be made. Bearing in mind that scabies has an incubation period of 4–6 weeks and that the patient may not have reported the condition at once, such inquiries may have to cover a previous period of up to 6 months.

It is useful to know what previous treatment the patient has had since it may influence the physical condition and presentation. If an antiscabietic has been used, inquiry should be made to ascertain which one, how it was applied, at what interval and for how long. This will help to decide whether a patient may have had scabies, has been correctly treated and is suffering from a post-scabietic pruritus (Dubreuilh and Beille 1895); whether he has been inadequately treated and still has scabies; whether he has been overtreated and is suffering from a contact eczema caused by medicament; or whether he has been treated for scabies when he did not in fact have that disease (Dubreuilh and Baille 1895; Bacon 1944).

On the other hand, the patient may actually have scabies but have been treated for some other disease. Eczema is the most likely condition to be so treated and topical corticosteroids are the most likely to have been used. These drugs aggravate scabies (McMillan 1972). Should the patient happen to have eczematised scabies, it would be valuable to know that the application of a topical corticosteroid did not produce the expected alleviation of symptoms. This is particularly important to remember in infants, who are often eczematised when they have scabies (see Figs. 15.7, 15.16) and treated without the underlying disorder being suspected. Elmers and Hornqvist (1981) apparently treated a patient for scabies, but an existing seborrhoeic eczema of the scalp continued actively until it was found that sarcoptic mites were proliferating there under the influence of the topical corticosteroid being used. Tables 15.3 and 15.4 summarise the data required from the history.

The necessity for careful examination of the whole body of a suspected scabietic in a good light with a lens (see p. 228) must be reiterated. This is important for most skin disorders but absolutely essential for scabies (MacCormac 1918, 1943; Stokes 1936; Dixon 1941; Lunn 1942). Particular attention should be paid to *all* those sites where burrows might be expected, the fingers and interdigital webs being inspected individually. Without a lens small burrows and the papules and vesicles produced by immature mites are easily overlooked and certain physical appearances such as tiny scratch marks or the edges of fine desquamation could easily be mistaken for burrows. Examination of the feet is especially important since they are often overlooked and may show evidence of scabies which is absent elsewhere (see Fig. 15.3). Burrows on the feet are much commoner, even in adults, than is generally taught, but deliberate search must be made for them.

Of special diagnostic importance are the papular lesions on the penis and scrotum (see Fig. 15.5) in men and less commonly the areolar lesions in women, the latter often being eczematous (see Fig. 15.15). Numerous uncomplicated lesions are often found on the palms and soles of hemiplegics (Nayler 1866; Mapother 1872; personal observation).

Occupation sometimes appears to influence the situations of scabietic lesions. Hebra (1854) noted that whilst pustular lesions on the buttocks in those whose occupations compelled them to sit for long periods (e.g. tailors) were pathognomonic of scabies, such lesions were never seen in those who stood at work. Similarly Nayler (1866) observed that in blacksmiths the hands were spared, presumably because of hardening of the skin of the palms and fingers (Shoemaker 1902). The latter also pointed out that burrows were not found on the hands in those patients who constantly immersed them in hot water containing washing chemicals.

Table 15.3. Data required about itching in scabies

Duration
Severity
Localisation:
If localised, which areas?
If generalised: a) At onset?
b) Delayed?
Timing, nocturnal or otherwise
Contacts:
Familial
Others
Absent but present in contacts

Table 15.4. Data required about previous treatment in scabies

Was medicament an antiscabietic? If so, which?
Was medicament a topical corticosteroid? If so, which?
How was it applied?
Where was it applied?
How often was it applied?
Over how long a period was it used?
Did it help?

Borda (1954) observed this phenomenon in professional laundrywomen.

Difficulty in making a diagnosis of scabies may be encountered in the very clean and in those whose rash is complicated by other skin lesions. The difficulties in persons whose hygiene is excellent have been well described by Fox (1875) and by Stokes (1936). Lesions may be so few or even absent that diagnosis is heavily dependent on history and family history, whilst complications may completely mask the specific lesions of scabies. Meticulous examination is particularly important in these persons. There may be only a few linear lesions on the abdomen or hips or perhaps a pustule on the elbow or genitalia (Farkas 1974), or the only skin lesions may be papules on chest or flank (Levenson 1974). In one pregnant patient seen by the present writer a patch of eczema on one breast raised the possibility of scabies. There were no lesions of any kind elsewhere, except for three burrows on one little toe, from which a *Sarcoptes* was removed.

Quite apart from the morphology of the actual lesions their distribution is of diagnostic value. In order to appreciate this better the examining physician is advised to stand back a little from the patient (Stokes 1936). An uncomplicated scabies will be seen to have lesions distributed over the areas described in the clinical section, whilst in those whose scabies is complicated by eczema or secondary infection the scabietic lesions will still be seen to be most prominent in the same areas. (see Fig. 15.8), especially those in which burrows commonly occur. The features to be looked for on examination of the patient suspected of having scabies are summarised in Table 15.5.

Table 15.5. Points to be noted when examining a patient for suspected scabies

Good light, preferably daylight
Lens or loupe
Examine whole patient, undressed, in detail
Look for burrows and associated papules and vesicles
Look at the distribution of the eruption
Never forget to examine the feet
Note the areas where there are no lesions

After history taking and examination of the patient the microscopic demonstration of the *Sarcoptes* at any stage of its development is convincing proof of the diagnosis. Such confirmation is advisable even in obvious cases, if only to convince a doubting patient. Neither of the two techniques available takes more than a few minutes.

The first method, succinctly described by Kavli (1978), requires a loupe, a needle (e.g. a disposable intravenous needle) and good light. The burrow is gently opened with the needle, working towards the blind end. When the latter is opened the mite will adhere to the tip of the needle, just visible as a shiny whitish object less than 0.5 mm long. It should be placed on a glass slide inside a ring of ink (Sneddon and Church 1979) for convenience of subsequent location. It may be mounted temporarily in 80% lactic acid or 30% potassium hydroxide for confirmation of the morphological features.

Alternatively, the suspected burrow or other lesion—usually from a preferred site on a hand or foot and by its nature practically confined to the stratum corneum—can be scraped off with a *round*-bodied scalpel blade (No 15 or 20 disposable is best). The blade, held between finger and thumb with the edge vertically against the stretched skin, is drawn firmly along the burrow (or the lesion) removing it entirely as a small scale. Blood should not be drawn. The specimen is placed in a drop or two of potash, a cover glass applied, the whole gently warmed for a few seconds (not boiled), the cover glass lightly pressed and the preparation examined microscopically with the low power for evidence of the *Sarcoptes* in any form (eggs, faecal matter etc.). This is the more reliable method, especially in doubtful cases. Variations in concentration of the potash have been recommended (Howell 1950; Mikhail and Krull 1973). Wilson (1971) advised saline instead of potash but it does not soften and clear keratin and has no advantages. Others (Muller et al. 1973; Levenson 1974; Orkin 1975; Hansen and Lynch 1976; Muller 1977) have advocated using mineral oil instead of potash because it has a different refractive index from the *Sarcoptes* and its products, which are thus easier to see. It does not dissolve faecal pellets; however, it does not soften or clear keratin either. In the opinion of the present writer, it bears no comparison with potash for clarity of preparation. The immersion oil which Hoke (1973) advised is no better.

The examination of scrapings from beneath the free edge of fingernails would also seem to be a useful diagnostic procedure. Scher (1983) found a *Sarcoptes* in the parakeratotic debris in a nail biopsy, quite by chance. This prompted him to order thorough nail paring of all patients, staff and other contacts in an intractable epidemic of scabies in two nursing homes; there was subsequently a remarkable improvement in the epidemic.

Woodley and Saurat (1981) described the burrow ink test (BIT), as used at the Hôpital Saint-Louis in Paris for generations. It involves rubbing an ink pen (a ballpoint pen seems suitable) over the suspected burrow and wiping the ink off at once with an alcohol swab. The ink penetrates the burrow and outlines it clearly. Although up to 36% of false negative findings may occur, the authors clearly state that a positive burrow by this technique can be found in scabies, an opinion which can be accepted in view of the vast experience involved. However, it may take 20–30 min to find a positive burrow. The present writer finds the scraping method preferable. Estes (1982) noted that a liquid tetracycline preparation, applied generously, left on for a few minutes and then the excess wiped off with an alcohol swab, revealed burrows fluorescing bright yellow-green under Wood's light.

Carpenter (1948) used a Skeet's eye curette and said, "as the mite is quite deep in the epidermis proper curetting should include some of the elastic and fibrous tissue of the upper cutis". This is incorrect and not recommended. Hand (1946) and Itani (1970) recommended shaving off the burrow and surrounding skin with a sharp blade held parallel to the surface. The specimen was treated subsequently in the same manner as scrapings.

The most convincing and beautiful means of demonstrating a *Sarcoptes* actually in the burrow together with its eggs is to open the burrow with a needle under direct vision with a dissecting microscope. It is an exercise well worth trying by anyone interested and is very instructive for students. It is not difficult, merely requiring a cooperative patient, a well-illuminated dissecting microscope, a sharp sterile needle (large intravenous size) and a steady hand. More can be learnt about the appearance of the mite and its behaviour and movements in and around the burrow in 15 min than in several hours' reading. At a magnification of 25 times the beauty of the *Sarcoptes* has to be seen to be believed. Its movements can be observed, and every seta and the row of tiny glistening eggs lying in the burrowlike peas in the pod can be seen.

Differential Diagnosis

Scabies must be differentiated from eczema, impetigo and furunculosis (all of which may also complicate it) and from other itching skin disorders such as lichen planus, pityriasis rosea, dermatitis herpetiformis, papular urticaria, animal scabies and other parasitoses, including pediculosis and phthiriasis pubis, sabra dermatitis, symptomatic pruritus, delusion of parasitosis and the itching dermatoses of pregnancy.

Eczema

Unless eczema is complicating scabies, it does not have the latter's typical distribution. There are no burrows and scabietic scratch marks are not seen. Most plaques of eczema are easily distinguished, but the vesicles seen on the fingers in contact eczema or in generalised sensitisation eczema may be impossible to differentiate individually from the tiny pearly vesicles occurring near immature forms of *Sarcoptes*. The latter are usually smaller than eczematous vesicles, tend to occur in small clusters in the vicinity of burrows and seldom extend the full length of the finger. Eczema occurs on the face, neck and back, whereas scabies does not (except on the face in babies). Oedema of the eyelids may accompany an eczematous sensitisation. Eczema tends to itch all the time and is not characteristically nocturnal. The family history of itch is negative in eczema, although if the latter were secondary to a fungal infection there might be a family history of this with localised itching on the feet.

Impetigo

When it is not associated with scabies, impetigo tends to affect the limbs and face. It may be familial. It is usually an acute disorder. It lacks any of the features of scabies except that it may occasionally itch slightly. It may present with crusts or with seropurulent bullae.

Furunculosis

In the absence of scabies furunculosis has no set distribution and lacks any of the features of scabies.

Lichen Planus

Apart from itch, symmetry and the occurrence of penile lesions, this disease does not resemble scabies. Lesions may also occur on the lower back and oral mucosa. The lesions are flat, shiny, violaceous papules.

Pityriasis Rosea

This condition presents with an abrupt onset following a herald patch. The lesions are scaling maculopapules, which occur principally on the trunk, both back and front, but may affect the head and neck. The palms and soles are never affected. The itch is not specifically nocturnal. Family history is lacking and spontaneous resolution occurs in

3–6 months. This never happens in scabies (Fox 1864), although both Hebra (1868) and Mellanby (1943) said that it could if the only active parasites happened to be removed by scratching.

Dermatitis Herpetiformis

The itching dermatosis known as dermatitis herpetiformis is frequently mistaken for scabies, although the reverse seldom happens (but see Ackerman et al. 1975). It is characteristically a chronic, symmetrical, itching, vesiculopapular eruption in which the lesions go through a regular progression of changes from erythema, urtication to vesiculation. It has its own distribution, chiefly affecting the forearms, scapular areas, the intergluteal cleft and the knees. The hands and feet are only very rarely affected. It itches at any time of the day, persists indefinitely and shows none of the features of scabies. There may be malabsorption or a family history of malabsorption.

Papular Urticaria

This disorder is almost confined to children and is often confused with scabies, especially in infants. It presents with scattered, excoriated, papular urticated lesions, sometimes surmounted by a vesicle, often scratched and sometimes secondarily infected. The lesions occur principally on the forearms, lower legs and around the waistline. Their distribution is otherwise haphazard. The soles may be affected in babies, but burrows are never found. There is no general familial itch, although occasionally more than one child in a family is affected. The disease, caused mainly by flea bites, is somewhat seasonal and clears up when the child is admitted to hospital. As Lyell (1967) has said, children with papular urticaria leave their parasites at home but scabietics take theirs with them.

Animal Scabies

Animal scabies and other ectoparasitic diseases caused by mites may be mistaken for human scabies. More than one member of a family may be affected, as may a colleague doing similar work or exposed to the same source of infestation. A history of such source should be obtained if suspected. The lesions resemble those of papular urticaria but are distributed according to areas of contact. For example, men carrying bundles which are infested with *Pyemotes tritici* on their backs will have these lesions on the back of the neck, on the forearms and around the waist, whereas children handling a dog infested with scabies tend to get the lesions on the forearms, the anterior abdominal wall and the front of the thighs. All such ectoparasitic infestations also tend to produce lesions in the vicinity of constrictive bands of clothing, such as round the waist. None of the parasites make burrows on humans and none affects the hands. All spontaneously clear when the source of the infestation is dealt with.

Pediculosis Corporis

Pediculosis corporis may accompany scabies (rarely) but usually only when both are known to be epidemic, as, for example, in the trenches in World War I. Occasionally vagrants with exceedingly poor hygiene and living in squalid conditions may also suffer from both diseases. Uncomplicated pediculosis corporis is typically severely itchy and this itch is not confined to the time spent in bed. Gross linear excoriations are a feature on the trunk. Vesicles are never seen, but there is pigmentation on the trunk and flexures in longstanding cases. The hands and feet are seldom involved. Burrows are never found but lice are present in the clothing.

Phthiriasis Pubis

In the condition of phthiriasis pubis there is generalised itch, but it is more usually confined to the lower trunk, the groins and perineum. Lesions which are in the same areas are hard to see and usually consist of scratch marks. Lice can be seen with difficulty amongst the pubic hair and extending to the umbilical area and axillae. Nits on the hairs in these areas are rather easier to see. There is no evidence of scabies.

Sabra Dermatitis

Persons handling prickly pears (*Opuntia* species) for any reason are liable to contract this condition. The lesions are produced by the barbed glochidia, which cause spherical pinhead vesicles and papules and pea-sized papules and occasionally crusts, pustules or even tiny ulcers, without adenopathy or fever. The lesions occur on the interdigital webs, on the wrists, arms, chest, abdominal wall, buttocks and genital area. Confusion with scabies will obviously arise. However, there are no burrows, the lesions also occur on the nose, oral mucosa and palate and there may be conjunctivitis and keratitis. Patients complain of a burning itch and pain. This disease has been reported from Israel, South America, Mexico, Morocco and Italy (Shanon and Sagher 1956) from South Africa (Whiting and Bristow 1975) and in California (A. Lyell 1976, personal communication).

Itching Dermatoses of Pregnancy

In pregnancy scabies may be temporarily diagnosed in a patient developing herpes gestationis because of the severe itch, but the acute bullous nature of the condition will soon reveal itself and the true diagnosis. More confusing is the papular pruritic dermatosis of pregnancy, which only shows non-specific excoriated papules. There are no features of scabies and the disorder disappears when the pregnancy terminates.

Symptomatic Itch

The only lesions are scratch marks and very rarely secondary infection. The marks are widespread and haphazard. There are no scabietic lesions. There may be evidence of underlying systemic disease such as jaundice, diabetes mellitus, thyroid or hepatic disease, tumours etc.

Delusion of Parasitosis

Here again the only lesions are indiscriminate scratch marks. Patients complain that they are infested with "insects" and produce "a small crumpled piece of paper for the doctor's inspection containing 'the parasites'; it holds a collection of heterogenous debris such as scales, crusts, bits of hair, crumbs, nail clippings, sugar grains" (Lyell 1967). In spite of the likely diagnosis of an obsession, it is essential to examine the patient carefully to exclude scabies.

Syphilis

The nodulopapular penile lesions of scabies have to be distinguished from the primary chancre of syphilis. Other evidence of syphilis, such as a bubo, fever and possibly a secondary rash, and of scabies must be looked for. It should be remembered that the two conditions can coexist and that scabietic papules can be the portal of entry for the pallid spirochaete (Stokes 1936).

Finally it must be emphasised that scabies should not be diagnosed on inadequate grounds, and especially not just because no other cause for itch can be found.

Norwegian Scabies

The condition first described in lepers by Boeck and Danielssen [1848] was called Norwegian scabies (NS) in their honour by Hebra in 1852. It has subsequently been suggested by many others that scabies crustosa is a preferable name, but the condition is better known by its eponym, which is quite acceptable. NS has such a remarkable clinical appearance that the large majority of examples seen have been recorded. There are over 300 reports. The details which follow have been culled from a representative sample of this literature and include all the important features.

The onset is usually insidious. In some instances NS starts as ordinary scabies but changes its character gradually. In other patients scabies is never suspected as the diagnosis, the progressive condition being regarded as chronic eczema or neurodermatitis. It is generally held that patients with NS do not itch. This is misleading; at least 50% do itch. In some itch is a minor feature and, although present, is mild; in others the itch is marked initially but diminishes with time; whilst in many others there is pronounced, often intense itch throughout, even to the extent of making the patient's life totally miserable (Beatty 1913).

There are two principal components of the eruption, localised horny plaques and a more diffuse erythematosquamous appearance. The plaques are composed of hyper- and parakeratotic crusts. They vary in thickness from about 3 to 15 mm and in colour may be creamy, grey, yellow, yellow-brown or yellow-green. They are adherent and firm but when removed and teased apart they have a porous appearance like a sponge or pumice stone. They are found chiefly over extensor surfaces liable to pressure or over small joints. Because of their situation and skin movements they show deep fissuring (Fig. 15.22). When they are large and very thick the whole surface may be broken up into slabs by these fissures (Dubreuilh and Sainte-Marie 1924), rather like a mud flat which is drying out. The outer surface may be smooth or rugose. If they are removed by forceps the undersurface is smooth, red, somewhat moist and velvety in appearance. Such crusts are usually found on the dorsal surface of the hand, the wrists, the fingers, over the metacarpophalangeal joints (Fig. 15.23), on the palms, on the extensor aspect of the elbows, on the scalp and ears, the soles of the feet and the toes. Hubler and Clabaugh (1976) notes that these exact areas were affected in all of their mentally defective child patients with NS, and the sites have been involved in most other patients. Many other

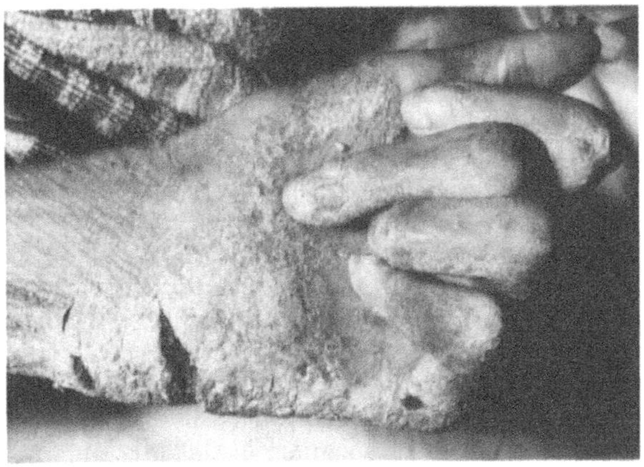

Fig. 15.22. Norwegian scabies in a patient suffering from 70% burns. Showing deep fissuring in the hyper-/parakeratotic epidermis. Note the probable burrows on the dorsum of the ring finger.

thick and involving the fingers and palms they may prohibit movement, as was seen in the third of Boeck and Danielssen's original patients (Hebra 1868) and also in a patient seen by the present writer (see below).

The erythematosquamous component of the eruption is more diffuse. It is composed of similar horny crusts, which are more scaly and thin (Fig. 15.24). The erythema is more evident. The surface beneath the scales is the same as that under the thick crusts. Sometimes only the trunk or the limbs are involved. In other patients the whole body may be affected (Dubreuilh and Sainte-Marie 1924; Ingram 1951). The appearance of the patient described by Dubreuilh and Sainte-Marie gradually developed over a year from small pinpoint papules on the back of each hand to a "veritable shell" of crusts covering the whole body.

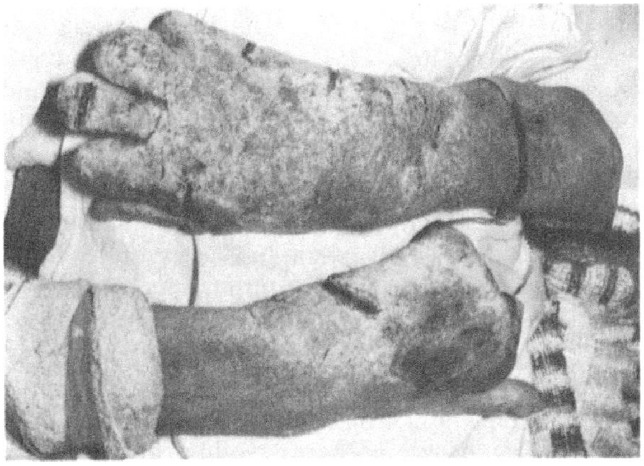

Fig. 15.23. Norwegian scabies in the same patient as in Fig. 15.22. Showing the gross, adherent hyper-/parakeratotic epidermis on the dorsum of the hands and fingers.

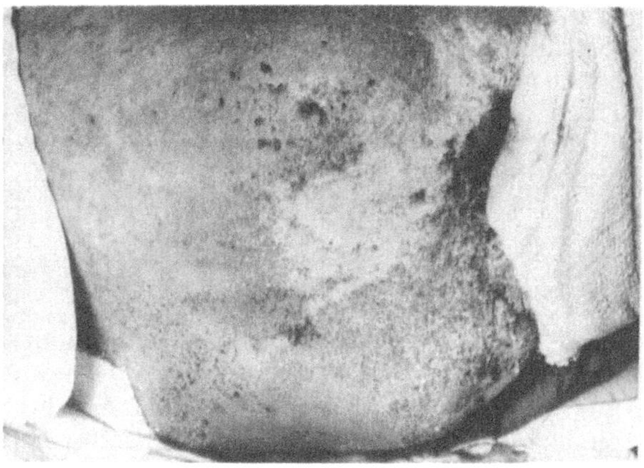

Fig. 15.24. Diffuse erythroderma with hyperkeratosis and crusting in Norwegian scabies. Same patient as Fig. 15.22.

areas have thick crusts in individual patients and include the points of the shoulders, the neck, the eyebrows, the tip of the nose, the scapular areas, the buttocks (not uncommonly), the hips, outer thighs, front of the knees and around the ankles. The occurrence of plaques may be conditioned by pressure, as in Beatty's (1913) patient. This man had a congenitally deformed leg and was a taxi driver. As a result of the deformity undue pressure was put on the other buttock when sitting. This region was the site of a particularly thick plaque, as were the palms, which were in constant contact with the steering wheel while driving. Martin-Scott (1957) had a similar patient who was a lorry driver and had plaques on the buttocks. Plaques may sometimes be sharply circumscribed, as in the patient of Short and Derrick (1948). When very

The involvement of all parts of the head and neck distinguishes NS from the ordinary variety of scabies. Not all the skin is necessarily affected and sometimes only a few very localised areas are involved, e.g. Dowling's (1929) patient had lesions confined to the feet and hands.

The nails are often involved and show two types of change. The commonest appearance rather resembling onychomycosis (Burks et al. 1956) involves the nail bed and nail plate (Fig. 15.25). They become thickened, rough, laminated, soft, friable and discoloured (Hebra 1852; Brug et al. 1930) and often become elevated 1 cm or more and unrecognisable as nails. In the other type of change seen the nail plate seems to escape involvement and retains its hard smooth appearance, but the underlying nail bed and surrounding nail fold are

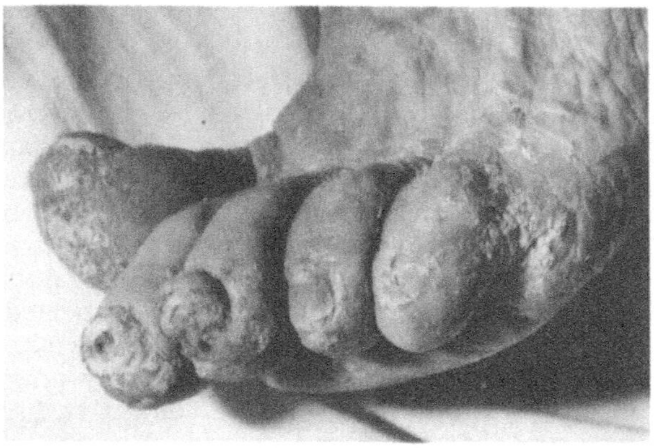

Fig. 15.25. Gross hyper-/parakeratosis of toenails in Norwegian scabies. (Courtesy of Dr. Malcolm Young, Greenock Royal Infirmary)

grossly keratotic and elevate the nail plate (Dubreuilh and Sainte-Marie 1924; Short and Derrick 1948; Boas 1952). In one patient recorded by Saruta and Nakamizu (1978) the only evidence of scabies was a single grossly thickened nail in which many *Sarcoptes* were found. Borda (1954) observed partial or complete alopecia and sometimes vitiligo as complicating features of NS.

NS may begin as ordinary scabies with burrows, papules and vesicles in the usual places (or unusual sites, see Fig. 15.26), only to have this appearance overshadowed by the keratotic reaction, so that the diagnosis is not evident when the patient is first seen. On the other hand, burrows may be discernible on careful examination at the margin of horny plaques or on areas which are not keratotic (Hebra 1852), such as the penis, hands and feet, when they have no horny plaques. At a rough estimate from the literature about 25% of patients have evident burrows.

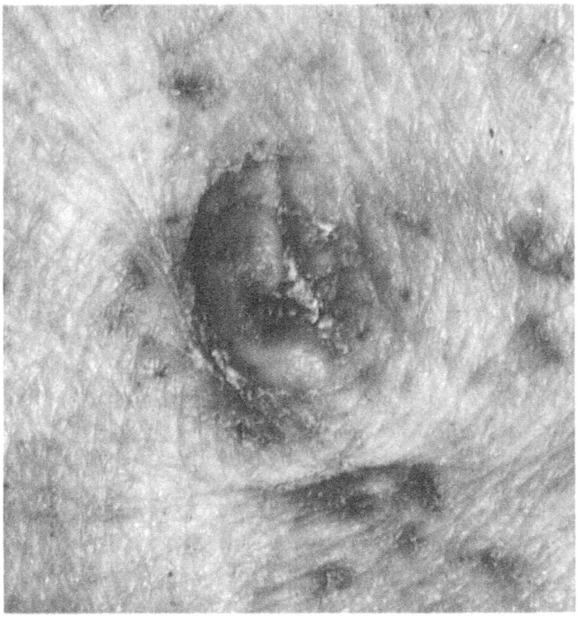

Fig. 15.26. Multiple burrows on the anterior abdominal wall in Norwegian scabies. Same patient as in Fig. 15.25. (Courtesy of Dr. Malcolm Young, Greenock Royal Infirmary)

Patients suffering from NS are frequently inmates of long-stay institutions (i.e. closed communities), and when presented to the dermatologist appear to be suffering from chronic exfoliative eczema, the common diagnosis. They have often been confined to bed for some time and present a pitiable picture of misery, accompanied on occasion by a very disagreeable odour variously described as "evil" (Baranova 1927), "like sour dough" (Cherikover 1937) or "musty" (Boas 1952). Many patients seen outside such institutions appear to be in a state of extreme neglect. Cachexia and hypovitaminosis were emphasised as accompanying features by Borda (1852); the former could have been due to other associated factors (see below), whilst the latter could have been a consequence of general neglect not infrequently occurring with NS, although vitamin A deficiency has been held to be a predisposing factor by some (see Table 15.7.). Strobel et al. (1982) have added kwashiorkor with its gross protein, iron, folate and pyridoxin deficiency to the list of diseases in which NS occurs.

Another feature of patients with NS is the association with mental or physical defects or other circumstances. In fact, Wells (1952) remarked that it was almost unknown in physically and mentally normal persons. This is not strictly correct, since Piers and Tims (1946), Burks et al. (1956), Martin-Scott (1957) and Konstantinov and Stanoeva (1976) have all described the disease in otherwise normal healthy people. The commonest associated condition is Down's syndrome, but other mental deficiency states, dementia, diseases of the central nervous system such as syringomyelia, cerebrovascular accidents and spinal injury, leprosy, reticulosis and, more recently, immunosuppression have all been recorded in association with NS. Bearing in mind that immunosuppressive therapy is a fairly recent innovation and that a higher proportion of recent reports is involved, the accompanying Table 15.6 shows the approximate incidence of associated conditions in 100 recorded examples. To these could be added a patient of the present writer. He developed NS after being accidentally burned (70%) in a factory explosion. During his treatment he was observed to have retained a human skin homograft for 8 weeks instead of the

Table 15.6. Relative numbers of conditions associated with Norwegian scabies (100 samples)

Down's syndrome	46
Leprosy	9
Mental deficiency	9
Neurological disorders	8
Immunosuppression	9
"Autoimmune disease"	4
Topical corticosteroids	2
Reticuloses	4
Others	9

expected 2 or 3 weeks. Some 4–5 months after his accident he was noted to have widespread 'eczematous' lesions with erythema and scaling on the limbs and trunk and enormous hyperkeratotic plaques on his hands and fingers (see Figs. 15.22 and 15.24) and, to a lesser extent, on the forearms and buttocks. He was miserable with itch. A mistaken diagnosis of neomycin sensitivity was corrected a day or two later when several members of the nursing staff were found to have ordinary scabies.

When patients with NS, especially in closed communities, are seen the diagnosis is rarely made until an outbreak of scabies occurs. In this respect Heid et al. (1974) noted that contagion is favoured by two factors: rapid proliferation of the *Sarcoptes* and misdiagnosis. In approximately 70 randomly chosen references from the literature at least 32 reported associated epidemics of ordinary scabies. In many the number of affected contacts was not disclosed but in at least seven instances over 30 cases of scabies occurred. In one example 104 persons were infested (Bricklin and Musgnug 1978). In some cases associated with Down's syndrome many of the contacts were also suffering from that disorder. In Hubler and Clabaugh's (1976) series 22 of 25 contacts developed NS. In Calnan's (1950) patients those contacts who had Down's syndrome developed NS and those who did not developed ordinary scabies, whilst in Wilkinson's (1953) outbreak several of the contacts who developed ordinary scabies had Down's syndrome. Additional to these types of patients must be included conditions occurring in tropical countries, particularly in primitive villages where most of the population have scabies. Some of these conditions have the appearance of NS and have local names such as *craw-craw* in Sierra Leone (Blacklock 1924) or *kas kas* in New Guinea (Backhouse 1929). The implications of the findings mentioned will be discussed later.

The pathology of NS is discussed on pp. 252–254. A pronounced eosinophilia is often present and some patients are febrile. The changes all clear up when the NS is cured.

Diagnosis

Once a suspicion of the correct diagnosis has been raised it is relatively easy to confirm. If a burrow should be found, a mite can be extracted and identified microscopically. However, it is even easier to examine a scale placed in potassium hydroxide under the low power of the microscope. Very large numbers of *Sarcoptes* in all stages will be seen (Fig. 15.27; present writer's patient described above). As many as a dozen or more mites, parts of mites or eggs can be seen in one low-power field. By extrapolation from the content of three small scales from the patient, with an area of no more than 50 mm^2 and containing 550 mites and eggs, it was calculated that a reasonable estimate would put the total number of parasites and eggs on the patient's skin at between five and ten million. An idea of the vast number occurring in NS was given by Dubreuilh and Sainte-Marie (1924), who said "with a lens this surface (after removing the crusts) appears chequered and honey-combed and when the eye has become accustomed to recognition, one can see that it is dotted with *Sarcoptes*, appearing as ovoid bodies, whitish and brilliant, covering the surface in extraordinary numbers often as many as 6 to the square mm, walking here and there, reminiscent of a flock of sheep at pasture". They also noted that a large number of the mites seen were immature (Figs. 15.28, and 15.29). Fig. 15.28 gives a most vivid impression of what a tiny fragment of crust from NS looks like by scanning electron microscopy.

Treatment

The treatment of NS is the same as for ordinary scabies, with the necessary addition of some measures to soften and remove the crusts with starch poultices or salicylic acid ointment for a day or two. In the present writer's patient 1% gamma-benzene hexachloride applied three times a day for 3 days sufficed. Within 3 weeks all evidence of NS had disappeared (Fig. 15.30), with only burn scars remaining. Patients described in the literature have all cleared with sulphur ointment, benzyl benzoate emulsion or gamma-benzene hexachloride, some as quickly as the present writer's patient, some even sooner and some after 2 or 3 months' intensive therapy. There are no sequelae, but if treatment is stopped too soon in difficult cases there will be a relapse sooner or later. It goes without saying that all contacts should be treated simultaneously with the patient.

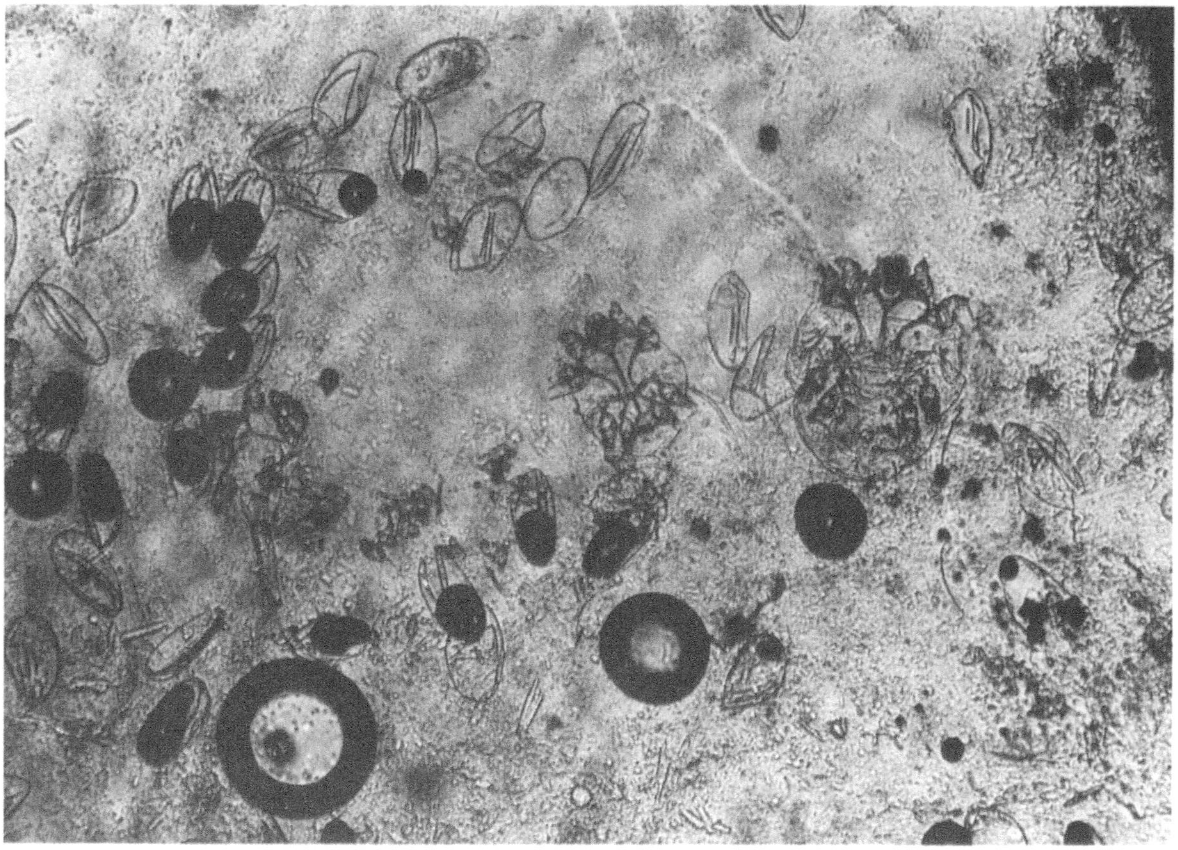

Fig. 15.27. Norwegian scabies. Low-power microscopic view of a fragment of scale from the same patient as in Fig. 15.22, showing male and female *Sarcoptes*, innumerable egg shells and fragments of exuvia. The dark spherical objects are air bubbles. Specimen mounted in 30% potassium hydroxide.

Aetiology

Carslaw et al. (1975) pointed out that many lesions in the contacts were of the papular variety caused by immature forms of *Sarcoptes*. Persons infested by such forms would develop ordinary scabies if sufficient numbers of these immature forms survived on their skin to reach the adult stage and begin reproduction. Thus scabies would appear in such contacts, especially if they were bedridden, in 2 or 3 weeks at the earliest. Others, of course, would produce typical lesions in 2 or 3 days (Haydon and Caplan 1971) by being infested with ovigerous adult female *Sarcoptes*. Carslaw and his colleagues (1975) emphasised that persons associated with NS patients could develop scabies either by direct contact or through the medium of contaminated clothing, dressings and scales from these patients on account of the enormous numbers of mites involved. They said that control of epidemics in hospital wards housing a patient with NS required isolation of the patient, environmental and then personal disinfestation. They showed that airborne dissemination of the mites occurred in these situations (although the mites were not necessarily alive). Lerche et al. (1983) noted that amongst the cases of ordinary scabies secondary to a case of NS admitted to hospital, the distribution of lesions was unusual. The hands and feet were spared, the lesions occurring chiefly on the legs, abdomen, arms and back, in that order of frequency. This suggests indirect (?airborne) rather than direct contact as the cause of the spread and supports the views of Carslaw and his colleagues.

Why do certain people develop NS rather than ordinary scabies? Hebra (1852) said it was because the "soil" was altered rather than because there was a different species of *Sarcoptes* involved. There has been much argument about the latter, which it is not proposed to repeat. Some entomologists and acarologists have maintained that there are morphological differences between the *Sarcoptes* causing NS and that causing ordinary scabies. Fain (1978) said that the only difference that he could

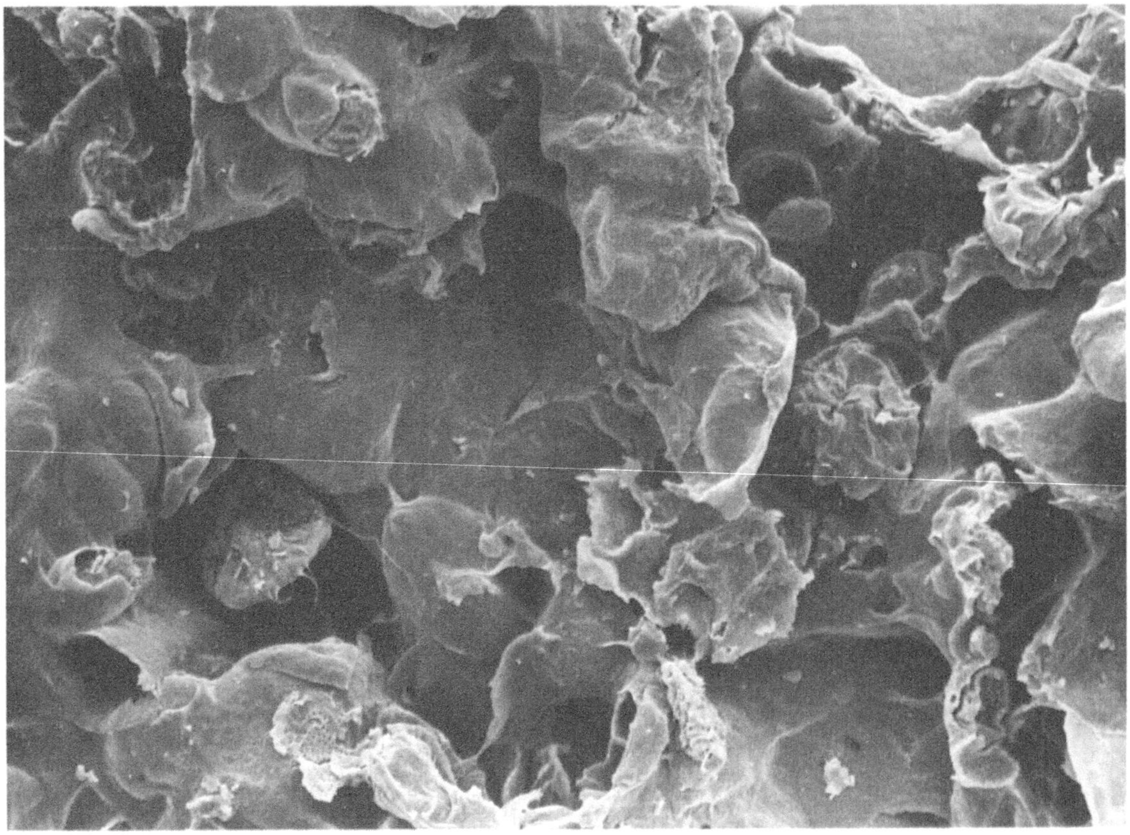

△ **Fig. 15.28.**

Fig. 15.29. ▽

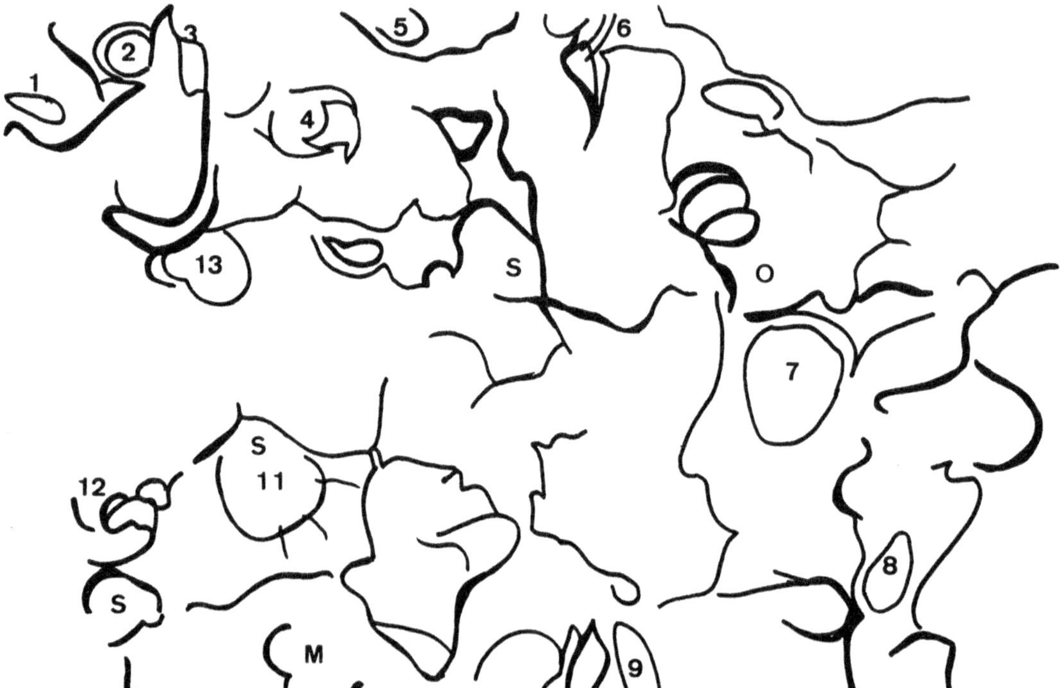

Fig. 15.28. Scanning electron micrograph of crusty scale in Norwegian scabies showing numbers of *Sarcoptes* in all stages and eggs in the burrows. (From Van Neste et al. 1981, by kind permission of Dr. Van Neste and the Editor of *Annales de Dermatologie et de Syphilographie, Paris*)

Fig. 15.29. Key to Fig. 15.27. The parakeratotic horny mass is invaded by numerous parasites (*1, 2, 3, 5, 6, 7, 8, 9, 10, 11, 13*) and hollowed with burrows (*S*). Hatching of eggs (*4, 12*) leave mature larvae and empty shells (*O*) which remain attached to the horny wall. Moults (*M*) are left during development of larvae into nymphs and then into sexually distinct adults. (From Van Neste et al. 1981, by kind permission of Dr. Van Neste and the Editor of *Annales de Dermatologie et de Syphilographie, Paris*)

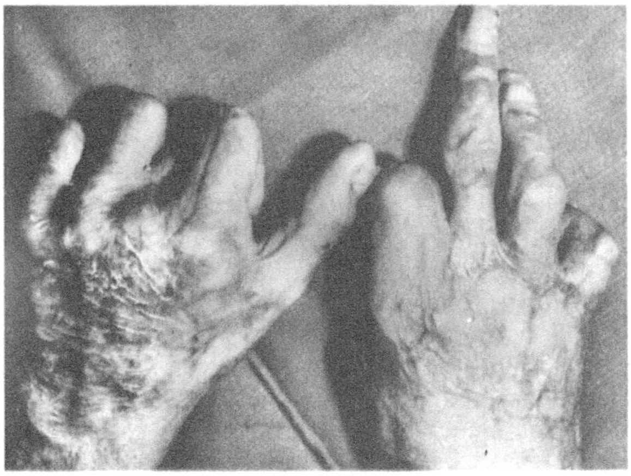

Fig. 15.30. Hands of the same patient as in Fig. 15.22, 3 weeks after treatment for Norwegian scabies. No trace of infestation to be seen, only residual burn scars remaining.

Table 15.7. Various factors which may play a part in the aetiology of Norwegian scabies

1. *Reduced itch*:
   a) Skin anaesthesia to itch
   b) Increased tolerance to itch
2. *Reduced scratching*:
   a) Because of (1) above
   b) Result of immobility or paralysis
   c) Result of patient apathy
3. *Predisposition*:
   a) Liability to keratosis
   b) ? Vitamin A deficiency
4. *Altered immunity*:
   a) Result of inborn or acquired disease
   b) Induced by drugs

detect was in the size of the so-called bare area on the dorsum of the female in the centre of the area of scales. It was somewhat larger in mites from NS, but he attributed this to the effect of the (relative) absence of burrows in NS, the scales serving the function of holding the mite against the burrow roof during the process of digging. Nevertheless, innumerable numbers of contacts of NS develop ordinary scabies, unless they are persons with conditions which seem to predispose them to develop NS, when they will develop the latter, as reported by Hubler and Clabaugh (1976) and by Calnan (1950). Herridge (1963) recorded the instance of a demented woman admitted to a ward where scabies was already rife. She was declared to be free of scabies on admission. She developed an eczematous eruption which was aggravated by oral prednisolone. This proved to be NS. It is difficult to see in the face of these facts how it can be argued that different species of *Sarcoptes* are involved in the two clinical varieties of scabies.

We therefore come back to Hebra's "soil". Do patients with NS differ in some way from those who suffer ordinary scabies? Table 15.7 summarises various factors which have been considered as being involved. Skin anaesthesia certainly seems to be involved in some cases. Brug et al. (1930) noted that the crusted lesions in their patient were on the anaesthetic patches. Rook (1979) pointed out that lack of appreciation of pruritus has been suggested as a factor favouring heavy infestation, as in patients with Down's syndrome. There are several reports of NS in hemiplegics. Both Wells (1952) and Boas (1952) noted that arthritic immobility played an important part in lack of scratching in their patients. An effect of the crusts on the fingers and hands is to immobilise them and this may have an aggravating effect. Patients with Down's syndrome are known to be susceptible to dry ichthyosiform scaling, which may also increase their susceptibility to NS. Vitamin A deficiency also causes a tendency to excessive keratosis. Patients with NS have been shown to have reduced vitamin A levels, as originally suggested by Kitchevatz (cited by Bommer 1955) and by Burks et al. (1956), although George (1958) found normal levels in his patient. More recently there has been an increasing emphasis on altered immunity as the reason behind the development of NS. Immunosuppression may be either the result of circumstances (e.g. in the present writer's patient, whose immunity was evidently depressed by his burns because he tolerated homografts for nearly three times the normal period), or be caused by drugs such as corticosteroids or azathioprine (Herridge 1963; Paterson et al. 1973; Heid et al. 1974; Anolik and Rudolf 1976; Espy and Jolly 1976; Briklin and Musgnug 1978; Chouvet et al. 1979). Ferguson (1973) recorded an instance associated with radiotherapy and corticosteroids. Even topical fluorinated corticosteroids can suppress itch to the extent of allowing the *Sarcoptes* to multiply rapidly on babies and others. Three patients with NS had a history of having had such potent applications to their skin as treatment for itching in the early stages of undiagnosed scabies. This treatment was continued for the subsequent eczema (Millard 1977) and even extended to oral corticosteroids later (Hay 1974; Clayton and Farrow 1975). It seems very likely therefore that altered immune status plays an important part in the development of NS and could be invoked to explain its occurrence in many patients with some of the associated conditions mentioned above. Ward (1971) quoted J. D. Matthews as pointing out that "Australian antigen" occurs with great regularity in the serum of institutionalised patients with Down's syndrome and in relatively high frequency in lepers. This trait may be due to a defect in cellular immunity. Many consider this antigen to be a virus and its presence to denote a lowering of immunity. Matthews said that it was also found in patients with chronic leukaemia, chronic renal disease and sometimes in patients with poor sanitary living conditions in tropical countries but without any disease to account for the presence of the antigen. Kobayashi et al. (1982) described a scabietic with *Pneumocystis carinii* pneumonia. This disease only occurs in patients whose immunity is compromised. There did not seem to be any skin disease present except for florid scabies, possibly the onset of NS. There was no detectable immunological abnormality, but the authors suggested that the simultaneous occurrence of these two disorders indicated some as yet undisclosed abnormality. The subject of immune status in scabietics is discussed fully later (see pp. 265–267).

Histopathology

Ordinary Scabies

Heilesen (1946) outlined the findings up to the start of the twentieth century. He noted that Torok [1889] had always found the burrow confined to the stratum corneum and that papules, vesicles and pustules were the combined result of scratching and irritation from the mite secretions, the latter, he presumed, because of vascular dilation and endothelial changes with oedema of the corium. Unna [1894] had added that vesicles beneath the burrows were the result of inter- and intracellular oedema with slight leucocytic invasion attributed to the chemotactic effect of these secretions. Other vesicles in isolation, often found in scabies, were, said Unna, due to bacterial infection. Heilesen also pointed out that Schischa [1900] had observed that whilst the body of the mite was confined to the burrow in the stratum corneum, its gnathosome frequently penetrated into the stratum mucosum, especially where the horny layer was thin. Volk [1904] had added that the scabies eruption was a mixture of pyoderma and an eczema-like eruption caused by the mite and its secretions.

Heilesen confirmed that the gnathosome of the *Sarcoptes*, whether adult or immature, was usually embedded in the upper stratum granulosum. Van Neste and Lachapelle (1981) added that it could even reach the dermoepidermal junction. Heilesen concluded that this situation was the objective of the burrowing mite and that it secreted a digestive fluid to dissolve epidermal cells. Van Neste and his colleague confirmed this, observing epidermal cell cytolysis some 30–80 μm in advance of the mite's body. The resultant amorphous material forms the nutrient medium for the mite. The mouthparts become embedded in it and the eggs adhere to it (see Fig. 15.38). This cytolysis interfered with keratinisation, causing parakeratosis, initially beneath the advancing burrow but ultimately surrounding it. Eczematous changes may occur, and Heilesen (1946) and Van Neste and Lachapelle (1981) all observed mild changes in the underlying dermis, which the latter authors said was mainly lymphohistiocytic. Heilesen emphasised that epidermal changes leading possibly to vesicle formation occurred beneath these burrows in thick epidermis such as is found on the hands and feet, whilst in those regions such as the penis and axillary folds where the epidermis was thin, there was a much more marked dermal reaction, producing papular lesions. In some instances these reactions could be found beneath small moulting burrows in which remains of shed integument indicated the source of irritation.

Hejazi and Mehregan (1975) and Fernandez et al. (1977) also published detailed accounts of the histopathological appearances in scabies. Ackerman (1977) reiterated the findings of the latter authors but also included the results of his own investigations. In general the changes seen can be divided into epidermal and dermal and the following description includes the known and generally agreed information to date.

Epidermal Changes

When a *Sarcoptes* at any stage is present it is found lying in the stratum corneum (Fig. 15.31). If the

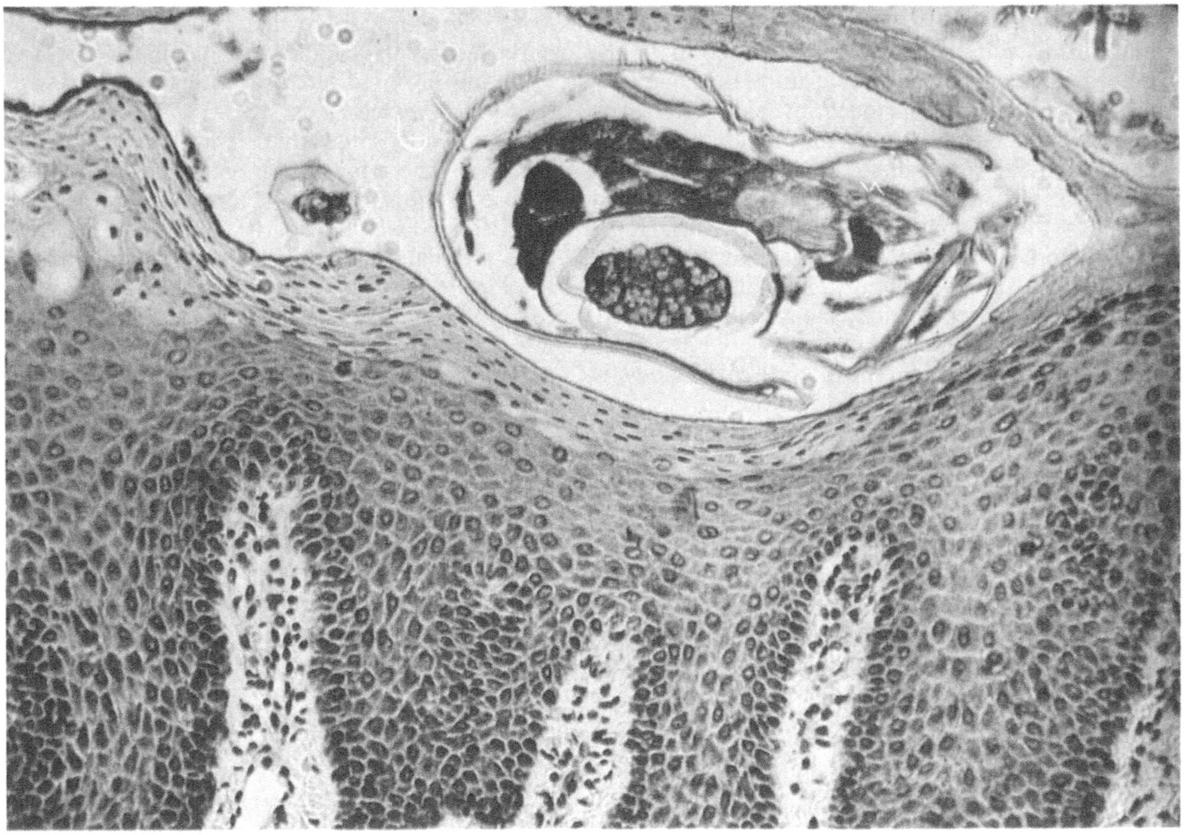

Fig. 15.31. Adult female *Sarcoptes* in situ in burrow, the mouthparts (to the *right* of the picture) having reached the granular layer of the epidermis. Note the parakeratotic stratum corneum beneath the older portion of the burrow. (From Van Neste and Lachapelle 1981, by kind permission of Dr. Van Neste and the Editor of the *British Journal of Dermatology*)

capitulum happens to be in the section examined it will almost certainly be embedded in the upper layers of the stratum mucosum. Fragments of shed integument left behind after moulting will be found in the superficial stratum corneum. New papules or vesicles are covered by normal keratin, but other older lesions have a heaped-up parakeratotic surface, which may also show evidence of excoriations with crust formation. There is usually some reactionary acanthosis beneath the burrow. In the stratum mucosum there are one or more foci of spongiosis, which may have reached the stage of vesicle formation. If a mite is present it always overlies such a focus. Neutrophils and eosinophils may migrate into the spongiotic areas and occasionally they collect in large numbers in the vesicles producing superficial intraepidermal microabscesses. There is no evidence of either pyoderma or bacterial colonies in the early lesions (Hejazi and Mehregan 1975). Occasionally a mite or an egg may be seen in the infundibulum of a hair follicle.

Dermal Changes

Dermal changes extend from the papillary layer through to the junction between dermis and subcutaneous fat. There is a perivascular infiltrate of variable intensity composed of lymphocytes, histiocytes and eosinophils. Some of the latter are also sometimes found scattered amongst the collagen bundles and even in the subcutaneous fat. Papillary oedema may occur, especially when intraepidermal vesicles form. There may also be collections of neutrophils and even a few extravasated erythrocytes in the same area (Fernandez et al. 1977), whilst Hejazi and Mehregan (1975) have observed foci of breaking-down eosinophils in this region. The blood vessels may show endothelial swelling with the deposition of fibrinoid material in and around the vessel walls. The lumina of the vessels may show narrowing or even partial occlusion.

According to Hejazi and his colleague (1975), these findings are specific for scabies. These authors consider the appearance to be like erythema multiforme and the result of sensitisation to the mite and its products. They claimed to have confirmed this in one instance by skin tests with sarcoptic material. Ackerman and his colleagues (1975), on the other hand, think the changes are not those of erythema multiforme (by which they mean erythema multiforme exudativum of Hebra or the epidermal type of erythema multiforme), because there are no neutrophils and eosinophils present and the epidermal changes are not necrotic. Hejazi and Mehregan appear to have been referring to the dermal type of erythema, known in the United Kingdom as "toxic erythema".

Nodular Scabies

The histology resembles that of a lymphoma (Barale et al. 1971; Thomson et al. 1974; Fernandez et al. 1977; Garcovitch et al. 1978). There is moderate parakeratosis and acanthosis. There is spongiosis and occasional vesiculation in early lesions. Similarly, there may be dermal oedema in early lesions with dilation of papillary blood vessels, and fibrinoid necrosis with thrombi down to the deep vessels (Fig. 15.32). Fernandez et al. (1977) noted some thickening of the papillary collagen. There is a dense inflammatory infiltrate, diffuse in the superficial layers and perivascular in the deeper layers. In early lesions the infiltrating cells are mainly lymphocytes and eosinophils, but in older lesions histiocytes, fibroblasts and plasma cells predominate (Konstantinov and Stanoeva 1973; Fig. 15.33). Mast cells are increased in the pigmented macules (this may account for the urtication). Various stages of the *sarcoptes* or its faecal scybala have been seen in early lesions (see Fig. 15.32).

Norwegian Scabies

It is generally agreed that there is gross thickening of the stratum corneum as the result of hyperkeratosis and parakeratosis, the latter often being

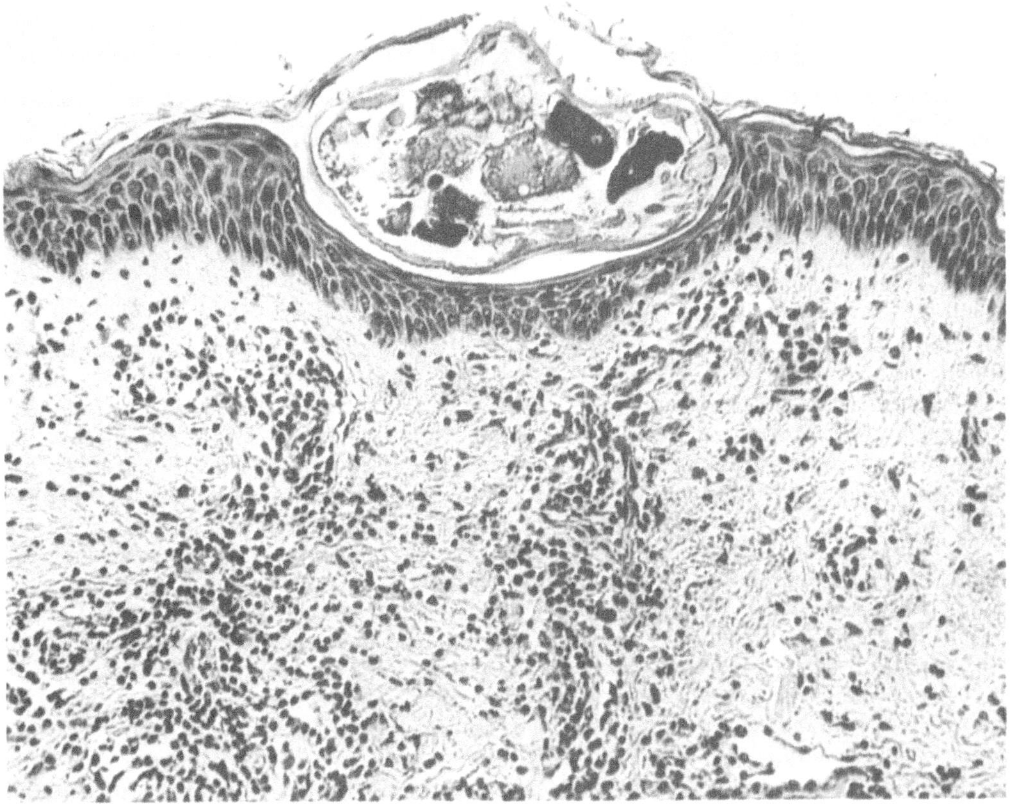

Fig. 15.32. Histology of nodular scabies. A section of *Sarcoptes scabiei* is seen in the keratin layer of the epidermis. In the dermis there is a pleomorphic infiltrate, which is predominantly perivascular, extending from the papillary to the deeper layers. (From Thomson et al. 1974, by kind permission of the authors and the Editor of the *British Journal of Dermatology*) H&E, x 64

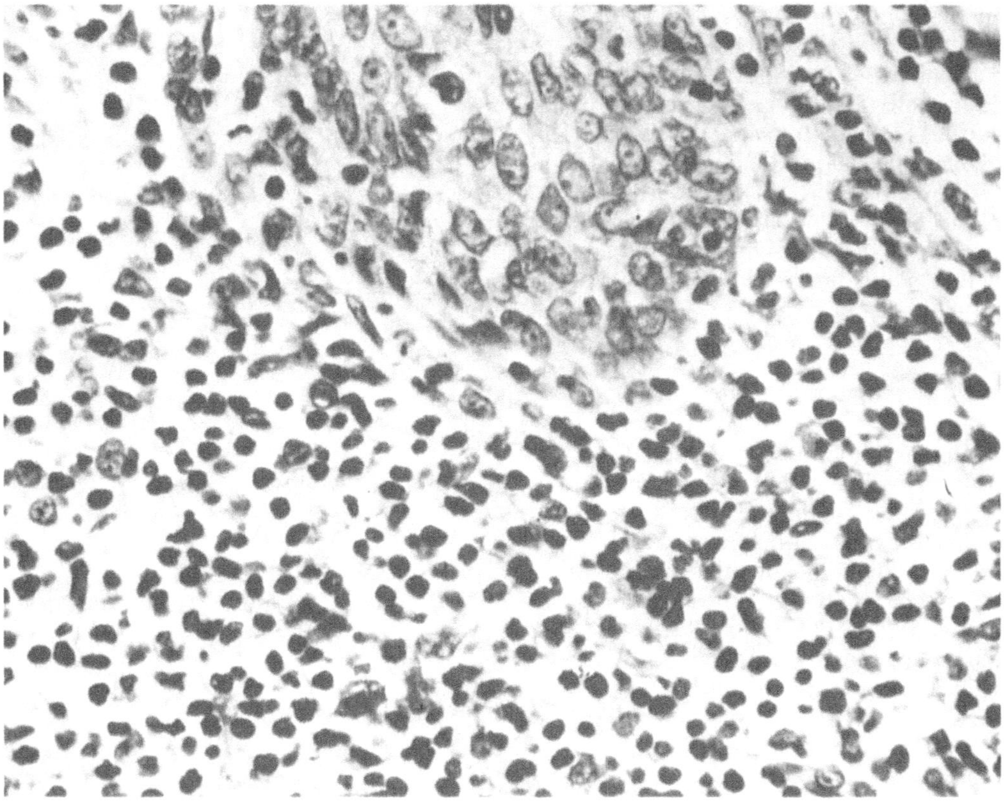

Fig. 15.33. Histology of persistent nodular scabies, showing pleomorphic dermal infiltrate with some large cell forms, nuclear hyperchromatism and occasional mitotic figures. (From Thomson et al. 1974, by kind permission of the authors and the Editor of the *British Journal of Dermatology*) H&E, × 400

patchy (Piers and Timms 1946). This layer is honeycombed with tunnels and galleries, the walls of which Ingram (1951) described as being composed of thin partitions of keratin. In these cavities vast numbers of *Sarcoptes* in all stages of development can be seen. Dubreuilh and Sainte-Marie (1924) noted collections of neutrophils and a few erythrocytes in the horny layer, and in addition to these features Ingram added that there was sometimes noted an increase in thickness of the stratum granulosum, a finding confirmed by Piers and Timms (1946). All workers have observed acanthosis; Dubreuilh and Sainte-Marie (1924) remarked that this was primarily due to a great increase in size of the interpapillary rete pegs, which was accompanied, as they and Konstantinov and Stanoeva (1976) agreed, by elongation of the dermal papillae and thinning of the stratum mucosum overlying the papillae. Dubreuilh and Sainte-Marie (1924) pointed out that the epidermis could be as thick as the dermis. There could also be spongiosis of a patchy nature (Bonaduce 1927), which Konstantinov and Stanoeva (1976) said was to be found beneath a burrow. Migration of inflammatory cells into the epidermis could cause tiny microabscesses in the mucosal layer (Cherikover 1937; Hay 1974).

In the dermis the papillae, in addition to being elongated, showed dilated and hyperaemic capillaries (Konstantinova and Stanoeva 1976). Cherikover (1937) and Konstantinov and Stanoeva (1973) agreed that there was papillary oedema associated (according to the former) with a lymphocytic and histiocytic infiltrate. Dubreuilh and Sainte-Marie (1924) said that eosinophils were uncommon in the papillary infiltrate, whilst Piers and Timms (1946) noted a marked inflammatory reaction in the papillae. Deeper in the dermis Bommer (1955) noted vascular changes, which he said had been described by Grutz, consisting of endothelial swelling, dilation of the vessels, complete or partial occlusion of some vessels by vesicular nucleated cells and even thrombi in some venules. He said the appearance resembled localised granulomata in or on the vessel walls, like those seen on nodular mesarteritis. A variety of cells were described around these deeper vessels: eosinophils and lymphocytes (Wishart 1972), lymphocytes and plasma cells (Bonaduce 1927; Ingram 1951), plus histiocytes (Konstantinov and Stanoeva 1976) and a polymorphic picture (Dubreuilh and Sainte-Marie 1924). Dubreuilh and Sainte-Marie (1924) and Piers and Timms (1946) emphasised the great preponderance of eosinophils in the infiltrate, matching the greatly increased number of circulating eosinophils.

Morphology of *Sarcoptes scabiei*

The itch mite of humans is zoologically classified as being in the order Acarina, suborder Sarcoptiformes, cohort Acaridae, family Sarcoptidae, subfamily Sarcoptinae, genus *Sarcoptes*, species *scabiei*. Those interested in the detailed minute anatomy of the *Sarcoptes* in all its stages are recommended to read Fain (1968) and Heilesen (1946), where full reference will be found to this aspect of the scabies mite. The following description, which is based on the papers of these two authors (and personal observation), should serve as a useful practical guide. The reader is also advised to consult pp. 11–14 for a definition of descriptive terms.

Adult Female

The adult female, the form commonly found when searching in burrows to confirm the clinical diagnosis (Fig. 15.34), has an ovoid body, which is flattened dorsoventrally and measures 300–500 μm long by 230–340 μm broad. Lunn (1944–1945) has pointed out that the size of *Sarcoptes* appears to vary and he attributed this to differing techniques of mounting specimens. For example, specimens measuring a mean of 368 μm long on a dry slide may increase to 373 μm on mounting in gum arabic; after covering with a coverslip this measurement increased on average to 415 μm, and compression of this coverslip increased this to 457 μm.

It has a creamy white-coloured body with brown legs and gnathosome (capitulum), the latter being the sclerotised parts. Viewed microscopically in potassium hydroxide the integument of the dorsal surface is finely striated more or less all over (Fig. 15.35). There are a large number of small triangular scales on the hysterosome area and also a small lateral and a small ventral group just posterior to legs III and IV. A number of short stout spines are arranged symmetrically on the dorsal surface. The most prominent of these, which

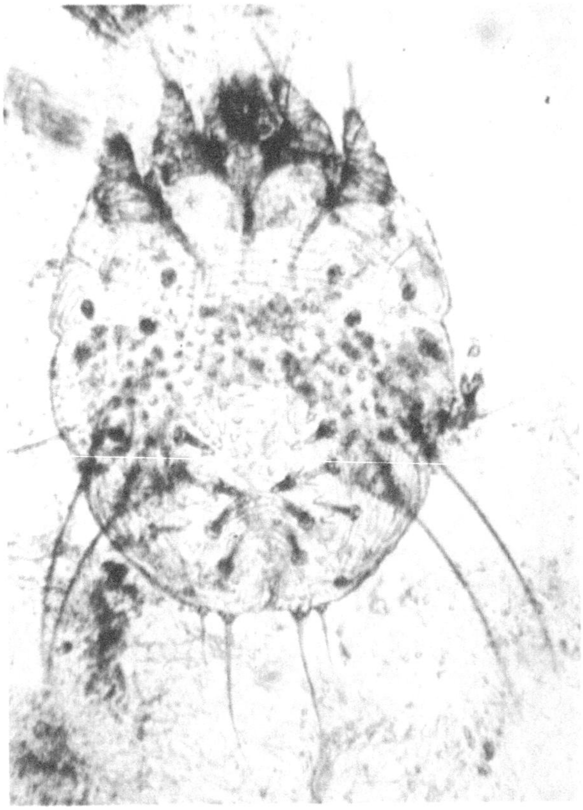

Fig. 15.34. Adult female *Sarcoptes scabiei* extracted from burrow and mounted in 30% potassium hydroxide.

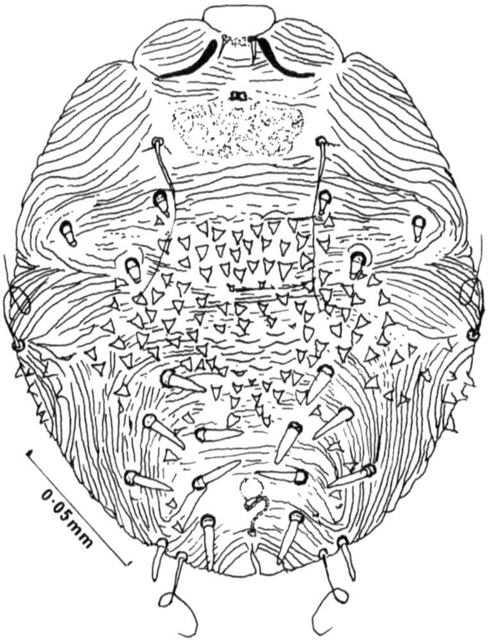

Fig. 15.35. Dorsal view of female *Sarcoptes scabiei* showing particularly the dorsal scales and spines. (After Fain 1968, by kind permission of the author and the Editor of *Acta Zoologica et Pathologica Antverpiensia*)

resemble inverted carpet tacks, are a group of 14, in two rows of three and four respectively, on either side of the midline posteriorly. There is a long posterior seta on each side, lateral to the anal opening. A vitally important structure, very difficult to see, is the minute copulatory bursa lying in the midline and opening dorsally anterior to the anal margin. It is not present in any of the immature forms.

In the midline at the anterior end, better seen on the ventral surface (Fig. 15.36), is the gnathosome. ("Gnathosome" is the correct modern nomenclature but the term "capitulum" is commonly used in clinical parlance.) It has a complicated symmetrical structure. There is a short jointed pedipalp curving slightly medially around an inner chelicera on each side. Each chelicera has two segments, the smaller being hinged to the larger. Both have an undulating surface like molar teeth and are used for chewing epidermal cells when burrowing and feeding. Lying medially and slightly ventrally to the chelicerae are the centrally fused mouthparts.

The four pairs of legs are arranged symmetrically. Legs I and II lie lateral to the gnathosome, whilst legs III and IV are situated laterally

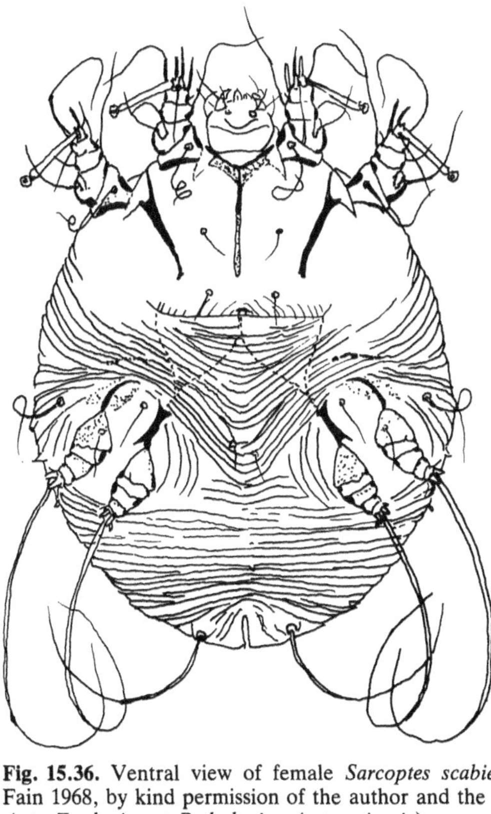

Fig. 15.36. Ventral view of female *Sarcoptes scabiei*. (After Fain 1968, by kind permission of the author and the Editor of *Acta Zoologica et Pathologica Antverpiensia*)

on the ventral surface on the anterior portion of the hysterosome. Each leg has five segments, the tarsus, tibia, genu, femur and trochanter, which appear as if telescoped into each other, an adaptation for living in an epidermal burrow. The tarsus of legs I and II terminates in an elongated peduncle tipped with a small sucker—which Heilesen (1948) described as a small flap rather like a minute piece of wash leather—beautifully illustrated in the scanning electron micrographs taken by Dr. Van Neste of Brussels (Figs. 15.37, 15.38). The tarsus of legs III and IV ends in a long seta. All four legs are supported at their base by sclerotised, exoskeletal structures called epimeres. Those for leg I are centrally fused into a common Y-shaped structure but the epimeres for the other legs are independent. There is a single transverse slit in the midline of the ventral surface mid-way between the epimeres of legs I and II and those of legs III and IV. This is the genital opening through which the egg is extruded (see also Pascual et al. 1977 for further details).

Adult Male

The male *Sarcoptes* (see Fig. 15.27) is much smaller than the female, measuring 213 μm long by 162–210 μm broad (Fain 1968). Dorsal striation is less well developed (Fig. 15.39). In common with all the immature forms it has only 12 spines in the posterior group. There are very few dorsal scales. The most obvious differences from the female are the legs III and IV and the genital apparatus (Fig. 15.40). The epimeres for these legs are fused into an inverted U shape. Leg IV has an elongated peduncle on the tarsus instead of a seta. In the midline there is a complicated chitinous structure housing the male genital organ.

Larval Stage

The larva (Figs. 15.41, 15.42) differs from all the other stages of *Sarcoptes* in having only six legs; leg IV is absent. In size it is about 215 μm long by 156 μm broad (Fain 1968). It is well striated and scales are present but less numerous than in the adult female.

Nymphal Stage

The nymph forms are seldom found clinically except in Norwegian scabies. They have also been observed by Heilesen (1946) in his experimental scabies where the mites were confined by restrictive apparatus. The first nymph measures 270 μm long by 196 μm broad (Fain 1968). The second nymph, studied almost exclusively by Heilesen

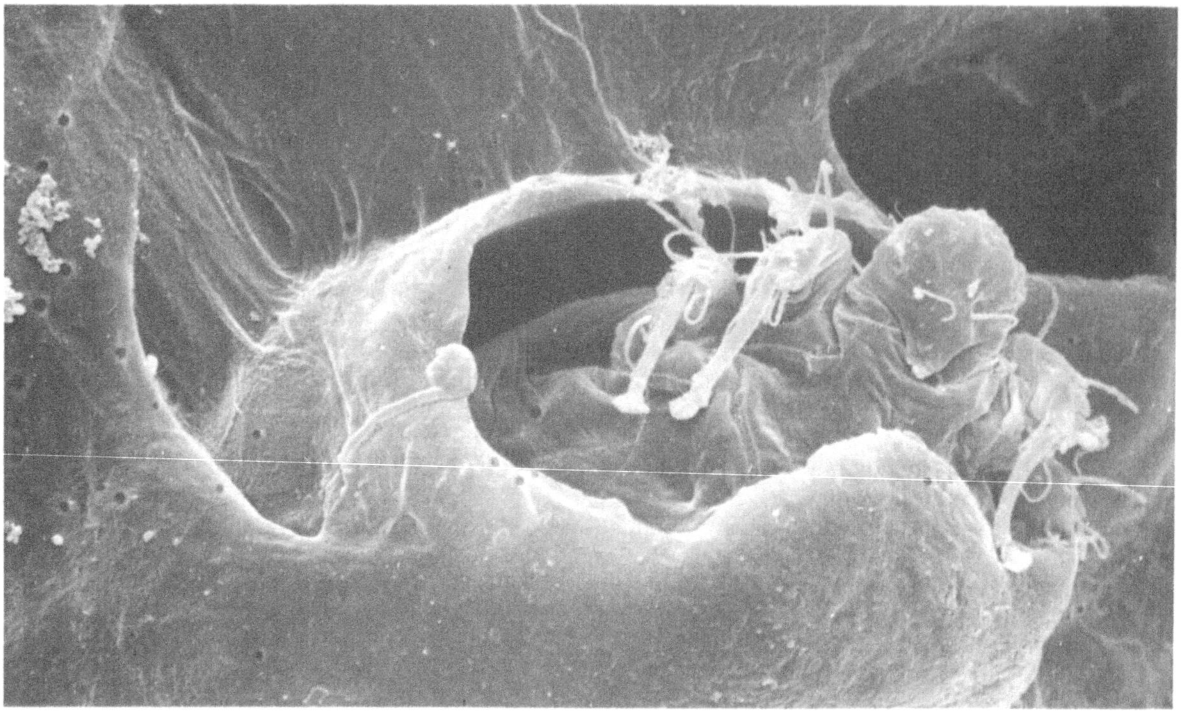

Fig. 15.37. Scanning electron micrograph of *Sarcoptes* larva emerging from the egg, from a case of Norwegian scabies. Showing the elongated ambulacrum and sucker-like pulvillus of legs I and II. (From Van Neste and Lachapelle (1981), by kind permission of Dr. Van Neste and the Editor of the *British Journal of Dermatology*)

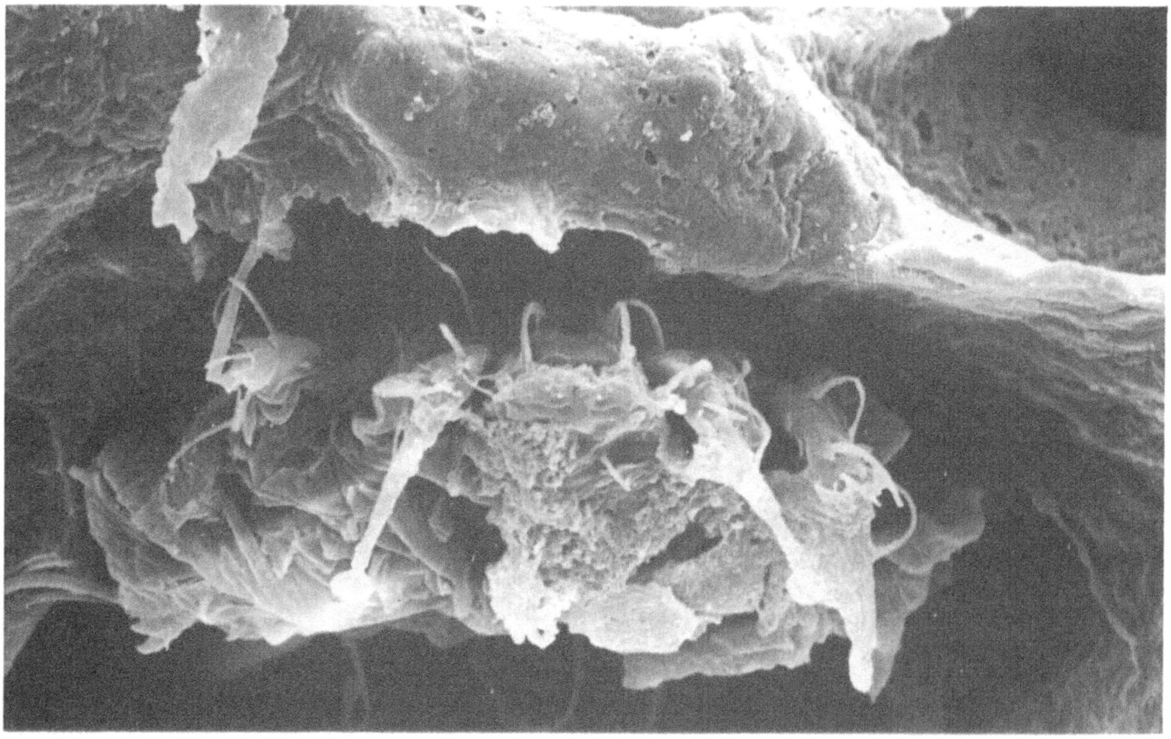

Fig. 15.38. Head-on-view of *Sarcoptes scabiei* (female) in burrow in Norwegian scabies. Showing mouthparts embedded in amorphous epidermal debris. (From Van Neste 1981, by kind permission of the author and the Editor of the *International Journal of Dermatology*)

(1946), measures 243 μm by 200 μm. The third nymph, equivalent to the adult female but lacking the copulatory bursa, is 340 μm by 270 μm (Fain 1968).

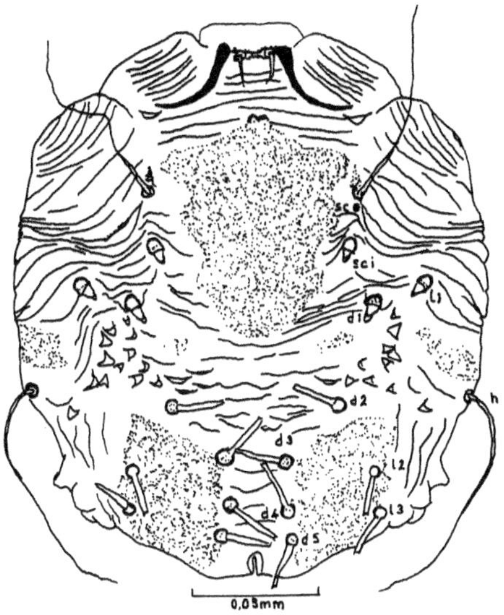

Fig. 15.39. Dorsal view of *Sarcoptes scabiei*, male. (After Fain 1968, by kind permission of the author and the Editor of *Acta Zoologica et Pathologica Antverpiensia*)

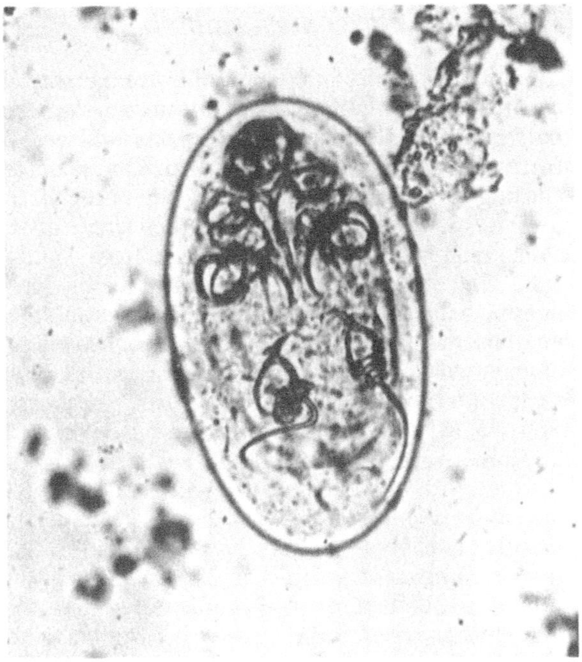

Fig. 15.41. Scabies egg with enclosed embryo, showing the six-legged larva in the "fetal" position. Taken from crusts from same patient as in Fig. 15.22 and mounted in 30% potassium hydroxide.

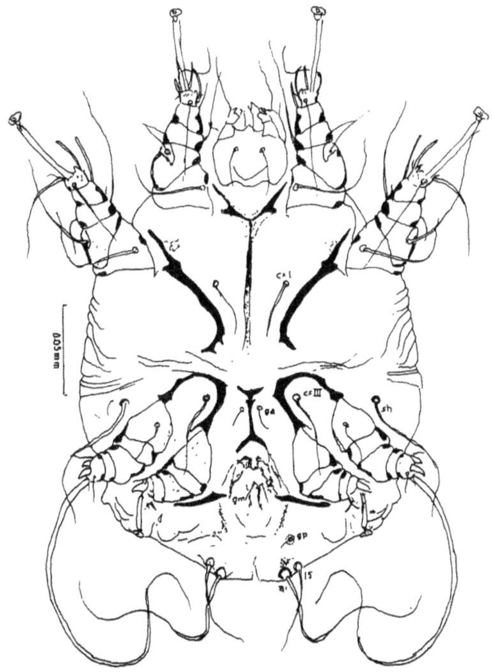

Fig. 15.40. Ventral view of male *Sarcoptes scabiei*. (After Fain 1968, by kind permission of the author and the Editor of *Acta Zoologica et Pathologica Antverpiensia*)

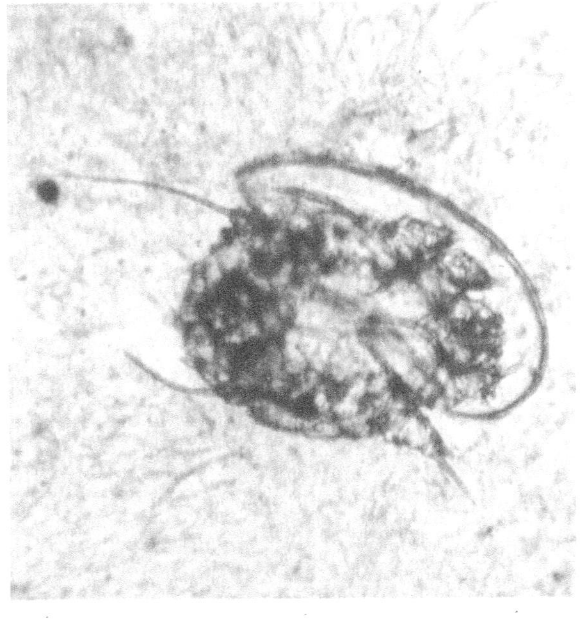

Fig. 15.42. *Sarcoptes scabiei* larva emerging from the egg. Taken from a scraping of scabies burrow and mounted in 30% potassium hydroxide. (From Alexander 1969, by kind permission of the Editor of *Clinical Pediatrics*)

Biology of *Sarcoptes scabiei*

The human scabies mite is an obligate parasite. It can thrive and multiply only on human skin. An ovigerous female placed on the skin will seek a furrow in which it rests for up to 30 min before starting to excavate a burrow. It chews the horny layer of the epidermis with the chelicerae, at the same time moving its gnathosome from side to side. Tiny fragments of epidermis are dislodged and the scale thus formed is levered upwards by the gnathosome. The digging process is continued and augmented by hook-shaped spines on the distal segments of the two pairs of front legs (see Figs. 15.36, 15.37, 15.38). These are used one side at a time, rather like a hen scratching in the dust. As the burrow is enlarged the mite will gradually disappear into it. According to Heilesen (1946) this usually takes about 20 min, but Munro (1919) said that it could take as little as $2\frac{1}{2}$ min. The boring rate is dependent on the ambient temperature. Once it has entered the burrow it lengthens it by about 2–3 mm daily. Forward movement is accompanied by side-to-side motion as if the creature is elbowing its way along. The hind legs assist by pressing the body against the roof of the burrow and then they are extended. The dorsal spines prevent backward movement (see Figs. 15.34, 15.35). Anderson (1894) considered that the general direction of the burrow was slightly downwards towards the granular layer and this, combined with the regular outgrowth of the epidermis, resulted in a tunnel parallel to the surface.

Bourguignon (1852) stated that the egg-laying female never left the original burrow, an opinion shared by many others. On the rare occasions on which it did so in Heilesen's experiments it at once began to make a new burrow. The burrows often show minute perforations in the roof, which Bourguignon attributed to the necessity for a supply of fresh air. Warburton (1920) and Heilesen (1946) both noted that larvae escaped from the parent burrow by boring through the roof, and this seems a rather more likely explanation for the holes.

Egg laying commences when the burrow is about 1 mm long and, according to Munro (1919), it alternates with burrowing. The latter goes on during the night when the host is warm in bed. During the daytime, when conditions are cooler for the skin, the mite rests. Then one or two eggs are deposited and the cycle is repeated the next night. A cycle of this type results in eggs being deposited in pairs with a space of empty burrow between. Faecal matter is also deposited in the vicinity of the eggs. If for any reason the burrowing is interrupted, e.g. by change of temperature, the next clutch of eggs will be found in close proximity to the previous ones. If egg laying and burrowing proceed at an even pace the interval between eggs is even (Fig. 15.43). Friedman (1942) depicted one such burrow in which no fewer than 38 eggs could be discerned. The female lives approximately 4–6 weeks and lays on average 40–50 eggs.

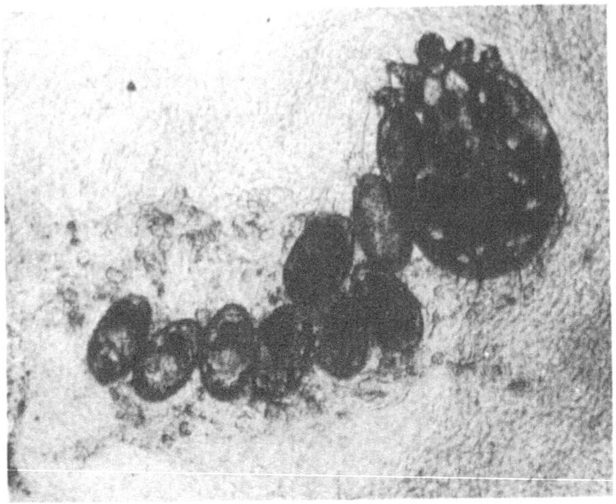

Fig. 15.43. Female *Sarcoptes scabiei* and eggs in burrow. From a scraping of a scabies burrow mounted in 30% potassium hydroxide. (From Alexander 1969, by kind permission of the Editor of *Clinical Pediatrics*)

The eggs hatch after 72–96 h. Gerlach (1857) estimated the time to be between 67 and 76 h, with which Munro (1919) and Heilesen (1946) agreed. Munro, however, pointed out that unfavourable conditions, e.g. cold, could temporarily halt development of the embryo, which would be resumed when the conditions returned to normal. The six-legged larva which emerges is very active. It may excavate a pocket just off the parent burrow or it may leave the parent burrow and at once dig a new burrow in the near vicinity, just large enough to conceal itself. This has been called a "moulting pocket" by Gordon and Lavoipierre (1962; Fig. 15.44). The larva sometimes leaves the pocket almost at once and makes another, but usually remains there until its transformation into a first nymph. Moulting involves the whole interior of the animal becoming a granular mass, from which an entirely new creature emerges, leaving only the empty external integument (the exuvium) as evidence of its previous existence. This stage in development also takes some 72–96 h. The first nymph behaves in a similar manner and after a further 72–96 h a second moult may give rise to an adult male or a second nymph. The latter has to go through a third moult to produce a young adult

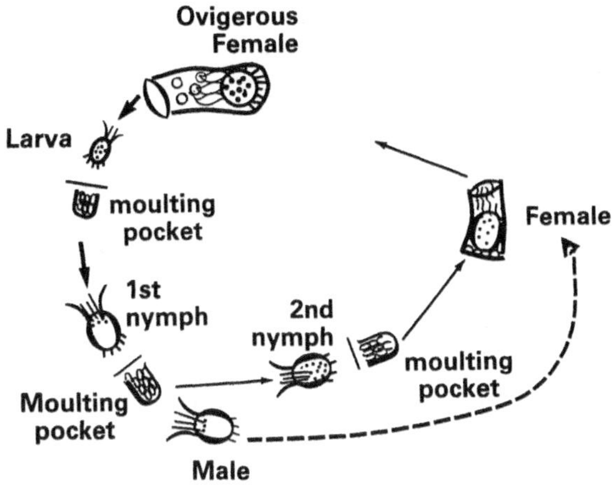

Fig. 15.44. Life cycle of *Sarcoptes scabiei*. (After Gordon and Lavoipierre 1962, by kind permission of Prof. M.M.J. Lavoipierre and the publisher, Blackwell Scientific Publications)

female. Each moulting stage requires a fresh burrow to be excavated. The male is the most active of all forms (Heilesen 1946) and immediately begins to search for an adult female. Success may be achieved within the hour or may take several days and involve much travelling about, with rests in tiny pockets. In the neighbourhood of an adult female it becomes agitated, running to and fro and even in circles before suddenly boring into the female burrow. Heilesen (1946) noted that once inside the short burrow it climbs on top of the female, wedging itself between the latter and the roof of the burrow. When in position just over half the male mite will be on the back of the female. It then turns through 180° and remains in this copulating posture for several minutes. This 180° turn is evidently necessary, as Heilesen observed it on several occasions. Copulation only occurs inside the female burrow and only with an adult female. Second nymphs are ignored (Heilesen 1946). Buxton (1921) pointed out that the second nymph does not possess a copulatory bursa and fertilisation is impossible without this minute structure.

It is generally agreed that the female only copulates once. Friedman (1947) quoted Bourguignon (1852) to the effect that a male could fertilise several females, but Heilesen (1946) observed that after copulation the male shrivelled up and died within 48 h. Once fertilisation has occurred, the female continues vigorously to enlarge her burrow and start the whole cycle over again.

Tiny vesicles occur beneath the burrows of all stages of the developing *Sarcoptes*, although only Heilesen has observed this phenomenon in relation to second nymphs. It is probably the result of chemical irritation by a fluid said by Bourguignon (1852) to be secreted to assist in the digestion of horn cell material. There is a reactionary flow of intercellular fluid to the irritated area. By the time enough has collected to form a visible vesicle (usually 2–4 days), the burrowing mite will have moved forward. It will thus be just visible at the blind end of the burrow, to one side of the vesicle. That this is a delayed reaction was confirmed by Heilesen (1946), who saw a vesicle appear beneath an empty burrow after it had been vacated by its occupant.

The general belief is that scabies is spread by a gravid female *Sarcoptes* transferring to a new host and burrowing there. In support of this contention Mellanby (1944a) cited instances in which men who had never previously had scabies showed burrows containing an egg within 3 days of exposure. This could only have come about by an adult fertilised female transferring to the new host. Similar occurrences have been reported in contacts with Norwegian scabies who contracted scabies within 3 days of contact. Mellanby added that experimental infestation could easily be achieved by the transference of fertilised adult females, but transfer of immature mites very seldom resulted in scabies developing. However, the spread of scabies by adult female mites which have been fertilised does not accord with the observed fact that the ovigerous female rarely leaves her original burrow. There is no evidence to suggest that this habit changes in order to transfer to another host. On the other hand, all the immature stages actively move about on the skin surface, moulting in special short burrows. The number of mites maturing from 40 to 50 eggs produced by the female usually considerably outnumber the parent, although many perish. The wandering propensity of the immature forms places them in a very favourable situation for transfer to another host. Munro (1919) placed four larvae on the skin of a non-scabietic and in due course the burrow of an ovigerous female appeared, thus indicating that at least one of each sex developed from the larvae and established scabies in the new host. It seems most likely that this is what often occurs naturally and would seem to vindicate the view expressed by Pye-Smith (1893) and Hyde (1905). It would also explain why spread occurs less frequently through clothing and bedding, because these would probably only contain immature forms (usually very few) and they do not survive for much more than 24 h away from the human body. In Norwegian scabies, where the number of mites is enormously increased, such means of spread is very likely even through clothing (see p. 247).

Parasitology

Johnson and Mellanby (1942) and Bartley and Mellanby (1944) collected in two consecutive and meticulous searches all the adult female mites (considered by them to comprise at least 95% of those present) from 886 men and from 119 women and 18 children respectively. The number on each individual they called the "parasite rate", which they regarded as a reliable indicator of the degree of infestation. Heilesen (1946) made similar collections from 123 men and 152 women but from only a single examination. The parasite rates for Mellanby's patients were 11.3 for men, 12.1 for women and 19.7 for children. Heilesen's rates for men were 6.3 and for women 7.3. Figure 15.45 shows that about 50% of Mellanby's patients had from 1 to 5 mites and a further 20% between 6 and 10. Only an occasional patient had a parasite rate in excess of 100, the highest record being 511. Detailed figures for children were not given. Table 15.8 shows the comparative distribuion of mites in various sites. The great majority were higher in women. Children had many more mites on the feet and ankles than did adults. In Heilesen's (1946) patients relatively very few mites were found in the latter areas. On the other hand, he found more on the genitalia than did Mellanby and his colleagues. The other striking feature was the paucity of mites on the palms in men; in fact Mellanby did not find any.

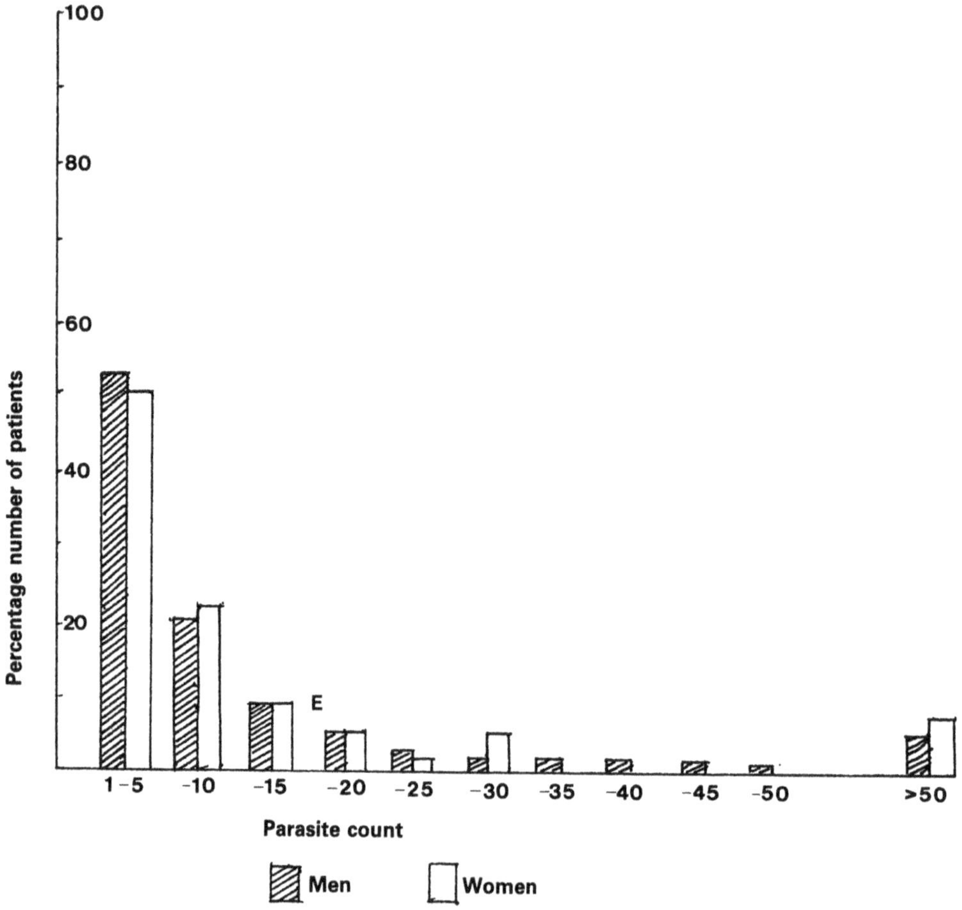

Fig. 15.45 Histogram showing parasite rates as percentages in 886 men and 119 women. (From Johnson and Mellanby 1942 and Bartley and Mellanby 1944, by kind permission of Prof. K. Mellanby and the Permissions Controller, Cambridge University Press)

Table 15.8. Comparison of distribution of parasites in men, women and children[a]

	Men		Women		Children
Sites	Johnson and Mellanby (1942)	Heilesen (1946)	Bartley and Mellanby (1944)	Heilesen (1946)	Bartley and Mellanby (1944)
Hands and wrists (not palms)	63.1%	68.3%	74.3%	77.6%	55.5%
Palms	—	1.4	7.5	5.6	6.8
Elbows	10.9	—	5.9	—	4.8
Feet and ankles	9.2	5.6	8.8	6.7	20.3
Penis and scrotum	8.4	14.3	—	—	3.6
Buttocks	4.0	0.6	1.1	—	3.2
Axillary folds	2.4	3.3	0.9	2.1	1.3
Knees	0.7	0.1	0.3	0.1	2.3
Umbilicus	0.4	2.4	0.1	0.5	0.6
Chest	0.1	—	0.1	—	—
Breasts	—	—	0.5	1.5	—
Other sites	0.8	2.4	0.5	1.0	1.6

[a] Figures taken from Johnson and Mellanby (1942), Bartley and Mellanby (1944) and Heilesen (1946) by kind permission of Prof. K. Mellanby and the Permissions Controller, Cambridge University Press, and by kind permission of Dr. B. Heilesen and the Editor of *Acta Dermato-venerologica* (*Stockholm*)

Although the figures are difficult to compare, the frequency with which individual sites were affected differed considerably in the various groups (Table 15.9). The percentage of individuals with at least one burrow on the hands and wrists was very high (100% in children), but noticeably higher in women than in men. There were several discrepancies in the figures for men between those given by Heilesen (1946) and those by Johnson and Mellanby (1942). These were unexplained. In general the distribution of mites in children was more diffuse that in adults, but the number of children examined was relatively very small. All the figures reinforce the necessity to examine the whole body in anyone suspected of having scabies.

Johnson and Mellanby (1942) pointed out that the number of parasites by no means always showed a steady increase as the disease progressed, rapid falls in the parasite rate being frequent (see p. 262). They noted that severe cases with widespread lesions did not always have many parasites and, conversely, that patients with few lesions often had many mites. Heilesen (1946), on the other hand, thought that there was a fairly good correlation between the parasite rate and the severity of the eruption.

Table 15.9. Frequency with which various sites are infested with *Sarcoptes*[a]

	Men		Women	Children
Sites	Johnson and Mellanby (1942)	Heilesen (1946)	Heilesen (1946)	Bartley and Mellanby (1944)
Hands and wrists (not palms)	84.8%	82.1%	93.4%	100.0%
Palms	—	—	—	44.4
Elbows	40.5	18.7	24.3	33.3
Feet and Ankles	37.0	8.1	25.6	77.8
Penis and Scrotum	36.0	33.3	—	44.4
Buttocks	15.8	2.4	—	33.3
Axillary folds	14.7	18.7	9.2	22.2
Knees	6.4	0.8	0.7	22.2
Umbilicus	3.0	8.1	3.9	11.1
Breasts	—	—	8.6	—
Other sites	up to 2.5	8.1	7.2	up to 5.6

[a] Figures taken from Johnson and Mellanby (1942), Bartley and Mellanby (1944) and Heilesen (1946) by kind permission of Prof. K. Mellanby and the Permissions Controller, Cambridge University Press, and by kind permission of Dr. B .Heilesen and the Editor of *Acta Dermato-venereologica* (*Stockholm*)

Mellanby (1944a) examined the parasite rate, by counting burrows, repeatedly over periods varying between 50 and 200 days in 55 individuals with no previous history of scabies during a voluntary first experimental infestation, repeating this exercise on the same volunteers after they had been cured and subsequently re-infested. Heilesen inspected 172 persons with a first infestation and 62 different individuals with re-infestation, each apparently on a single occasion. Mellanby found the parasite rate in general to be much higher during the primary infestation than in subsequent attacks. His results are illustrated in Figs. 15.46 and 15.47. The graphs in Fig. 15.46 show clearly the steady increase in rate with a peak reach in 80–115 days and then a fall. The re-infested patients (Fig. 15.47) did not show the same type of rise and fall, although the rate in some did reach as high as 40 at times. Nevertheless, comparing individuals in the two attacks the rate was always much higher in the first attack. Heilesen's figures at first sight appear in direct contradiction to this, as he found parasite rates in the two groups to be much the same. It should be remembered, however, that he was not discussing the same patients with two attacks but two different groups of patients, so that the two sets of figures are not strictly comparable. Secondly, Mellanby's patients were volunteers whom he watched under conditions over which he had control, whilst Heilesen's patients were attending as ordinary hospital outpatients. Mellanby has pointed out in this respect that such patients would include many who had endeavoured to treat themselves before coming to hospital, and treatment, though insufficient for cure, would reduce the number of parasites. Secondary infection, when it occurs, also reduces the number of mites and would have been more likely in Heilesen's patients than in those of Mellanby because of the absence of control. Nevertheless, Heilesen did observe that the number of re-infested patients with low parasite rates was rather higher than the corresponding number with first attack.

Mellanby recorded in his study that almost every mite which burrowed could be identified in its burrow for the first 5 or 6 weeks during a first attack. The second generation of ovigerous females was never found earlier than on day 21 after infestation, although it was theoretically possible for them to appear in 10–14 days. He regarded this

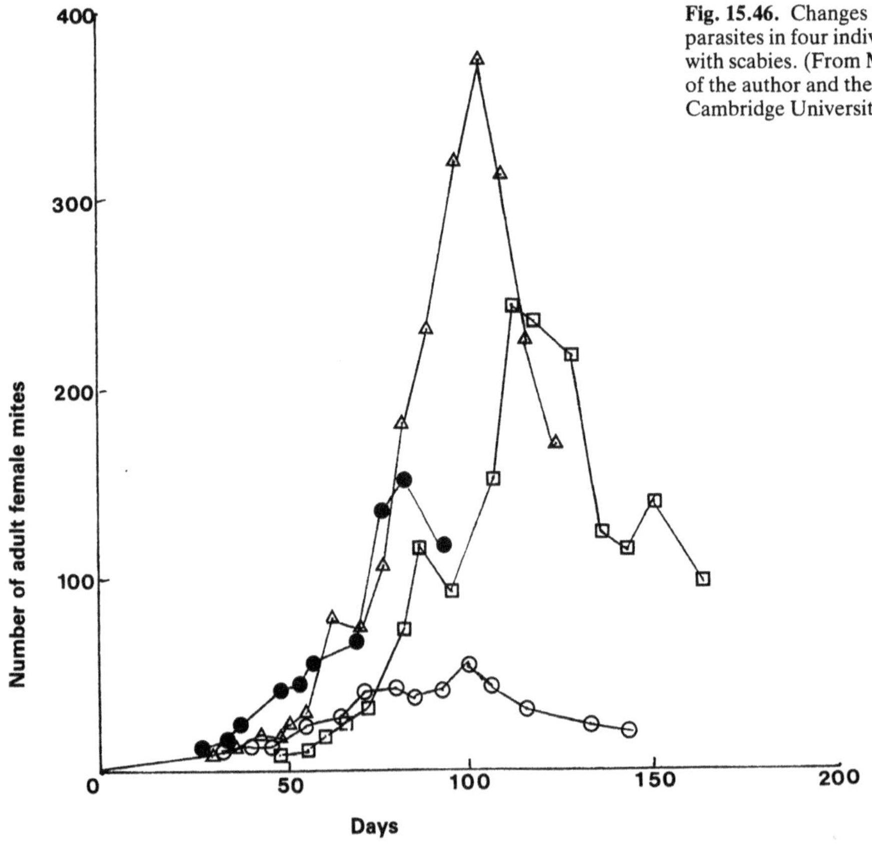

Fig. 15.46. Changes in the number of adult female parasites in four individuals infested for the first time with scabies. (From Mellanby 1944, by kind permission of the author and the Permissions Controller, Cambridge University Press)

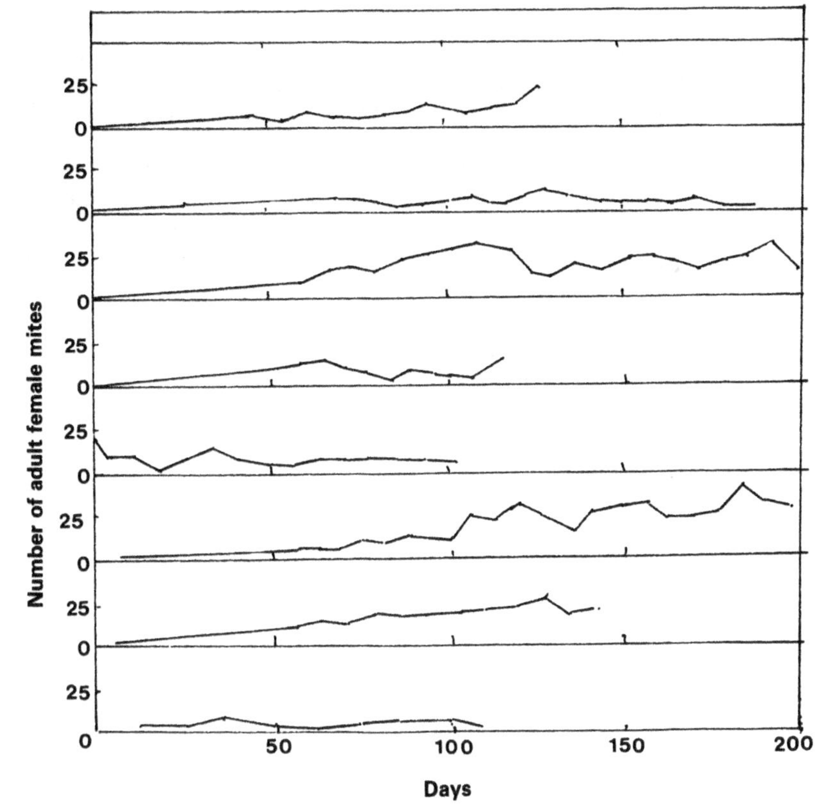

Fig. 15.47. Changes in the parasite rate of adult female parasites in eight persons infested with scabies who had all previously had scabies. (From Mellanby 1944, by kind permission of the author and the Permissions Controller, Cambridge University Press)

as an indication of general wastage during development. He said that the lower parasite rate in re-infested persons could be accounted for by the dual effects of scratching and the unfavourable environment created by host reaction induced by the first infestation.

Immunology

Hebra (1868) first observed that the eruption and itch in scabies extended beyond the areas where the *Sarcoptes* burrowed. Noting that some physicians considered that scabietics might have a predisposition to the disease he remarked that "everyone can afford the accommodation needed by the acarus", adding that the infesting mite should be a gravid female. He also considered that the different clinical picture in Norwegian scabies could be due to an alteration of the "soil" in which the mite developed.

According to Dubreuilh and Beille (1895), Hardy induced reactive itching in the skin by the inoculation of the products of eight mites, control test results being negative. Sezary (1934) using an alcoholic extract of crushed mites obtained negative results. Kitchevatch and Pochtich (1934) tested 146 scabietics with an alcoholic extract from the crusts of a patient with Norwegian scabies with immediate-type response and also in some cases a partial delayed response to intradermal injections, all control test results being negative. (Both references were cited by Prakken and van Vloten 1949).

Mellanby noted (1941a) that the less the host reaction the better the conditions for the parasites to multiply. He emphasised (1942) what Adams had observed in 1807, namely that there was a symptomless period of about 3–4 weeks in scabies before symptoms occurred, which could sometimes be shortened to 1 week if the initial infestation was very heavy (Mellanby 1943). Then a widespread papular eruption accompanied by increasingly severe itch would suddenly appear. This he regarded as a true sensitisation (Mellanby 1943), thus confirming a suggestion made by Warburton (1920) that the eruption was a secondary phenomenon in the disease. Histologically he noted that there was an eczematous reaction with vascular congestion and dilation beneath an area of spongiosis and neutrophil polymorphonuclear exocytosis. This sometimes produced clinically visible vesicles lying beneath the burrow and just behind the burrowing *Sarcoptes* (Mellanby 1943; 1944a). Heilesen (1946) also noted spongiosis immediately below the point where the mite's gnathosome was buried in the upper stratum mucosum (see p. 250). Mellanby also observed (1943) that re-infestation of a cured patient evoked an instant response with localised erythema and weal around the invading mite and a recrudescence of rash and severe itch within 24 h. The mite quickly disappeared, he said, because the oedematous reaction produced an unfavourable environment for it (Mellanby 1944a). He regarded this as evidence of previous sensitisation and antibody production and thought the antigen responsible for this was in the sarcoptic digestive juices. He observed that when re-infestation occurred the number of mites which succeeded in establishing themselves was usually very small, perhaps three to four. Nevertheless, he pointed out, this number was sufficient to maintain the antigenic effect and the clinical rash. It was noted that when all the mites were removed the reaction could persist for some time after this removal. In addition, he declared that, whereas in experimental infestation of volunteers success was the rule, about 60% of attempts to re-infest cured scabietics failed. Using intradermal injections of a watery extract of *Sarcoptes* he demonstrated an immediate weal and flare reaction in six of seven patients who had been infested with scabies for more than 3 months. Patients who had been cured of scabies responded to the tests with generalised irritation, which was most marked in those areas where lesions had previously been. Mellanby concluded that in clinical scabies antibody formation occurred, but only became evident after 4–6 weeks, increasing in strength thereafter but only reaching sufficient concentration to react to intradermal tests after about 6 months.

Heilesen (1946) agreed that there was a shorter incubation period for subsequent experimental infestation than for the initial attack and that the reaction seemed to be stronger. However, in patients he found the incubation period to be much the same for first and subsequent infestations and he found that there was no difference in the number of mites found on those infested for the first time compared with those in re-infested patients (see under Parasitology, p. 262).

Mellanby, however, made repeated examinations of the same persons, whilst Heilesen's figures are based on single examinations. Heilesen could not confirm Mellanby's results with intradermal tests except for a few positive results. This could have been because almost all his patients had itched for less than 3 months. The three markedly positive reactions either had a severe eruption or a history of more than one attack previously.

Prakken and van Vloten (1949) confirmed Mellanby's intradermal tests by using an extract made from the crusts of a patient with Norwegian scabies. With serum from the same patient they obtained positive passive transfer reactions (Prausnitz–Kustner reaction), but when they used serum from patients with ordinary scabies the results were always negative.

Barthelmes and Barthelmes (1974) agreed with Mellanby's conclusions but repeated the intradermal tests using an extract of *Notoedres alepis*, a sarcoptic mite found on laboratory rats. This extract cross-reacted with extract of *Sarcoptes scabiei* but, unlike the latter, contained no antigenic material of human origin. They showed that about 50% of scabietics gave a positive immediate response to the tests, the results indicating that the older the patient, the longer the duration of the eruption, and the more extensive and eczematised the eruption, the more likely the reaction was to be positive, and vice versa. Secondary infection tended to make the tests unreliable. They confirmed these results in a second series of 23 patients, all with marked scabies. All showed strongly positive reactions. In a third series they showed that the technique had a certain diagnostic value in difficult or doubtful cases. They also noted that three patients with persistent nodules had marked immediate-type reaction when tested intradermally.

In the past 6 or 7 years most investigators have concentrated on studying immunoglobulin levels in the serum of scabietics. Hancock and Milford-Ward (1974) found serum IgA levels to be significantly below normal in scabietics, irrespective of the duration of the disease. Randazzo et al. (1977) also found reduced serum IgA values in scabietics, especially in young children; in two patients the levels were raised and this he attributed to scratching. Falk (1980) measured serum levels of IgA during the stage of active disease and found them to be significantly lower than the levels at 6 and 9 months after successful treatment. The latter values were not significantly different, suggesting that return to normal occurred fairly quickly after the scabies was cured. Both Randazzo and Falk found IgG levels to be increased in scabies, noting that the value returned to normal slowly over the next 9 months. Frentz et al. (1977) demonstrated positive IgM immunofluorescence along the basement membrane zone in two of 11 patients, but only in lesions which contained a *Sarcoptes*.

Hancock and Milford-Ward (1974) found normal levels of serum IgE in 200 scabietics regardless of the duration of symptoms, and Randazzo et al. (1977) found the values to be elevated in 20% of their patients. Araujo-Fontaine et al. (1977) noted raised levels in only 15% of their patients, which they attributed either to liver disease or to the affected persons being atopic. Larregue et al. (1976) found increased serum IgE levels in 13 of 20 children with scabies but free of any other parasitic disease. The average figure for these 13 was 1442 units/ml compared with the upper limit of normal for their laboratory of 80 units/ml. All the 13 children had had scabies for over 2 months, all were under 6 years of age and many had nodular lesions. The high values persisted for up to 1 month after cure.

Falk (1980) noted raised serum IgE levels in 39 of 94 scabietics investigated at the time of presentation. Falk and Bolle (1980a) obtained similar results in 45% of 135 patients with scabies; 35% of the same group had positive radioallergosorbent test (RAST) reactions to *Dermatophagoides pteronyssinus* (DP) antigen, and 23% of 120 who completed a questionnaire were atopic. In a matched control group the respective percentages were 4%, 2% and 9%. The authors said that this indicated that scabies stimulated IgE production even in non-atopic persons. The same workers (1980b) tested 12 persons cured of scabies, seven less than and five more than 1 year previously. IgE value was raised in only two. These patients were tested by intradermal injection of extract of *Sarcoptes*. The seven more recently infested had positive immediate reactions, the others were negative. Prick tests were negative in all 12, presumably because the antigen was too weak. Intradermal tests with commercial DP extracts gave the same results, and five of the seven with positive intradermal tests had positive prick test reactions to DP extract. Four of the seven had positive RAST reactions to *Sarcoptes* antigen. Three control patients, all with a history of atopy, also had positive reactions to *Sarcoptes* antigen. The *Sarcoptes* extract and DP extract had been shown to cross-react, and these latter results in control patients with atopy confirmed this.

Van Neste et al. (1979) obtained immediate type I reactions in one patient with ordinary scabies and one with Norwegian scabies. The latter also gave a positive basophil degranulation test result against material containing scales and sarcoptic material but not against scales alone. This, the authors stated, indicated involvement of IgE associated with scabies antigenic material. Rantanen et al. (1981) confirmed this when they found IgE antibodies specific to scabies in two of five patients examined and elevated serum IgE levels in eight of 16 patients.

Frentz et al. (1977) demonstrated immunofluorescent C3 deposits in the basement membrane zone in two biopsies containing a *Sarcoptes* and in one lesion which contained no mite. Van Neste and Lachapelle (1981) confirmed this in one patient with Norwegian scabies. Salo and Reunala (1977) and Salo et al. (1982) noted positive immunofluorescent C3 deposits in the blood vessels of the corium in biopsies of papules from eight of 11 scabietics, which they considered to be a further indication that immunological factors played a part in the formation of scabies lesions.

Van Neste and Salmon (1978) found circulating immune complexes in the serum, as measured by C1q binding, in 29 scabietics, the results in 52 controls being negative. The patients examined had already been treated and the authors claimed that the treatment had released antigenic material in the skin, which lead to the formation of the complexes. Salo et al. (1982) also found IgM and IgA deposits around the dermal blood vessels in three and two patients respectively. They could not detect circulating immune complexes but found circulating IgM antibodies of a rheumatoid type in five of 32 sera using a special technique, suggesting that local complement activation and perhaps immune complex deposition was important in the pathogenesis of papular and nodular lesions of human scabies.

Discussion

The findings which have been described afford strong, but as yet inconclusive, evidence that the clinical features of scabies have an immunological basis. Mellanby regarded the generalised eruption as a sensitisation phenomenon and there is now general agreement with his view. He pointed out that the slowly developing immune reaction could have accounted for the cyclical occurrence of scabies in the Middle Ages, producing population immunity, an idea which was revived and emphasised by Shrank and Alexander (1967). In 1977, when Mellanby was reviewing the immunological position of scabies, he noted that transmission was most likely to be effected by those with large numbers of mites, and these individuals were expected to be found in populations in which few cases had recently been seen and in which the majority would in all probability never have had scabies. The major cause of periodicity of outbreaks of scabies he attributed to the difference between the reactions of the unsensitised and the re-infested (Mellanby 1977c).

Marples (1965), on the other hand, suggested that the sensitivity reaction might in fact be a reaction to staphylococci in scabietic burrows and not to the sarcoptes. She said that when infection (i.e. with staphylococci) was established, synergism, which existed between the mites and the bacteria in the burrows at first, ceased and antagonism began. It is true that *Sarcoptes* do not flourish in the presence of pus, which indicates the establishment of bacterial infection, and are never found in burrows where there is clinically obvious infection. The corollary to this suggestion, however, is that widespread secondary infection should cause the scabies to disappear along with the mites. If this were so, heavily infected scabies could be cleared by antibiotics alone, whereas all clinical experience is to the contrary. Secondary infection in scabies cannot be cured until antiscabietic treatment has first been used.

Shrank and Alexander pointed out that the increased incidence of scabies observed in 1967 was not due to resistance to treatment, as had been suggested, since none had really been encountered. Supporting Mellanby's theory of population immunity, they felt that the upsurge of scabies in the United Kingdom—and noted a year or two later in the United States (Orkin 1971)—was due to some loss of this immunity through the rarity of scabies for some years. Indeed the writer of an Editorial (1976a) in the *British Medical Journal* doubted whether there were in fact a sufficient number of cases in the United Kingdom to produce any of the so-called herd immunity at all. This is a somewhat false argument since there are always many more cases in the community than is revealed by hospital statistics. Any immunity which does occur is only partial; herd immunity is merely the sum of the immunity of the members of the herd and therefore is also likely to be only partial at best. If the Editorial writer were correct, then one would not expect scabies to persist in tropical areas where anything from 20% to 100% of the population, whether rural or urban, are constantly infested. Herd immunity seems to have no effect in these areas, but in fact scabies is present in such vast numbers because there is constant re-infestation after treatment. Even mass treatment in confined areas fails to get rid of scabies (Nair et al. 1973). It would seem that if immunology factors are at work in these countries they are heavily outweighed by other factors, such as gross overcrowding, which are conducive to the spread of the disease. In the United Kingdom, where such overcrowding does not occur to the same extent, the influence of immunity is felt and the incidence of scabies is low.

The special forms of scabies pose their own problems. Prakken and van Vloten (1949) suggested that in Norwegian scabies there was an especially strong allergy (i.e. antibody formation) because the serum from their patient gave positive Prausnitz–Kustner reactions, whereas the serum from cases of ordinary scabies did not. It has been suggested that Norwegian scabies is the only form of scabies in which an "immunity" (i.e. asymptomatic response) exists—although Orkin (1975a) has more correctly described Norwegian scabies as being an anergic form of scabies—so that the patient did not react and the *Sarcoptes* proliferated. This seems to be a paradoxical statement since immunity in the immunological sense means antibody production. When the antigen is present there is a reaction, and Mellanby has quoted such a reaction as being one of the reasons for the disappearance of the mites on re-infesting a cured patient. However, there is no reaction of this kind in Norwegian scabies. In those cases where Norwegian scabies is precipitated by immunosuppressive therapy it is understandable, since the suppressing agents prevent such reaction even if antibodies are present. Burgess (1973) has stressed this very point. It is possible also to explain the disease in those with impaired sensations or with mental deficiency as they also have impaired immune status. But there are instances of Norwegian scabies occurring in otherwise normal persons (see p. 245), where the reasons why they develop this particular form of scabies cannot as yet be explained on immunological grounds.

In nodular scabies there is marked pleomorphism of the cellular reaction extending deeply into the dermis (Thomson et al. 1974, confirmed by Barthelmes and Barthelmes 1974) which could well be immunological in origin. It starts beneath a burrow and persists long after the mite has disappeared. Barthelmes and his colleague found positive reaction to intradermal tests, which is probably related to the high IgE levels in those patients found by Larregue et al. (1976) and the finding of IgE deposits around the blood vessels by Frentz et al. (1977).

As far as immunoglobulins are concerned, it seems to be established that IgE antibodies play a part in the production of lesions in scabies. Dockhorn (1974) noted that the reactions to "insect" bites are of the IgE type and that some allergic eczemas are similarly mediated, as well as the type I reaction in atopic persons.

The writer of an Editorial (1976b) in the *Lancet* pointed out that parasites were a potent stimulus for the induction of IgE antibodies, that they could potentiate a pre-existing antibody response to an unrelated antigen and that there appeared to be a relationship between allergy and parasitic infestation. Although some of the authors already quoted above did not find elevated IgE levels, those who examined the matter in more detail found raised values (tenfold or more) in the very young and in those with an atopic history. A lesser number of other patients also showed such increases in serum IgE levels but many had normal levels. The results of Falk and Bolle (1980a, b) suggested that there might be a correlation between the IgE levels and the degree of RAST response. The latter indicated allergy to a different, although in the present instance cross-reacting, antigen, which bears out the opinion of the Editorial writer referred to above. The value of positive intradermal tests against the *Sarcoptes* antigen as a possible aid to diagnosis in difficult cases (Barthelmes and Barthelmes 1974) has been greatly reduced by the demonstration by Falk and Bolle of positive reactions in atopic persons who have never previously had scabies. The ubiquitous mite, *Dermatophagoides pteronyssinus*, is responsible for this. The contention that atopics have a predilection for scabies is rather tenuous. The present writer's experience has given him the impression that this is not the case. Certainly scabies in patients with atopic eczema is not a common occurrence and the writer of the Editorial (1976b) in the *Lancet* noted that, for example, asthma and hay fever were rare in those areas where parasites were abundant. Falk and Bolle (1980b) claimed that the positive reactions to intradermal tests represented specific immunological reactions in scabies and this, they said, had been confirmed by the Prausnitz–Kustner tests which they performed. However, they added that the IgE antibody measured could be either to *Sarcoptes scabiei* or *Dermatophagoides pteronyssinus*. Negative RAST reactions and two negative Prausnitz–Kustner reactions were explained by suggesting that the IgE in those cases was localised and not circulating, a suggestion supported to some extent by the findings of Frentz and his colleagues (1977).

The role played by other immunoglobulins is much less important. That associated with changes in IgM and IgG levels is nebulous. The fall in IgA is undoubted but not adequately explained. Falk (1980) has indicated that if IgA is not synthesised locally in the skin then a possible reason for the decreased serum levels during scabies infestation could be that the infestation causes a transfer of IgA from the serum to the lesions. That such a transfer occurs has yet to be verified. The significance of the findings on C3 and C1q binding have also to be explained. Van Neste (1981) pointed out that the changes in the levels of various immunoglobulins indicated B cell activity in both types of scabies. This suggestion of B cell activity fits well with the presence of circulating C1q binding immune complexes found in the serum of some scabietics. He further suggested that precipitation of the immune complexes and subsequent activation of the complement system may have caused the C3 deposition at the dermoepidermal junction. Van Neste et al. (1979) considered that the various disparate results of the findings with regard to immunoglobulins could be due to a combination of inadequately extracted scabies antigen and the variation in duration and severity of the scabies. New and more refined techniques are required. There is a considerable amount of further work to be done to elucidate and explain the immunological changes in scabies. Perhaps when they are more fully understood it may be possible to consider the question as to whether therapeutic immunisation is feasible. Such a step would seem to hold out the best practical means of eradicating the disease altogether.

An anomalous effect of a drug on scabies was reported by Ward (1971). He treated eight patients with Down's syndrome who had Norwegian scabies with methotrexate in a dosage of one tablet daily for 6 days, followed by 6 days' rest and then repeated. The treatment was successful. Burrows et al. (1975) reported on the effect of methotrexate in a patient with acute lymphatic leukaemia. This patient was being treated with several other potent immunosuppressive drugs as well as radiotherapy. Scabies appeared as a fine papular eruption about 3 days after finishing a 4-day course of oral methotrexate. It quickly faded but recurred similarly at the end of or within 3 days of finishing each of two subsequent courses of the same drug orally. Burrows and his colleagues had suggested that the larvae may have been suppressed but could find no evidence to support this. Van Aerssen (1968) may, in fact, have provided the answer because he showed that methotrexate killed the mite *Demodex folliculorum* and was effective as a treatment for rosacea (not, however, to be recommended as a treatment for that disease). It could be, therefore, that the effect of methotrexate on scabies is that of an antimitotic and fatal to the *Sarcoptes* (but evidently not to unhatched eggs), as Burrows and his colleagues suggested, and not due to any anomalous effect of immunosuppression.

Treatment

The treatment of scabies is as important as the correct diagnosis. Just as it is wrong to treat a patient for scabies without proof or virtual certainty of the diagnosis, so it is wrong to be casual or incorrect in the treatment of those with scabies. A number of principles must be observed if these patients are to be treated properly and they are enumerated in Table 15.10.

Table 15.10. Principles of treatment of scabies

1. Choose a suitable medicament
2. Prescribe a limited amount
3. Avoid overtreatment
4. Treat the whole body from neck to toes. Treat the head and face as well in babies
5. Treat all household contacts simultaneously
6. Trace and treat other contacts
7. Give detailed verbal and written instructions
8. Have a follow-up inspection at 1 and 4 weeks
9. Launder underclothing and bedding after completion of treatment. Do not use again for 3 days

An effective medication is one which will quickly kill the *Sarcoptes* in the adult, immature or egg form (Bazin 1858; Mellanby 1943). It was realised long ago (Turner 1725; Mead 1751; Wilson 1867; Hebra 1868) that topical preparations alone are enough to treat scabies, although there have recently been renewed attempts at oral treatment (discussed on pp. 273–274). Topical therapy should be effective after one application, although a second dose is usually applied as a precaution, in case of inadequate use. The preparation used should not irritate normal or inflamed skin and should not be absorbed in sufficient quantity to produce systemic effects in the patient. It must be borne in mind that many patients are infants, who are particularly susceptible to very small quantities of toxic substances. The preparation should be cheap and simple to apply and, preferably, should be cosmetically acceptable, although as Epstein (1977) has pointed out, efficiency is more important than elegance. However, if an efficient remedy is cosmetically unacceptable it may not be used at all by patients and may therefore be unsuitable. The choice of preparation is discussed on pp. 270–274.

To reduce the risk of overtreatment Orkin et al. (1976, 1977) prescribed only a limited quantity of medicament, so that the patient would be obliged to obtain a further prescription to continue the treatment, thus enabling the physician to exercise control. Topical medicaments other than antiscabietics should be withheld until completion of antiparasitic therapy (Bazin 1858; Wilson 1867; Orkin et al. 1977). This will avoid confusion and minimise the risk of overtreatment and of contact reactions, the dangers of which were emphasised by Hebra (1868) and by Kaposi (1895). Persistent itch often encourages both patient and doctor to continue far too long with antiscabietics. The informed physician should explain to his patients why only one or two applications are necessary (Orkin et al. 1976, 1977). The use of too much medicament at a time, which is also risky, can be avoided by knowing how much to prescribe. A reasonable guide to quantities per adult patient is 100 g for sulphur ointment, 50 g for proprietary ointments and creams, 100 ml for lotions and 200 ml for emulsions.

If domiciliary self-treatment is indicated it is vital that the treatment should be thorough (Green 1835; Hardy 1886; Mellanby 1943; Lyell 1967; Orkin et al. 1977) and that clear instructions be given (Stokes 1936; Orkin et al. 1976, 1977). Lack of instruction is a recipe for failure. Instructions should be written but also given verbally to the patient or parent. A suggested format is given in Table 15.11. Steps should be taken to ensure that the patient or parent fully understands what is to be done. In the past many of the experts who had great influence on the profession (e.g. Wilson 1847;

Table 15.11. Sample instruction sheet for the treatment of scabies. It can be modified to suit whichever treatment is chosen

Instructions for the Treatment of Scabies

Scabies is caused by a minute parasitic mite burrowing in the surface of the skin. It is easily curable if instructions are carefully followed.

1. Start with a warm bath. (If this is not required you will be told.) Be sure to dry thoroughly afterwards.
2. The ointment (cream/lotion/emulsion) provided should be thoroughly rubbed into (painted over) all the skin of your body and limbs whether there are any spots to be seen or not. No part of the skin from the chin downwards should be left untreated. The face, head and neck must also be treated in babies.
3. Treatment is best done at night before going to bed. Wear your usual nightclothes. Repeat the treatment next night.
4. Change your underclothing and sheets (or blankets) next day.
5. Do not have another bath until 24 hours after the last treatment.
6. You may itch for a few days. Do not repeat the treatment but use simple calamine lotion until you see your doctor again.
7. Launder soiled underclothing and bedding in the usual way. Do not use it for at least 3 days after laundering.
8. *Everyone* without exception, living in your house, whether a relative or not, should be treated as above at the same time. Any frequent visitors (babysitters/close friends/relatives) should all be treated as well.
9. Report to your doctor 1 week after treatment is finished.

Bazin 1858; Hebra 1868; Greenhough 1886; Dubreuilh 1918) either deliberately treated only visible lesions or failed to emphasise the necessity to treat the whole body. Their influence still exists and is responsible for many so-called failures after treatment. Dubreuilh (1918) later corrected his omission, and whole body treatment has been re-emphasised by many others, including Mellanby (1943), Clayton (1943) Bradshaw (1944), Wooldridge (1948), Chowdhury and Hati (1975) and by Rook (1979). Personal experience over more than 40 years has shown that it is not enough to tell the patient to apply the medicament to the whole body from the chin to the toes. Even this simple instruction is frequently misinterpreted, the principal mistake being to think that it applies only to lesions. It has therefore been the present writer's practice to instruct patients as follows:

Apply the remedy to the whole body below the collar line. Start with the fingers, the spaces between the fingers, the hands and the wrists and rub in (or paint on) the medicament thoroughly. Then do the same to the forearms, the upper arms, the armpits, axillary folds, shoulders and back and front of the trunk. Women should pay particular attention to the breasts and nipple areas and men and boys to the external genitalia. The buttocks, thighs, lower legs, soles of the feet and the toes should finally be treated. All these areas should be treated whether there are any spots to be seen or not so that no part of the body mentioned is left untreated.

This may seem tedious and unnecessary but in fact it takes only half a minute and the results in terms of success fully justify the time spent.

Secondary infection, especially if the organism involved is a beta-haemolytic streptococcus (see p. 238), should be treated simultaneously by means of the appropriate oral antibiotic.

Item 8 in Table 15.11 should also be emphasised, as it has been by many in the past (e.g. Hunt 1865; Wilson 1867; Hardy 1886; Dubreuilh and Baille 1895; Dubreuilh 1918; Geffen 1944; Burckhardt and Rymarowicz 1946; Erskine 1967; Danby et al. 1967; Gourley 1967; Keczkes et al. 1967; Lyell 1967; Hernandez-Perez 1976; Verbov 1976; Orkin et al. 1977). In an instance seen by the present writer scabies persisted in a family, despite protestations that the whole family had been treated, until a visit to the house unveiled a bedridden grandmother in a back bedroom who had been "overlooked" as a member of the family! Her treatment resolved the problem. It can sometimes be difficult to persuade all contacts (who may have no obvious lesions or symptoms) to accept treatment. Fathers and teenagers are the worst offenders in this respect. Practical demonstration may sometimes convince them of the necessity to comply. Graham (1943) noted a 3% relapse rate in patients transported and treated at a special scabies treatment centre, which was traced to untreated, unsuspected contacts. He inferred that professional surveillance of patients and contacts was necessary to eradicate scabies. Mellanby et al. (1942) emphasised that the 1.7% recurrence rate in the 1500 persons they treated represented re-infestation (presumably from untreated contacts).

Follow-up inspection, as advocated by Hardy (1886) and by Knowles (1918), is of great value; it enables the physician to check the results of his treatment. If this is apparently unsuccessful he can ascertain whether medicaments were used correctly and whether contacts have been treated. At the same time he can curb overtreatment. A second follow-up inspection by health visitors after a further month is ideal.

Should clothing be disinfested? Up to the early years of World War II this was regarded as imperative (Dubreuilh 1918; Da Costa 1918; MacCormac 1918, 1943; Munro 1919 and many others). Mellanby (1943) showed (see p. 279) that this was a matter of minor importance and the expenditure of much time and money on disinfestation was wasteful. In practice all that is necessary is to tell the patient that he should continue to wear the same clothing and use the same bedding as before during the period of treatment. This will ensure that a small proportion of the medicament will be transferred to these items and will exert an antiparasitic effect on any mites of adult or immature form which might happen to be on them. The day after the last treatment, clothing worn next to the skin and bedding immediately covering the body should be changed and laundered in the usual way. They should not be used for at least 3 days. This will avoid any possible chance of spread of the disease through these articles because no active mites could survive this laundering. (With ordinary scabies eggs are never transferred to clothing.) However, Percival (1941) has pointed out a social complication of this procedure: It may be economically impossible for the poorer members of the community, especially those with large families. Nevertheless, whenever it is possible it should be carried out, and community help should be sought in cases of difficulty. Reasons for lack of success in treatment are summarised in Table 15.12. Some patients may occasionally fail to respond to correct treatment because of the presence of intercurrent disease (Borda 1954).

Hernandez-Perez (1983) thought that mite resistance might be developing to lindane because 6% of his patients in El Salvador still had active mites present after treatment. Taplin (1983) felt that this might be the result of failure of the medicament to penetrate crusts, a point emphasised by Anderson (1863) when he said that no (topical) medicament should be condemned until it had been used on a crust-free area.

Table 15.12. Reasons for failure of treatment of scabies

1. Inadequate application of the chosen medicament
   a) Carelessly applied
   b) Applied only to obvious lesions
   c) Applied less often than recommended
   d) Washed off too soon
   e) Other topical measures used simultaneously
   f) Incompletely used because of intolerance
2. Medicament too dilute for effectiveness
3. Re-infestation
   a) From untreated household contacts
   b) From other unsuspected source

Choice of Medicament

Innumerable remedies have been advocated for the treatment of scabies over the years. Detailed study has shown that only five of these are really adequate and suitable for large-scale use. Medicaments not now recommended (with references for those interested) are flowers of sulphur (Hebra 1868), betanaphthol (Shoemaker 1902), balsam of Peru (Dubreuilh and Beille 1895), pyrethrum extract (Sweitzer and Tedder 1935; Eddy 1944), derris root (Saunders 1941), rotenone (Thomson and Miller 1940; Epstein 1942; Mellanby 1973), Mitigal (Mellanby et al. 1942), Dixanthogen (Heilesen 1948), sodium thiosulphate and hydrochloric acid (Ssutiejeff 1923; Demjanovic 1933; Percival 1941), Tenutex (Floden 1947) and NIBN, EAY and NTBB (Eddy 1946). The last three were parasiticidal combinations, denoted by initials, but are not now used.) NTBB contained DDT, which is ineffective in scabies (Hellier 1945) and against mites in general.

Sulphur

Sulphur is the oldest antiscabietic in use. The Chinese used it as long ago as 1111 A.D. (Hoeppli 1959). It has been recommended in a great variety of forms and techniques by countless authorities from the Middle Ages onwards. It is cheap, easy to apply and effective. If used too vigorously, for too long or in too high a concentration it can cause irritation (Anderson 1872), but the present writer has experienced no trouble with its use during his career. It is not absorbed in appreciable amounts and produces no toxic symptoms from its therapeutic use in scabies. Beek and Mellanby (1953) felt that "it might be absorbed by suckling children up to 2 years old" if their mothers were having it applied to their skin. Whether this is dangerous is doubtful, since sulphur was in regular use as a children's tonic 60 or 70 years ago without adverse effects (or benefit). Only in ointment form is it uniformly successful as an antiscabietic. Older prescriptions with complicated formulations and techniques were innumerable but had little or no advantage over simple 10% sulphur in yellow soft paraffin. Interested readers can find full details of these older measures in Hebra's book (1868).

The technique of using 10% sulphur ointment is very simple. A preliminary bath is unnecessary but is aesthetically pleasant. Borda (1954) advised preliminary bathing, but without soap or friction, which is contrary to the commonly accepted practice. The ointment is then thoroughly rubbed into the skin of the whole body (see p. 269) for 2 or 3 consecutive days. It is preferable for the patient to do this personally as this will ensure that the hands will be well impregnated with the ointment. Assistance may be required for inaccessible areas. The present writer agrees with Percival (1941) that ointments are more easily and more efficiently applied than other preparations. This is particularly important for unsupervised patients. Borda (1954) also advocated ointments in preference to other preparations because they induced anoxia in the mites. He claimed that immersion in water had the same effect, hence the value of a bath. Sulphur has the great advantage that at a reduced concentration of 2.5% it is well tolerated and very effective in infantile scabies, where it is also applied to the head and neck. Hellier (1941) has pointed out that he never encountered parasite resistance to sulphur in scabies, and none is recorded in the literature. Mellanby et al. (1942a) found that the mite could survive being stuck in sulphur ointment on a glass slide for several days, but it did not survive contact with the active products of sulphur ointment on the human skin. It is the treatment of choice on primarily economic grounds, apart from its efficacy.

Benzyl Benzoate

Benzyl benzoate (BB) is the antiscabietic ingredient in balsam of Peru. Although first suggested for use in scabies by Sachs in 1900, it was not given a full clinical trial until 1937, when Kissmeyer found it to be so effective that it was quickly adopted as a standard method of treatment. It is easy to apply, but Percival (1941) noted that it cost over twice as much as sulphur ointment. Mellanby found that a 20% concentration proved quite adequate, but it is now generally accepted that

25% aqueous emulsion gives more reliable results. Mellanby's (1943) technique consisted of a preliminary bath if possible, followed by thorough drying. (Borda 1954 said a bath should not be omitted when using BB.) The whole body (see p. 269) should then be painted with BB emulsion using a 5 cm (2 in.) paint brush and allowed to dry for at least 5–10 min before dressing. This painting should be repeated once, either the next day or one week later. Some workers give a total of three paintings. Borrie (1967) has suggested that BB should remain on the skin for 48 hours before a second bath is taken. Used correctly, BB is 100% effective.

BB has certain drawbacks. If dispensed as a 10% alcoholic solution it stings severely (even the standard emulsion can sting briefly) and for this reason is disliked by children (Bradshaw 1944). Although Gray (1942) and Bacon (1942) strongly denied it, the majority of workers agree that BB causes scrotal irritation and should not be used if there is any broken surface on the scrotum, whether from scratching or eczema. It is also a conjunctival irritant and should therefore never be used for infants and probably not in young children. In spite of these disadvantages, if properly used and with the above reservations it gives little trouble.

Nevertheless, a great deal of controversy over the efficiency of BB has arisen and many failures have been attributed to its use. Inadequate use (i.e. haphazard application, only one application or too weak concentration) is the commonest cause of failure (Franklin and Baker 1967; Gourley 1967; Keczkes et al. 1967; Mummery 1967; Lomholt 1972; Chowdhury and Hati 1975). The blame for this should be put where it belongs, on the shoulders of the physician for inadequate instruction of patients and failure to follow up patients. A vivid demonstration of this was reported by Gourley, who reduced the recovery period from scabies in his practice from 17 days to 10 days by the simple expedient of issuing printed instructions. BB is overused by patients more than any other antiscabietic. Many patients have developed contact reactions through the habit of applying it daily for months (Mummery 1967) and have complained bitterly about its failure to cure. This is the result of lack of supervision and follow-up, which is especially necessary in unsophisticated communities. Lomholt (1972), in fact, indicated that he always insisted on supervised treatment in his clinic before allowing the patient to go home. The third reason for failure to cure scabies with BB is not due to BB but to failure to treat contacts (Geffen 1944; Keczkes et al. 1967). Erskine (1967) added a fourth reason—that the *Sarcoptes* was becoming resistant to BB—but there is certainly no evidence to this effect in the literature. The addition of benzocaine, allegedly to prevent stinging, is to be condemned, as it is a well-known sensitiser. Compounds containing DDT for combined treatment of scabies and pediculosis (Carpenter et al. 1946) are not recommended because of the ecological objections to DDT.

Tetraethylthiuram Monosulphide (Monosulfiram B.P.; TETMS; Tetmosol)

Tetraethylthiuram monosulphide (TETMS) was first used as a treatment for human scabies by Percival (1942). His 100% success was confirmed by Clayton (1943) and by Bradshaw (1944), but Borda (1954) found it less effective. Clayton (1943) found the aqueous solution rather irritant, but Bradshaw (1944) used an emulsion which was well tolerated, especially by children, who much preferred it to BB. It is commercially supplied (Tetmosol) as a 25% w/w concentrated solution in industrial alcohol, which should be diluted with two or three times its volume of water to form an emulsion. After a warm soapy bath it is painted over the whole body (see p. 269) and rubbed in well once a day on 2 or 3 consecutive days. If applied without dilution it can produce an Antabuse effect with oedema of the skin, flushing, sweating and severe tachycardia if the patient imbibes alcoholic beverage during or soon after treatment (Gold 1966). TETMS is chemically related to Antabuse, which is a disulphide of tetraethylthiuram. It can thus be absorbed through the skin from the concentrated form. Its use in infants should therefore be avoided, and other persons should be warned about simultaneous alcohol intake. Morley (1967) recommended its suspension in coconut oil as a means of overcoming this complication. Landgren et al. (1979) used Tenutex minus DDT successfully. It contains 2% disulfuram and 22.5% benzyl benzoate.

Soap containing TETMS was used by Gordon et al. (1944) as a prophylactic measure in an infested community with a resultant reduction in the number of active cases and the prevention of the appearance of new cases. Mellanby (1945) confirmed this in a closed community. His control group of patients continued to develop new cases until Bartley et al. (1945), after observing them for a further 17 weeks, introduced the soap for 13 weeks, and the suppressive effect was again seen. Both these groups of workers observed mild irritation from the soap in some patients. Gordon et al. (1944) felt that a larger trial to exclude contact reactions was required before adopting the soap as a general measure. Mellanby (1944), on the basis of the results obtained in a trial using a quarter of a million school children who had BB applied to their hands daily, felt that treatment of actual infested patients was simpler because of the great difficulty in controlling contacts.

Crotamiton (*N*-ethyl-o-crotonotoluide; Eurax)

Crotamiton was first suggested for scabies by Domenjoz (1946) on the basis of its success in controlling *Psoroptes cuniculi* infestation in dogs. It was confirmed clinically in man by Burckhardt and Rymarowicz (1946). Used as an outpatient measure it was effective after two applications over a 24 h period, but the success was not 100%. Poor results were obtained by Balfanz (1978), by Cubela and Yawalker (1978) and by Konstantinov et al. (1979) on a similar basis; however, Konstantinov et al. attributed this to failure to treat contacts, because they obtained 100% success with 50 children treated in hospital. Crotamiton is dispensed as a cream and applied in the same manner as sulphur ointment. It is odourless, non-greasy, non-irritating and has antipruritic properties apart from its antisarcoptic effect. It has been advocated for children by Hurwitz (1973, 1977) but appeared to require prolonged application. Sneddon and Church (1979) recommended it for nodular scabies. Borda (1954) advised its use if facilities for bathing were not available. The present writer has not been impressed with crotamiton as an anti-scabietic on the few occasions which he has prescribed it. It is however, excellent for the persistent post-scabietic itch.

Gamma-benzene hexachloride (γBHC; hexachlorocyclohexane; Gammexane; Lorexane; lindane)

Although the parent substance (which is chemically hexachlorocyclohexane and not a benzene compound) was synthesised in 1825 by Faraday (Kornblee and Combes 1949), the pure gamma isomer was first prepared by Smart in 1943 (Solomon et al. 1977). The insecticidal properties were investigated by Thomas [1942], who found that they were entirely due to the gamma isomer (cited by Kornblee and Combes 1949). Slade (1945) pointed out that γBHC was chemically related to inositol (hexahydrocyclohexane) and that it probably owed its toxic properties to competitive inhibition of inositol in the insect tissues. Kornblee and Combes (1949) considered that the toxic effects on the insect central nervous system, producing increased excitability, convulsions and death, gave it its insecticidal value.

γBHC was first used in scabies by Wooldridge (1948) and its efficiency was confirmed by Cannon and McRae (1948), who found that three applications were 100% successful. Kornblee and Combes (1949) noted that this cure rate fell to 55% if the concentration of the medicament was reduced to 0.5% (from 1%). In a recent trial with 1% cream, Amer et al. (1981) only achieved 85% cure. Its efficiency against the *Sarcoptes*, its non-irritating quality, cleanliness and ease of application made it a popular treatment. It was felt to be especially suitable for infants and children, a view which the present writer shared with many others. Hurwitz (1973) recommended it especially for children, but again prolonged treatment was required. He attributed its slow action to the greater number of mites present on the skin of this age group. This reasoning is as illogical as that of the British wartime submarine cook who boiled 50 eggs for 150 min on the grounds that they required 3 min each. It is more likely that the children were repeatedly re-infested by untreated contacts. Niedelman (1948) also thought it safe for children. Verbov (1976) recommended it for inflamed and secondarily infected scabies. Farkaš (1974) thought it should be reserved for abortive (scabies in the clean), papular and eczematised scabies.

Toxicity. Suspicions about the safety of γBHC were roused when Hans (1976) drew attention to the fact that 11 instances of aplastic anaemia and two of leukaemia caused by γBHC had been published and that there was a definite temporal relationship between exposure to γBHC and the development of these toxic complications. Two of these patients had been handling dogs to which γBHC had been repeatedly applied. Hans pointed out that it was well known that this compound could be absorbed through unbroken skin.

Orkin et al. (1976) noted that toxic levels could be built up and also advised that medicaments containing γBHC should be kept away from the eyes and mucosae. Lee et al. (1976) and Lee and Groth (1977) reported nine instances of systemic toxic effects in humans caused by γBHC, seven of which resulted from its therapeutic application to the skin. A girl aged 8 years developed convulsions after 18 daily applications, a boy aged 10 after only one application and a boy aged 4 some $8\frac{1}{2}$ h after a single application. This last child then stopped breathing but recovered in hospital. A 13-month-old boy had a grand mal seizure after 14 daily applications of 100 mg γBHC followed by one oral dose of 50 mg. A child aged 7 had convulsions 48 h after a single application which had been left in situ for 36 h, whilst a man aged 37 experienced dizziness and amblyopia after three applications at 12-h intervals. A mother of five children suffered an increase of nervousness, irritability, anxiety and insomnia for several days after shampooing her children's scalps with γBHC. Both of the last two patients had relapses after re-exposure. Two further adults had convulsions after accidentally ingesting the compound in mistake for meat tenderiser.

Pramanik and Hansen (1979) reported two more scabies patients with convulsions. One was a 4-month-old premature infant, also suffering from pneumonia, whose symptoms occurred after one application. The other was a boy aged 2 with a severely excoriated scabies which was treated by the application of 80 ml of 1% γBHC lotion over a 2-week period. Pramanik and his colleague measured the blood levels of γBHC in these two children and found 0.1 μg and 0.012 μg/ml respectively, compared with the expected levels of 0.005 μg/ml in infants so treated and a background level of 0.0005 μg/ml in unexposed adults. Davies et al. (1983) measured a blood level of 0.206 μg/ml after ingestion of 392 g of 1% γBHC cream, falling to 0.001 μg/ml 25 days later in a 16-year-old mental defective. They found 0.110 μg/ml in the brain of a 2-month-old boy, dead within hours of the excessive application of 1% γBHC lotion. Blood levels were one-third of brain concentration.

These cases with toxic symptoms arising from the therapeutic use of γBHC indicate that it is not as safe as was originally supposed. It is known to be absorbed through intact skin, especially through inflamed or damaged skin and in very young children. Solomon et al. (1977) have also pointed out that scrotal skin offers no barrier in its absorption through the skin. High blood levels of γBHC can be attained by percutaneous absorption. The principal toxic effects following absorption in humans are on the central nervous system and gross absorption has caused death (Solomon et al. 1977), as it does in arthropods.

Rasmussen (1981) and Shacter (1981) reviewed γBHC and agreed that its benefits probably outweighed its risks. Rasmussen felt that the toxic effects derived either from its ingestion or its misuse in therapeutic application and that such instances were very small compared to the overall use (assessed as equivalent to 30 million tubes of 50 g each over a period of 5 years). Shacter on the whole agreed but considered it should be avoided in pregnancy, in small children and in the presence of heavy excoriation. Both indicated that the evidence produced had failed to show that γBHC *at therapeutic dosage* had any carcinogenic or teratogenic effects. Both made suggestions as to precautions to be taken, which are incorporated in those outlined below. Although γBHC is an efficient scabiecide, it must therefore be prescribed with caution in the knowledge of its potential effects. Restrictions governing its use in scabies (or pediculosis for that matter) are suggested as follows:

1. It should be applied to a cool dry skin (Solomon et al. 1977). A preliminary hot soapy bath may increase absorption. Should soap be inadvertently left on the skin, γBHC may be decomposed (Wooldridge 1948).
2. Theoretically one 30-min application is adequate (Maibach and Orkin 1977a). Toxic effects can occur if it is left on the skin for 24 h. Pramanik and Hansen (1979) advised that it be washed off after 6 h.
3. Do not use in infants, in small boys or in pregnancy.
4. Do not use on inflamed skin (eczematised) or secondarily infected or heavily excoriated skin.
5. Do not repeat its use within 8 days (Solomon et al. 1977).
6. Do not use in a concentration above 1%. It is also less effective at a lower concentration.
7. Use as little as possible concomitant with efficient and adequate treatment.
8. Do not use γBHC as a household spray.
9. If in any doubt do not use it for treating scabies. This is especially applicable if there is doubt as to whether instructions are understood. It is all very well to inform the patient (or parents) of potential hazards of misuse (as suggested by Rasmussen 1981), but the very people to whom this applies are those who would not or could not comprehend such explanations. There are persons who cannot grasp even simple instructions.

Oral Treatment

Sulphur preparations by mouth were found to be useless for treating scabies (Hebra 1868). Oral thiabendazol, an anthelminthic, was first used for scabies by Hernandez-Perez et al. (1969) with reasonably good results. Using 50 mg/kg daily for 5 days at a time they cured two of five patients in 5 days; however, one was not free of infestation after

20 days' treatment. At a dosage of 25 mg/kg for 10-day periods, six of seven patients were cured in 10 days, the seventh requiring a further 10 days' treatment. The side-effects were nausea, diarrhoea and dizziness. De Mello and Uthad-Tanaka (1970) treated a closed community of 55 persons, which included 37 carrying scabies; 18 patients (48.6%) were cured. The preparation was better tolerated in syrup than as tablets. Side-effects were mainly digestive. One case of photosensitivity occurred. Martins-Castro et al. (1974) also used thiabendazol to treat a severe outbreak of scabies in a community of patients with South American pemphigus foliaceus. The results were very moderate, but as no figures were given conclusions cannot be drawn.

Topical thiabendazol was used with considerable success as a 5% cream daily for 5 days by Biagi and Delgardo-y-Garnica (1974) and Hernandez-Perez (1976). No complications were reported, although Biagi and his colleague pointed out that it caused dermatitis when used against larva migrans.

Barranco et al. (1976) cured 29 out of 30 patients with resistent scabies within 4 weeks using oral metrefonate (2-2-2-trichloro-hydroxyethyl-phosphone) in a dosage of 10 mg/kg daily for 2 days each week. Four patients developed transitory nausea and vomiting.

These methods of treating scabies orally are very interesting, not because the treatment is likely to replace the much cheaper topical therapy but because in certain circumstances (e.g. in South American pemphigus foliaceus) topical treatment might not only be difficult but even hazardous for an already ill patient. So far, however, the preparations have been insufficiently used to warrant recommending them. The search for such a treatment should go on, because in theory a cheap, brief, simple oral therapy which is non-toxic to humans could hold out a hope of eradicating scabies altogether. With regard to South American pemphigus foliaceus, it might be worth trying the effect of oral methotrexate. This might be beneficial in combating the basic disease and could also possibly alleviate the scabies (see p. 267).

Summary of Available Treatment

There are obviously several good measures to choose from when treating scabies. The choice may depend on whether the sufferer is an adult, child or infant, whether the scabies is complicated by secondary infection or eczematisation, and, if a woman is involved, whether she is pregnant or not. Sulphur ointment, 10% for adults and $2\frac{1}{2}$% for infants, can be used for any case of scabies and is recommended as the first choice. It is cheap and reliable. Aqueous emulsion of 25% benzyl benzoate is also reliable but should be avoided for infants and males with scrotal eczema. Gamma-benzene hexachloride is effective with one proper application but is contraindicated for infants, small children, in pregnancy and in those with extensive inflammatory lesions. Tetmosol is also reliable if properly used and seems to be particularly suitable for children; however, it should be avoided in infants as it can be absorbed through the skin and is also contraindicated in those likely to imbibe much alcohol and in pregnancy. Crotamiton is a good medicament if properly used and is safe for all scabietics, but results have not been so convincing as with the other substances mentioned.

Epidemiology

Scabies has played a modest but not insignificant role in human history (Rook et al. 1979). For example, scabies probably affected about 400 000 men in the French army in the Napoleonic wars and was the second or third commonest cause of casualties (Friedman 1941, 1948). In more recent times Crewe (1955) has indicated that the 72 000 military cases in the United Kingdom in 1942 were equivalent to a battalion of 800 strong being *hors de combat* for that year. Careful perusal of the literature of the morbidity of scabies throughout the globe suggests that a figure of 300 million people infested is probably a very conservative estimate. Such numbers cannot in any way be regarded as of little significance.

Human scabies is worldwide, affecting all races and social classes in every climate from arctic to equatorial, and is constantly with us. Except in a very few enlightened areas it is not a notifiable disease. Figures for the incidence of scabies are therefore very variable. In some instances they are based on cases among school children (Wilson 1969); in many other instances on its percentage incidence among skin disease patients (e.g. Shrank and Alexander 1967; Sehgal 1977; Desai 1972 and many more); on its incidence at clinics for veneral diseases (Hutfield, 1967); on its occurrence in closed communities (Pierce 1951); and on its morbidity in the whole population (Christopherson 1978) or in the population in a selected area (Yarrow 1967; Nair et al. 1973). Whilst only figures based on total populations can give an accurate assessment of the actual number of cases, those based on hospital populations give an idea of the incidence of scabies in relation to other diseases, and it is possible from such figures to estimate whether the disease is on the increase or declining. Such figures are revealing when used to compare different regions of the world. For example, in the United Kingdom an incidence of 2% among the patients attending a skin clinic in a large hospital means perhaps 80–100 patients seen annually with scabies, which is regarded as a substantial number. The incidence in a hospital in Korea was shown to average 3.2% of all skin clinic patients over 15 years, with a peak of 4.5% in 1975 (Han et al. 1983). In a tropical or semitropical country the proportion is more likely to be 20% of a very much larger total. In Bombay, for example, Desai (1972) reported the average number of patients with scabies seen annually over a 10-year period in the K.E.M. hospital to be 9824, about half of whom were new patients. The figures given for Bombay are representative of what happens elsewhere in India, Southeast Asia, South and Central America and probably China (although information from there is not available). Most of these countries have similar climates and large populations, often concentrated in large cities with extensive slums and shanty towns, are relatively poor and have inadequate medical services to cope with a problem of such magnitude, when many other equally pressing problems also have to be overcome. In spite of these other problems, however, scabies should be high on the list for urgent attention because it is , at least theoretically, capable of being eradicated or reduced to negligible proportions.

A study of the incidence of scabies in developed countries, where it still remains a considerable problem, reveals its behavioural characteristics and allows the importance of the many factors involved in its spread and management to be assessed.

It was well known that the number of patients with scabies rapidly increased in time of war, during periods of human migration and following natural disasters such as floods and earthquakes. Friedman (1948) concluded after a detailed study that war was the principal cause of scabies epidemics and he attributed the continued huge increase of the disease after World War I to the influence of that war. He noted the enormous number of soldiers in all wars who suffered from scabies. (Incidentally he observed that in military conflicts in the eighteenth and nineteenth centuries the prevailing view was that scabies was of internal origin. Treatment was in consequence singularly ineffective.)

In World War I the view was generally held that soldiers were responsible for the spread of scabies, bringing it with them from the trenches. However, Parkinson (1918) said that in fact the reverse was true and that new cases originating in the fighting zones were unusual. Mellanby (1943, 1977b) said that civilians were much more commonly affected (see p. 277). Crewe (1955) said that the estimated incidence among civilians in Britain was four or five times that in the army. Epstein (1955) drew attention to the virtual disappearance of scabies from dermatological clinics in North America in the early 1950s. In his own practice the fluctuating incidence for the years 1937–1953 is shown in Table 15.13. The increased incidence associated with World War II began well before the outbreak of hostilities, which suggested to many that it might have a periodicity. A dramatic fall after the 1946 peak persisted until 1963, when it began to rise again. This led Shrank and Alexander (1967) to postulate a 15-year cycle. This rise was confirmed worldwide (Fergusson 1967; Keczkes et al. 1967; Hernandez-Perez 1971; Banerjee and Chowdhury 1972; Rigatos and Kappos-Rigatou 1976; Petitt 1976; Ferencei et al. 1976; Lomholt 1977; Christopherson 1978; Andrews 1979). It was noticeable, however, that the increase was not synchronous throughout the world. The increase in the United Kingdom preceded that in the United States by over a year (Hellier 1966). Scabies was subsiding in Malaysia but spreading in Vietnam and the Philippines towards Hawaii (Petitt 1976). Amongst Glasgow school children the periodicity was irregular, there being 10-year cycles in the 1920s and 1930s, a peak emphasised by war in 1943 and further peaks in 1959 and 1968 (Wilson 1969). In Denmark, where scabies became notifiable in 1900, 850 629

Table 15.13. Incidence of scabies in a private practice, based on percentage of new patients[a]

Year	Incidence percentage	Year	Incidence percentage
1937	2.5	1951	0.45
1938	4.4	1952	0.40
1939	3.6	1953	0.15
1940	2.5	1954	0.48
1941	3.3	1955	0.00
1942	3.7	1956	0.32
1943	3.3	1957	0.025
1944	4.5	1958	0.30
1945	5.4	1959	0.00
1946	8.2	1960	0.039
1947	4.2	1961	0.052
1948	2.6	1962	0.068
1949	1.1	1963	0.067
1950	0.95	1964	0.038

[a] From Epstein E (1966) Arch Dermatol 93: 60–61, by kind permission of the author and publisher, American Medical Association. Copyright 1966, American Medical Association

scabietics were treated between 1900 and 1975. There were peaks of incidence accentuated by war in 1918 and 1945, but in each instance the rise began before the respective wars. A further rise commenced in 1968. The post-war fall in Denmark also occurred in neutral countries (Christopherson 1978). The infestation rate in Denmark in 1975 was almost the same as in 1900, in spite of the improvement in health and living standards.

Shrank and Alexander (1967) suggested that herd immunity would account for the periodicity. During an epidemic rise in incidence scabies would be contracted by many persons, most of whom would be under 16. After several years the population in this group would, these authors claimed, have a relatively high immunity. Consequently, many fewer people would be at risk and the rate of spread would fall until, after about 15 years, a new non-immune population would appear, become infested and start a new cycle. Nair K.P.B. (1973) apparently confirmed this view: 6% of the 19 000 population of a fishing village surveyed for scabies were infested, and 81% of these scabietics were below 14. Since mass treatment had been undertaken in the village 16 years ealier, those susceptible according to the theory would be under 16—as was the case.

On the other hand, the morbidity rate in Denmark is uniform for all ages up to 45; with major epidemics lasting 15 years, this would give a cycle of 60 years (Christopherson 1978), which does not conform to actual records. The persistence of a very high morbidity rate year after year without any apparent fluctuation in many communities in tropical and subtropical countries is difficult to explain by the herd immunity theory. Many of these scabietics relapse after treatment, often more than once and after a long interval. This relapse rate does not suggest immunity, although it must be conceded that even in these communities the very young seem to be the group most involved. Cyclical incidence is not yet satisfactorily explained.

Seasonal Incidence

Almost all authorities are agreed that the incidence of scabies rises in the autumn and winter. In such centres as Vienna, Paris and Copenhagen this was attributed to crowding together for warmth in cold winters (Friedman 1948), a theory which was shared by Beek and Mellanby (1953) and which probably explained the increase of scabies in the wet season in India (Banerjee 1972; Sehgal 1977; Sehgal et al. 1972). In France Degos (1953) noted that the autumnal rise coincided with the return home of school children infested at their summer holiday camps, whilst in Glasgow schools the spring and summer decline has been attributed to continued inspection and supervision throughout the academic year, with resurgence in the autumn after the unsupervised long summer holiday. In contrast Rycroft and Calnan (1977) observed that in the localised outbreak amongst Thames watermen the incidence fell in the winter only to rise again in the spring, when pleasure-craft activity increased and the crew lived in cramped quarters. Han et al. (1983) noted the highest incidence in January in their clinic but did not find any definite seasonal fluctuation.

Age

The relationship of age to scabies incidence varies. Some workers recorded the greatest incidence below 16 (Palicka and Merka 1971; Ellis et al. 1971; Sehgal et al. 1972; Nair et al. 1973; Gulati et al. 1977b; Desair and Nair 1978), some below 19 (Church and Knowlesden 1974; Zukowski 1976; Han et al. 1983), some between 16 and 30 (Golebiowska–Podgorczyk 1968; Chang et al. 1983), some in the postpubertal period (Olin 1942) and some noted a uniform rate up to the age of 45 (Nathan 1945; Christopherson 1978). Nair et al. (1973) and Masawe and Nsanzumuhire (1975) observed a steady decline in incidence with increase in age. The figures given in many of the papers quoted are not comparable with each other, being based on different circumstances such as local or national surveys, attendances at skin clinics or even at special scabies clinics. In general, scabies is commonest in the very young, remains frequent in older children and young adults and thereafter declines sharply.

Sex

Opinions differ about the incidence of scabies in the two sexes. Hebra (1868) attributed the 7:1 predominance amongst males in the clinics to the habit of young male apprentices of sleeping in communal beds. Mellanby (1977b) found women to be twice as frequently infested as men in the United Kingdom during World War II for a similar reason and thought their habit of fondling young children and babies was also a factor. There is no sex difference in the occurrence of scabies in babies and young children, a fact confirmed in a survey of over 25 000 school children in Chile by Lolio et al.

(1975). Nair et al. (1973), Masawe and Nsanzumhire (1975) and Gulati et al. (1977a) found no sex difference at any age, whilst Olin (1942) said that the same applied to the overall incidence in Finland but that scabies was commoner in women between the ages of 16 and 20 and in men between 21 and 25. Nathan (1945) and Church and Knowlesden (1974) found postpubertal women more often infested, whilst Marchand et al. (1975) found men predominated in the same age group. Han et al. (1983) and Chang et al. (1983) found male predominance—3:1 and 2:1 respectively.

The probability is that there is little difference in incidence between the sexes, such differences as are reported being due to varying circumstances. Another factor is the time over which figures are collected. The present writer well remembers his own experience regarding the sex incidence of alopecia areata. Some textbooks held that it was much commoner in males, and other books were equally adamant that the exact opposite was true. All the cases seen at the Skin Clinic of the Glasgow Royal Infirmary over a 20-year period were enumerated, totalling 3001. Of these, 1501 were male and 1500 were female. In any one year the incidence could be 2:1 in favour of one sex or the other. Thus to take the figures for 1 year only would give a completely misleading impression, which emphasises the need for care in interpreting statistical information, unless very large numbers are collected over a long period. In Denmark, where statistics covering the whole country for 75 years are available, it was shown that up to the age of puberty girls with scabies outnumbered boys in the proportion of 1.4:1. Thereafter there was no sex difference in incidence at any age.

Ethnic Type

Whilst no ethnic group is immune to scabies, Friedman (1948) has said that the yellow and black races appear to be more prone to it than others. This seems doubtful, since he also said that all groups were equally affected amongst the civilian population of the United States and in World War II it was three times as common in Causasoids as in Negroids in the American Army. On the other hand, Alexander (1978) recorded that only one of 37 patients with scabies seen at his Maryland clinic was Negroid, whereas 48% of the population was Negroid. This was apparently representative of the situation elsewhere in the United States. By contrast, in Africa Negroids have a higher incidence rate than other races (Hersch 1967). Andrews (1976) observed a 50% incidence of scabies amongst Bantus in Pretoria. Race is important in regard to secondary infection in South Africa. Acute glomerulonephritis of streptococcal origin (see p. 238) was found by Hersch (1967) to be secondary to infected scabies in the Bantu race. Sehgal et al. (1972) thought Moslems were more prone to scabies than were Hindus, whilst Andrews (1979) found Polynesian immigrants had a higher incidence than Maoris, who in turn were more affected than those of European extraction in New Zealand. All these racial differences are likely to be due to differences in customs, habits, housing and overcrowding and not to ethnic origin.

Familial Incidence

Intrafamilial spread of scabies has not always been recognised as important. Little was made of it until Hyde's paper in 1905. The opinions of Parkinson (1918) and Mellanby (1977a) regarding spread from military sources have been noted. The difficulties of controlling outbreaks because of the recalcitrance of some family contacts in obtaining treatment have been emphasised by Geffen and by Sehgal et al. (1972), who stressed that in India treatment involving loss of a day's work by the family breadwinner could mean no food for his family for that day. The importance of contagion within the family has been reiterated by Ingram (1967), by Church and Knowlesden (1978), by Hernandez-Perez (1971), who remarked on its progress through a family, the so-called ping-pong scabies, and by Palicka and Merka (1971) in Czechoslovakia, where the intrafamilial incidence was 22% compared with 1.3% in the general population. High familial incidence has been noted in many centres in India (Sehgal et al. 1972; Desai 1972; Nair K.P.B. 1973; Nair et al. 1973). In Kerala, Nair K.P.B. (1973) reported that 56% of all households in a representative village were affected, whilst throughout the province 38% of the population of 14.4 million had scabies. This represents 5.5 million scabietics. In Korea, Han et. al. (1983) observed that nearly 60% of patients had a family history, although nearly 50% were unable to ascertain the source of infestation.

Two school epidemics in the United States were found by Herman et al. (1975) and by Blumenthal (1976) to have had domestic rather than school origin. The habits of overnight week-end visiting and of exchanging clothing was much commoner amongst those with than those without scabies.

Nair et al. (1973) found that the number with scabies in a family was closely related to the degree of overcrowding of sleeping accommodation.

Spread is less likely among the well-to-do, who have many more individual sleeping quarters, but still occurs.

The frequency and importance of intrafamilial contact in the spread of scabies was stressed by Bagnall and Rook (1977). The close-knit family life of Maoris was said by Andrews (1979) to accentuate the spread of the disease. The intimate contacts between mother and child and between those family members sharing the same bed are especially important (Hyde 1905). Such prolonged intimate contact is more important in disseminating scabies than is the casual often brief contact of sexual promiscuity.

Overcrowding

Intrafamilial spread is inextricably bound up with overcrowding, poor hygiene and poverty, but these factors can operate outside the family circle. Overcrowding is most frequently due to accommodation being far too small for the numbers of persons involved. The importance of single housing in this respect has been emphasised over and over again (Rayer 1835; Degos 1953; Nair et al. 1973; Desai and Nair 1978), especially in rapidly expanding cities with shanty towns burgeoning on the periphery, such as Caracas (Ochoa 1977), and in much older cities with huge populations such as Bombay and Calcutta (Desai and Nair 1978). In the more prosperous developed countries such slum areas are rapidly being replaced. Even in more sparsely populated localities scabies is relatively commoner in the few areas where the population is densest (Grant 1967). In underdeveloped countries overcrowding is common in all communities regardless of size, and the incidence of scabies is high (Masawe and Nsanzumhire 1975).

Temporary overcrowding may be induced in a number of ways. War obviously may cause this by attacks on large towns and especially by creating hordes of refugees, as for example in the recent influx of fleeing population into Eastern India from Bangladesh (Banerjee and Chowdhury 1972). The movement of populations as government policy in time of war, as with evacuation of children from town to country in the United Kingdom in World War II, brings the same problem. Scabies increases in the reception areas. Similarly, the influx of visitors to trade fairs brings scabies with it (Hyde 1905; Friedman 1948), as may crowds of tourists on holiday (Bagnall and Rook 1977; Fain 1978).

In the past, permanent population changes by immigration spread scabies. There was often gross overcrowding of the transportation accommodation, causing a rapid increase in the scabies present. When this scabietic leviathan disembarked in the land of its dreams it was often housed temporarily in overcrowded dwellings where it gathered strength before bursting forth to ravage the unsuspecting area chosen by the immigrants for their final settlement. In the great immigrations to the United States in the latter half of the nineteenth century scabies thus became known variously as "the Polish itch", "the Italian itch", etc. (Stelwagon 1904).

Internal migrations, e.g. to the great cities of northeastern Brazil from the rural areas (Ramos y Silva and Olivi 1970) or those of migrant workers within the EEC (Fain 1978), the same surge in scabies incidence occurred. However, migrants are not the only ones who bring scabies with them. Orkin (1975), Björnberg (1975) and Fain (1978) have warned that those who adopt orphans from the war zones of Southeast Asia run the same risk because these children are very often scabietic.

Occupation

The occupational risks of catching scabies have already been referred to in association with overcrowding (apprentices, pleasure-craft, p. 276). An occupation which is constantly at risk from scabies is nursing. Scabies is not infrequent amongst hospital inmates, especially geriatric patients, psychiatric long-stay patients and hemiplegics. The close bodily contact inevitable in the proper nursing of such patients exposes nurses, particularly if working in short sleeves, to the risk of infestation from unsuspected scabietics. The present writer witnessed two nurses assisting a convalescent patient by supporting her, with their forearms bare, beneath her armpits, both of which had numerous burrows on the folds.

Sexual Promiscuity

Many authorities (Darier 1918; Degos 1953; Hutfield 1967a, b, c, d; Orkin 1975a; Schroeter 1977) have held that sexual intercourse is a common cause of spread of scabies. Those who believe this theory base their conclusions on figures obtained from biased sources, such as clinics for sexually transmitted diseases (Shrank 1967). Children are completely ignored in these statistics, although they are the group with the highest incidence. The alleged association between the increase of scabies and of syphilis and gonorrhoea is misleading, since Olin (1942), Parish (1975) and

Christopherson (1978) have all shown that there are clear differences between the epidemiology of scabies on the one hand and the venereal diseases on the other. However, Munkvad et al. (1982) found that 8% of 234 female scabietics and 1.4% of 436 male scabietics had asymptomatic gonorrhoea (but no other venereal disease). Whilst this was lower than the 12% for women with scabies reported by Nielsen et al. (1976), it was markedly above the incidence found in gynaecology clinics (1.3%–2.8%) and contraceptive clinics (1.5%–3.1%) and led them to conclude that females with scabies (but not males) were a high risk group for contracting gonorrhoea. Conversely, they concluded in general that scabies was a high risk in a promiscuous population. Whilst this conclusion is acceptable, it should be reiterated that sexual intercourse is not the common mode of scabies transmission. This is in accord with Mellanby (1941c). Indeed, Chang et al. (1983) found no association with sexually transmitted disease in their patients. Rollier (1969) recorded a concomitant epidemic of scabies and syphilis in Morocco between 1966 and 1968. The secondary infection associated with the scabies concealed the early secondary syphilitic eruption.

Cohen (1982) noted that the long incubation period of scabies may make contacts through alleged promiscuous intercourse difficult to trace.

Poverty and Poor Hygiene

Poverty and poor hygiene are factors in the spread of scabies because they are nearly always associated with overcrowding. However, there is little evidence to suggest that they spread scabies per se. Olin (1942) noticed a diminished incidence during periods of general prosperity, which may be due to less overcrowding and better housing. Mere squalor does not spread scabies (except in overcrowded conditions). Greenhough (1886) made the point that vagrants, who frequently live in squalid conditions, are conspicuous by their absence from lists of scabietic patients, although often infested with lice.

Water Supply

Ochoa (1977) felt that absence of an internal water supply was an important factor in spreading scabies. Munro (1919) stated that frequent washing tended to remove many immature mites from the skin of those infested and so might reduce spread. Pierce (1951), on the other hand, reported a severe internal epidemic (27% infested) amongst the inmates of a correctional home for men and an associated home for the indigent. The water supply and washing facilities were excellent, but the scabies spread rapidly, because of gross overcrowding, until diagnosed. This applies to other closed communities such as boarding schools, geriatric and long-stay psychiatric wards and overcrowded prisons, where close proximity resembling family contact will facilitate the spread of the disease if it appears.

Clothing and Bedding

The prime sources of infestation up to the end of World War I (MacCormac 1918) were considered to be clothing and bedding, but little importance is now attached to them. Munro (1919) noted that clothing after exposure to the air posed little risk. Mellanby, between 1941 and 1943, demonstrated conclusively that whilst scabies could be contracted by contact with these items it was the exception not the rule (Mellanby 1941a, b, 1942, 1943). He succeeded in infesting four volunteers after prolonged trials in which the men wore the clothing of scabietics and slept in the bedding just vacated by them. The chance of infestation was about one in two hundred. Pierce (1951) claimed that three of his patients contracted scabies by sleeping for 4 weeks in the bedding of scabietics, but all three lived in a closed community and were exposed to scabies in other ways as well. The risk from these items, although present, is small.

Other Factors

Inaccurate diagnosis and poor treatment must be recognised as factors in the spread of scabies. As long ago as 1886 Greenhough declared that scabies "ought to be diagnosed", thereby implying that it was frequently overlooked. Mention has already been made (p. 238) of the reasons for poor diagnosis. Pillsbury and Livingood (1947) blamed lack of foresight in the teaching of Dermatology in the United States. Epstein (1955) emphasised the low index of suspicion as a prime cause for failure in diagnosis, an opinion supported by Hellier (1966), Hare (1967), Hernandez-Perez (1971), Orkin (1971), Juranek and Schultz (1977) and Bagnall and Rook (1977). Added to this is the increasing number of atypical cases (Fain 1978).

Inadequately treated patients are also potent sources of further spread (Hare 1967; Grant 1967; Nair et al. 1973; Witkowski and Parish 1978).

Wrong diagnosis, resulting in the use of unsuitable medicaments such as topical corticosteroids, can have an equally unfortunate result.

Finally, Norwegian scabies must be mentioned as the known cause of many localised outbreaks of ordinary scabies, usually in closed communities. This has already been discussed when considering that special form of scabies (see p. 246). Bagnall and Rook (1977) have even suggested that unsuspected foci of Norwegian scabies may be responsible for keeping the disease alive in times when its incidence seems to be low. This seems to be rather doubtful, since there is no evidence to indicate that increased morbidity of scabies on a worldwide basis, such as occurs in the cycles discussed above, is related to the uncovering of instances of Norwegian scabies. The latter is a disease of special circumstances, and, when uncovered, the cases of ordinary scabies are quickly and energetically brought under control. This does not seem to influence the general incidence.

Large-Scale Management

On whatever scale scabies has to be combated, in the end management will depend on individual treatment. Thus the problems implicit in the treatment of individuals will be added to those of the logistics of coping with very large numbers of people and to those involving the prejudices and inevitable objections of individuals (see Geffen 1944) and sectional interests, when dealing with scabies on a large scale. Percival (1941) has admirably summed up the problem, which is as difficult now as when he made his remarks. He said, "the management of scabies presents so many deficiencies that it almost deserves a pinnacle all to itself as a deficiency disease . . . the whole subject is a vast waste—a waste of consultant's time, G.P.'s time, ointment, school time, working time". In this day and age it seems ridiculous, if not scandalous, that a disease so easy to treat as scabies should still flourish more or less unchecked.

The most important first step is to ensure widespread dissemination of information about scabies, in particular what its symptoms are, what causes it and how it is spread. Any steps taken without this are, as Percival said, a waste of time. Those responsible for medical and nursing curricula must be convinced that instruction in dealing with dermatological conditions is important in order to secure adequate time for this instruction. Every effort must be made to ensure that all medical *and nursing* students can recognise scabies, know how to confirm the diagnosis, what are the alternative treatments available and what is the correct method of application of each. Proof of the efficacy of an educational programme with proper back-up was afforded by the efforts of the Canadian Armed Forces medical staff in World War I. McPhail (1925) recorded how the disease yielded to concerted treatment on a large scale, spear-headed by the establishment of a special school of instruction on scabies for the entire Canadian Army at Hazebrouck.

Public health authorities should be made fully aware of the implications of neglecting scabies, especially with the added risk of acute glomerulonephritis in tropical countries, and should be equipped to undertake treatment on whatever scale is required. In this respect Da Fonseca (1969) advocated an education committee for public health authorities. Borda (1954) stressed the importance of interprofessional cooperation. Administrative authorities, both local and central, should be left in no doubt of the economic cost of doing nothing and the financial advantages to be gained from action to eradicate scabies. Percival (1941) said that one of the reasons for the ineffectiveness of measures then in use was that the problem had not been adequately presented, the authorities had not been given proper guidance and not enough had been asked for. A number of writers (Mellanby 1942a; Da Fonseca 1969; Richardson 1972; Nair K.P.B. 1973; Nair et al. 1973; Ochoa 1977), most of whom had first-hand experience of dealing with scabies in very large numbers of people, advocated better education of the general public in this regard. Instructional leaflets should be distributed and classes should be arranged, but, above all, judicious and intelligent use of television for communication could be of inestimable value. When people know something about the infestation from which they are suffering or which they may acquire they are much more likely to cooperate in measures to get rid of it. Ignorance is the greatest obstacle of all to the eradication of scabies.

Shrank and Alexander (1968) expressed doubt about the value of education and early diagnosis being sufficient to prevent the spread of scabies. They were quite right. Although education is essential, it is not enough; it must be backed up by action, which can take various forms, as follows:

Surveys

Public health authorities, with the guidance of an experienced dermatologist, should conduct regular surveys of the incidence. This could be achieved through channels presently available such as school health services and venereology clinics, where reasonably accurate figures are recorded. Equally valuable information could be obtained from local dermatology clinics and by means of questionnaires to general practitioners. Scabies is notifiable in some countries, e.g. Denmark, Norway and Poland. Ideally it should be universally notifiable, but it has frequently been stated, at least in the United Kingdom, that this is not justifiable or would be unacceptable in peacetime. If the general public were in possession of the full facts, including the fact that scabies is curable, there is little doubt that notification would be perfectly acceptable as a small price to pay to get rid of a great nuisance.

Treatment

Treatment should be pursued with vigour at all times, whether scabies is on the increase or not. Full details of treatment have already been given (pp. 268–274). Nair et al. (1973) have emphasised that when facilities are adequate, home treatment is perfectly satisfactory. The tracing of contacts is very important in the control of scabies. Senior nursing health visitors trained in the recognition and management of scabies should visit the homes of confirmed cases to check upon the treatment of the patient and other occupants. It should be repeated that written instructions should always be given to patients and the treatment used for children should never cause pain.

Treatment Centres

Percival (1941), Crewe (1955), Fergusson (1967) and Da Fonseca (1969) all stressed the value of treatment centres. In those mainly tropical countries where scabies abounds such centres are essential if the disease is to be controlled. In other areas where the numbers are relatively small the necessity for permanent centres is less certain. Contingency plans for their establishment, equipping and staffing should always be available, so that if the incidence suddenly increases they can be set up. Treatment centres can cope with large numbers of patients, provide facilities which may not otherwise be available and enable supervision of treatment where this is regarded as necessary. The requisites for a treatment centre, as recommended by Percival (1941), include adequate facilities for bathing, treatment, waiting, laundry and disinfestation. The last facility will only be needed for disinfestation of clothing and bedding in severe cases or, especially in poorer countries, whenever changes of bedding and clothing may not be economically possible. In the majority of instances disinfestation of clothing is unnecessary. Centres should be so designed that when their need is no longer required they can be put to some other useful purpose. For remote or primitive communities a well-designed mobile centre could be very valuable.

Mass Treatment

Ideally a worldwide mass treatment campaign should eradicate scabies, but this is obviously impossible as long as there is not even unanimity about the best treatment. Nevertheless, a concerted effort would be worthwhile, even if it only reduced the incidence by half. Borda (1954), in fact, recommended mass simultaneous treatment. Unfortunately, those countries with the highest incidence are also amongst the relatively poorest. Perhaps a start could be made by the World Health Organisation instituting a "Year of the Mite".

Soap impregnated with TETMS has been shown to be effective in reducing the incidence of new cases of scabies in a community (see p. 271). This prophylactic measure is expensive, but it would be worthwhile for wealthy groups to sponsor a trial in a sizeable community of about 20 000 population (e.g. one of the Kerala villages in India) for a period of 1–2 years. If it could significantly reduce the number of patients developing scabies in that period it would be a most valuable contribution to the control of the disease.

Animal Scabies

Sarcoptes scabiei attacks many other mammals as well as human beings. Many of the infestations of animals have been transferred to man from time to time but they result in a different clinical picture with no burrows. Sometimes the mite can be found on the human skin but often not. The disease is self limited, indicating that the *Sarcoptes* does not propagate on the human skin in such instances. There has long been debate as to the zoological position of these mites. To the ordinary observer they seem to be morphologically identical with the mite of human origin. Entomological experts have long argued about alleged differences, which appear mainly to concern the extent of dorsal scales, occasional chaetotaxic variations and other minutiae. Physiologically the *Sarcoptes* from each animal is host specific. Fain (1978) has summarised the position and given an explanation beyond which it is not proposed to go. Pointing out that *Sarcoptes scabiei* produces scabies in 40 different hosts belonging to 17 families and seven orders of mammals he said that this might be explained by phylogeny. The Sarcoptidae is composed of four subfamilies. The genus *Sarcoptes* belongs to the subfamily Sarcoptinae, containing the four most evolved genera of the family Sarcoptidae. He has proposed that the genus *sarcoptes* has derived from one of the three genera of Sarcoptinae parasitic on monkeys (*Pro-sarcoptes*, *Co-sarcoptes* and *Pithe-sarcoptes*). *It seems that man is the original primary host for sarcoptes scabiei*, and that domestic animals acquired the mite from man. Later these mites infested wild carnivores and Bovidae. To adapt to these new hosts the mite developed slight differences (morphological and others) which have lessened its ability to re-infest man efficiently. However, these differences, according to Fain, have never become sufficient to prevent occasional interbreeding with strains from man and other animals.

Pillars (1931) stated that "Sarcoptic mange in animals tends to disappear gradually with the approach of summer and to recur as the winter returns. This I believe bears relation to the requirements of the parasite and to their differences in the length of coat and other seasonal variations of host function. In these circumstances it is possible for a lethargic and tolerant animal to infect its attendant whilst not being itself actually regarded as infected." This is particularly applicable to farmyard and zoological park animals.

Canine Scabies

Human cases of infestation by canine scabies were first described by Sauvages in 1763 (cited by Toomey 1922).

In the dog no breed is immune (Smith and Claypoole 1967) and no age exempt, although scabies is commonest in undernourished puppies. According to Schwartzmann (1977), the incidence of scabies in dogs is increasing in the United States. The onset is rapid, although Schwartzmann maintains that there is an incubation period of 4–6 weeks, less for heavy initial infestation, as in human scabies. The first lesions may appear on the muzzle, around the eyes and the edges of the ears (Toomey 1922), also in the axillae and groins (Smith and Claypoole 1967), or on the sternal area, hocks or root of the tail (Jubb and Kennedy 1970). It spreads from these areas in severe cases to the underside of the neck, the sides of the face, the belly and legs. This spread may occur in a matter of days (Tannenbaum 1965), especially if the animal is in poor condition (Schwartzmann 1977).

The lesions are pale or reddish papules, which are discrete but very numerous. Smith and Claypoole (1967) noted that burrowing occurred, but the burrows are not clinically visible. These lesions quickly become excoriated by scratching and biting, leading to crusting. There is a reactionary thickening of the skin, causing a lichenified wrinkled and fissured appearance. The hair tends to become matted together and often falls out in localised or widespread areas. There is a characteristic mousey odour (Smith and Claypoole 1967). Schwartzmann (1967) noted lymphadenopathy and fever. If the animal is untreated, secondary infection, cachexia and death ensues in 2–3 months (Toomey 1922). Smith and Claypoole (1967) have drawn attention to a diagnostic sign—the induction of paroxysmal scratching by rubbing the ears gently. Parasites are usually found fairly easily in the scales and crusts by using correct techniques (see p. 240) but sometimes are not discovered until a biopsy is examined (Schwartzmann 1967). Treatment consists of removing scales and crusts and applying antiscabietic preparations (e.g. sulphur ointment or γBHC) and is promptly curative, especially when used early.

The infestation is transferred to man by direct contact and also sometimes indirectly by the dog sleeping on chairs and beds used by its owners (Madison 1965). Outbreaks in man tend to occur in families who have just acquired an infested dog. All those in contact are usually affected. Elgart and Higdon (1972) have observed that the itch usually begins simultaneously in all affected members of the family. Any infested member of the family who leaves home for a period rapidly recovers, only to relapse on return home if the dog has not been treated (Madison 1965; Charlesworth and Johnson 1974).

Canine scabies in man was said by Tannenbaum (1965) to be relatively uncommon, but nowadays Orkin (1975a, 1977) maintains that it is becoming much commoner in the United States. Carillo and Carillo (1976) reported that 19 of 700 patients with scabies were proven to have acquired their infestation from dogs and appeared to have animal rather than human scabies. The onset is usually rapid, within a few hours of the first contact (Degos 1953; Hewitt et al. 1971), although Beck (1965) and Norins (1969) both observed a delay of 3–4 days. The first indication is itching, which, according to Madison (1965), is worse in the daytime and paroxysmal in character. Beck (1965), on the other hand, found it to be more pronounced in the evening. The lesions always appear first on the areas of contact with the dog. Charlesworth and Johnson (1974) emphasised that there was no relation between the degree of contact and the severity of the eruption. The areas commonly first affected are the forearms, the chest, the anterior abdominal wall and the front of the thighs, which are those areas in contact with the dog when it is held on the lap. To these areas Smith and Claypoole (1967) add the face in children, which Hewitt and his colleagues (1971) said was often affected. The neck is said to be initially involved in women who allow their small pet dogs to sit on their shoulders (Sequeira 1925; Martin 1938), whilst Williamson (1938) said that the *Sarcoptes* gained access on the wrists and ankles. Madison (1965) noted that the covered areas were those principally involved, and Hewitt et al. (1971) have pointed out that the mites can easily penetrate clothing. Secondary spread to other areas quickly occurs. Table 15.14 shows the frequency of involvement of the various areas in 22 cases (Smith and Claypoole 1967). The interdigital webs are very rarely affected (Beck 1965; Smith and Claypoole 1967).

Table 15.14. Frequency of involvement of different areas in 22 human patients with canine scabies. (After Smith and Claypoole 1967)

Area	Frequency
Belt line	20
Chest	15
Forearms and wrists	15
Back	13
Groins and upper thighs	12
Axillary folds	11
Sacrum	7
Lower leg and ankles	5
Face	3
Nipples	2
Finger webs	1
Genitalia	1

The lesions are papular, about 3 mm in diameter (Tannenbaum 1965), often becoming vesicular at the tip. There may be an underlying urticarial weal (Toomey 1922) and occasionally the base of the lesions may be telangiectatic (Madison 1965). They are discrete but tend to group and, if undiagnosed, continue to appear in crops so that early and late lesions are present simultaneously (Degos 1953). Although Toomey (1922) stated that very short burrows were present, all other authors agreed that burrows were not found. Excoriations quickly give rise to exudation and crust formation, and lichenification appears if the duration exceeds a few weeks. Treatment or removal of the infested dog results in gradual subsidence of the eruption. New lesions as a rule stop appearing. The outbreak may clear in from 6–10 days (Degos 1953) to 4–5 weeks (Smith and Claypoole 1967). The latter authors said that lesions will appear for as long as the mite can survive on human skin; in this respect Schwartzmann (1971) said that the canine *Sarcoptes* could survive away from the normal host for 2–3 weeks in dry conditions and for up to 8 weeks in humid conditions. Muller and Kirk (1971) quoted Parrish as suggesting that where canine *Sarcoptes* had multiplied on humans the dog in question had been, in fact, harbouring human mites which on return to their human host flourished normally. Whether this is correct is doubtful, since such patients could transmit the disorder to other humans and this has not been recorded as such. Dominguez et al. (1977), however, have reported from Mexico that a dog was successfully infested with a *Sarcoptes* (said to be var. *canis*) from a man with scabies of 8 years' duration. As long ago as 1928 Vitzhum asserted that canine scabies, in contrast to other animal strains, could multiply on the human skin.

Diagnosis depends on the history of contact, the distribution and character of the lesions and the identification of the *Sarcoptes*, either from human skin or more commonly from canine scrapings. In the last resort the diagnosis may be inferred if human patients recover on successful treatment of the dog. Newton and Gerrie (1966) have pointed out that diagnosis may be delayed if the technique of confirmation is inadequate and if symptomatic shotgun therapy including oral corticosteroid is used either for dog or man.

Although canine scabies is a self-limiting disease, Smith and Claypoole (1967) showed that the use of antiscabietics reduces the average duration from 18 to 4 days. Sulphur ointment and γBHC are both effective.

Equine Scabies

The equine form of scabies is less common than heretofore because of the diminishing use of the horse for military, agricultural and transport purposes. Nevertheless, it is still a risk. The first human cases of equine scabies were reported by Sik in 1791 (Toomey 1922). Engelberting (1920) thought it was commoner than was generally realised. Pillars (1931) noted that he suspected it whenever he saw a stablehand standing about scratching both arms simultaneously.

Affected horses are usually neglected or debilitated (Imes 1926). According to Jubb and Kennedy (1970), the eruption usually starts on the head and neck or the withers, but in severe cases large areas may be affected. In the latter case the number of parasites may be very great (McDonald 1922).

The condition is acquired, as a rule, by grooming or riding affected horses. McDonald's patients were six veterinary students who had performed a post-mortem on an infested animal. The equine variant of the *Sarcoptes* does not thrive on man, although Pick (1917) had observed an adult female with two eggs in scrapings from a human patient. Once the source of contagion is removed, the condition begins to subside.

In the early stages the lesions in man consist of pinhead-sized, usually follicular, slightly raised fiery red papules (McDonald 1922), whereas in lesions of longer duration than 1 or 2 days there is erythema and urtication with some infiltration and crust formation following scratching (Toomey 1922). The urtication may give rise to residual staining. Toomey claims to have seen tiny burrows in the papules.

The first lesions appear in the areas of contact within a matter of a few hours, on the forearms, in the groins, on the inner thighs in riders, and, in the students mentioned above, on the forearms, ankles and calves. Other areas such as shoulders, upper arms, thighs, neck and trunk and, to a lesser degree, the buttocks are secondarily involved. Axillae, breasts and interdigital webs are not involved (Toomey 1922), although one of McDonald's students had interdigital lesions. The face, scalp and genitalia are seldom affected. All lesions itch, especially when warm, but not excessively.

The plentiful use of carbolic soap and water after contact is an effective inhibitor of the condition (Pick 1917; McDonald 1922). The diagnosis depends on the history and the distribution and on finding the parasite in scrapings from the human or animal contact. Toomey (1922) said it may only be distinguished from trombidiasis or tarsonemidosis by the distribution—the lower legs and thighs in the former and the trunk and general asymmetry in the latter.

Treatment consists of removal from and treatment of the source; sulphur ointment is used for the lesions. In the very early stages tincture of iodine applied to the lesions is apparently adequate (McDonald 1922).

Camel Scabies

Camel drivers and zoological attendants are liable to develop a skin eruption if in contact with mangy camels. The first confirmed cases were recorded by Biett in 1827 (Toomey 1922). In man the eruption consists of exceedingly irritating follicular papules, many of which are excoriated and secondarily infected (Dyson 1921). It usually commences on the arms and spreads to the legs and chest (the areas of contact). Dyson noted that belts or other constrictive bands sharply limited the involved area (cf. flea bites, *Pyemotes* infestation etc). Toomey (1922) claimed that it closely resembled human scabies, but the absence of burrows and the character and distribution of the lesions show that he was incorrect.

The diagnosis is made by identifying the mite in scrapings from the papules, since the parasite tends to conceal itself in hair follicles. Examination of scales from the camel is more reliable.

Treatment consists of avoiding the camel and applying antipruritic preparations. The disease is self limited. Treatment of the camel will prevent recurrence.

Goat Scabies

Goat owners and their families and possibly other contacts, especially those who milk the goats, are the most likely victims. The goat itches severely, relieving itself by rubbing on hard surfaces, and shows multiple small papules, sometimes excoriated and often lichenified (Jubb and Kennedy 1970). Some lesions may be perifollicular and scale profusely; the hair becomes matted and may fall out and sometimes there is a foul smell with blood-stained discharge. Mostly the lesions occur on the head and neck but may spread to the trunk. The condition responds to Tetmosol soap and sulphur ointment (Chakravorty 1953).

In human patients the itch is severe, especially in the young. According to Panja and Ghosh (1952), the lesions are tiny papules and blisters, but Chakravorty et al. (1953) found mostly pustules with a few papulovesicles. There were no burrows. The affected areas varied according to contact. In some the back and palm of the hands was the chief site, whilst Chakravorty's patients were affected on the inner aspect of the upper arms, the forearms, the elbows, lower abdomen, groins and the buttocks.

The diagnosis depends mainly on the history of contact and the nature and distribution of the lesions. Confirmation by finding mites in scrapings from the papules can often be obtained. Sulphur ointment may help. The disease is self limiting, but itch often persists after cure.

Cat Scabies

Cat scabies is uncommon. When it does occur it resembles canine scabies and when transmitted to man it presents the same picture (Degos 1953).

Sheep Scabies

Only the hairy areas (i.e. the face and feet) are involved in sheep, not the woollen areas of the skin (Muller and Kirk 1969). The condition can affect man on rare occasions. It is very tenacious and apparently does not clear spontaneously (Degos 1953).

Pig Scabies

Scabies is not uncommon in pigs; usually it is generalised, but sometimes localised to the ears (Muller and Kirk 1969). According to Toomey, only eight cases in man had been recorded up to 1922 and usually localised. One case quoted persisted for 40 days and was not transmitted to the patient's wife, although she shared his bed during the period of his illness. Burrows were not found, but there were disseminated small, intensely itchy vesicopapules with a diffuse urticarial reaction. The condition responded to simple glycerine of starch dressings.

Cattle Scabies

Muller and Kirk (1969) stated that the condition of cattle scabies is similar to that in horses. Huynen (1926) reported scabies exclusive to cattle which did not affect horses but which could be transferred to humans. One case he described occurred in a woman who milked an affected cow and developed lesions on her arms and whole of the trunk. The eruption cleared quickly with a preparation containing balsam of Peru. Huynen noted that in the cattle the disease disappeared in the summer but recurred in the winter (see Pillars 1931, referred to on p. 282).

Monkey Scabies

Goldman and Feldman (1949) described an outbreak in ten gibbons in a zoological park, all of which were scratching. When put into their quarters they were noted to be weak and to have lost weight. The skin was extensively involved, with scaling over the limbs and trunk, and was infiltrated and hairless. Seven died fairly quickly and two more after treatment with sulphur dips. There were huge numbers of parasites and histologically the skin resembled that of Norwegian scabies. Five helpers became infested with a condition indistinguishable from human scabies, even to the extent of having burrows on the hands and genitalia, and one patient developed a persistent nodule on the scrotum. They were successfully treated with benzyl benzoate or γBHC.

References

Ackerman AB (1977) The pathology of scabies. In: Orkin M, Maibach HI, Parish LC, Schwartzman RM (eds) Scabies and pediculosis. Lippincott, Philadelphia, pp 88–95

Ackerman AB, Stewart R, Stillman M (1975) Scabies masquerading as dermatitis herpetiformis. JAMA 233: 53–54

*Adams J (1807) Observations on morbid poisons, chronic and acute, 2nd edn. Callow, London, pp 293–310

Alexander AM (1978) Role of race in scabies infestation. Arch Dermatol 114: 627

Alexander JO'D (1967a) The scabies epidemic. Br Med J I: 766

Alexander JO'D (1967b) Infectivity of scabies. Br Med J II: 683

Alexander JO'D (1968) Scabies and pediculosis. Practitioner 200: 632–644

Alexander JO'D (1969) Scabies in children. Clin Pediatr 8: 73–85

Allen BR (1972) Scabies and acute glomerulonephritis. Lancet I: 434

Amer M, El-Bayoumi M, Rizk MK (1981) Treatment of scabies; preliminary report. Int J Dermatol 20: 289–290

Anderson TMcC (1863) A practical treatise upon eczema, including the lichenous, impetiginous and pruriginous varieties. Churchill, London

Anderson TMcC (1872) On treatment of diseases of the skin. Macmillan, London, pp 32, 102, 125

Anderson TMcC (1894) A treatise on diseases of the skin. Griffin, London, pp 143, 209, 228, 613, 616, 617

Andrews JRH (1979) Scabies in New Zealand. Int J Dermatol 18: 545–552

Andrews MLA (1976) The life that lives on man. Faber and Faber, London, pp 75–165

Anolik MA, Rudolph RI (1976) Scabies simulating Darier's disease in an immunologically suppressed patient. Arch Dermatol 112: 73–74

*Anthony BF, Perlman LV, Wannamaker LW (1967) Skin infections and acute nephritis in American Indian children. Pediatrics 39: 263–279

Araujo-Fontaine A, Thiery R, Heid E (1977) Les IgE sèriques dans la gale. Étude sur 100 cas. Ann Dermatol Venereol 104: 203–205

Aterman K, Krause VW, Ross JB (1976) Scabies masquerading as Letterer-Siwe disease. Can Med Assoc J 115: 434–444

Ayres S, Anderson NP (1932) Persistent nodules in scabies. Arch Dermatol Syphilol 25: 485–493

Backhouse TC (1929) Sarcoptic skin disease in the natives of Territory of New Guinea. Trans R Soc Trop Med Hyg 23: 173–178

Bacon LJ (1942) Scabies. Br Med J II: 266

Bacon LJ (1944) Diagnosis of scabies. Med Officer 71: 101–103

Bagnall B, Rook A (1977) Arthropods and the skin. In: Rock A (ed) Recent advances in dermatology 4. Churchill, Edinburgh, pp 59–90

Balfanz U (1978) Antipruriginosum auch bei Skabies effektiv. Artz Praxis 30: 245–247

Banerjee AK, Chowdhury D Sur Roy (1972) Epidemic of scabies in 1971. Bull Calcutta School Trop Med 20: 12–14

Barale Th, Bidard de la Noe A, Agache P (1971) Nodule post-scabieux. Bull Soc Fr Dermatol Syphiligr 78: 449–451

Baranova O (1927) Scabies norvegica (in Russian). Medicinskaya 4: 49–52. Extracted by Zentralbl Haut Geschlechtskr (1928) 27: 72–73

Barranco DG, Trujillo VM, Mallen MS, Llamas OO (1976) Tratamento del enfermo escabiosico resistente a los medicamentos. Med Cutan Iber Lat Am 4: 149–152

Barthelmes H, Barthelmes R (1974) Untersuchungen zur Zunahme der Scabies-Erkrankungen IV: ? Scabies, Allergie und persistieren Noduli. Dermatol Monatsschr 160: 573–586
Bartley WC, Mellanby K (1944) The parasitology of human scabies (women and children). Parasitology 35: 207–208
Bartley W, Unsworth K, Gordon RM (1945) Incidence of scabies in a community using ordinary soap, and its subsequent fall on the substitution of 5% Tetmosol soap. Br Med J I: 332–333
Bateman T (1813) A practical synopsis of cutaneous diseases, 2nd edn. Longman, Hurst, Rees, Orme and Brown, London, pp 197–201
Bateman T (1819) A practical synopsis of cutaneous diseases, 5th edn. Longman, Hurst, Rees, Orme and Brown, London, pp 190–206
Bateman T (1829) A practical synopsis of cutaneous disease, 7th edn. Longman, Rees, Orme, Brown and Green, London
Bazin E (1858) Lécons thèoriques et cliniques sur les affectious cutanées parasitaires. Delahaye, Paris, pp 217–235
Bean SF (1974) Bullous scabies. JAMA 230: 878
Beatty W (1913) A case of Norwegian or crusted scabies. Br J Dermatol 25: 56–60
Beck AL Jr (1965) Animal scabies affecting man. Arch Dermatol 91: 54–55
Beek CH, Mellanby K (1953) Scabies. In: Simon RDGP (ed) Handbook of tropical dermatology and medical mycology. Elsevier, Amsterdam, pp 875–888
*Beeson DB (1927) *Acarus scabiei*: a study of its history. Arch Dermatol Syphilol 16: 294–307
Biagi F, Delgado-y-Garnica R (1974) First therapeutic trial in the treatment of scabies with thiabendazole cream. Int J Dermatol 13: 102–103
Bible II Kings 15, verses 9–27
Leviticus 5, verses 2–13
Björnberg A (1975) Ricidiverandi pustulos hos adoptivbarn fran Sud-och Ostasien. Lakartidningen 72: 5142
Blacklock B (1924) Craw-Craw in Sierra Leone. Ann Trop Med Parasitol 18: 253–262
*Blumberg RW, Feldman DB (1962) Observations on acute glomerulo-nephritis associated with impetigo. J Paediatr 60: 677–685
Blumental DS, Taplin D, Schultz MD (1976) Am J Epidemiol 104: 667–672
Boas H (1952) Scabies norvegica—a case. Hautarzt 3: 40
Bommer S (1955) Scabies Norvegica (Norwegian Scabies). Arch Dermatol Syphilis 200: 433–436
Bonaduce F (1927) Sintomatologia rara da acaro della scabbia. G Ital Dermatol Sifil 68: 887–888
Boog-Watson WN (1971) Notes on collection and research—"The Scotch fiddle". Off Scot Stud 15: 141–145
*Borda JM (1954) Sarna Humana. Arq Argent Dermatol 4: 101–133, 255–286
Borrie P (1967) Roxburgh's common skin diseases, 13th edn. Lewis, London, pp 123–146
Bourguignon M (1852) Traité entomologique et pathologique de les gales de l'homme. Paris. Cited by Heilesen (1946)
Bradshaw DB (1944) Tetraethyl thiuram monosulphide in the treatment of scabies. Lancet II: 273–274
Bricklin AS, Musgnug RH (1978) Norwegian scabies; a new complication of immunosuppressive therapy. Cutis 22: 81–89
Brug SL, Haga J, Joost RPACh van, Verbunt JAM (1930) Scabies crustaso s. norvegica (in Dutch). Geneesk Tyijdschr Ned Indie 70: 576–587. Cited in Zentralbl Haut Geschlechtskr (1931) 35: 522
Burckhardt W, Rymarowicz R (1946) Ehrfahrungen mit dem neuen Antiscabiosum 'Eurax'. Schweiz Med Wochenschr 47: 1213–1214
Burgess I (1973) Unusual features of scabies associated with topical fluorinated steroids. Br J Dermatol 88: 519–520
Burkhart CG (1983) Scabies; an epidemiological reassessment. Ann Intern Med 98: 498–503
Burks JW, Jung R, George WM (1956) Norwegian scabies. Arch Dermatol 74: 131–140
Burrows D, Bridges JM, Morris TCM (1975) Reactivation of scabies by methotrexate. Br J Dermatol 93: 219–222
Buxton PA (1921) The external anatomy of the *Sarcoptes* of the horse. Parasitology 13: 114–145
Calnan CD (1950) Crusted scabies. Br J Dermatol 62: 71–78
Cannon AB, McCrae ME (1948) Treatment of scabies; report of one hundred patients treated with hexachlorocyclohexane in vanishing cream base. JAMA 138: 557
Carillo JM, Carillo D (1976) Acariasis estudio de 700 cases. Actas Dermosifiliogr 67: 195–206
Carpenter CC (1948) A rapid technique for the diagnosis of scabies. US Navy Med Bull 48: 566–568
Carpenter CC, Henlein JA, Sulzberger MB, Baer RL (1946) Scabies and pediculosis treated with benzyl benzoate, D.D.T., benzocaine emulsion. J Invest Dermatol 7: 93–98
*Carslaw RW, Dobson RM, Hood AJK, Taylor RN (1975) Mites in the environment of cases of Norwegian scabies. Br J Dermatol 92: 333–338
Chakravorty AN, Ghosh S, Banerjee AK (1953) Case notes of scabies in a family transmitted from goats. Indian Med Gaz 88: 153–154
Chang KH, Lee WH, Chun SI, Koh CJ (1983) The clinical study of scabietic patients (in Korean with English summary). Korean J Dermatol 21: 23–27
Charlesworth EN, Johnson JL (1974) An epidemic of canine scabies in man. Arch Dermatol 110: 572–574
Charmes JP, Bonnet-Blanc JM, Roux J, Benevent D, Leroux-Robert C (1978) Scabies and acute glomerulonephriitis Lancet I: 499
Cherikover YA (1937) Norwegian scabies (in Russian). Clin Med (Moscow) 15: 739–743
Chouyet B, Ortonne JP, Perrot H, Thivolet J (1979) La gale norvègienne: circonstances étiologiques. Ann Dermatol Venereol 106: 569–574
Chowdhury DSR, Hati AK (1975) Treatment of scabies. Indian J Dermatol 20: 33–35
*Christopherson J (1978) The epidemiology of scabies in Denmark. Arch Dermatol 114: 747–750
Church R, Knowlesden J (1974) Scabies in the city of Sheffield. Br J Dermatol 9, Suppl. 10: 13–14
Church RE, Knowlesden J (1978) Scabies in Sheffield: a family infestation. Br Med J I: 761
Clayton R, Farrow S (1975) Norwegian scabies following topical steroid therapy. Postgrad Med J 51: 657–659
Clayton TM (1943) Treatment of scabies by T.E.T.M.S. Br Med J I: 443–445
Cohen HB (1982) Scabies continues. Int J Dermatol 21: 134–135
Crewe FAE (1955) Army Medical Services Administration vol II: Medical history of the Second World War. HMSO, London, pp 207–212
Cubela V, Yawalkar SJ (1978) Clinical experience with crotamiton cream and lotion in treatment of infants with scabies. Br J Clin Pract 32: 229–231
Cumston CG (1924) Some remarks on the history of the discovery of the *Acarus scabiei*. Br J Dermatol Syphilol 36: 13–18
Da Costa SM (1918) Scabies. Ned Tijdschr Geneeskd 1: 1281. Extracted in JAMA (1918) 71: 502
Da Fonseca (1969) An effective public health programme for combating cutaneous parasitoses. Dermatol Int 8: 63–65
Danby PR, Church RE, Sneddon IB (1967) Eradicating scabies. Br Med J I: 496

Darier J (1918) In discussion on scabies and pediculosis. Med Bull Am Red Cross Soc Fr 1, 4: 223–233
Davies JE, Dadhia HW, Morgade C, Barquet A, Maibach H (1983) Lindane poisoning. Arch Dermatol 119: 142–144
DeGeer C (1778) Memoires pour servir, à l'histoire des insectes. Stockholm
Degos R (1953) Dermatologie. Flammarion, Paris, pp 946–960
De Mello ET, Uthida-Tanaka AM (1970) Escabiose e tiabindazole. Rev Paul Med 73: 77–79
Demjanovic M (1933) Methode der beschleinigten Scabiesbehandlung (in Russian). Sov Vest Venereol Dermatol 2: 254–260. Cited by Zentralbl Haut Geschlechtskr (1933) 46: 343
Desai SC (1972) Infections and communicable dermatoses. Reflections on the massive morbidity of scabies, pyoderma and mycotic infections. In: Marshall J (ed) Essays on tropical dermatology. Excerpta Medica, Amsterdam, pp 296–300
Desai SC, Nair SS (1978) Ecology and epidemiology of scabies in India. Indian J Dermatol Venereol Leprol 44: 197–203
Dixon CW (1941) Scabiės: a golden opportunity. Public Health 55: 10–14
Dockhorn RJ (1974) Classification of immune tissue reaction in dermatological disease. Cutis 13: 1063–1068
Domenjoz R (1946) Ueber ein neues Antiscabiosum. Schweiz Med Wochenschr 76: 1210–1212
Dominguez OJ, Ruiz-Maldonaldo R, Tamayo SL, Auro SR (1977) Transmission esperimental del hombre al pero de escabiosis por *Sarcoptes scabiei* var. *canis*. Veterinaria (Mexico) 8: 37–41
Dowling GB (1929) Norwegian scabies. Proc R Soc Med 23: 355
Dubreuilh W (1918) Scabies. J Med Bordeaux 89: 183. Cited in JAMA (1918) 71: 858
*Dubreuilh W, Beille L (1895) Parasites animaux de la peau humain. Masson et Cie, Paris, pp 1–177
Dubreuilh W, Sainte-Marie F (1924) Un cas gale norvègienne. Bull Soc Fr Dermatol Syphiligr 31: 45–56
Dyson W (1921) Camel itch. Br J Dermatol 33: 107–108
Eddy GW (1944) A treatment for head lice, crab lice and scabies. War Med 6: 319–322
Eddy GW (1946) A combination treatment for lice and scabies. J Invest Dermatol 7: 85–91
Editorial (1976a) Whither scabies. Br Med J I: 357
Editorial (1976b) IgE, parasites and allergy. Lancet I: 894
Elgart ML, Higdon RS (1972) Canine scabies: a report of a family outbreak. South Med J 65: 375–376
Ellis T, MacDougall JA, Reeves RM, Fisher D (1971) Scabies—Maine. Morbid mortal weekly rep 20: 445
Elmers T, Hornqvist R (1981) Infestation of scabies in the scalp area. Acta Derm Venereol (Stockh) 61: 360–362
Ely PH (1977) Estar gel for nodular scabies. Schoch Let 27: 11
Engelberting (1920) Die Uebertragung der Rande des Pferdes auf den Menschen. Dtsch Tieraerztl Wochenschr 28: 501–502
Epstein E (1942) Rotenone in the treatment of scabies. Arch Dermatol Syphilol 45: 950–952
Epstein E (1955) Incidence of scabies. Dermatologica 110: 126–132
Epstein E (1977) Traditional methods of treatment. In: Orkin M, Maibach HI, Parish LC, Schwartzman RM (eds) Scabies and pediculosis. Lippincott, Philadelphia, pp 105–107
Epstein E, Orkin M (1977) Scabies—clinical aspects. In: Orkin M, Maibach I, Parish LC, Schwartzman RM (eds) Scabies and pediculosis. Lippincott, Philadelphia, pp 17–22
Erskine D (1967a) Eradication of scabies. Br Med J I: 699
Erskine D (1967b) A skinful of alcohol. Lancet I: 54
Espy PD, Jolly HW (1976) Norwegian scabies, occurrence in a patient undergoing immunosuppression. Arch Dermatol 112: 193–196
Estes SA (1982) Diagnosis and management of scabies. Med Clin North Am 66: 955–963
*Fain A (1968) Étude de la variabilité de *Sarcoptes scabiei* avec une revision des Sarcoptidae. Acta Zool Pathol Antverp No 47: 1–196
*Fain A (1978) Epidemiological problems of scabies. Int J Dermatol 17: 20–30
Falk ES (1980) Serum immunoglobulin values in patients with scabies. Br J Dermatol 102: 57–61
Falk ES, Bolle R (1980a) IgE antibodies to house dust mite in patients with scabies. Br J Dermatol 102: 283–288
Falk ES, Bolle R (1980b) *In vitro* demonstration of specific immunological hypersensitivity to scabies mite. Br J Dermatol 103: 367–373
Farkaš J (1974) K problematike swabi. Cesk Dermatol 49: 343–349
Ferencei M, Holanová J, Farkaš J (1976) Epidemiologiká analýza vizokylii u Bratislava za Voky 1972–1974. Cesk Dermatol 51: 124–130
Ferguson AJA (1973) Norwegian scabies during immunosuppressive therapy. Br J Dermatol 89, Suppl 4: 485–486
Fergusson AG (1967) Eradication of scabies. Br Med J I: 628
Fernandez N, Torres A, Ackermann AB (1977) Pathologic findings in human scabies. Arch Dermatol 113: 320–324
Floden CH (1947) Tenutex, a new compound containing DDT for the treatment of scabies and lice. Acta Derm Venereol (Stockh) 27: 1–12
Forsbeck M, Werner Y, Kolmodin-Hedman B (1977) Treatment of scabies. Opuscula Med 22: 124–126
Fox T (1864) Skin disease. Hardwick, London
Fox T (1875) Clinical lecture on itch in private practice and its treatment. Br Med J I: 102–103
Franklin JL, Baker JA (1967) Benzyl benzoate. Br Med J I: 766
Frentz G, Veien NK, Eriksen K (1977) Immunofluorescence studies in scabies. J Cutan Pathol 4: 191–193
Friedman R (1941) Scabies—civil and military. Its prevalence, prevention and treatment. Froben, New York
Friedman R (1942) Biology of *Acarus scabiei*. Froben, New York
Friedman R (1943) Atypical scabies—diagnosis by the scrape and smear method. Penn Med J 47: 39–41
*Friedman R (1948) The story of scabies. Froben, New York
Garcovitch A, Capizzi R, Garcovitch M (1978) La scabbia nodulare. G Ital Dermatol Minerva Dermatol 113: 349–354
Geffen MW (1944) Observations on scabies at the St. Pancras Bathing Centre. Br Med J II: 825
George WM (1958) Norwegian scabies. Arch Dermatol 78: 320–324
Gerlach AC (1857) Krätze and Räude. Berlin. Cited by Heilesen (1946)
Gold S (1966) A skinful of alcohol. Lancet II: 1417
Goldman L, Feldman MD (1949) Human infestation with scabies of monkeys. Arch Dermatol Syphilol 59: 175–178
Golebiowska-Podgorczyk I, Szarmach H (1968) Czy epidemia swierzbu? Pol Tyg Lek 23: 1931–1933
Gordon RM, Lavoipierre MMJ (1962) Entomology for students of medicine. Blackwell, Oxford
Gordon RM, Davey TH, Unsworth K, Hellier FF, Parry SC, Alexander JRB (1944) Control of scabies by use of soap impregnated with tetraethyl-thiuram monosulphide. Br Med J I: 803–806
Gourley CA (1967) Eradicating scabies. Br Med J I: 112
Graham JR (1943) Scabies treated with one application of benzyl benzoate. Br Med J I: 413–414
Grant PW (1967) Scabies. Br Med J I: 246
Grant PW, Keczkes K (1964) Persistent nodules in scabies: a case report with a review of the literature. Arch Dermatol 89: 239–242
Gray AMH (1942) Treatment of scabies. Br Med J 2: 170
Green J (1835) Diseases of the skin. Whittaker, London, pp 63–68
Greenhough FB (1886) Clinical notes on scabies. Boston Med

Surg J 115: 269–272
Gulati PV, Singh KP, Braganza C (1977a) Role of socio-cultural and environmental factors in the cause of scabies. Int J Dermatol 16: 281–283
Gulati PV, Braganza C, Singh KP, Borker V (1977b) Scabies in a semi-urban area of India: an epidemiologic study. Int J Dermatol 16: 594–598
Haber H (1963) In discussion on Samman (1963) Br J Dermatol 73: 35
Han EH, Kwan KS, Chung TA (1983) Clinical study of scabies for 15 years (In Korean with English summary). Korean J Dermatol 21: 7–17
Hancock BW, Milford-Ward A (1974) Serum immunoglobulins in scabies. J Invest Dermatol 63: 482–484
Hand EA (1946) Diagnosis of infestation with *Sarcoptes scabiei* var. *hominis*. US Nav Med Bull 46: 834–844
Hans R (1976) Aplastic anaemia associated with gamma benzene hexachloride JAMA 236: 1009–1010
Hansen RC, Lynch PY (1976) Scabies; problems in physician recognition. Ariz Med 33: 366–368
Hardy A (1886) Traité pratique et descriptif des maladies de la peau. Baillière, Paris, pp 427–470
Hare PJ (1967) Eradicating scabies. Br Med J I: 699
Hay RJ (1974) Norwegian scabies in a patient with a cutaneous vasculitis. Guys Hosp Rep 123: 177–185
Haydon JR, Caplan RM (1971) Epidemic scabies. Arch Dermatol 103: 168–173
Hazelrigg DE, Jarratt M (1975) Diagnosis of scabies. South Med J 68: 549–551
Hebra F von (1852) Über eine in Norwegen beobachte neue Form der Krätze. Z Gesellschaft Aerzt Wien I: 390
*Hebra F von (1868) On disease of the skin including the exanthemata, vol II. Translated by Fagge CH and Pye-Smith PH The New Sydenham Society, London, pp 164–252
Heid E, Samsoen M, Strobel M, Grosshans E, Oberling F (1974) Gales florides et déficits immunitaires. Rapport avec la gale croûteuse. Bull Soc Fr Dermatol Syphiligr 81: 584–587
*Heilesen B (1946) Studies on *Acarus scabiei* and scabies. Acta Derm Venereol (Stockh) 26 Suppl 14: 1–370
Heilesen B (1948) Treatment of scabies with dixanthogen liniment. Acta Derm Venereol (Stockh) 28: 515–517
Hejazi N, Mehregan AH (1975) Scabies: histologic study of inflammatory lesions. Arch Dermatol 111: 37–39
Hellier FF (1941) In discussion on prevention and treatment of parasitic disease; some recent works on the louse. Br J Dermatol 53: 157
Hellier FF (1945) Scabies and DDT. Br Med J II: 255
Hellier FF (1966) Incidence of scabies. Arch Dermatol 93: 634
Hellier FF (1976) Whither scabies? Br Med J I: 772
Herman P, Jacobs M, Smith B, McClintock B, Martz A, Farrar W, Holder W (1975) Scabies: Florida, New Mexico. Morbid Mortal Weekly Rep 24: 118–123
Hernandez-Perez E (1971) Escabiosis: Una parasitosis que vuelva. Arq Col Med El Salvador 24: 92–99
Hernandez-Perez E (1976) Topically applied thiabendazole in the treatment of scabies. Arch Dermatol 112: 1400–1401
Hernandez-Perez E (1983) Resistance to antiscabietic drugs. J Am Acad Dermatol 8: 121–122
Hernandez-Perez E, Bechelli CA (1969) Tiabendazol oral en escabiosis Dermatol Iberolat 4: 427–432
Hernandez-Perez E, Santos LR, Bechelli CA (1969) Thiabendazol en escabiosis. Med Cutan 3: 509–511
Herridge CF (1963) Norwegian scabies (crusted scabies) Br Med J I: 239–240
Hersch C (1967) Acute glomerulonephritis due to skin diseases with special reference to scabies. S Afr Med J 41: 29–34
Hewitt M, Walton GS, Waterhouse H (1971) Pet animal infestations and human skin lesions. Br J Dermatol 85: 215–225
Hoeppli R (1959) Parasites and parasitic infections in early medicine and science. University of Malaya Press, Singapore
Hoke AW (1973) Scabies scraping. Arch Dermatol 108: 424
Howell JB (1950) Office diagnosis of scabies. Arch Dermatol Syphilol 62: 144–147
Hubler WR, Clabaugh W (1976) Epidemic Norwegian scabies. Arch Dermatol 112: 179–181
Hunt T (1865) A guide to the treatment of diseases of the skin, 8th edn. Richards, London, pp 118–123
Hunter RL (1972) Of prophets, kings, worms and things. Cutis 9: 317–324
Hurwitz S (1973) Scabies in babies. Am J Dis Child 126: 226–228
Hurwitz S (1977) Scabies in infants and children. In: Orkin M, Maibach HI, Parish LC, Schwartzman RM (eds) Scabies and pediculosis. Lippincott, Philadelphia, pp 31–38
Hutfield DC (1967a) Incidence of scabies. Lancet I: 844
Hutfield DC (1967b) Scabies and promiscuity. Int Med Trib 2: 5
Hutfield DC (1967c) Rise of scabies. Int Med Trib 2:
Hutfield DC (1967d) Scabies and promiscuity (2). Int Med Trib 2:
Huynen E (1926) De la gale sarcoptique chex le bête bovine. Sa transmission à l'homme. Ann Med Vet 71: 56–60
Hyde JN (1905) Scabies in the United States of America and Canada. Am J Med Sci 129: 453–465
Imes M (1926) Lice, mange and ticks of horses and methods of control and eradication. US Dept of Agriculture Farmers Bulletin No 1493. US Govt Printing Office, Washington DC, pp 1–22
Ingram JT (1951) Ward epidemic from Norwegian scabies. Br J Dermatol 63: 311–317
Ingram JT (1967) The scabies epidemic. Br Med J I: 506
Itani Z (1970) Scabies—diagnostik, Z Haut Geschlechtskr 45: 617–624
Ive FA, Marks R (1968) Tinea incognito. Br Med J 3: 149
Johnson CG, Mellanby K (1942) The parasitology of human scabies. Parasitology 34: 285–290
Jubb KVF, Kennedy PC (1970) Pathology of domestic animals, 3rd edn. Academic, New York
Juranek DD, Schultz MG (1977) Epidemiologic investigations of scabies in the United States. In: Orkin M, Maibach HI, Parish LC, Schwartzman RM (eds) Scabies and pediculosis. Lippincott, Philadelphia, pp 64–72
Kaposi M (1895) Diseases of the skin. Translated by Johnson JC Baillière, Tindall and Cox, London
Kavli G (1978) Diagnosis of scabies. Arch Dermatol 114: 798
Keczkes K, Innes ID, Haywood CP (1967) Eradication of scabies. Br Med J 1: 628
Kissmeyer A (1937) Rapid ambulatory treatment of scabies with benzyl benzoate lotion. Lancet I: 21
Kitchevatz M, Pochtich Z (1934) Reaction allergiques cutanées dans la gale. Bull Soc Fr Dermatol Syphilogr 41: 989. Cited by Prakken and van Vloten (1949)
Knowles FC (1918) Scabies in military and civil life. JAMA 71: 1657–1658
Kobayashi M, Miyoshi I, Sonobe H, Taguchi H, Kubonishi (1982) Association of *Pneumocystis carinii* pneumonia and scabies. JAMA 248: 1973
Kocsard E (1976) Crude coal tar for nodular scabies. Schoch Lett 26: 3
Kolmodin-Hedman B, Borglund E, Werner Y (1979) Percutaneous absorption of DDT from a parasiticide used for treatment of scabies. Acta Derm Venereol (Stockh) 59: 276–278
Konstantinov D, Stanoeva I (1973) Persistent scabious nodules. Dermatologica 147: 321–327
Konstantinov D, Stanoeva I (1976) Norwegian scabies in

homozygous twins. Dermatologica 152: 55–59
Konstantinov D, Stanoeva I, Yawalkar SJ (1979) Crotamiton cream and lotion in treatment of infants and young children with scabies. J Int Med Res 7: 443–448
Kornblee LV, Combes EC (1950) Gammexane in the treatment of scabies. Arch Dermatol 61: 407–412
Landgren J, Borglund E, Storgards K (1979) Treatment of scabies with disulfiram and benzyl benzoate emulsion: a controlled study. Acta Dermat Venereol (Stockh) 59: 274–276
Lane JE (1928) Bonomo's letter to Redi. An important document in the history of scabies. Arch Dermatol Syphilol 18: 1–25
Larregue M, Gompert P, Levy Cl, Gallet Ch, Raj J-P (1976) Elevation des IgE dans le gale chez l'enfant. Bull Soc Fr Dermatol Syphiligr 83: 54–56
Lasch EE, Frankel V, Vardy PA, Bergner-Rabinowitz S, Ofek I, Rabinowitz K (1971) Epidemic glomerulonephritis in Israel. J Inf Dis 124: 141–147
Lee B, Groth P (1977) Scabies—transcutaneous poisoning during treatment. Paediatrics 59: 643
Lee B, Groth P, Turner W (1976) Suspected reaction to gamma benzene hexachloride. JAMA 236: 2846
Lerche NW, Currier RW, Juranek DD, Baer W, Dubny NJ (1983) Atypical crusted "Norwegian" scabies. Report of a nosocomial transmission in a community hospital and an approach to control. Cutis 31: 367–384
Levenson I (1974) Scabies. Arch Dermatol 110: 463
Lolio M, Schenone H, Saavedra T, Banda R, Villarrael F, Rojo M, Subiabre V, Arias B, Rujas A, Vicent P, Grinspun M, Sudy E, Caneilo J, Sepulveda A, Salas L (1975) Prevalencia actual de sarna y pediculosis capitis en alumnos de la ensenanzo basico de Santiago, Chile (Junio–Junio de 1975). Bol Chil Parasitol 30: 50–53
Lomholt G (1972) Dermatology in Uganda. Int J Dermatol 11: 156
Lomholt G (1977) Scabies in Norway. In: Orkin M, Maibach HI, Parish LC, Schwartzman RM (eds) Scabies and pediculosis. Lippincott, Philadelphia, pp 81–83
Lunn HF (1942) Recognition of scabies by army medical officers. J R Army Med Corps 79: 203–206
Lunn HF (1944–1945) Observations on the *Sarcoptes* of man. Parasitology 36: 67–68.
Lyell A (1967) Diagnosis and treatment of scabies. Br Med J II: 223–225
MacCormac H (1918) In discussion on scabies and pediculosis. Med Bull Am Red Cross Soc Fr 1, 4: 223–233
MacCormac H (1943) Three skin diseases in wartime. Br Med J II: 667–669
MacDonald RAS (1922) Observations on an extensive human infection by sarcoptic mange of the horse. Lancet I: 738–739
MacMillan AL (1972) Unusual features of scabies associated with topical fluorinated steroids. Br J Dermatol 87: 496–497
McPhail A (1925) History of the Canadian forces 1914–1919: medical services. Acland, Ottawa
Madison JF (1965) Human infestation with canine scabies. J Maine Med Assoc 56: 131
Madsen A (1970) Mite burrows in crusts from young infants. Acta Derm Venereol (Stockh) 50: 391–392
Maibach HI, Orkin M (1977a) Adverse reactions to treatment. In: Orkin M, Maibach HI, Parish LC, Schwartzman RM (eds) Scabies and pediculosis. Lippincott, Philadelphia, pp 117–124
Maibach HI, Orkin M (1977b) Scabies: therapy on the horizon. In: Orkin M, Maibach HI, Parish LC, Schwartzman RM (eds) Scabies and pediculosis. Lippincott, Philadelphia, pp 125–129
Mallen KC (1942) Benzyl benzoate in treatment of scabies. A comparison of the effects of aqueous and spirit emulsions. Br Med J II: 452–453
Mapother ED (1872) The treatment of chronic skin diseases. Baillière Tindall and Cox, London
Marchand JP, Renault-Steens, Baquillon G, N'Diaye B (1975) La gale. À propos d'une épidemie actuelle au Sénégal et de ses complications. Bull Soc Med Afr Noire Lange Fr 20: 74–82
Marples MJ (1956) The incidence of certain skin diseases in Western Samoa; a preliminary survey. Trans Soc Trop Med Hyg 44: 319–332
Marples MJ (1965) Ecology of the human skin. Thomas, Springfield, Ill
Martin HM (1938) Parasitic skin diseases of domesticated animals and their importance to dermatologists. J Invest Dermatol 1: 313–324
Martins-Castro R, Proença N, Salles-Gomes LF (1974) On the association of some dermatoses with South American pemphigus foliaceus. Int J Dermatol 13: 271–275
Martin-Scott I (1957) Norwegian scabies. Br J Dermatol 69: 326
Masawe AEJ, Nsanzumuhire H (1975) Scabies and other skin diseases in pre-school children in Ujamaa village in Tanzania. Trop Geogr Med 27: 288–294
Mead R (1751) The medical works of Richard Mead M.D. Alexander Donaldson and Charles Elliott, Edinburgh, pp 416–417
Mellanby K (1941a) Transmission of scabies. Med Officer 66: 190–191
Mellanby K (1941b) The transmission of scabies. Br Med J II: 405–406
Mellanby K (1941c) Treatment of scabes. Br Med J II: 669–670
Mellanby K (1942) The transmission and prevention of scabies. Public Health 55: 150–151
*Mellanby K (1943) Scabies, Oxford University Press, London
*Mellanby K (1944a) The development of symptoms, parasitic infection and immunity in human scabies. Parasitology 35: 197–206
Mellanby K (1944b) Experiments on scabies prophylaxis. Br Med J I: 689–690
Mellanby K (1945) Scabies prophylaxis using "Tetmosol" soap. Br Med J I: 38–39
*Mellanby K (1973) Human guinea pigs. Merlin, London
Mellanby K (1977a) Biology of the parasite. In: Orkin M, Maibach HI, Parish LC, Schwartzman RM (eds) Scabies and pediculosis. Lippincott, Philadelphia, pp 8–16
Mellanby K (1977b) Epidemiology of scabies. In: Orkin M, Maibach HI, Parish LC, Schwartzman RM (eds) Scabies and pediculosis. Lippincott, Philadelphia, pp 60–63
Mellanby K (1977c) Immunology of scabies. In: Orkin M, Maibach HI, Parish LC, Schwartzman RM (eds) Scabies and pediculosis. Lippincott, Philadelphia, pp 84–87
Mellanby K, Johnson CG, Bartley WC (1942) The treatment of scabies. Br Med J II: 1–4
Mellanby K, Johnson CG, Bartley WC, Brown P (1942) Experiments on the survival and behaviour of the itch mite, *Sarcoptes scabiei* DeG var. *hominis*. Bull Entomol Res 33: 267–271
Mikhail GR, Krull EA (1973) Scabies. Arch Dermatol 108: 424
Millard LC (1977) Norwegian scabies developing during treatment with fluorinated steroid therapy. Acta Derm Venereol (Stockh) 57: 86–88
Morley D (1967) A skinful of alcohol. Lancet I: 275
Moulin G, Bouchet B, Berthoux F (1977) Glomerulo-nephritis post-scabieuse. Ann Dermatol Venereol 104: 81
Muller GM (1977) Laboratory diagnosis of scabies. In: Orkin M, Maibach HI, Parish LC, Schwartzman RM (eds) Scabies and pediculosis. Lippincott, Philadelphia, pp 99–104
Muller GM, Kirk RW (1969) Small animal dermatology. Saun-

ders, Philadelphia, pp 146–147
Muller GM, Jacobs PH, Moore NE (1973) Scraping for human scabies. Arch Dermat 107: 70
Mummery MB (1967) The scabies epidemic. Br Med J I: 766
Munkvad JM Nielsen AO, Secher L (1982) Venereal disease in patients with scabies: a five year survey. Acta Derm Venereol (Stockh) 62: 274–275
*Munro JW (1919) Report of scabies investigation. J R Army Med Corps 33: 1–41
Nair BKH (1973) Scabies—a retrospect. Indian J Dermatol Venereol 39: 29–32
Nair BKH, Joseph A, Narayanan PI, Chacko KB (1973) Epidemiology of scabies. Indian J Dermatol Venereol 39: 101–105
Nair KPB (1973) Scabies eradication: national policy needed. Indian Paediatr 10: 749
Nathan HA (1945) Some observations on scabies and its treatment. Lancet I: 95–98
Nayler G (1866) Practical and theoretical treatise on disease of the skin. Churchill, London, pp 209–224
Neligan JM (1852) A practical treatise on diseases of the skin. Fannin, Dublin; Churchill, London
Newton DK, Gerrie W (1966) Sarcoptic scabies in a dog (with human involvement). Can Vet J 7: 43
Niedelman ML (1948) Treatment of common skin diseases. J Paediatr 32: 566–579
Nielsen AO, Secher L, Seier K (1976) Gonorrhoea in patients with scabies. Br J Venereol 52: 394–395
Norins AL (1969) Canine scabies in children. Am J Dis Child 117: 239–242
Ochoa GR (1977) Epidemiologic and health education measures in Venezuela. In: Orkin M, Maibach HI, Parish LC, Schwartzman RM (eds) Scabies and pediculosis. Lippincott, Philadelphia, pp 78–80
Olin TE (1942) The epidemiology of scabies with particular attention to its relationship to venereal diseases. Acta Derm Venereol (Stockh) 23: 14–34
Orkin M (1971) Resurgence of scabies. JAMA 217: 593–597
Orkin M (1975a) Today's scabies. Arch Dermatol 111: 1431–1432
Orkin M (1975b) Today's scabies. JAMA 233: 882–885
Orkin M (1977) Special forms of scabies. In: Orkin M, Maibach HI, Parish L, Schwartzman RM (eds) Scabies and pediculosis. Lippincott, Philadelphia, pp 23–30
Orkin M, Maibach HI (1978a) Scabies in children. Paediatr Clin North Am 25: 371–386
Orkin M, Maibach I (1978b) Current concepts in parasitology. The scabies pandemic. N Engl J Med 298: 276–278
Orkin M, Epstein E, Maibach HI (1976) Treatment of to-day's scabies and pediculosis. JAMA 236: 1136–1139
Orkin M, Epstein E, Maibach HI (1977) Treatment of to-day's scabies. In: Orkin M, Maibach HI, Parish LC, Schwartzman RM (eds) Scabies and pediculosis. Lippincott, Philadelphia, pp 108–116
Palicka P, Merka V (1971) Contemporary epidemiological problems of scabies. J Epidemiol Microbiol Immunol 15: 457–461
Panja D, Ghosh S (1952) Scabies in goats and rabbits communicable to man. Indian Med Gaz 87: 449–450
Parish LC (1975) Scabies again. Int J Dermatol 14: 115–116
Parkinson Capt (1918) In discussion on scabies and pediculosis. Med Bull Am Red Cross Soc Fr 1, 4: 223–233
Parlette HL (1976) Scabies in man. Arch Dermatol 112: 409
Pascual AM, Asensio A, Vazquez R (1977) Morphologie du *Sarcoptes scabiei* (variété *hominis*) au microscope electronique à balayage. Ann Dermatol Venereol 104: 719–723
Paterson WD, Allen BR, Beveridge GW (1973) Norwegian scabies during immunosuppressive therapy. Br Med J 4: 211–212
*Percival CH (1941) Organised treatment for scabies. Br J Dermatol 53: 346–350
Percival GH (1942) The cure of scabies and a new remedy. Br Med J II: 451–452
Pettit JHS (1976) Scabies in Malaysia. Arch Dermatol 112: 1324
Pick W (1917) Ueber Pferderäude beim Menschen. Wien Klin Wochenschr 30: 849–850
Pierce HE Jr (1951) Scabies: epidemiology and management at correctional institution. J Natl Med Assoc 43: 107–112
Piers F, Timms GL (1946) Scabies Norvegica in native of East Africa. Br J Dermatol 58: 61–66
Pillars AWN (1931) In: Scabies and ringworm as transmissable between animals and man. Br J Dermatol 43: 438–455
Pillsbury DM, Livingood CS (1947) Experience in military dermatology. Arch Dermatol Syphilol 55: 441–462
Pillsbury DM, Scully JP (1948) Subacute lupus erythematosus disseminatus and non-pruritic scabies. Arch Dermatol Syphilol 57: 409–410
*Poon-King T, Mohammed I, Cox R, Potter EV, Simon NM Siegal AC, Earle DP (1967) Recurrent epidemic nephritis in South Trinidad. N Engl J Med 277: 728–733
Poon-King T, Potter EV, Svartman M, Achong J, Mohammed I, Cox R, Earle DP (1973) Epidemic of acute nephritis with reappearance of M-type 55 streptococci in Trinidad. Lancet I: 475–479
Potter EV, Ortiz JS, Sharrett AR, Burt EG, Bray JP, Finklea JF, Poon-King T, Earle DP (1971) Changing types of nephritogenic streptococci in Trinidad. J Clin Invest 50: 1197–1205
Potter EV, Mayon-White R, Svartman M, Abidh S, Poon-King T, Earle DP (1977) Secondary infestations in scabies and their complications. In: Orkin M, Maibach HI, Parish LC, Schwartzman RM (eds) Scabies and pediculosis. Lippincott, Philadelphia, pp 39–50
Prakken JR, van Vloten TJ (1949) Allergy in scabies: Positive intracutaneous tests with antigen from scabies norvegica: passive transfer of antibodies (Prausnitz–Kustner). Dermatologica 99: 124–131
Pramanik AK, Hansen RC (1979) Transcutaneous gamma benzenehexachloride absorption and toxicity in infants and children. Arch Dermatol 115: 1224–1225
Pye-Smith BH (1893) Diseases of the skin. Churchill, London, pp 65–75
Ramos y Silva J (1977) Sarna nodular e sarna papulosa, sua diferenciacao. An Brasil Dermatol 52: 407–414
Ramos y Silva J, Olivi WR (1970) Endemo-epidemiologia da escabiose no Rio de Janiero. An Bras Dermatol 45: 241–247
Randazzo SD, Guaneri B, Panizza E (1977) Movimento anticorporale nella scabbia. G Ital Dermatol Minerva Dermatol 112: 561–563
Rantanen T, Björksten F, Reunala T, Salo OP (1981) Serum IgE antibodies to scabies mite. Acta Derm Venereol (Stockh) 61: 358–360
Rasmussen JE (1981) The problem of lindane. J Am Acad Dermatol 5: 507–516
Rayer P (1835) Diseases of the skin, 2nd edn. Translated by Willis R. Baillière, London, pp 336–350
Rayer P (1845) A theoretical and practical treatise on the diseases of the skin (English translation). Carey and Hart, Philadelphia, p 36
Richardson BD (1972) *Sarcoptes scabiei*: the almost forgotten parasite. Lancet I: 839
Rigatos GA, Kappos-Rigatou I (1976) Scabies in Greece. Arch Dermatol 112: 1466
Rollier R (1969) À propos d'une épidemie conjointe de gale et de syphilis. Lyon Med 222: 953–954
Rook A (1979) In: Rook A, Wilkinson DS, Ebling FJC (eds) Textbook of dermatology, 3rd edn. Blackwell, Oxford,

pp 911–954
Russell B (1964) Parasitic infections of the skin. Practitioner 192: 621–628
Ryecroft RJG, Calnan CD (1977) Occupational scabies. Br Med J II: 303–304
Sachs R (1900) Beitrag zur Behandlung der Scabies. Dtsch Med Wochenscr 26: 631–634
Salo OP, Reunala T (1977) The demonstration of C3 in the vessel walls of scabies papule. Proceedings of the XVth international congress on dermatology, Mexico, 16–21 October 1977
Salo OP, Reunala T, Kalimo K, Rantanen T (1982) Immunoglobulin and complement deposits in the skin and circulating immune complexes in scabies. Acta Derm Venereol (Stockh) 62: 73–76
Samman PD (1963) Persistent scabious nodules. Br J Dermatol 75: 35–38
Saruta T, Nakimazo Y (1978) Usual scabies with nail infestation. Arch Dermatol 114: 956–957
Saunders L (1941) The derris root treatment of scabies. Br Med J 1: 624
Scher RK (1983) Biopsies of nails; subungual scabies. Am J Dermatol 5: 187–189
Schroeter A (1977) Scabies—a venereal disease. In: Orkin M, Maibach HL, Parish LC, Schwartzman RM (eds) Scabies and pediculosis. Lippincott, Philadelphia, pp 56–59
Schwartzman RM (1967) Clinico-pathological conference. J Am Vet Assoc 150: 217–223
Schwartzman RM (1977) Scabies in animals. In: Orkin M, Maibach HI, Parish LC, Schwartzman RM (eds) Scabies and pediculosis. Lippincott, Philadelphia, pp 96–98
Sefton L (1947) Some experience in a skin department of a prisoner-of-war camp hospital in Singapore 1942–1945: Part II. Br J Dermatol 59: 159–168
Sehgal VN (1977) Scabies—ecology and epidemiology. Indian J Dermatol Venereol Leprol 43: 266–269
Sehgal VN, Rao TL, Rege VL, Vadiraj SN (1972) Scabies: a study of incidence and a treatment method. Int J Dermatol 11: 106–111
Sequeira JH (1925) Skin affections transmissable from animals to man. Proc R Soc Med 28: 45–56
Sezary A, Ducourtioux M, Felsenwalb E (1931) Recherches experimentales sur la gale. Bull Soc Fr Dermatol Syphiligr 38: 820. Cited by Prakken and van Vloten (1949)
Shacter B (1981) Treatment of scabies and pediculosis with lindane preparations; an evaluation. J Am Acad Dermatol 5: 517–527
Shanon J, Sagher F (1956) Sabra dermatitis: an occupational dermatitis due to prickly pear handling simulating scabies. Arch Dermatol 74: 269–275
Shelley WB, Wood MG (1976) Larval papule as a sign of scabies. JAMA 236: 1144–1145
Shoemaker JV (1902) A practical treatise on diseases of the skin, 3rd edn. Appleton, New York
Short B, Derrick EH (1948) A remarkable case of scabies. Med J Aust 1: 621
Shrank AB (1967) Scabies and V.D. clinics. Int Med Trib 2, April 27: 415
Shrank AB, Alexander SL (1967) Scabies: another epidemic. Br Med J I: 669–671
Shrank AB, Alexander SL (1968) More cases of scabies. Br Med J I: 445
Slade RE (1945) Gamma isomer of hexachlorocyclohexane (Gammexane) Chem Ind 64: 314–319
*Smith EB, Claypoole TF (1967) Canine scabies in dogs and humans. JAMA 19: 95–100
Sneddon IB, Church RE (1979) Practical dermatology, 3rd edn. Arnold, London, pp 93–95
Solomon LM, Fahrner L; West DP (1977) Gamma benzene hexachloride toxicity. Arch Dermatol 113: 353–357
Ssutiejeff GO (1923) Treatment of scabies by Rossini's method (translated from Russian). Mosk Med J 61, No 1. Extracted in Zentralbl Haut Geschlechtskr (1924) 12: 181
Steigman AJ (1967) Incidence of scabies. Lancet I: 1329–1330
Stelwagon HW (1904) Treatise on diseases of the skin, 3rd edn. Saunders, Philadelphia, pp 1069–1075
*Stokes JH (1936) Scabies among the well-to-do. JAMA 106: 674–678
Strobel M, Ball M, Moreira C, Fall M (1982) Gale croûteuse et kwashiorkor Ann Dermatol Venereol 109: 87–88
Svartman M, Potter EV, Finklea JF, Poon-King T, Earle DP (1972) Epidemic scabies and acute glomerulonephritis in Trinidad. Lancet I: 249–251
Sweitzer SE, Tedder JH (1935) Pyrethrum in the treatment of scabies. Minn Med 18: 793–795
*Symonds BER (1960) Epidemic nephritis in South Trinidad. J Paediatr 56: 420–424
Tannenbaum MH (1965) Canine scabies in man. A report of human mange. JAMA 193: 321–322
Taplin D (1983) Resistance to antiscabietic drugs. J Am Acad Dermatol 8: 121–122
Thomas CC, Miller E (1940) Rotenone in the treatment of scabies. Am J Med Sci 199: 670–674
Thomson J, Cochrane T, Cochran R, McQueen A (1974) Histology simulating reticulosis in persistent nodular scabies. Br J Dermatol 90: 421–429
*Toomey N (1922) Scabies of animal origin. Urol Cutan Rev 26: 473–489
Turner D (1726) De morbis cutaneis. A treatise of disease incident to the skin, 2nd edn. Rivington, Lacey and Clarke, London
Van Aerssen RGL (1968) Demodicidosis and its therapy. Dermatologica 136: 412–413
Van Neste D (1981) Immunologic studies in scabies. Int J Dermatol 20: 264–269
Van Neste D, Lachapelle JM (1981) Host-parasite relationship in hyperkeratotic (Norwegian) scabies. Pathological and immunological findings. Br J Dermatol 105: 667–678
Van Neste D, Salmon J (1978) Circulating antigen-antibody complexes in scabies. Dermatologica 157: 221–224
Van Neste D, Salmon J (1980) Immune complexes in scabies. *In vitro* study of the serum Clq fixation in the presence of mites and unparasitised human scale extracts. Dermatologica 160: 131–134
Van Neste D, Lachaier L, Desmons F, Dessant JP (1979) Sensibilisation au *Sarcoptes scabiei* dans la gale commune et la gale Norvègienne. Bull Actual Ther 24, 78: 2372–2378
*Van Neste D, Mrena E, Marchal G (1981) Le cycle evolutif du *Sarcoptes scabiei* (*var. hominis*): un étude en microscope élèctronique à balayage. Ann Dermatol Venereol 108: 355–361
Verbov JL (1976) Skin problems in children. Practitioner 217: 403–415
Vitzhum H (1928) Zoologische Acarusstudien. Z Parasitärkr 1: 1–23
Warburton MA (1920) Sarcoptic scabies in man and animals. A critical survey of our present knowledge regarding the acari concerned. Parasitology 12: 265–300
Ward WH (1971) Scabies norvegica. Treatment with methotrexate. Australas J Dermatol 12: 44–51
Wells GC (1952) Norwegian scabies. Br Med J 2: 18–20
Whiting DA, Bristow JH (1975) Dermatitis and keratoconjunctivitis caused by a prickly pear (*Opuntia microdasys*). South Afr Med J 49: 1445–1448
Whittle HG, Abdullahi MT, Fakunle F, Parry EHO, Rajkovic AD (1973) Scabies, pyoderma and nephritis in Zaria, Nigeria.

A clinical and epidemiological study. Trans R Soc Trop Med Hyg 67: 349–363
Wilkinson DS (1953) Norwegian (crusted) scabies. Br J Dermatol 65: 31
Williamson GS (1938) In discussion of Martin (1938) J Invest Dermatol 1: 313–324
Wilson E (1867) Diseases of the skin, 6th edn. Churchill, London
Wilson JW (1971) Scabies. Arch Dermatol 104: 223
Wilson TS (1969) A study of the incidence of scabies in Glasgow from the early nineteen twenties. Med Officer 122: 125–129
Wishart J (1972) Norwegian scabies, a Christchurch epidemic. Australas J Dermatol 13: 127–131
Witkowski JA, Parish LC (1978) Scabies update 1978. Int J Dermatol 17: 401–402
Woodley D, Saurat I (1981) The burrow ink test and the scabies mite. J Am Acad Dermatol 4: 715–722
Wooldridge WE (1948) The gamma isomer of hexachlorocyclohexane in treatment of scabies. J Invest Dermatol 10: 363–366
Yarrow A (1967) Scabies. Br Med J I: 245–246
Zukowski K (1976) Human scabies in Poland in the years 1966–1970 (in Polish). *Przegl Epidemiol* 30: 225–233. Abstracted in Rev Appl Entomol 65: 585 (Abstract No 2017)

16 Hair Follicle Mites in Man

Demodex folliculorum was discovered in 1841 in cerumen by Henle and independently described in detail as an inhabitant of the pilosebaceous follicle by Simon in 1842 (Lawrence 1916). Owen named the genus *Demodex* in 1843 (Hirst 1916). Erasmus Wilson described its appearance and possible pathogenicity in 1843, and since then it has been regarded by most dermatologists as a fairly harmless saprophyte. In dogs, however, it has long been known that *Demodex* is associated with a serious and sometimes fatal pustular mange and causes serious lesions in many other domestic animals (Martin 1913). Skin changes in man have been attributed to it by De Amicis (1918), Majocchi (1918), Dubreuilh (1901), Lawrence (1916) and Ayres (1930), and more recently this link has been re-inforced by studies by Grosshans et al. (1972). A small but growing body of opinion is now inclined to concede that *Demodex* may be pathogenic under certain circumstances.

Morphology and Biology

With the usual basic structure of a mite, *Demodex folliculorum* has adapted itself to life in a hair follicle by assuming an elongated worm-like shape; its legs have an almost rudimentary appearance. Hirst (1919) considered that it was probably phylogenetically related to the cheyletiellid fur mites. In his original description Simon had noted shortened forms and this was confirmed by Lawrence (1921), Fuss (1933) and Norn (1970), all of whom considered there might be two separate species. Lawrence and Brodie (1931) observed that the numerous mites found in scrapings from "pityriasis folliculorum" were all shortened forms, in contrast to the longer mites found in the hair follicles of nearby normal skin. Akbulatova (1963), in fact, proposed two subspecies, *D. folliculorum* and *D. brevis*. Desch and Nutting (1972) showed conclusively that there were two species, which were morphologically and biologically distinct. The species, which they named *D. folliculorum* and *D. brevis*, are fully described in their paper; Fig. 16.1, which derives from their microphotographs, shows the superficial differences between the species. *D. folliculorum* is much longer than *D. brevis*. Some of the finer details in the morphology of *Demodex* in man are shown in Hirst's drawings (Fig. 16.2), most of which appear to be of *D. folliculorum*.

Spickett (1961) recorded an incubation period of 60 h and first, second and third moults after 60, 40 and 72 h respectively, plus an adult life of 4–6 days, giving a life span of 14–16 days; however; these figures were considered to be obsolete following the paper of Desch and Nutting (1972). No new data for the two species is yet forthcoming.

There have been several papers which have estimated the incidence of *Demodex* colonising the pilosebaceous follicle in man at from 23.6% to 100% (Daniel et al. 1959; Vanston 1957; Baksht 1965; Riechers and Kopf 1969; Norn 1970; Bøge-Rasmussen et al. 1982). However, the most comprehensive investigation by Fuss (1933) showed quite clearly that with a good technique *Demodex* mites could be found in some, if not all, follicles of the entire population, with the exception of neonates. Fuss used a comedo extractor to exert firm but very localised pressure on the follicles and found mites at the first attempt in 95% of persons, only requiring a second or further attempt in the remaining 5%. The mites are commonest on the forehead, malar areas of cheeks, nose and nasolabial fold, but can occur anywhere on the face or around the ears and occasionally elsewhere. They lie with the head end directed inwards (Fig. 16.3). Crosti et al. (1983) noted that only the opisthosomal end of *Demodex* was visible at the orifice of the hair follicle when examined by scanning electron microscope (seen in normal skin in 18 of 20 persons of varying age.) They also remarked on the annular striation on the surface of the integument resembling fingerprint markings.

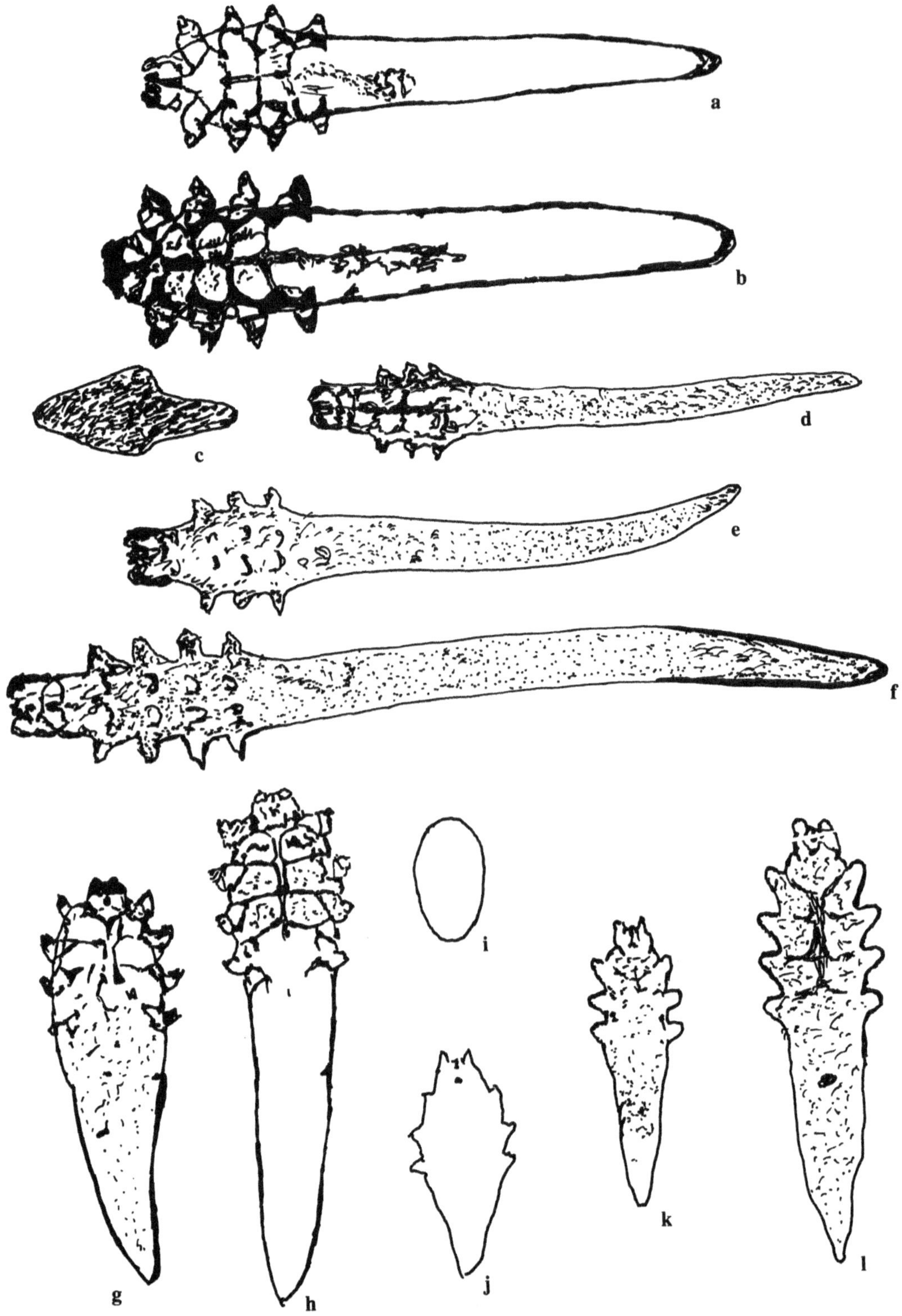

Fig. 16.1a–f. *Demodex folliculorum*. Ventral views of **a** male, **b** female, **c** ovum, **d** larvae, **e** protonymph and **f** nymph. **g–l** *D. brevis*. Ventral views of **g** male, **h** female, **i** ovum, **j** larva, **k** protonymph and **l** nymph. All originally × 325 and therefore to the same scale. Tracings of photographs (After Desch and Nutting 1972, by kind permission of the authors and the Editor of the *Journal of Parasitology*)

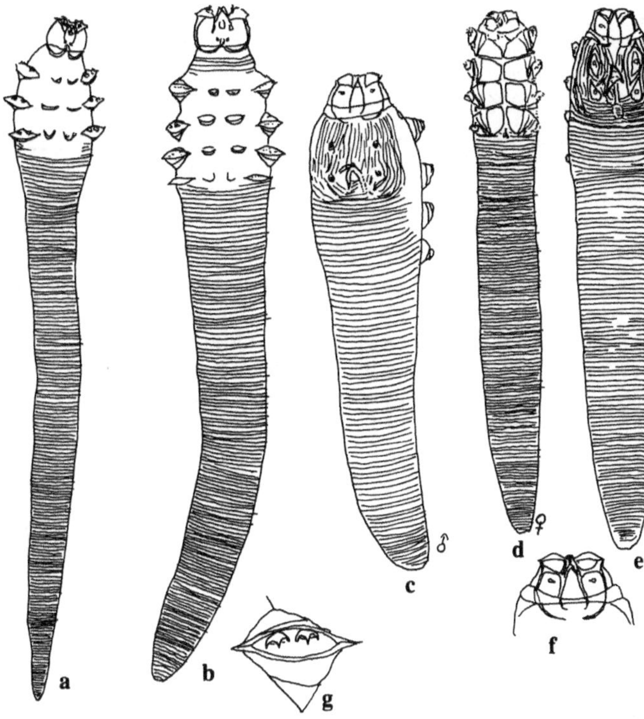

Fig. 16.2a–g *Demodex folliculorum*. **a** Elongated larval form; **b** elongated nymph; **c** short form of male; **d** female, ventral view; **e** male, dorsal view showing dorsal, backward-pointing penis; **f** capitulum from above; **g** appendage of adult. [After Hirst 1919, by kind permission of the Trustees of the British Museum (Natural History)]

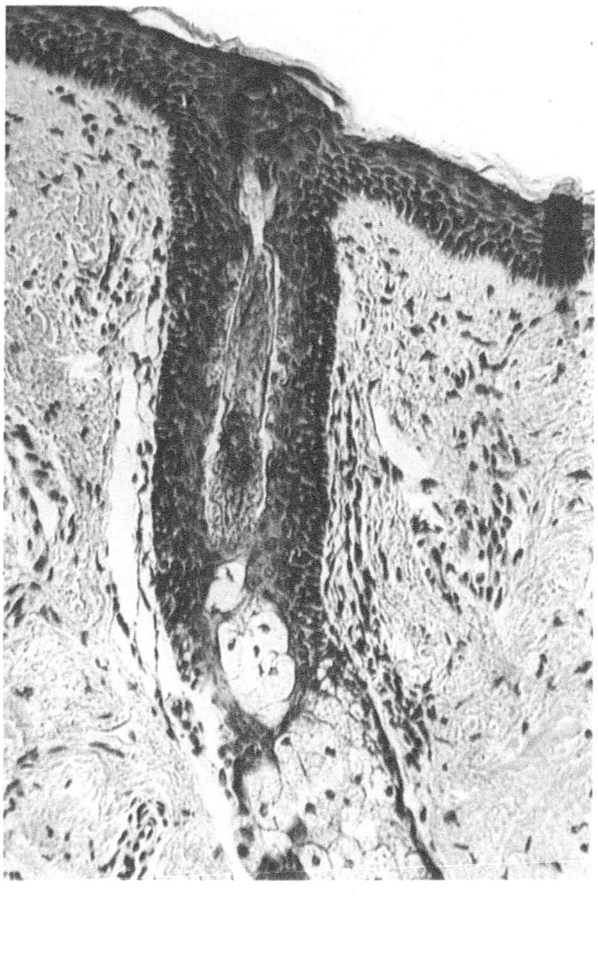

Fig. 16.3. *Demodex folliculorum* in the hair follicle. Note the head end directed downwards. (Courtesy of Dr. Brian Russell, Saffron Walden, Essex)

D. folliculorum lives in the hair follicle and *D. brevis* in the sebaceous gland (Desch and Nutting 1972). They are also found, often in considerable numbers, in the eyelash follicles. Dubreuilh and Beille (1895) found up to 200 in a meibomian gland. They occur equally in either sex, although Baksht (1965) thought they were commoner in men because of the reduced sebum secretion in women. Nutting and Green (1974) noted that *Demodex* was much commoner in men than in women amongst the Australian aborigines. Their numbers increase with the age of the host and are greatest in those with "seborrhoeic" skins (Fuss 1933). Reproduction may be either oviparous or viviparous, and it has been observed that when examined in vegetable oil they are surprisingly active (Fuss 1937). Norn (1971) has estimated their motility at 8–16 mm/h. They migrate from follicle to follicle, especially at night. Spickett (1961) alleged that this was because of their dislike of light, but Norn stated that they could do so equally in the daytime, whilst Baksht (1965) stated that they were not observed outside the hair follicle. They probably first colonise infants through close contact with their mother. Ku Quizun (1982) noted the total absence of *Demodex* in the follicles of 150 neonates and surmised that infestation occurred during household (especially maternal) contacts. Euzeby (1970) thought that this transfer occurred in the active nymphal stages of their development when they are more often found on the surface. Both species feed on the cells of their habitat (Nutting 1976). Akbulatova (1959) noted that *D. folliculorum* was found most often and in the greatest numbers in the springtime, when all stages could be seen and were very active, whereas in summer and winter only a few fully mature mites could be seen. Baksht (1965) also noted an increased number of *D. folliculorum* in nasal follicles in the warm months of the year. Chambers and Somerset (1925) observed that secondary infection was frequently fatal to the *Demodex*. Kaufman-Wolf (1925), on the other hand, noted two reports where an adult and children had acquired pustular lesions containing many *Demodex* mites on the hands, forearms, chest and abdomen after sleeping with a mangy goat and an infested cat respectively!

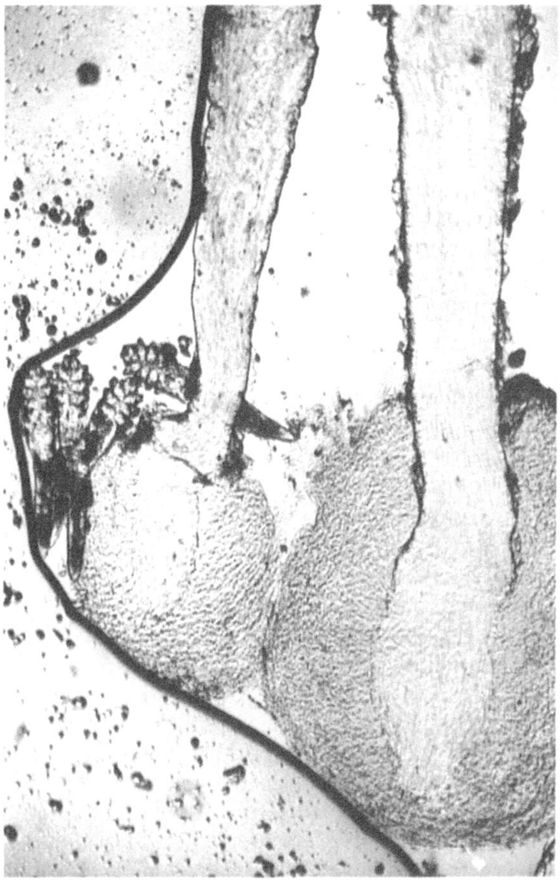

Fig. 16.4. Two hair roots with attached *Demodex folliculorum*, mounted in 40% potassium hydroxide. Note that because of the trauma of removal, mounting and movement of the preparation on the slide the normal downward orientation of the mites' heads has been lost, but they are all pointing more or less in one direction. (Courtesy of Dr. Brian Russell, Saffron Walden, Essex)

Parasitology

The average number of 2–6 *Demodex* mites per inhabited follicle (Fig. 16.4) is regarded as harmless. In some persons, however, this number may be increased to 15–16 or more (Fig. 16.5), the individual follicles then becoming densely packed with mites. Such numbers may of themselves induce reactions in the skin (Agostini 1939). Nutting and Beerman (1983) suggested that 10 or more mites per follicle was markedly above what they regarded as normal.

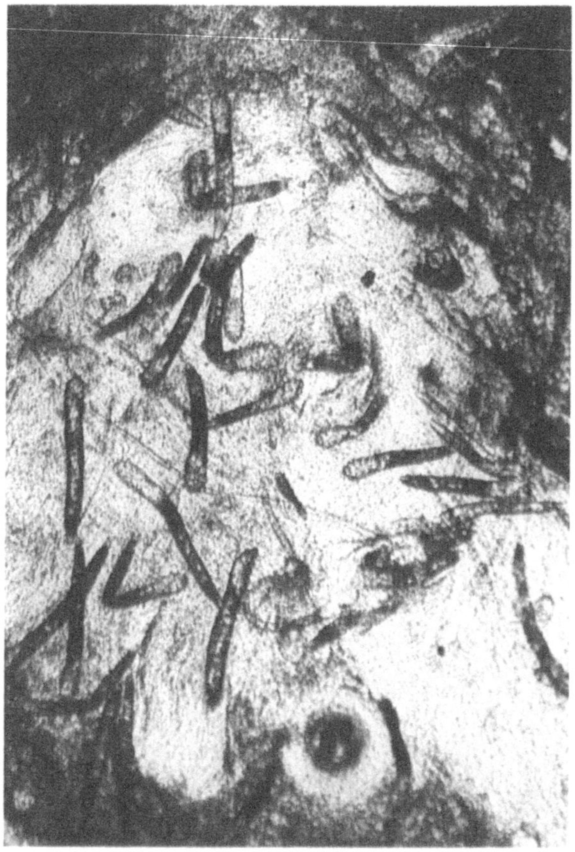

Fig. 16.5. Large numbers of *Demodex folliculorum* expressed from a hair follicle and mounted in 40% potassium hydroxide. This technique tends to destroy the normal orientation of the mite. Over 50 can be seen in the picture. (Courtesy of Dr. Brian Russell, Saffron Walden, Essex)

It has been claimed (Stcherbatchoff 1903; Post and Juhlin 1963; Morgan and Coston 1964; Coston 1967; Smith and McCulloch 1969) that *Demodex* activity could cause blepharitis in some instances. Norn (1970), on the other hand, in an exhaustive study, concluded that whilst there might be an association between increased numbers of *Demodex* in the eyelids and blepharitis, he did not regard it as significant. However, Byun et al. (1983), in a very recent study of *Demodex* in eyelashes, found a significantly higher incidence in persons with blepharitis than in controls, and Coston (1967) did demonstrate that in some cases removal of excess numbers of *Demodex* from the eyelashes by means of ether soaks (under local anaesthesia) greatly improved the blepharitis.

Clinical Appearances on the Skin Caused by *Demodex*

The skin does not react to the presence of a few *Demodex* mites in the hair follicles. However, if the follicles become overpopulated, reaction may occur. Should the mite escape into the surrounding dermis, for whatever reason, a reaction will occur.

With an increase in *Demodex* numbers the patient may present with a persistent, dry, rough, fine scaly skin on the cheeks, forehead and chin, which on close inspection may show a faint redness (Ayres 1930). Ayres' patients, all women, complained of irritation of the skin and sometimes of heat or burning on the face. He noted that the skin, which looked normal from a distance of 1.5 m (5 ft), showed a finely stippled appearance and he found large numbers of *Demodex* in the scales around lanugo follicles. He named the condition "pityriasis folliculorum (*Demodex*)". Although at first it was not generally accepted by other dermatologists, after a review of 303 patients with this condition Ayres and Ayres (1961) persuaded more of their colleagues to agree with them. Andrews and Domonkos (1971) accepted it as an entity. A scaly circinate eruption on the face with a similar aetiology had previously been described by Lawrence (1916) in Australia.

A rare manifestation of increased numbers of *Demodex* is hyperpigmentation. De Amicis (1918) described a woman who presented with a *café au lait*-coloured plaque of several years' duration on her chin. The smooth, shiny surface showed several prominent follicular openings. There were no subjective symptoms. Examination of scrapings of fine scaly material from the surface revealed large numbers of *Demodex*. At the same meeting Majocchi recorded two instances of a similar eruption in patches of atrophic "lupus". Dubreuilh (1901) and Agostini (1939) also observed similar cases.

Rosacea presents with small, red papules 1–4 mm in diameter, many of which may develop central pustules, with crusting if the latter discharge (Fig. 16.6). The background skin has an erythematous flush; the lesions usually occur on the

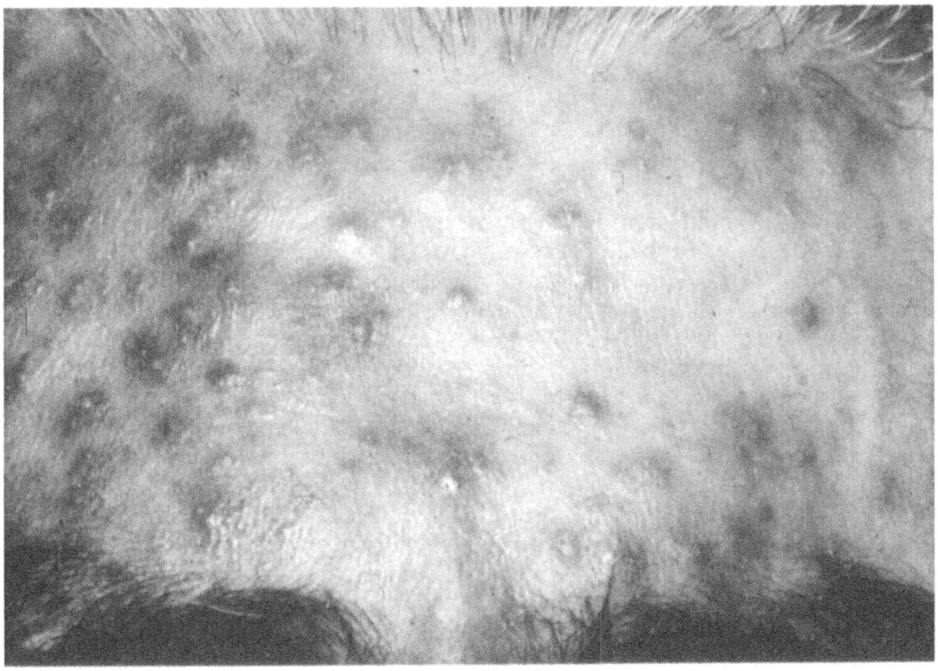

Fig. 16.6. Lesions of rosacea showing papules and papulopustules on the forehead.

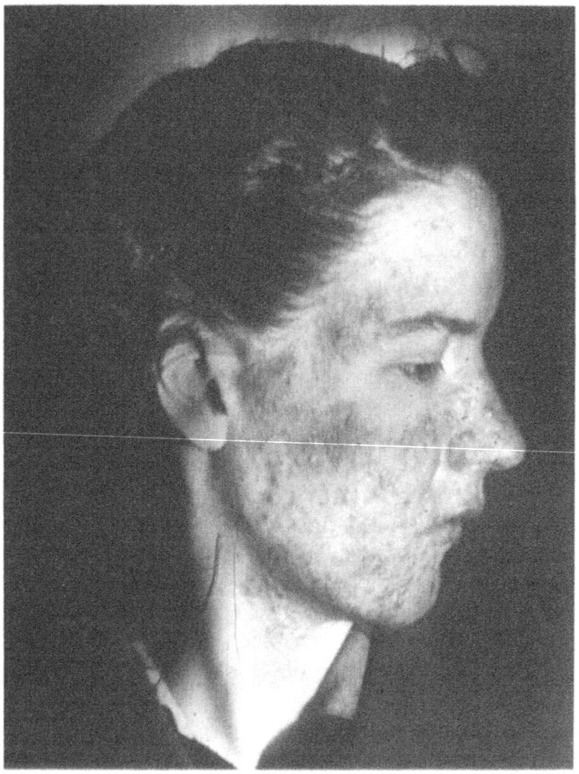

Fig. 16.7. Distribution of lesions in rosacea.

forehead, nose, cheeks and chin but may extend to the neck (Fig. 16.7), bald scalp and rarely to the upper trunk. In some instances the condition has been regarded as being caused by *Demodex*. Ayres and Anderson (1932) presented 17 patients with rosacea in whom examination of surface scales revealed considerably increased numbers of these mites. Miskjian (1951) described rosacea-like dermatitis in which an increased number of demodices were found. He also described as characteristic of this infestation an eruption on the bald area of the scalp of a middle-aged man. (Yue Xiu-Xia et al. 1982 held a similar opinion.) The affected skin was faintly red all over and studded with a large number of very small, intensely red, more or less acuminate papules, 1–2 mm in diameter. The papules terminated in a white pinpoint summit from which an oily liquid could be expressed. This contained many specimens of *Demodex*. Vanston (1957), in a study of 400 patients with acneiform or rosaceous lesions, diagnosed 40 as belonging to a group he designated "demodicidosis" with lesions similar to those described by Miskjian. He regarded these as "oil retention vesicles" in the epidermis (although he presented no proof of their being vesicular), which gave rise to scaling after the oil was discharged. He found many demodices in these scales. Kinugawa (1925) had described many of these mites in what he termed "acne demodicidi", but not in acne vulgaris. Steigleder and Strumpfel (1968) and Steigleder (1969) described under the name "rosacea-like dermatitis" a papulopustular eruption affecting the nasolabial fold, chin and adjacent areas of cheeks, the glabella, forehead and eyelids. The primary lesion of this eruption was a firm red papule with a yellowish-white tip. Although *Demodex* was not specifically mentioned, these authors suggested that an outside agency (unspecified) was the cause. It is possible they may have been discussing perioral dermatitis, but the eruption seemed too extensive for that condition. Ayres (1963) and Ayres and Mihan (1967) emphasised that what they called "rosacea-like demodicidosis" was a dry scaly eruption involving the sides of the face as well as the central area. The papulopustular lesions occurred more in the central area and in one patient were prominent on the eyelids. Ordinary rosacea was, they said, associated with a more oily skin and confined more to the centre of the face. Baksht (1965) found that *Demodex* occurred very frequently in the contents of the small pustules in rosacea and was noticeably more numerous in follicles of rosaceous patients than in those of normal persons. Russell (1962) observed a heavy infestaion with *Demodex* in rosacea (see Fig. 16.5), which he thought could cause an inflammatory reaction. This overpopulation could rupture the follicle, thus causing the inflammation (B. F. Russell 1981, personal communication).

An inflammatory reaction to the presence of *Demodex* in the dermal tissues outside the hair follicle has been seen in occasional instances by many dermatologists and histophathologists but has generally been regarded as a chance finding of no special significance. The clinical lesions caused by such a reaction are discrete, red nodulopapules, usually from 1 to 4 mm in diameter. A number of facial eruptions, which have had different names applied to them in the past, produce such lesions. For example, lupus miliaris facei disseminata (LMFD) presents with many such discrete encrusted papular lesions along the cutaneous border of the lower eyelids and adjacent upper cheek, the groove between the nose and cheek and sometimes the central forehead. These lesions are usually of uniform size, about 1–2 mm across. The so-called rosaceous tuberculid of Lewandowsky (RTL) presents with nodulopapules or nodulopustules mainly around the chin and sides of the mouth. These lesions may appear to have a necrotic centre. Conditions referred to as "micropapular tuberculids of the face" and some cases of rosacea may present with similar lesions. All of this group of conditions have one thing in common—a tuberculoid granulomatous histopathology but no evidence of a tuberculous aetiology.

Immunology

Grosshans et al. (1980) examined 31 patients (24 with papulopustular rosacea and seven with granulomatous rosacea shown to be related to the presence of *Demodex* in the granuloma) for antibodies to *Demodex*. The antigen had been prepared from goat *Demodex* because of the technical difficulty of obtaining sufficient mites from human sources. Antibodies to *Demodex* were demonstrated in the serum of 22 of the patients with rosacea as well as in the serum of goats and of rabbits sensitised to *Demodex*. Cross-reactivity to the mite *Tyroglyphus putrescentiae* (in house dust) was frequent. The granulomatous reaction in the dermis to *Demodex* would also seem to be an immunological reaction. Scott et al. (1974) noted that there was T-cell depression indicating cell-mediated immune deficiency in 14 of 20 dogs with generalised demodectic mange (cf. Norwegian scabies, see pp. 265–267).

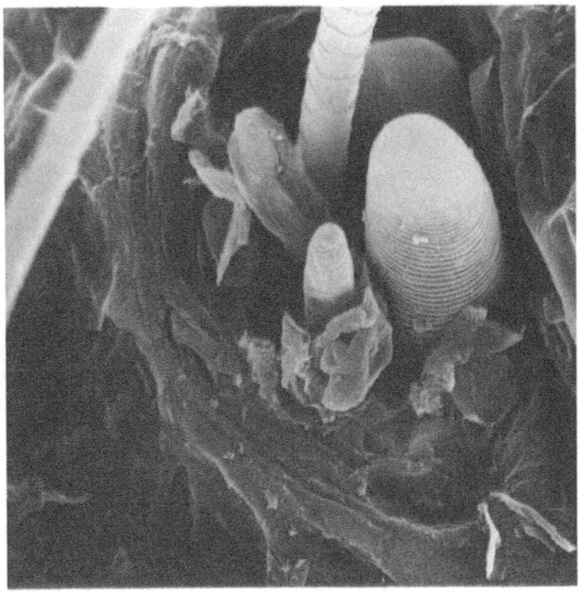

Fig. 16.8. Scanning electron micrograph of follicular opening with one hair and the opisthosomas of three *Demodex* protruding. (From Crosti et al. 1983, by kind permission of Dr. C. Crosti and the Editor of the *Journal of Cutaneous Pathology*.) Originally × 710

Aetiological Role of *Demodex* in Facial Eruptions

There are two kinds of facial eruption in which *Demodex* has been incriminated as the aetiological agent: (1) those in which an excessive number of mites overflow onto the skin surface and (2) those in which *Demodex* appears to have penetrated into the dermal tissues.

The evidence to support the first concept that pityriasis folliculorum, certain superficial pigmentary facial plaques and a fine papulopustular rosaceous eruption are caused by *Demodex* is threefold. Firstly, large numbers of these mites are present on the skin surface or at the mouth of the affected follicles (Fig. 16.8). Both numbers and situation of the mites are unusual, but the authors concerned (Crosti et al. 1982, 1983) were unanimous in their findings. In discussing the cases presented by Ayres and Anderson (1932), Weidman said that in the specimens shown the *Demodex* mites were all pointing in one direction, which was strong evidence that the scales in which they were found originated in follicles, since the mites in the latter were always orientated head downwards, i.e. in the same direction, in the follicles. He regarded this, together with the large numbers of mites as very suggestive of a pathogenic role for the mites. Secondly, Ayres and his colleagues (Ayres 1930, 1963; Ayres and Anderson 1932, 1933; Ayres and Ayres 1961) and Steigleder and Strumpfel (1968) all observed that a common factor in their patients was avoidance of soap and water for washing the face (even for months continuously) and the substitution of cosmetic creams, powders and skin foods. Such a regimen seems to favour multiplication of the mites. Thirdly, the response to treatment consisting exclusively of restoring the use of soap and water, banning cosmetics and the brief use of antiparasitic preparations such as Danish ointment, was singularly successful in producing simultaneous clearing of the lesions and disappearance of the excess of the mites (Ayres and Anderson 1933). This applied to all of the conditions discussed under this heading. As a corollary to this, B. F. Russell (1981, personal communication) observed that, regardless of their opinion on the aetiological role of *Demodex*, all of his colleagues at St. John's Hospital for Diseases of the Skin in London used sulphur in the preparations prescribed for rosacea.

The second concept of *Demodex* escaping into the dermal tissues is quite different. In these lesions the evidence for the involvement of *Demodex* is histological. Laymon and Schoch (1948) and Laymon (1951) drew attention to the histological

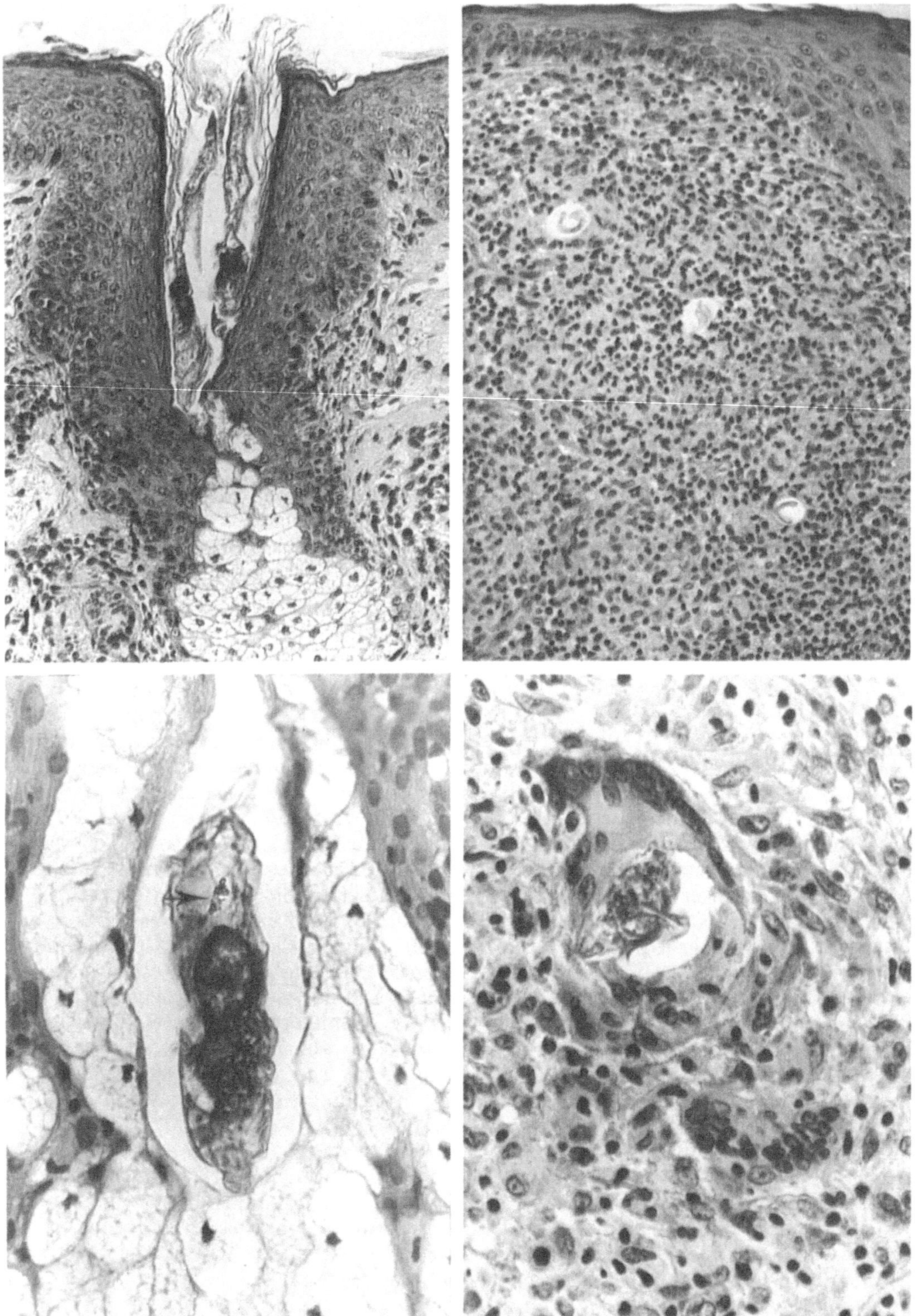

Fig. 16.9. **a** *Demodex folliculorum* in hair follicle. **b** *Demodex* (? *D. brevis*) in sebaceous gland. **c** *Demodex* or fragments of *Demodex* in tuberculoid granuloma of the face. **d** Higher magnification of *Demodex* portion in the centre of a facial tuberculous granuloma. Note the giant cell *above* and *below* the *Demodex*. (From Grosshans et al. 1974, by kind permission of Prof. E. M. Grosshans and the Editor of *Hautazt*)

similarity between RTL, LMFD, micropapular tuberculids of the face and some cases of rosacea, all of which showed a tuberculid granulomatous picture. They called the whole group "lupoid rosacea". This did not imply a tuberculous aetiology, because, as Rothman (1948) noted, a tuberculous focus and a hypersensitivity to the bacillus would have to be demonstrated, which was rarely if ever successful. Dermatologists obviously did not believe in a tuberculous cause since they did not adopt antituberculous therapy (Michelson 1951). *Demodex* was not mentioned as an aetiological factor, but rupture of the hair follicle near the granuloma was seen in two sections.

Marks and Harcourt-Webster (1969), in a study of 108 biopsies from patients with rosacea, found a ruptured follicle in 20% of 78 biopsies of papular rosacea; all but one of these follicles contained fragments of *Demodex*, although none had penetrated into the dermis, where the inflammatory reaction occurred. This evidence, they held, was against a role for *Demodex* in rosacea, although they did suggest that perhaps the reaction might be due to the effect of diffusion of *Demodex* antigen into the tissues, even though there was no evidence for this. Grosshans et al. (1972, 1974) examined biopsies from 53 patients with a rosaceous picture which included LMFD and micronodular "tuberculid". In ten patients they found a characteristic tuberculoid granuloma, in the centre of each of which they found, by examining serial sections, a *Demodex* or part of a *Demodex* (Fig. 16.9). The only distinction between this picture and the histology of rosaceous nodules in the other 43 biopsies was the absence of *Demodex* fragments in the latter. They pointed out that rosacea-like dermatitis lacked this granulomatous histology. Pinkus and Mehregan (1976) agreed with their conclusion that *Demodex* may cause a tuberculoid granulomatous reaction if it escapes into the dermis. This reaction is indistinguishable from that produced by keratin or free fatty acid in the dermis. An interesting comparison was made by Grosshans and his colleagues (1972, 1974) concerning acute pustular demodectic mange in dogs. In these cases it appears that the follicles become so heavily populated by mites that they burst. The mites can also bore through the follicle wall and in either case get into the dermal tissues. The reaction produced is a pseudotuberculoid granuloma exactly like that seen by Grosshans and his team in their cases. Nutting and Beerman (1965) have shown that in marsupial mice the *Demodex* on its own can induce the production of giant cells (ectodermal giant cells) from follicular epithelium without any inflammatory reaction. Penetration into tissues other than the skin, as occurs in the dog (Martin 1913; French 1964), has not been seen in man. However, it could be postulated that penetration is not essential to induce a reaction to *Demodex* when large numbers are present and the follicle becomes distended. It is perfectly feasible, as Marks and his colleague (1969) suggest, that antigens might diffuse through the follicle into the dermal tissues. Evidence that this may well occur is furnished by the finding of antibodies to *Demodex* in the serum of rosaceous patients (Grosshans et al. 1980). This finding will require much elaboration and confirmation but is valuable supportive evidence for a pathogenic role for *Demodex* under favourable circumstances. Another very curious finding in support of the role of *Demodex* in rosacea comes from the reported success of Van Aerssen (1968) in treating two patients with severe rosacea by using methotrexate under carefully controlled conditions. This killed the *Demodex*, which were present in large numbers, and cleared the rosacea at the same time without any other treatment.

It should be emphasised that, in general, *Demodex* is a harmless saprophyte. It is only exceptionally that it appears to exercise a pathogenic influence, as, for example, when excessive amounts of cosmetics prepare the ground for its proliferation or when it escapes into the dermis. It may be that with better techniques for its clinical identification and more frequent examination of serial sections of rosacea *Demodex* may be shown to play a greater role than is accepted at present.

Treatment by good general hygiene with soap and water and the simple applications of sulphur preparations or Danish ointment seems adequate for all the various conditions mentioned above.

References

Agostini A (1939) La questione del *Demodex folliculorum* in dermatologia: a proposito di un caso pigmentazioni circoscritte del volto. Il Dermosifilografo 14: 421–448

Akbulatova LKh (1959) Discovery of the *Demodex folliculorum* mite in pruritic dermatosis patients (in Russian). Vestn Dermatol Venereol 3: 63–65

Akbulatova LKh (1963) Cited by Desch and Nutting (1972)

Andrews GC, Domonkos AN (1971) Diseases of the skin, 6th edn. Saunders, Philadelphia, p 390

Ayres S Jr (1930) Pityriasis folliculorum (*Demodex*). Arch Dermatol Syphilol 21: 19–24

Ayres S Jr (1963) Rosacea-like demodicidosis. Cal Med 98: 328–330

Ayres S Jr, Anderson NP (1932) *Demodex folliculorum*: its role in the etiology of acne rosacea. Arch Dermatol Syphilol 25: 89–98

Ayres S Jr, Anderson NP (1933) Acne rosacea: response to local treatment for *Demodex folliculorum*. JAMA 100: 645–647

Ayres S Jr, Ayres S III (1961) Demodectic eruption (demodicidosis) in the human. Arch Dermatol 83: 816–827

Ayres S, Mihan R (1967) Rosacea-like demidicidosis involving the eyelids. Arch Dermatol 95: 63–66

Baksht BP (1965) On the role of *Demodex folliculorum hominis* mite in the human skin pathology (in Russian). Vestn Dermatol Venereol 7: 31–36

Bøge-Rasmussen T, Christensen JD, Gluud B, Kirstensen G Norn MS (1982) *Demodex folliculorum hominis* (Simon). Incidence in a normomaterial and in patients under systemic treatment with erythromycin or glucocorticoid. Acta Derm Venereol (Stockh) 62: 454–456

Byun DG, Kim HO, Cho BK (1983) A study of *Demodex* of the eyelashes (in Korean with English summary). Korean J Dermatol 21: 13–19

Chambers A, Somerset AM (1925) Breast disease and the *Demodex folliculorum* Lancet I: 172–173

*Coston TO (1967) *Demodex folliculorum* blepharitis. Trans Am Ophthalmol Soc 65: 361–392

Crosti C, Menni S, Piccinno R, Sala F (1982) Aspetti ultrastrutturali della infestazione demodecica del volto in soggetti sani ed affetti da acne rosacea. G Ital Dermato P Venereol 117: 277–281

Crosti C, Menni S, Sala F, Piccinno R (1983) Demodectic infestation of the pilo-sebaceous follicle. J Cutan Pathol 10: 257–261

Daniel M, Bozdech V, Moucka C (1959) Vyskyt .trudnika tukoveho (*Demodex folliculorum hominis* Owen 1843) u liki a jeho epidemiologie. (The occurrence of *Demodex folliculorum* (Owen 1843) in man and its epidemiology.) Cesk Dermatol 8: 52–60

De Amicis T (1918) *Demodex folliculorum* e ipercromia cutanea. G Ital Malatta Venereo Pelle 33: 205–207

*Desch C, Nutting WB (1972) *Demodex folliculorum* (Simon) and *D. brevis* Akbulatova of man; re-description and reevaluation. J Parasitol 58: 169–177

Dubreuilh W (1901) Cited by Kaufman-Wolf (1925)

Dubreuilh W, Beille L (1895) Parasites animaux de la peau humaine. Masson et Cie, Paris

Euzeby J (1970) Les infections parasitaires des follicules pilosebacés en médecine vétérinaire. Rev Med Vet 121: 981-1012

French FE (1964) *Demodex canis* in canine tissue. Cornell Vet 54: 271–290

*Fuss F (1933) La vie parasitaire du *Demodex folliculorum hominis*. Ann Dermatol Syphiligr (Paris) (7th ser) 4: 1053–1062

Fuss F (1937) Nouvelle contribution à l' étude de *Demodex folliculorum hominis*; sexe et reproduction. Ann Dermatol Syphiligr (Paris) 8: 224–229

Grosshans E, Kremer M, Maleville J, Wanner R (1972) Du rôle des *Demodex folliculorum* dans l'histogenese de la rosacée granulomateuse. Bull Soc Fr Dermatol Syphiligr 79: 639–641

*Grosshans EM, Kremer M, Maleville J (1974) *Demodex folliculorum* und die Histogenese der granulomatosen Rosacea. Hautarzt 25: 166–177

Grosshans E, Dungler T, Kien TT, Kremer M (1980) *Demodex folliculorum* und Rosacea: experimentelle und immunologische Studien. Z Hautkr 55: 1211–1218

*Hirst S (1919) Studies on Acari No 1. The genus *Demodex* Owen. The Trustees of the British Museum (Natural History), London

Kaufman-Wolf M (1925) Über regelmässiges Vorkommen von *Demodex folliculorum* in der Pusteln von Rosacea pustulosa. Dermatol Wochenschr 81: 1095–1103

Kinugawa C (1925) Acne caused by *Demodex folliculorum*. Jpn J Dermatol Urol 25: 21

Ku Quizun (1982) An epidemiological investigation of human demodicidosis. Chin J Dermatol 15: 89–93

Lawrence H (1916) On a skin eruption association with the presence of great numbers of *Demodex folliculorum*. Med J Aust 2: 555–556

Lawrence H (1921) The pathogenicity of the *Demodex* (Owen) in the human being. Med J Aust 2: 39–40

Lawrence H, Brodie R (1931) Pityriasis folliculorum (*Demodex*). Med J Aust 1: 529–530

Laymon CW (1951) Lupoid rosacea. Arch Dermatol Syphilol 63: 409–418

Laymon CW, Schoch EP (1948) Micropapular tuberculid and rosacea. Arch Dermatol Syphilol 58: 286–300

Majocchi (1918) In discussion of De Amicis (1918). G Ital Malatta Venereol Pelle 33: 205–207

Marks R, Harcourt-Webster JN (1969) Histopathology of rosacea. Arch Dermatol 100: 683–691

Martin A (1913) La gale démodecique des herbivores. Rev Vet 38: 321–328, 389–397

Michelson HE (1951) In discussion of Laymon (1951). Arch Dermatol Syphilol 63: 409–418

Miskjian HG (1951) Demodicidosis (*Demodex* infestation of the scalp). Arch Dermatol Syphilol 63: 282–283

Morgan RJ, Coston TO (1964) *Demodex* blepharitis. South Med J 57: 694–699

*Norn MS (1970) *Demodex folliculorum*: incidence and possible pathogenic role in the human eyelid. Acta Ophthalmol [Suppl] (Kbh) 108: 7–85

Norn MS (1971) *Demodex folliculorum*; incidence, regional distribution, pathogenicity. Dan Med Bull 18: 14–17

Nutting WB (1976) Hair follicle mites (*Demodex* species) of medical and veterinary concern. Cornell Vet 66: 214–231

Nutting WB, Beerman H (1965) Atypical giant cells in *Antechinus stuartii* due to demodicid mites. J Invest Dermatol 45: 504–509

Nutting WB, Beerman H (1983) Demodicidosis and symbiophobia status, terminology and treatment. Int J Dermatol 22: 13–17

Nutting WB, Green AC (1974) Hair follicle mites (Acari: Demodicidae) from Australian aborigines. Austr J Dermatol 15: 10–14

Pinkus H, Mehregan AH (1976) A guide to dermatohistopatholgy, 2nd edn. Appleton-Century-Crofts, New York, pp 275, 298

Post CF, Juhlin E (1963) *Demodex folliculorum* and blepharitis. Arch Dermatol 88: 298–302

Riechers R, Kopf AW (1969) Cutaneous infestation with *Demodex folliculorum* in man. J Invest Dermatol 52: 103–106

Rothman S (1948) In discussion of Laymon and Schoch (1948). Arch Dermatol Syphilol 58: 286–300

Russell BF (1962) Some aspects of the biology of the epidermis. Br Med J I: 815–820

Scott DW, Farrow BHH, Schultz RD (1974) Studies on the therapeutic and immunologic aspects of generalised demodectic mange in the dog. J Am Anim Hosp Assoc 10: 233–244

Smith S, McCulloch C (1969) *Demodex folliculorum palpebrarum*. Can J Ophthalmol 4: 3–15

Spickett SG (1961) Studies on *Demodex folliculorum* Simon (1842). Parasitology 51: 181–192

Stcherbatchoff (1903) Cited by Post and Juhlin (1963)

Steigleder GK (1969) Die Rosacea-artige Dermatitis: ein neuartiges Krankheitbild. Dtsch Med Wochenschr 94: 1393–1398

Steigleder GK, Strumpfel A (1968) Rosacea-artige Dermatitis des Gesichts 'Periorale Dermatitis'. Hautarzt 19: 492–494

Van Aerssen RGL (1968) Demodicidosis and its therapy. Dermatologica 136: 412–413

Vanston WJ (1957) Demodicidosis—*Demodex* infestation in man. Pa Med J 60: 624–628

Yue Xiu-Xia et al. (1982) Report of one case of *Demodex* infestation of the scalp (in Chinese). J Clin Dermatol 11: 192

17 Infestation with Gamasid Mites

Attacks on man by members of the family Gamasidae (suborder Mesostigmata) have been recorded on a worldwide basis. They not only cause irritating skin eruptions but are also known or suspected vectors of several rickettsial and viral diseases (Table 17.1). Hirst (1922) enumerated five species which attacked humans. The nomenclature of this group in the literature is very confusing because of the necessity for periodic revision of classification as new species and facts are discovered. Suffice it to note that the various species of the genus *Ornithonyssus* have previously been included as *Leiognathus*, *Liponyssus* or *Bdellonyssus*, whilst *Liponyssoides sanguineus* has been termed *Dermanyssus* or *Allodermanyssus sanguineus* (Ewing 1923; Oudemans 1937; Da Fonseca 1948).

The characteristic features of this family are given in Table 17.2, which is best studied in conjunction with Figs. 17.4, 17.6, 17.7, 17.8 and 17.10. A similar skin eruption is produced by all the species. Diagnosis of the cause of the lesions is therefore greatly assisted by an understanding of the differing life cycles, habits and hosts of the respective mites, which are discussed in detail later.

Table 17.2. Main characteristics of the gamasid group of mites. (After Da Fonseca 1948)

1. *Mandibles*—fixed and moveable arms; no armature in females.
2. *Palps*—bifid seta on fifth segment
3. *Dorsal shield*—entire or divided in adult female
4. *Sternal plate*—two or three pairs of setae
5. *Genital plate*—not enlarged in female; 1–3 pairs of setae
6. *Holoventral shield*—entire or divided in male
7. *Haematophagous*
8. Oviparous; ovoviviparous; sometimes facultative parthogenetic
9. Permanent ectoparasite on mammals, birds or reptiles

Clinical Features

Persons of any age, of either sex and regardless of ethnic origin may be affected. Children tend to

Table 17.1. Viral and rickettsial diseases for which gamasid mites are said to be vectors

Species	Disease	References
Ornithonyssus bacoti	Endemic typhus	Shelmire and Dove (1930, 1931); Dove and Shelmire (1931, 1932); Audy (1938); Pang (1941); Liu (1947)
	Relapsing fever	Morisita (1938)
	Q fever[a]	Burnet and Freeman (1939)
	St. Louis encephalitis	Reeves et al. (1947)
	Western equine encephalitis	Hammon et al. (1948)
	Rickettsialpox[b]	Philip and Hughes (1948)
O. sylviarum	Western equine encephalitis	Reeves et al. (1947)
	St. Louis encephalitis	Hammon et al. (1948)
O. bursa	Q fever[a]	Smith et al. (1939)
	Western equine encephalitis	Ferguson (1954)
Dermanyssus gallinae	Fowl tick fever	Sanders (1944) etc.
	Endemic typhus	Finnegan (1945)
	St. Louis encephalitis	Smith et al. (1946)
Liponyssoides sanguineus	Rickettsialpox	Huebner et al. (1946); Skaliy and Hayes (1949)

[a] Suspected only.
[b] Experimental only.

react more severely, but in general the response is as much dependent on individual susceptibility as on the number of attacking mites (Spencer 1936). Itch, often severe, is the principal complaint. It is nocturnal in infestation by *Dermanyssus gallinae*, usually beginning 30 min to 1 hour after retiring to bed (Frenken 1962; Sulzberger and Kamenstein 1936; Touraine 1947; DeOreo 1958; Gross 1959). In the patients described by Hill and Gordon (1945) it was usually nocturnal, but some of the soldiers only experienced itch after getting out of bed in the morning, often several hours later. Attacks by *Ornithonyssus sylviarum* may cause itch but no rash (Moniez 1893) and the same may occur with *D. gallinae* (Touraine 1947; Shaw and Pommerening 1950; Sexton and Haynes 1975, whilst laboratory personnel bitten by *O. bacoti* experienced neither pain nor itch (Hetherington et al. 1971). Some writers have noted the bites to be painful rather than itchy (Shelmire and Dove 1931; Anderson 1944; Browning 1950; Berndt 1952; Lodha 1969), whilst Lowell (1946) thought that the itch was due to the crawling of the mites and not to bites. The itch is often intermittent (Rothman and Niederman 1947; Shaw and Pommerening 1950; Fairburn and Frain-Bell 1956; DeOreo 1958; Dowlati and Maguire 1970; Hetherington et al. 1971; Hidano and Asanuma 1976) because of the periodic liability to attack in some instances (Cole and Driver 1937). At times it could be due to the nocturnal habits of the particular parasite (Spencer 1937), but Weber (1940) has pointed out that *O. bacoti* actively searches for food both day and night. *D. gallinae* is usually nocturnal in its feeding habits, but those who handle infested poultry and work in infested chicken houses get bitten in the daytime. Charlesworth and Cleghern (1977) noted a mild pyrexia in their patients, but this is exceptional. These infestations are not transmitted directly from person to person. Familial incidence is common only because of simultaneous exposure to attack.

The eruption appears soon after exposure, within 24 h as a rule, the primary lesion being a small urticated papule from 1 to 5 or 6 mm (or even 1 cm; Fox 1982) in diameter (Fig. 17.1). Many of the lesions have a small central punctum, which may be haemorrhagic (Rothman and Niederman 1947), but the latter feature is usually conspicuous by its absence. Vesicles occasionally occur in the centre of the papules (Riley 1940; Rothman and Niederman 1947; Shaw and Pommerening 1950), especially in children (Anderson 1944). Polano (1962) noted that whereas flea bites in most persons caused haemorrhagic papules, in those liable to strophulus the result was a *vesicle* surmounting a papule. This might explain why vesicles occur in some Gamasid bites. Excoriation with the formation of tiny serous crusts is frequent (Fig. 17.2). Sometimes secondary infection with pustule formation occurs. Haggard (1955) observed that any combination of macules, papules, weals, pustules or crusts could be presented, including a varicelli-

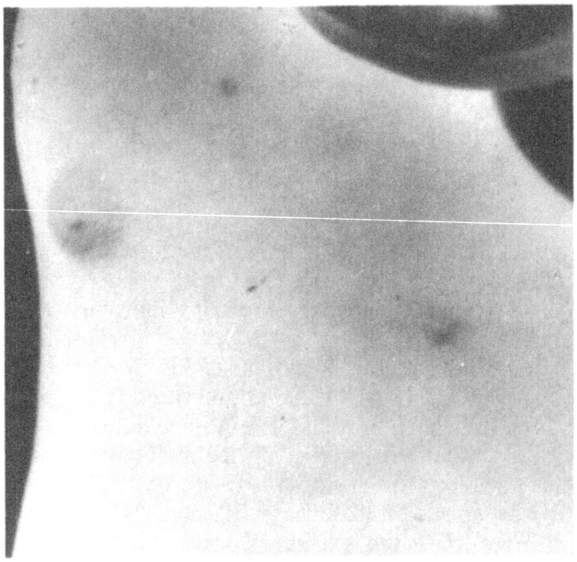

Fig. 17.1. Rat mite bite in a child. (From Theis et al. 1981, by kind permission of the authors and the publisher, the American Medical Association. Copyright 1981, American Medical Association)

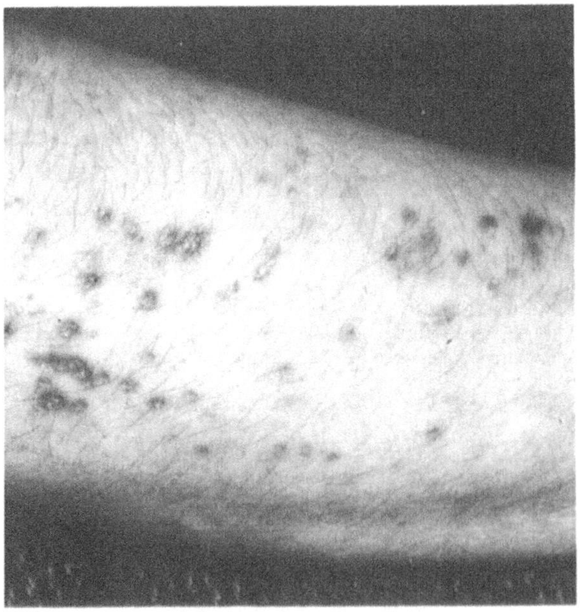

Fig. 17.2. Bites, probably from *Dermanyssus gallinae*, in a turkey plucker. (Courtesy of Dr. M. Young, Greenock, and Dr. A. Lyell, Glasgow)

form appearance. In contrast, the patient of Charlesworth and Cleghern (1977) had a monomorphic rash of papules 1 or 2 mm in diameter with an erythematous halo. Individual lesions fade in a few days, variously estimated at between 2 and 7 days (Frederick 1951; Haggard 1955; Hetherington et al. 1971; Nadchatram and Ramalingam 1974). There is a distinct tendency to grouping in clusters of from two to six lesions, attributed by Shelmire and Dove (1931) to piecemeal feeding. There was a tendency to linear arrangement in the patients of Fox (1982). There may be residual pigmentation (Lowell 1946; Pirila and Kilpio 1949). The eruption may be scanty or extensive but the lesions are always discrete. Sulzberger and Kamenstein (1936) pointed out that their patients infested with *D. gallinae* all exhibited dermographism. In the majority of patients mites were actually seen on the skin, sometimes in considerable numbers, but lesions akin to burrows were never seen. One patient was found to have a mite below the edge of the fingernail after scratching (Pirila and Kilpio 1949). In the discussion of Sulzberger and Fisher (1948a), Fisher categorically declared that mite bites left scars, but no other author before or since has seen this result. It seems from his description that he may not have been describing the true eruption of rat mite bites.

There is no preferred distribution. Exposed areas appear to be attacked more severely but not necessarily, depending on how and when the bites were acquired. Poultry handlers tend to get bitten on the hands and forearms (Fig. 17.2), whilst those acquiring lesions when in bed would have a different distribution. Both Anderson (1944; *O. bacoti*) and Laird (1950; *D. gallinae*) noted a preference for hairy regions such as the axillary and pubic areas, whilst Dowlati and Maguire (1970) felt that the flexor surfaces were more likely to be attacked. In general, however, any parts of the limbs, the shoulders, upper back, umbilical area, breasts in women and the groins may be affected (Fig. 17.3). The hands (palms and interdigital webs), soles of the feet, face and head are nearly always spared (Sulzberger and Kamenstein 1936; Anderson 1944; Shaw and Pommerening 1950; Frenken 1962; Hidano and Asanumo 1976). Areas where there is tight clothing such as in the region of a belt or brassière are particularly liable to be bitten.

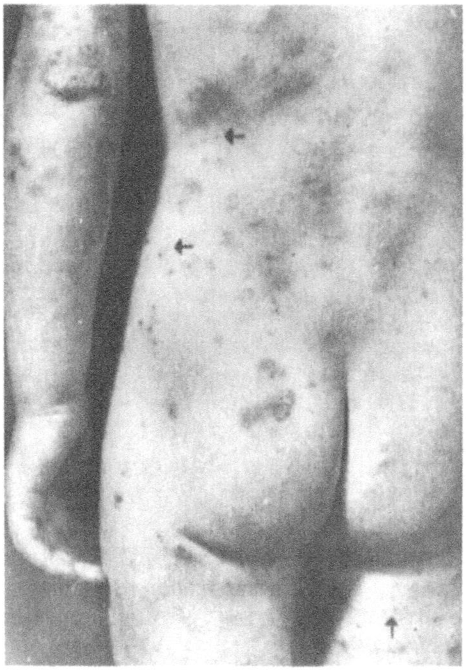

Fig. 17.3. *Dermanyssus* dermatitis eruption resembling excoriated papular urticaria. (From Frenken 1962, by kind permission of the author and the Editor of *Dermatologica*)

Diagnosis

The diagnosis of gamasid infestation depends primarily on the history of onset, the occurrence of groups of cases and the environmental associations, inquiry for which is prompted by the indication given by the clinical appearance of an ectoparasitic cause. The clinical picture itself is more or less common to many other ectoparasitic attacks, such as by fleas, chiggers and other mites. Przybilla et al. (1983) indicated that infestations with *D. gallinae* (or other arthropod) should always be considered a possible cause of pruritus of unknown origin. Scabies can be distinguished by its characteristic distribution, the presence of burrows, its chronicity and interfamilial spread. In patients with pediculosis the lice can be found either in the clothing or on the body, depending on which species is involved. Eczema, lichen planus and dermatitis herpetiformis each has its own peculiar features and none has any parasitic connection, unless perhaps eczema occurs as a secondary complicating phenomenon of an infestation. Some instances closely resemble papular urticaria which is now regarded as ectoparasitic in origin. Rickettsialpox can be very difficult to distinguish on clinical appearance, but there is a history of prodromal bite or bites and the sudden appearance 4 days or so later of the characteristic eruption with fever and systemic upset. It may be associated with *O. sylvarium* or *L. sanguineus* as vectors, which makes the differential diagnosis that much more difficult. Elevated antibody titres to the appropriate rickettsial organisms will settle the diagnosis.

Treatment

New lesions cease to appear when biting stops. All the patient needs is a warm soapy bath or shower followed by the application of simple antipruritic lotions or creams such as 0.5% phenol in oily calamine lotion or crotamiton cream. Oral antihistamines may give relief from the itch. Disinfestation of contaminated clothing and bedding can be done by steam heat or more conveniently by dusting with gamma-benzene hexachloride or malathion powders. Destruction of hosts and other mites is discussed under each separate species.

Dermanyssus gallinae DeGeer 1778

D. gallinae is the best known of the gamasid mites which attack men. It is a common parasite of domestic and wild birds and has been found associated not only with poultry but also with pigeons, sparrows, swallows, wrens (Hirst 1922), with starlings, parakeets, canaries and tiger finches (Frenken 1962) and with birds of the seashore (Laird 1950). Occasionally, according to Hirst, it attacks horses and other domestic animals. Its anatomical features are shown in Fig. 17.4. Ewing (1936) gave the dimensions of the adult female as 0.87 mm long by 0.46 mm wide (Fig. 17.5). These measurements increase after engorgement. The minute details of the anal plate shown in Fig. 17.4c are helpful in distinguishing *D. gallinae* from other gamasids.

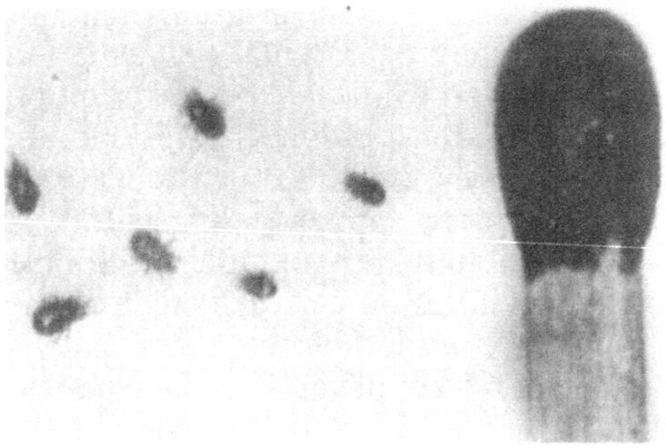

Fig. 17.5. *Dermanyssus gallinae* compared with the head of a match (From Frenken 1962, by kind permission of the author and the Editor of *Dermatologica*)

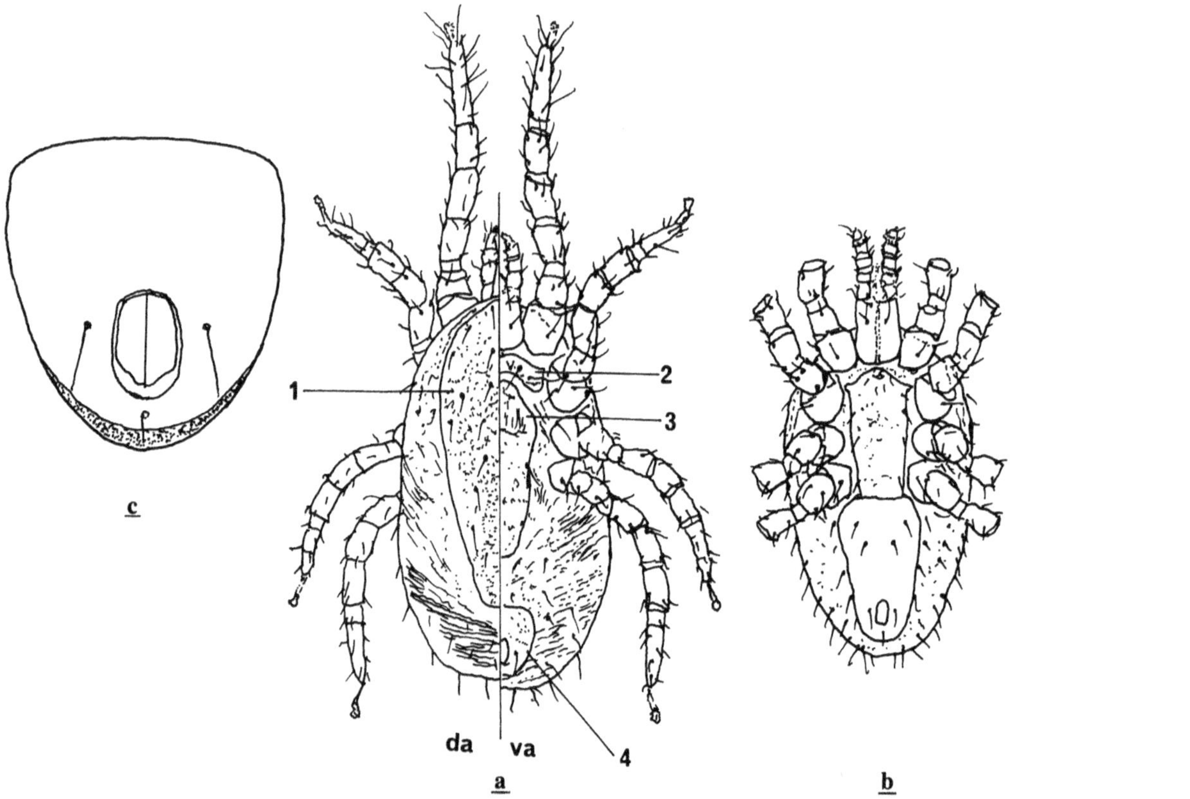

Fig. 17.4a–c. *Dermanyssus gallinae* (DeGeer 1778). **a** compound drawing of adult female; **b** ventral aspect of male; **c** anal plate of female. *da*, dorsal aspect; *va*, ventral aspect; *1*, dorsal shield; 2 sternal plate; *3*, ventral plate; *4*, anal plate. (**a** and **b** after Hirst 1922, by kind permission of the Trustees of the British Museum; **c** after Ewing 1923, by kind permission of the Smithsonian Institution Press)

Table 17.3. Life cycle of *Dermanyssus gallinae* (see text). (After Bishopp and Wood 1931)

	Time
1. Emergence of adults, mating, engorging and ovipositing	Within 2 days
2. Larvae emerge	Within 2 days
3. Larvae moult to protonymphs	Within 1–2 days
4. Protonymphs engorge, moult to deutonymphs	Within $1\frac{1}{2}$–2 days
5. Deutonymphs engorge and moult to adults	Within 1–2 days
Total	10 days

Details of the life cycle are given in Table 17.3. DeOreo (1958) has pointed out that the duration of the life cycle varies from 7 to 21 days according to the prevailing temperature and the environment. It can be seen from Table 17.3 that blood meals are not required until the protonymph stage is reached. *D. gallinae* is a nocturnal feeder. In the daytime the great majority of the parasites leave the host to hide in cracks in the floor and walls of the nest or poultry house, although a few mites, mostly immature forms, will remain in the feathers. Eggs are laid in batches of between 3 and 7 in the daytime hiding places. A fresh blood meal is required before each batch is deposited. Some seven or eight batches are laid in a life time of 4–5 months, with an average total of 25–35 eggs (Bishopp and Wood 1931). Rapid proliferation can quickly occur. High atmospheric humidity favours a longer life. Hirst (1922) has observed that adult females have survived for up to 113 days without food.

Bishopp and Wood (1931) have indicated that those who rear poultry on a commercial scale have little trouble with these mites because they are fully cognisant of their effects and how to avoid them. On the other hand, farmers and others who keep such birds as a sideline to their other operations are less aware of the risks and can find their poultry houses quickly overrun by hordes of the creatures, whose attacks may occur insidiously. In fact the first sign of infestation may be irritation of the farmer's skin. The constant loss of blood and disturbance of rest at night in the affected fowls causes a reduction in egg production, poor physical condition of the birds, desertion of the nest during hatching of eggs or even death of a sitting hen in situ after being attacked by swarms of mites. The black and white speckling of the acarine faeces around the nest may also indicate infestation.

Control of *Dermanyssus*

Fowl try to rid themselves of ectoparasites by taking dust baths (Banks 1915), a common sight in many farmyards. This, however, is an ineffective method, as is the adaptation of it by using miticides, since the majority of the mites are not found on the birds in the daytime. The correct management is to disinfest and if possible get rid of the daytime hiding places of the parasites. This will involve dismantling and disinfesting nesting boxes and roosts, burning nesting material and thoroughly disinfesting the premises using pressure sprays. The size and type of spray depends on the area to be disinfested. Parasiticides such as gamma-benzene hexachloride or malathion in concentrations of up to 10% can be used, but the operation must be carried out with caution: The operator must wear a gas mask and the procedure must be performed with open windows and doors. The floors, walls and ceiling should be sprayed, care being taken to penetrate all cracks and crevices, and then the premises should be briefly sealed. Afterwards it is essential to ventilate the premises well to get rid of toxic fumes before the poultry can be returned. Alternatively, carbolineums or high-grade anthracene oils can be used and are said to be very effective (Bishopp and Wood 1931). Although DDT has been recommended by several writers, its use is not advised, since it is by no means 100% effective against mites and has ecological disadvantages. The birds themselves should be treated once with a sulphur and soap dip as for *O. sylviarum* (see p. 311) to deal with larvae and protonymphs and the occasional adult mite which can be found in the feathers.

Liponyssoides sanguineus Hirst 1914

Known as the house mouse mite, *L. sanguineus* is parasitic on rats and mice. It has a fairly widespread distribution (Hirst 1926), although, according to Southcott (1978), it has not yet reached Australia. Figure 17.6 depicts its morphological features after Hirst (1914b). Its natural history does not seem to be very well known. Sulzberger and Fisher (1948b) recorded an outbreak of rickettsialpox in New York of which *L. sanguineus*

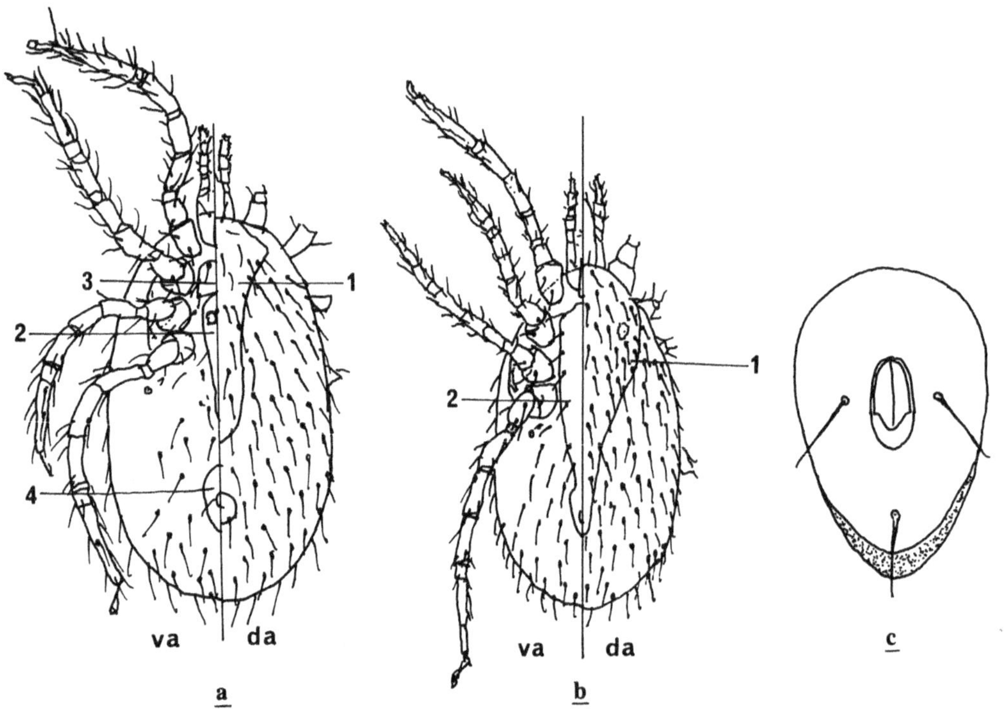

Fig. 17.6a–c. *Liponyssoides sanguineus* Hirst. **a** compound drawing of adult female; **b** compound drawing of male; **c** anal plate of female. *va*, ventral aspect; *da* dorsal aspect; *1*, dorsal shield; *2*, ventral plate; *3* sternal plate; *4*, anal plate. (**a** and **b** after Hirst, 1914, by kind permission of the Editor of the *Bulletin of Entomological Research*; **c** after Ewing 1923, by kind permission of the Smithsonian Institution Press)

was shown to be the vector (also confirmed by Philip and Hughes 1948). It does not appear to have attacked man otherwise than as a vector, although Baker et al. (1956) noted that it had been reported as occasionally doing so in some of the larger eastern American cities. In Iran, Semskaya and Neronov (1976–1977) found that it constituted about 10% of the gamasid mites found on small mammals.

Control

Infestation by *L. sanguineus* can only be controlled by control of its rodent hosts and disinfestation of the associated buildings by miticides such as gamma-benzene hexachloride or malathion.

Ornithonyssus bacoti Hirst 1913

O. bacoti is an important mite with a worldwide distribution. It has been recorded in Egypt and Abyssinia (Hirst 1913), Australia (Cleland 1908, cited by Holdsway 1926), the United States (Shelmire and Dove 1930 and many others, including Theis et al. 1981, who noted that it had been reported in 36 states of the United States), the United Kingdom (Browning 1950; Fairburn and Frain-Bell 1956), Germany (Oudemans 1936–1937), Japan (Ohmori 1938), Honolulu (Cole and Koepke 1947), Nigeria (Dipeolu and Ajayi 1976) and Iran (Semskaya and Neronov 1976–1977). It is probably a vector of murine typhus (Dove and Shelmire 1931, 1932; see Table 17.2) and is found principally as an ectoparasite of various species of rats, especially brown and black rats, also in mice, golden hamsters and guinea pigs (Olson and Dahms 1946; Lamb 1952) and rarely poultry (Evans 1938) and dogs (Ogata et al. 1976). It has been found not only on the animal hosts but also in and around their nests and in the floor dust (de Meillon and Lavoipierre 1944; Oshima 1964) and in clothing (Browning 1950). It was first recorded as attacking man by Cleland in 1908, although not under its present name (Holdaway 1926).

Figure 17.7 shows the anatomical details, as described by Hirst (1913). Skaliy and Hayes (1949) gave the length of the unfed male as averaging 764 μm, whereas in the fed state it measured 890 μm. An unfed female was 1153 μm long on average, rising to 1406 μm when fully engorged.

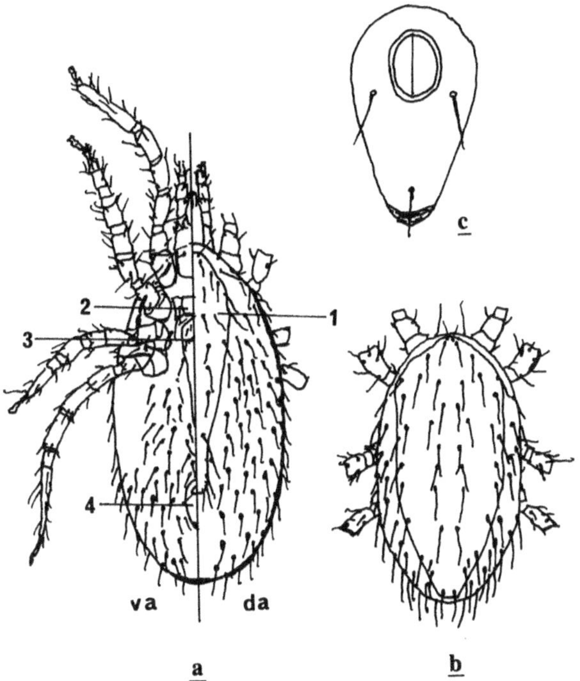

Fig. 17.7a–c. *Ornithonyssus bacoti* (Hirst 1913) **a** compound drawing of adult female; **b** dorsal aspect of male; **c** anal plate of female. *va*, ventral aspect; *da*, dorsal aspect; *1*, dorsal shield; *2*, sternal plate; *3*, ventral plate; *4*, anal plate. (**a** and **b** after Hirst 1914, by kind permission of the Editor of the *Bulletin of Entomological Research*; **c** after Ewing 1923, by kind permission of the Smithsonian Institution Press)

Unfed, the mite is a greyish colour and very active but when engorged it is red and sluggish in movement.

The life cycle has been estimated as 12 days (Dove and Shelmire 1932), 14 days (Skaliy and Hayes 1949) and $11\frac{1}{2}$ days (Bertram et al. 1946; Table 17.4). Both life cycle and survival are dependent on environmental temperature and relative humidity. Under favourable conditions the adult female feeds every 3 days, lays up to 9 eggs at a time (Holdaway 1926; Shelmire and Dove 1931; Bertram et al. 1946; Olson and Dahms 1946), lives for an average of 62 days and lays about 99 eggs in its lifetime (Skaliy and Hayes 1949). Egg laying occurs after an essential blood meal in excess of 0.1 mg (Sudd 1952) but is inhibited below 12°C. Adult mites can survive for a month at 6°–8°C but none above 36°C. Unfed larvae can survive 12 days (Pirila and Kilpio 1949), protonymphs 43 days (Hetherington et al. 1971) and adults for up to 63 days (Scott 1949) without food. *O. bacoti* will leave the host and travel long distances, up to several hundred feet, in search of a blood meal (Olson and Dahms 1946; Charlesworth and Cleghern 1977). Parthogenetic reproduction also occurs with these mites (Ohmori 1938). Eggs are laid in the nest or surroundings, the host only being visited for further meals. If the host is exterminated, man is often attacked as another source of food.

Control

Management of an infestation by *O. bacoti* consists of (1) destruction of the host animals, which may itself provoke further attacks at first; (2) simultaneous removal and burning of the nests of the hosts; (3) disinfestation of the area of the nest and its environment with gamma-benzene hexachloride or malathion spray, as for control of *D. gallinae*; and (4) similar disinfestation of clothing and furniture, domestic or office, which may have been contaminated. It is wise to repeat the spraying of the nest and its environment after an interval of 2–4 weeks.

Ornithonyssus sylviarum Canestrini and Fanzago 1877

The feather mite parasitises many domestic and wild birds (Hirst 1922) and has also been found on rats and mice (McGinnis 1959; Miller and Price 1977) and on dogs, cats, sheep, cockroaches, wallabies and kangaroos (McGinnis 1959). It can be

Table 17.4. Life cycle of *Ornithonyssus bacoti* as determined under optimal laboratory conditions by Bertram et al. (1946)

		Time
1. Adults emerge, mate and engorge		Within 3 days
2. Earliest eggs laid		Within 2 days
3. Larvae emerge		Within $1\frac{1}{2}$ days
4. Larvae moult to protonymph		Within 1 day
5. Protonymphs harden, feed and drop from the host		Within 2 days
6. Engorged protonymphs moult to deutonymphs		Within 1 day
7. Deutonymphs moult to adults		Within 1 day
	Total	$11\frac{1}{2}$ days

distinguished from the closely related *O. bursa* by the number and position of the setae on the sternal plate and posterior end of the dorsal shield, as in Fig. 17.8. Moniez (1893) gave its size as 0.55 mm long by 0.40 mm wide for the engorged female (Fig. 17.9). Its life cycle is not fully understood as it has not yet been reared in the laboratory and appears to lay only one egg at a time. It does not aestivate nor does it attack young chicks (Cameron 1938). The life cycle may be spent entirely in the feathers of the host, especially around the vent in poultry (Hirst 1922). It differs essentially from *D. gallinae* in that its eggs are deposited and hatched amongst the feathers, although, according to Cameron (1938), they may also be laid in the straw of the nest. The infested feathers have a dirty appearance around the vent and the irritation caused may produce a crusted state of the area (Bishopp and Wood 1931). According to Cutright (1929), the first evidence of infestation may be the presence of mites on the surface of the bird's eggs. Its presence may also be signalled by a reduction in egg yield. Miller and Price (1977) considered it to

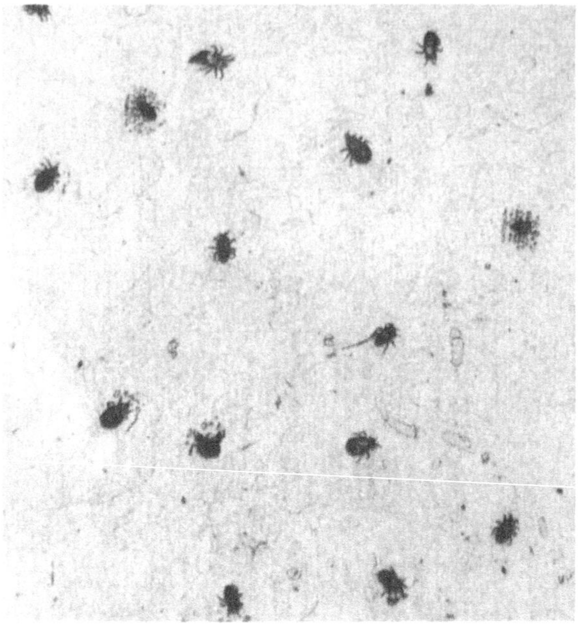

Fig. 17.9. *Ornithonyssus sylvarium* seen through Scotch tape. (From Braun 1979, by kind permission of the author and the Editor of *Cutis*) × 2

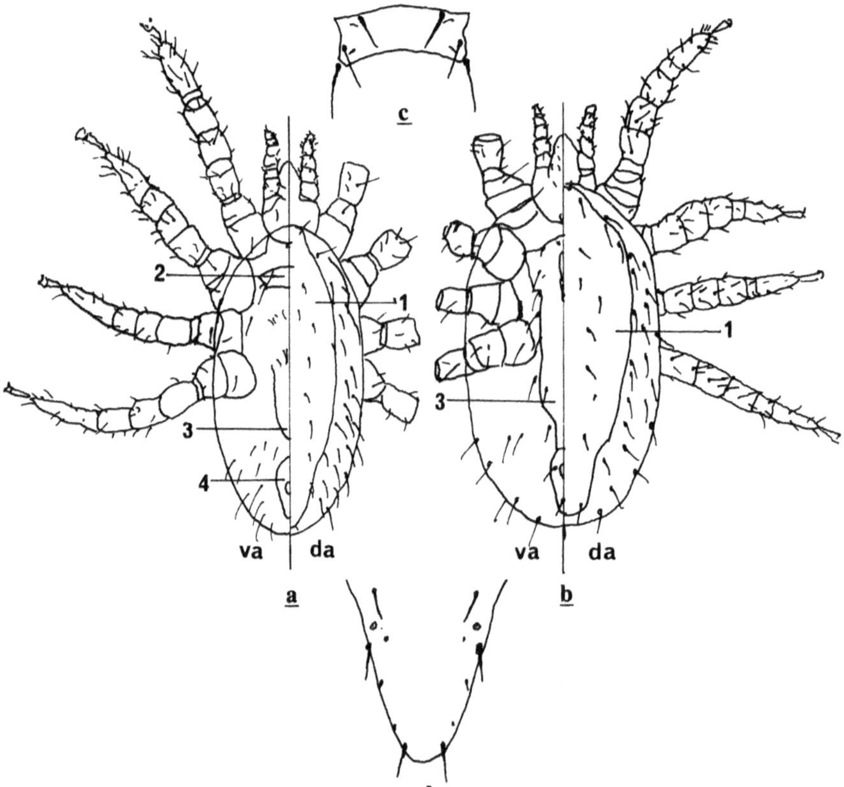

Fig. 17.8a–d. *Ornithonyssus sylviarum* (Canestrini and Fanzago 1877). **a** compound drawing of adult female; **b** compound drawing of male; **c** sternal plate of female; **d** posterior end of dorsal shield of female. *va*, ventral aspect; *da*, dorsal aspect; *1*, dorsal shield; *2*, sternal plate; *3*, ventral plate; *4*, anal plate. (**a** and **b** after Da Fonseca 1948, by kind permission of the Zoological Society of London; **c** and **d** after Hirst 1922, by kind permission of the Trustees of the British Museum)

be economically the most important ectoparasite of breeding and egg-producing poultry in the United States. It is not a serious pest in the United Kingdom.

Control

The birds themselves must be treated, since it is on them that the parasite resides. The treatment method chosen must ensure that the parasites are killed quickly, the birds are unharmed and their eggs uncontaminated. Preferably it should also be cheap and easy to use. Cutright (1929) advocated painting the roosts half an hour before shutting the birds up for the night, with a solution containing 40% nicotine sulphate. The vapour from this penetrates the feathers and kills the mites rapidly so that they fall from the bird; it is not toxic to the poultry and does not contaminate the eggs. It is wise to repeat this treatment in 2 weeks. Alternatively, the birds can be individually dipped in a mixture containing 60 g (2 oz) of flowers of sulphur and 30 g (1 oz) of soap in 4.5 litres (1 gal) of water. This soaks the birds to the skin and should be done outdoors on a warm and sunny day or indoors in a heated building. The nesting material should be simultaneously removed and burnt and the nesting boxes and house disinfested as an additional precaution, using gamma-benzene hexachloride or malathion.

Ornithonyssus bursa Berlese 1888

The tropical fowl mite *O. bursa* is widely distributed in all warm countries. According to Hirst (1922), it replaced *D. gallinae* in such climates and was closely related to *O. sylviarum*, perhaps even being a variant of that species. Details of its morphological characteristics are shown in Fig. 17.10. According to Cameron (1938), Hirst

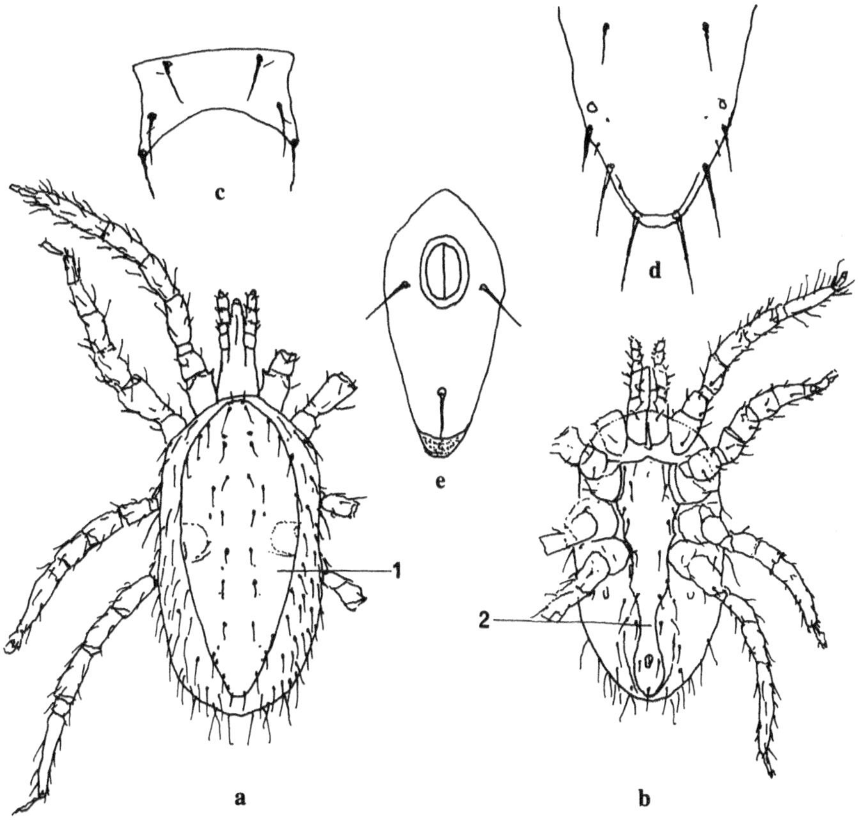

Fig. 17.10a–e *Ornithonyssus bursa* (Berlese 1888). **a** adult female; **b** male; **c** sternal plate of female; **d** posterior end of dorsal shield of female; **e** anal plate of female. *1*, dorsal shield; *2*, ventral shield. (**a** and **b** after Hirst 1915–1916, by kind permission of the Editor of the *Bulletin of Entomological Research*; **c** and **d** after Hirst 1922, by kind permission of the Trustees of the British Museum; **e** from Ewing 1923, by kind permission of the Smithsonian Institution Press)

stated that *O. bursa* infested nests and their surroundings, only attacking birds when it required food. In this respect it resembles *D. gallinae*, although Wood (1920) maintained that it could live and breed on both the host and its nest. Cameron also noted that when the host birds flew away, it could live for only about 10 days without food and did not breed, although Murray (1951) gave it a life of 5 weeks or more in the same circumstances. Apart from poultry, it parasitises many other birds (Hirst 1915–1916), including the common sparrow, which Hirst (1922) considered responsible for its dissemination. It has been recorded as attacking man in India (Hirst 1915–1916; Lodha 1969), in Formosa (Hirst 1921), Brazil, India and Africa (Da Fonseca 1947; de Meillon and Lavoipierre 1944), New Zealand (Murray 1951), Puerto Rico (Fox 1957) and California (Tarshis 1964). In these instances it was by no means always associated with poultry. H. L. Arnold (1981, personal communication) reported it was very troublesome in Hawaii, whilst Furumizo and Thomas (1977) had found it in house dust in Malaysia.

Control

Control is for *D. gallinae*. Murray said that gamma-benzene hexachloride killed this mite in 36 h.

Epidemiology

O. bacoti infestation has no preference for season, climate or country. However, it has a very strong association with rat infestation, which may be observed by patients but usually only emerges after specific questions or in the event of an obvious epidemic. Affected individuals may live in rat-infested houses (Riley 1940; Anderson 1944; Rothman and Niederman 1947; Pirila and Kilpio 1949; Dowlati and Maguire 1970; Hetherington et al. 1971; Charlesworth and Cleghern 1977) or more commonly work in premises where rats live. These premises vary greatly and include offices (McIntosh 1935; Riley 1940; Browning 1950; Lamb 1952), department stores (Shelmire and Dove 1930; 1931; Spencer 1937; Riley 1940; Weber 1940; Lowell 1946; Fairburn and Frain-Bell 1956), stationery stores (Holdaway 1926), laboratory animal house (Fox 1982), clinic buildings (Shelmire and Dove 1930, 1931), an orphanage (Haggard 1955) and a factory (Cory 1923). They have one common feature, however—an ample supply of paper, the favourite nesting material of the rat. Many also have an abundant food supply for rats. The mites wander from the infested nests over the surrounding walls, floor, ceilings, furniture, onto clothing, around warm radiators and to other rooms and levels in the building. This wandering is usually associated with rat extermination or nest desertion, but not invariably. Rat exterminators are very familiar with the parasites (Newton 1942). It should also be noted that whilst rat extermination often precipitates an outbreak of biting of humans, it is a necessary measure in control of the mites. Concurrent antiparasitic action should also be taken. If it is omitted, a period of 1–2 months may elapse before the epidemic dies down because of the capacity of the mites to survive for long periods without food, in the absence of the normal host.

In temperate zones *D. gallinae* infestation tends to have a seasonal incidence in the late summer and autumn (Frenken 1962) but also rather earlier, in relation to fledglings leaving their nests. This parasitosis is almost invariably associated with infested birds' nests in one way or another. Such nests are frequently found close to windows (Brendt 1952; Rockwell 1953; Frenken 1962; Hidano and Asanuma 1976; Przybilla et al. 1983), ventilators (Shaw and Pommerening 1950; Sexton and Haynes 1975), on or inside air-conditioner inlets (Cahn and Schechter 1958; Mercantini 1959; Gross 1959; Braun 1979), in attics (Brown 1953) or beneath a roof (DeOreo 1958). Mites from these nests wander, often in very large numbers, over windowsills, through cracks in walls and window frames onto the walls, floor, ceilings and pipes of the adjoining rooms, into cupboards and onto furniture, bedclothes, mats and carpets, around radiators and even onto clothing. They may be wind assisted in their dissemination, especially via air-conditioners. In one instance a patient with a fracture was bitten by a large number of mites inside a plaster of Paris splint. These mites have also been found in grass and mud flats, having been left there apparently by wild birds (Laird 1950). The rash produced by their bites quickly subsides after removal of the infested nests or if the patient moves away from the neighbourhood. There may be a short delay before all new lesions disappear after nest destruction unless the wandering mites are also attacked. Re-exposure to attack causes a rapid relapse.

Antiparasitic measures have been discussed above. One such measure which should be noted can be utilised for all the forms of parasite. It is the use of 4.7% ammonium fluosilicate in an aerogel silicate dust. This is applied with a dust blower at the rate of 1 kg to every 200 m^2 (approximately 1 lb for 1000 ft^2) and acts by virtue of its ability continuously to adsorb the lipid covering of the arthropod's chitinised exoskeleton. The mite dies of dehydration. The action is enhanced by the strong positive electrical charge which causes it to adhere to those surfaces with which it comes into contact. Because its action is physical rather than chemical, resistance to its effects will not develop. It is rapid and non-toxic to man and other animals and its curative effects are lasting (Ebeling 1960; Tarshis 1964).

Contact with *O. sylviarum*, *O. bursa* and *L. sanguineus* occurs in a manner similar to that for *D. gallinae*. Jo et al. (1983) found *O. sylviarum* in dust samples from both houses and henhouses of two poultry farmers in the Kyung Ki province of Korea. Three persons in one family had avian mite dermatitis.

Da Fonseca (1948) noted that *O. braziliensis* and *O. nagayoi* (alleged to be variants of *O. bacoti*), *O. theringi* from northeastern Brazil and *O. venezolarum* from Mexico, together with *Liponyssus lobatus* (which he called *Lepronyssus flavum*; see also Porta 1914), have all been recorded as biting man. Hidano and Asanuma (1976) claimed that *D. hirundis* caused a skin eruption, but Hirst (1920) regarded this species as another variant of *D. gallinae*. Schultz (1975) recorded lesions produced by the snake mite *Ophionyssus natricis*, whilst Keh (1974) reported that the mite *Chiroptonyssus robusti pes*, a parasite of Brazilian bats, has caused human lesions. The last report may have important relevance in the United Kingdom, where bats are now a protected species. The "rat mites" found in straw by Hill and Gordon (1945) were identified as *Haemogamasus oudemansii* (Hirst 1914a), *Hypoaspis fenilis*, *Eulaelaps stabularis* and *Cheyletus eruditus*. None had previously been identified specifically as biters (Ewing 1932 had claimed that *E. stabularis* was a biter), but the outbreak of dermatitis did clear when they were destroyed.

Immunology

Rook (1979) has suggested that these eruptions may be due to sensitisation. This would account for the severity of the itch, whereas the bites themselves are more likely to be painful because there may be an irritating proteolytic enzyme injected when they bite (cf. infestation by *Pyemotes*; see p. 321).

References

Anderson CR (1944) Rat mite dermatitis; acariasis caused by the tropical rat mite *Liponyssus bacoti* Hirst 1914. Arch Dermatol Syphilol 50: 90–95

Audy JR (1948) Natural history and scrub typhus. Malay Nat J 3: 114–129

Baker EW, Evans TM, Gould DJ, Hull WB, Keegan HL (1956) A manual of parasitic mites of medical or economic importance. National Pest Control Association Inc, New York

Banks N (1915) The acarina or mites. US Dept of Agriculture, Office of the Secretary Report No 108. US Govt Printing Office, Washington DC, pp 1–53

Berndt WL (1952) The chicken mite attacking children. J Econ Entomol 45: 1098

Bertram DS, Unsworth K, Gordon RM (1946) The biology and maintenance of *Liponyssus bacoti* Hirst 1913 and an investigation into its role as a vector of *Litomosoides carini* to cotton rats and white rats together with some observations on the infection of the white rats. Ann Trop Med Parasitol 40: 228–254

*Bishopp FC, Wood HP (1931) Mites and lice on poultry. US Dept of Agriculture Farmers Bulletin No 801. US Govt Printing Office, Washington DC, pp 1–25

Braun M III (1979) Avian mite dermatitis. Cutis 23: 680–682

Brown JH (1953) A chicken-mite infestation in a hospital. J Econ Entomol 46: 900

*Browning E (1950) On the occurrence of the tropical rat mite *Bdellonyssus bacoti* (Hirst 1913)—synonym *Liponyssus bacoti* (Hirst)—in Great Britain. Ann Trop Med Parasitol 44: 124–131

Burnet FM, Freeman M (1939) Note on a series of laboratory infestations with the Rickettsia of 'Q' fever. Med J Aust 1: 11–14

Cahn MM, Schechter FR (1958) Pruritus from an unusual source—bird mites; report of a case. JAMA 167: 724–726

*Cameron D (1938) The northern fowl mite (*Liponyssus sylviarum* C & F 1877). Can J Res 16: 230–254

Charlesworth EN, Cleghern RW (1977) Tropical rat mite dermatitis. Arch Dermatol 113: 937–938

Cole HN, Driver JR (1937) Gamasoidosis. Arch Dermatol Syphilol 38: 322–323

Cole LC, Koepke JA (1947) Problem of interpretation of the data of rodent ectoparasite surveys and studies of rodent ectoparasites in Honolulu, T.H., Savannah, Ga and Dothan, Ala. Public Health Rep Washington, Suppl 202

Cory EN (1923) *Liponyssus bacoti* Hirst. J Econ Entomol 16: 226

Cutright CR (1929) A valuable aid in the control of the feather mite *Liponyssus sylviarum*. J Econ Entomol 22: 422

Da Fonseca F (1948) A monograph of the genera and species of Macronyssidae Oudemans 1936 (Synan. Liponyssidae Vitzhum 1931) Acari. Proc Zool Soc Lond 118: 239–334

de Meillon B, Lavoipierre M (1944) New records and species of biting insects from the Ethiopian region. J. Entomol Soc S Afr 7: 38–67

DeOreo GA (1958) Pigeons acting as vector in acariasis caused by *Dermanyssus gallinae* (DeGeer 1778) Arch Dermatol Syphilol 77: 422–429

Dipeolu OO, Ajayi SS (1976) Parasites of the African giant rat *Cricetomys gambianus* Waterhouse) in Ibadan, Nigeria. East Afr Wild Life J 14: 85–89

Dove WE, Shelmire B (1931) Tropical rat mites *Liponyssus bacoti* Hirst, vectors of endemic typhus. JAMA 97: 1506–1511

Dove WE, Shelmire B (1932) Some observations on tropical rat

mite and endemic typhus. J Parasitol 18: 159–168
Dowlati Y, Maguire HC (1970) Rat-mite dermatitis; a family affair. Arch Dermatol 101: 617–618
Ebeling W (1960) Control of the tropical rat mite. J Econ Entomol 53: 475–476
Evans IBP (1938) Pasture, crop and insect problems of the Union. Annual report of the Division of Plant Industry. Farming S Afr 13: 519–538
*Ewing HE (1923) The dermanyssid mites of North America. Smithsonian Institution US National Museum Proceedings, vol 62 (art/13), Smithsonian Institution, Washington DC, pp 1-26
Ewing HE (1932) Early records and present known distribution in the United States of three recently introduced mites. Proc Entomol Soc Washington 34: 13–16
Ewing HE (1936) A short synopsis of the North American species of the mite genus *Dermanyssus*. Proc Entomol Soc Washington 38: 47–54
*Fairburn EA, Frain-Bell W (1956) *Bdellonyssus bacoti* as a causal agent of cutaneous disease. Br J Dermatol 68: 350–354
Ferguson FF (1954) Biological factors in the transmission of arthropod-borne virus encephalitis. Public Health Serv Bull No 372. (Public Health Monogr No 23). Cited by Fox (1957)
Finnegan S (1945) Acari as agents transmitting typhus in India, Australasia and the Far East. British Museum (Natural History) Economic Ser Br Museum No 16, London, Trustees of the British Museum, p 13
Fox I (1957) *Ornithonyssus bursa* (Berlese) attacking man in Puerto Rico. J Econ Entomol 50: 838
Fox JG (1982) Outbreak of tropical rat mite dermatitis in laboratory personnel. Arch Dermatol 118: 676–678
Frederick WG (1951) Rat mite dermatitis. Ind Med Surg 20: 382
*Frenken JH (1962) *Dermanyssus gallinae* (*D. avium*). Strophulus or "insect bites", diet or D.D.T. Dermatologica 125: 322–331
Furumizo RT, Thomas V (1977) Mites of house dust. Southeast Asian J Trop Med Public Health 8: 411–412
Gross ER (1959) Air-conditioning. A modern method for the transmission of parasites. Arch Dermatol 79: 355
Haggard CN (1955) Rat-mite dermatitis in children. Pediatrics 15: 322–324
Hammon WMcD, Reeves WC, Cunha R, Espana C, Sather G (1948) Isolation from wild bird mites (*Liponyssus sylviarum*) of a virus or mixtures of viruses from which St. Louis Western equine encephalitis viruses have been obtained. Science 107: 92–97
Hetherington GW, Holder WB, Smith EB (1971) Rat mite dermatitis. JAMA 215: 1499–1500
Hidano A, Asanuma K (1976) Acariasis caused by bird mites. Arch Dermatol 112: 882–883
Hill MA, Gordon RM (1945) An outbreak of dermatitis amongst troops in North Wales caused by rodent mites. Ann Trop Med Parasitol 39: 46–52
Hirst S (1913) On three new species of gamasid mites found on rats. Bull Entomol Res 4: 119–124
Hirst S (1914a) Preliminary list of the acari occurring on the brown rat (*Mus norvegica*) in Great Britain, with the description of a new species (*Haemogamasus oudemansii*). Bull Entomol Res 5: 119–124
Hirst S (1914b) On the parasitic acari found on the species of rodents frequenting human habitation in Egypt. Bull Entomol Res 5: 215–229
Hirst S (1915–1916) On a widely distributed gamasid mite (*Leiognathus morsitans* sp. n.) parasitic on the domestic fowl. Bull Entomol Res 6: 55–58
Hirst S (1920) Species of Arachnida and Myropoda injurious to man. Econ Ser Br Museum No 6, p 32
Hirst S (1921) On some new or little-known acari mostly parasitic in their habit. Proc Zool Soc Lond 25: 357–373
*Hirst S (1922) Mites injurious to domestic animals. Econ Ser Br Museum 13: 1–107
Hirst S (1926) The principal species of acari parasitic on rats, with brief notes on hosts and distribution. Ceylon J Sci 1: 273–276
Holdaway FG (1926) A note on the occurrence of the rat mite *Liponyssus bacoti* in South Australia, together with descriptions of certain stages. Trans R Soc S Aust 50: 85–88
Huebner RJ, Jellison WL, Pomerantz C (1946) Rickettsialpox—a newly recognised rickettsial disease. IV. Isolation of a *Rickettsia* apparently identical with the causative agent of rickettsialpox from *Allodermanyssus sanguineus*, a rodent mite. Public Health Rep 61: 1677–1682
Jo I, Cho BK, Lee WK (1983) Avian mite dermatitis (in Korean with English summary). Korean J Dermatol 21: 29–33
Keh B (1974) Dermatitis caused by the rat mite *Chiroptonyssus robustipes* (Ewing) in California. J Med Entomol 11: 498
Laird M (1950) Notes on the infestation of man by the chicken mite *Dermanyssus gallinae* (DeGeer) in New Zealand, NZ Med J 49: 22–23
Lamb KP (1952) The tropical rat mite *Bdellonyssus bacoti* (Hirst 1913) attacking man in New Zealand. NZ Med J 51: 320–322
Liu WT (1947) Isolation of typhus *Rickettsiae* from rat mites *Liponyssus bacoti*, in Peiping. Am J Hyg 45: 58–60
Lodha KR (1969) The occurrence of tropical fowl mite *Ornithonyssus* (*Bdellonyssus*, *Liponyssus*) *bursa* on a man in Ragasthan (India). Vet Rec 84: 363–365
Lowell ME (1946) Rat mite dermatitis. Acariasis caused by the tropical rat mite *Liponyssus bacoti* Hirst. Arch Dermatol Syphilol 54: 278–280
McGinnis GF (1959) Avian-mite dermatitis. N Engl J Med 261: 396–397
McIntosh A (1935) Tropical rat mite attacking man. Proc Helminthol Soc Washington 2: 62
Mercantini ES (1959) The transmission of parasites by air conditioning. Arch Dermatol 80: 587
Miller WV, Price FC (1977) The avian mite *Ornithonyssus sylviarum* on mammalian hosts with reference to transmission to poultry. J Parasitol 63: 417
Moniez R (1893) *Leiognathus sylviarum*. Rev biol Nord Fr 5: 408
Morisita T (1938) Transmission experiments in relapsing fever with tropical rat mite, *Liponyssus* sp. Jpn J Med 16: 551–555
Murray HD (1951) Tropical fowl mite, *Liponyssus bursa* (Berlese), infesting man in New Zealand. NZ Med J 51: 392–393
Nadchatram M, Ramalingam S (1974) Dermatitis caused by *Ornithonyssus bacoti* (Hirst 1913). Southeast Asian J Trop Med Public Health 5: 150
Newton HE (1942) Tropical rat mite infestation. Cal West Med 5: 143
Ogata M, Itagaki M, Ishida F, Nakai T (1976) A canine case of infestation with the tropical mite *Ornithonyssus bacoti* (Hirst 1913). J Jpn Vet Med Assoc 29: 442–444
Oudemans AC (1936–1937) Kritisch historisch Overzicht der Acarologie, vol 3. Brill, Leiden
Ohmori N (1938) Studies on the tropical rat mite; Second report on the sex ratio and parthenogenesis. Zool Mag Tokyo 48: 627–637
Olson TA, Dahms RG (1946) Observations on the tropical rat mite, *Liponyssus bacoti*, as an ectoparasite of laboratory animals and suggestions for its control. J Parasitol 32: 56–60
Oshima S (1964) Observations of floor mites collected in Yokohama. In the mites found in several schools in summer. Jpn J Sanit Zool 15: 233–244
Pang KH (1941) Isolation of typhus rickettsiae from rat mites during epidemic in an orphange. Proc Soc Exp Biol NY

48: 266–267

Philip CB, Hughes LE (1948) Tropical rat mite, *Liponyssus bacoti*, as experimental vector of rickettsialpox. Am J Trop Med 28: 697–705

Pirila V, Kilpio O (1949) Rat mite dermatitis. Acta Derm Venereol (Stockh) 29: 70–76

Polano MK (1962) In discussion on Frenken (1962) Dermatologica 125: 322–331

Porta A (1914) Dermatitis occasionale nell'uomo dovuta ad un acaro (*Liponyssus lobatus*). Zool Anzeiger (Berlin) 44: 481–482

Przybilla B, Ryckmans F, Postner M, Klöverorn W (1983) Epizootic durch die Milbe *Dermanyssus gallinae* (DeGeer 1778). Hautarzt 34: 335–338

Reeves WC, Hammon WMcD, Furman DP, McClure HE, Brookman B (1947) Recovery of Western equine encephalitis virus from wild bird mites (*Liponyssus sylviarum*) in Kern County, California. Science 105: 411–412

Riley WA (1940) Rat mite dermatitis in Minnesota. Minn Med 23: 423–424

Rockwell E (1953) Dermatitis due to *Dermanyssus gallinae* of pigeons. Arch Dermatol 68: 82

Rook A (1979) Skin diseases caused by arthropods and other venomous and noxious animals. In: Rook A, Wilkinson DS, Ebling FJG (eds) Text book of dermatology, 3rd edn. Blackwell, Oxford, p 947

Rothman S, Niederman D (1947) Rat mite dermatitis. Arch Dermatol Syphilol 55: 138–139

Sanders RN (1944) A blood sucking mite of poultry. Agric J Fiji 15: 27

Schultz H (1975) Human infestation by *Ophionyssus natricis* snake mite. Br J Dermatol 93: 695–697

Scott JA (1949) Longevity of tropical rat mites without food. J Parasitol 35: 434–435

Semskaya AA, Neronov VH (1976–1977) Some features of the gamasine mite fauna of small mammals in Iran (in Russian). Inst Epidemiol Mikrobiol AMN USSR, pp 187–188.

Sexton J, Haynes B (1975) Bird mite infestations in a University Hospital. Lancet I: 445

Shaw JW, Pommerening RA (1950) Avian mite dermatitis (gamasoidosis). Arch Dermatol 61: 466–469

Shelmire B, Dove WE (1930) Rat-mite dermatitis and the coincidental occurrence of *Liponyssus bacoti* and evidence of typhus in Texas. J Parasitol 17: 115 (Abstracted from Report to the Bureau of Entomology of the US Dep of Agriculture).

*Shelmire B, Dove WE (1931) The tropical rat mite *Liponyssus bacoti* Hirst 1914. The cause of a skin eruption of man and a possible vector of endemic typhus fever. JAMA 96: 579–584

Skaliy P, Hayes WJ Jr (1949) Biology of *Liponyssus bacoti* (Hirst 1913) (Acarina: Liponyssidae). Am J Trop Med 29: 759–772

Smith DJW, Brown HE, Derrick EH (1939) A further series of laboratory infection with the rickettsiae of 'Q' fever. Med J Aust 1: 13–14

Smith MG, Blattner RJ, Heys FM (1946) St. Louis encephalitis. Infection of chicken mites, *Dermanyssus gallinae*, by feeding on chickens with viraemia; transovarian passage of virus into the second generation. J Exp Med 84: 1–6

Southcott RV (1978) Australian harmful arachnids and their allies, Southcott, Mitcham, S. Australia

Spencer GJ (1936) The menace of rat parasites in Vancouver in 1936. Proc Entomol Soc Br Colombia 33: 44–45

Sudd JH (1952) Laboratory studies of adult female *Bdellonyssus bacoti* (Hirst 1916) (Acarina: Parasitiformes). Ann Trop Med Parasitol 46: 158–164

Sulzberger MB, Fisher AA (1948a) Rat mite dermatitis due to *Liponyssus bacoti*. Arch Dermatol Syphilol 57: 566–569

Sulzberger MB, Fisher AA (1948b) Rickettsialpox due to *Allodermanyssus sanguineus*. Arch Dermatol Syphilol 57: 767–769

Sulzberger MB, Kamenstein I (1936) Avian itch mites as a cause of human dermatoses. Canary birds' mites responsible for two groups of cases in New York. Arch Dermatol syphilol 33: 60–72

Tarshis IB (1964) A sorptive dust for control of the northern fowl mite, *Ornithonyssus sylviarum*, infesting dwellings. J Econ Entomol 57: 110–111

Theis JT, Lavoipierre MM, Lapierre R, Kroese H (1981) Tropical rat mite dermatitis. Arch Dermatol 117: 341–343

Touraine A (1947) Les traitements actuels des parasitoses animaux de la peau. Baillière, Paris

Weber LF (1940) Rat mite dermatitis. JAMA 114: 1442

Wood HP (1920) Tropical fowl mites in the United States. With notes on life history and control. US Dept of Agriculture Circular No 79. US Govt Printing Office, Washington DC, pp 3–8

18 *Pyemotes* Infestation

"Grain itch" has been known for a long time. Bernadino Ramazzini in 1700 noted unconfirmed reports of "lousiness" amongst bakers, millers and corngrinders (Glass 1948). Similar eruptions were recorded in the United States in 1829, 1830 and 1945, the earlier attacks being attributed to the wheat stem fly (Webster 1910).

Lagrèze-Fossat and Montané (1851) first showed that an outbreak of itching followed by a skin eruption amongst granary workers and dockers at Espalais, Bordeaux and Moissac, France, in 1850 was associated with a mite in wheat, which they described and named *Acarus tritici*. They were not able to see the reproductive cycle but only saw adults in the grain. Newport (1853) described the extraordinary gravid female and the whole reproductive cycle in mites which he found parasitising other parasites of solitary bees. Since then some 100 reports on the skin disorder have been published, many excellent ones being in relatively obscure journals. The condition has been variously known as "grain itch", "straw itch", "hay itch", "barley itch", "cereal itch", "prairie itch", *gale du blé, gale des cereales, acariasi da grano*, "Kiawe itch", "cotton seed dermatitis" and "acarodermatitis urticarioides", a name coined by Schamberg (1910).

Nomenclature of the mite has changed from time to time. Newport's name of *Heteropus ventricosus* was changed to *Pediculoides ventricosus* in 1878 by Tarzini and Tazzetti and in turn to *Pyemotes ventricosus* by Oudemans in 1937. Krczal (1959) named several different species of *Pyemotes*, but Moser (1975) reassessed the whole group and by cross-matching tests showed that those mites infesting straw and grain were all of one species, which he named *Pyemotes tritici* (Lagrèze-Fossat and Montané 1851). *Pyemotes ventricosus* was a different species parasitising wood-boring insects but also able to attack man. No other species were injurious to humans.

Outbreaks have been reported from numerous countries in Europe, from Africa, the United States and Canada, from Asia and from Australia. The eruption may be of brief duration and advice is often not sought. A physician may be baffled by the diagnosis and the patient may recover before one is made (Webster 1910; Rogers 1943). Many other outbreaks have involved huge numbers of people (Philippson 1914; Pantaleoni 1920; Booth and Jones 1952). Occasionally near panic may grip the population (Mariani 1952).

Clinical Manifestations

The *Pyemotes* mite will attack persons of either sex and any age or race. In some outbreaks the source is encountered at work, when adults are more likely to be attacked. The first indication of an attack is itching, which usually occurs within a few hours of contact with infested material. It may be evident within 15–20 min (Sergent and Alary 1916; Swan 1934b; Rogers 1943) or may be delayed for several days (Pascal 1900; Hung-Chiung and Sung-Nien 1958). It is very intense and aggravated by sweating and especially by warmth in bed. It prevents the majority of sufferers from sleeping and some are unable to continue at work. In farming communities threshing is anticipated with dread by previously attacked persons because of the itch (Webster 1910).

Cutaneous Symptoms

A few hours after the onset of itching a skin eruption appears. It consists initially of small urticarial papules, often with a tiny central vesicle about 0.5 mm in diameter. Schamberg (1910) regarded this as the characteristic lesion. The contents are clear at first but gradually become cloudy or even purulent over the next 24–48 h, the lesion enlarging up to 3 mm across. Fine and Scott (1963) observed that a central haemorrhagic punctum might precede the development of a vesicle, but most other observers said such lesions were notable for their absence. Most of these lesions become excoriated and the vesicle is rubbed off and replaced by a crust (sometimes blood-stained or purulent), which, when it falls off after a further 2 or 3 days, leaves a brownish stain which fades over the next few weeks. The urticarial element may be obviously oedematous and raised 1–2 mm, resembling papular urticaria, but sometimes the erythematous component is predominant. These lesions, whether raised or not, seldom exceed 3 mm in diameter, but Hudelo and Dumet (1924) described palm-sized plaques. The smaller lesions are round, oval or irregular. They have a warm rosy tint (Schamberg 1910) which gradually fades. Rarely there may be a pale centre and an erythematous halo like ordinary urticaria (Schamberg 1910; Micks 1963). When the genitalia are involved there may be diffuse oedema of the penis and scrotum. Philippson (1914) described extending lesions like erythema annulare centrifugum reaching several centimetres in diameter and persisting for up to 2 weeks.

The eruption may be profuse or scanty depending on the duration of the exposure and the nature of the contact (see under Epidemiology, p. 320), on the number of bites and the ambient temperature (Swan 1934a, b). The distribution of the eruption is also dependent on the circumstances of the contact and to some extent on the ambient temperature, which may determine the nature of the clothing worn at the time. Bearing these points in mind, it can be stated that the skin lesions usually start on the exposed areas such as the forearms, neck, shoulders, upper trunk or face and quickly spread over most of the trunk and the proximal portions of both upper and lower limbs and the genitalia in men. Glass (1948) noted that the eruption began on the covered areas and was often limited by the constriction around a belt or braces (Hudelo and Dumet 1924). The hands have been stated to be uninvolved (Hudelo and Dumet 1924; Kittredge 1933; Fine and Scott 1963), but others have specifically mentioned their involvement (Willis 1909; Hewitt et al. 1976). In fact, any area of the body can be affected, with the probable exception of the soles. Not infrequently the eruption may be very severe, with upwards of 10 000 individual lesions, either discrete or confluent (Schamberg 1910). Sometimes in the early stages, when the lesions are closely grouped and chiefly urticarial, the appearance of measles may be simulated (Thompson 1925). At other times, with very heavy exposure to dust, a scarlatiniform appearance may be presented (Pascal 1900). This was especially noticeable in the Italian epidemic recorded by Panteoloni in 1920 when thousands of persons were affected. The whole range of appearances was seen in this outbreak, with some patients having localised lesions on the forearms as a result of thrusting their arms into the grain heaps and others presenting with lesions confined to the buttocks as a result of sitting on infested sacks. With regard to the latter, Thompson remarked that "white men never sat on the sacks of grain twice". In very warm circumstances excessive sweating may increase the severity of the rash by increasing the amount of dust containing parasites which clings to the skin. In his comprehensive account Schamberg (1910) classified the eruption into three main types: (1) urticario-vesiculo-pustulosa type; (2) varicelloid, where the lesions were not too numerous and dominated by the rather larger central vesicle (2–3 mm); and (3) erythema multiforme type. The third type resembles the so-called dermal type of erythema multiforme or toxic erythema. Secondary infection leading to pyoderma or the development of eczema sometimes occurs (Schamberg 1910; Booth and Jones 1952; Mariani 1952; Hung-Chiung and Sung-Nien 1958.

Systemic Symptoms

Systemic symptoms are seldom pronounced and are to some extent dependent on the severity of the skin eruption. They consist of chilliness and occasional rigors, nausea and rarely vomiting (Schamberg 1910), epigastic discomfort (Hung-Chiung and Sung–Nien 1958). Malaise, anorexia, headache and backache are common. Hung-Chiung and his colleague recorded dizziness and transient amblyopia in one patient. There may be moderate pyrexia up to 39°C (102°F) or higher, with corresponding increase in pulse rate. A moderate superficial lymphadenopathy may also be present. Ancona (1923) observed asthmatic attacks in many of his patients. Grove (1926) demonstrated that these were not associated with increased reagin antibodies. Swan (1934b) noted that Storm van Leeuwen [1925] regarded the mite bites as the initiating factor in sensitisation and the subsequent inhalation as the stimulus for asthmatic attacks. Occasionally some people appear to be immune (Askins 1924; Rogers 1943), but the contrary picture of hypersensitivity has not been recorded.

Records of laboratory findings are scanty. An ill-defined eosinophilia was noted by Schamberg (1910) but was unrelated to the severity of the eruption. A mild leucocytosis was also recorded. Both these abnormalities quickly subsided when the rash disappeared. Mild transient albuminuria has been observed by some workers (Schamberg 1910; Rawles 1909; Booth and Jones 1952; Hung-Chiung and Sung-Nien 1958).

Histological Picture

In the early stages there is thinning and elevation of the epidermis with patchy parakeratosis and some increase in the stratum granulosum, together with flattening of the papillary body and shrinkage of the rete pegs and some diminution of the pigment cells of the basal layer (Katzenellenbogen 1947). The epidermal thinning proceeds over the central portion of the lesion to the point of virtual disappearance as the vesicopustule develops (Schamberg 1910; Doucas 1942; Booth and Jones 1952). Only a few strands of stratum corneum remain; the granular layer disappears along with malpighian cells, the latter being represented at the margins of the vesicopustule by stretched fusiform cells. The vesicopustule contains a few isolated epithelial cells intermingled with a densely packed polymorphonuclear mass of cells. At the sides of this structure there are small areas of spongiosis. Otherwise the epidermis is normal.

In the corium there is a perivascular infiltrate which is initially composed of lymphocytes (Katzenellenbogen 1947), but later, according to Booth and Jones (1952), it consists of a mixture of lymphocytes, histiocytes, neutrophils and eosinophils. The blood and lymph vessels are dilated (Schamberg 1910) but not noticeably so (Booth and Jones 1952). Schamberg (1910) found abundant mast cells, as did Doucas (1942), but this finding was refuted by Booth and Jones (1952). No mites or parts of mites were found by any of these investigators.

Course

When the source of infestation is removed the condition subsides quickly and there is little to see after 7–14 days. There are no scars or other after effects, although if the stains of lesions are rubbed vigorously there may be some temporary recrudescence (Swan 1934a). Re-exposure to *Pyemotes* results in a rapid relapse to the former state.

Diagnosis

Diagnosis is made on the following grounds:

1. The history of mode and place of onset and the nature of the occupation
2. The severe itch
3. The clinical appearance and behaviour strongly suggestive of bites
4. The finding of *Pyemotes* in the contaminated material thought to be responsible. Dust is usually the best source
5. Possibility of finding *Pyemotes* in skin scrapings or Sellotape strippings from the skin, although the mite is only a temporary resident (Micks 1963)
6. The occurrence of other similar cases in the locality

Differential Diagnosis

Isolated, unsuspected cases may be exceedingly difficult to diagnose. Schamberg (1910) included ordinary urticaria, chickenpox, scabies and pediculosis corporis in the differential diagnosis. To these should be added other infestations.

Urticaria has much greater variation in size of lesion but more uniformity of appearance. There is never any crusting, although rarely bullae may be present. The distribution is different and there is no association with ectoparasitic infestation. It may be recurrent or chronic, seldom seasonal and not epidemic.

Papular urticaria (strophulus) is a chronic recurring form of insect bite, usually due to fleas and commonly occurring in young children.

Chickenpox may superficially resemble the varicelloid type of *Pyemotes* infestation, but the lesions continue to appear after the patient is confined to bed, occur on the mucosae as well as on the skin, persist for up to 4 weeks and leave scars. Systemic symptoms may be marked. Children are predominantly affected. Katzenellenbogen (1947) recorded the simultaneous occurrence of the two conditions. Schamberg (1910) also mentioned an instance where the lesions of *Pyemotes* infestation were so numerous and confluent as to suggest a diagnosis of smallpox. Virological investigations give positive results in both smallpox and chickenpox, but not in *Pyemotes* infestation.

Scabies and other parasitic infestations have their own particular distributions and are much more chronic diseases as a rule. Burrows are characteristic of scabies, but no such lesions are seen in *Pyemotes* infestations. Sudden acute outbreaks of scabies amongst groups of workmen or hotel visitors etc. do not occur, and neither does scabies have a seasonal incidence of short duration.

The finding of the *Sarcoptes* or, in the case of pediculosis, of the louse helps to differentiate the condition. Fine and Scott (1965) emphasise that chigger bites (trombiculid mites) individually resemble those of *Pyemotes* but that the distribution is quite different, occurring under areas of tight clothing such as around the waist, in the groin and around the ankles. Moreover, the chigger is not infrequently seen in the centre of the lesion as a tiny red dot. Chigger bites are much less numerous than those of *Pyemotes*. The distribution of the latter was different in Fine and Scott's (1965) patient, but it must be remembered that the areas affected by the *Pyemotes* vary according to the circumstances of contact. The bites from gamasid mites are also indistinguishable from those of *Pyemotes* and the distribution may not be diagnostic. The history of the onset and the nature of the environment in which the disease was contracted, together with the finding of the offending mite, make the diagnosis certain. Flea bites can be very extensive and even vesicular but they tend to occur in small groups of two to four, especially around the waist and the distal parts of the limbs. They occur sporadically, although in some areas they may be endemic and have a tendency to recurrence if the flea has not been removed.

Epidemiology

Pyemotes infestation may occur in epidemic or in small circumscribed outbreaks. Although spread from person to person is not the rule in this infestation it has been recorded by Sergent and Alary (1916) and by Mandoul et al. (1950). Panteoloni (1920) noted its frequent familial incidence in the epidemic which he reported. The vast majority of patients contract the disease, however, by direct bodily contact with contaminated material. Katzenellenbogen (1947) observed five people who acquired it indirectly through their clothing being contaminated in a cloakroom.

Most of the recorded outbreaks have come from contact with infested grain, seeds or straw, which, as Moser (1975) has pointed out, are always infested with *P. tritici* and not *P. ventricosus* as now defined. A few less severe instances caused by the

Table 18.1 Various sources in which *Pyemotes* species reported as causing a skin eruption have been found

Source of parasites	References
Grain cargoes	
Barley	Pascal (1900); Wills (1909); Sergent and Alary (1916); Loir and Legangneux (1919); Askins (1924); Thompson (1925); Voukassovitch and Dojmi (1937); Mandoul et al. (1950)
Wheat	Lagrèze-Fossat and Montané (1851); Koller (1882); Flemming (1884); Gros (1908); Hone (1922)
Dried peas	Gros (1908); Hudelo and Dumet (1924); Mandoul et al. (1950)
Beans	Philippson (1915); Larson (1920); Doucas (1942); Mandoul et al. (1950)
"Corn"	Llambias and Lorenzo (1920)
"Cereals"	Mariani (1952)
Grain stores	Aoki and Hasegawa (1966)
Grain mills	Pantaleoni (1920); Ancona (1923)
Cotton seed	Willcocks (1914); Nixon (1915); O'Connor (1920); Mandoul et al. (1950)
Packed cereals	Micks (1963)
Wheat straw	
In general	Goldberger and Schamberg (1909); Rawles (1909); Webster (1910); Kittredge (1933)
As bedding	Goldberger and Schamberg (1909); Rawles (1909); Webster (1910); Kennedy (1924)
As packing	Webster (1910); Dorado and Vidal (1946)
Broom straw	Glass (1948)
Dried grass	Katzenellenbogen (1947)
"Hay"	Swan (1934a, b); Rogers (1943)
Bullrush flowers	Hung-Chiung and Sung-Nien (1958)
Tobacco	Mandoul et al. (1950)
Wooden house frames	Arnold and Haramoto (1962); Fine and Scott (1963, 1965)
Wicker furniture	Sampaio (1951)
Cherrywood	Hewitt et al. (1976)
Wood	Hickin (1969)

latter mite have been associated with wood-boring insects (Sampaio 1951; Fine and Scott 1963, 1965; Hickin 1969; Hewitt et al. 1976). These outbreaks were all of a sporadic nature involving relatively few persons. The epidemics involving *P. tritici*, however, often affected very large numbers and tended to occur in similar circumstances, that is to say by contact with heavily infested material. A list of the various sources of *Pyemotes* is given in Table 18.1. Contact can occur in a variety of ways. Lying on straw mattresses or loose straw bedding results in the back being chiefly involved. Handling straw used for packing causes the hands to be affected and sometimes the forearms. Carrying sacks of grain or seed exposes the forearms, neck and shoulders initially. Shovelling or sifting bulk grain in the holds of ships means working in an enclosed, very dusty atmosphere, which results in severe widespread biting and sometimes scarlatiniform eruptions. Stacking hay or unthreshed grain and the actual threshing of grain also involves working in a contaminated environment, often out of doors. Exposed areas are more liable to attack in these circumstances. In shops and storerooms contact may be close or casual, as with mere passers-by (Hung-Chiung and Sung-Nien 1958; Micks 1963; Aoki and Hasegava 1966). On at least one occasion infestation has been windborne to neighbouring houses (Askins 1924). Domestic animals can also be attacked simultaneously (Rawles 1909; Webster 1910; Davis 1950; Fine and Scott 1963). Schamberg (1910) recorded that a Dr. Collard in Algeria reported in 1887 that he developed *Pyemotes* infestation on entering a barley store to get grain for his mule. The mule developed asthma!

Apart from casual contact and contact associated with sleeping on infested straw, *Pyemotes* infestation has a definite bias towards workers in certain occupations, such as farm workers, flour mill workers, dock workers, warehousemen, cereal food processors, packers using infested straw and shopkeepers in certain circumstances. In all these occupations, and also in the manufacture of straw mattresses (if there is still such an industry), such infestation constitutes an industrial hazard. In the past workers have refused to continue under such conditions or have asked for much higher wages (Willcocks 1914), thus adding a further economic factor to the problem.

In farming communities, in particular, *Pyemotes* infestation tends to have a seasonal incidence. The factors determining this include such activities as threshing, harvesting or storing grain and straw and the weather, which may determine the ambient temperature and thus influence the behaviour of the mite and its insect host. The behaviour of the latter is probably the more important factor and is very influenced by the environmental temperature. Circumstances which are suitable for the metamorphosis of the insect are, at the same time, responsible for depriving the mite of its food source, and it is then liable to attack man and other animals.

Morphology of *Pyemotes*

Pyemotes is classified as belonging to the Pyemotidae, superfamily Tarsonemini, suborder Prostigmata. The mites are small, the male measuring 160 μm in length and the female 223 μm (see Figs. 18.1, 18.2). There are traces of segmentation laterally on the hysterosome. Tarsus I terminates in a single claw in both sexes, as does tarsus IV in the male. Between legs I and II near the lateral border on each side of the dorsal surface of the female arise the pseudostigmatic organs, which are characteristically stalked with a globular head. The hysterosome is twice as long as the propodosome, the whole mite having a rather slender appearance. The genital opening lies at the posterior extremity. The gnathosome is rounded, the chelicerae are stylet shaped and, according to Swan (1934a) are fused to form a tube. The segments of the pedipalps are indistinguishable from one another. This description is based on that given by Hughes (1961), who noted that tarsi II–IV in the female have bifid claws arising from a slender pretarsus, which is then expanded into a bilobed pulvillus. Legs I–III in the male are similar to those of the female just described, but legs IV have an elongated bent femur. The tarsus is short and terminates in a massive claw. The gravid female is described below.

Biology

Pyemotes is a parasite of the larval and nymphal stages of certain insects such as wheat stem worms, various seed weevils, wood-boring beetles etc. With the help of an entomologist and knowledge of the circumstances of the outbreak the host insects can be identified. All these insects deposit their eggs inside the stems or seeds of the plants on which they are parasitic. When the larval stages are reached they become the target of young female *Pyemotes* mites; these pierce the larval integument and undergo their development on the surface of the host body, consuming the contents of the latter as food. The process is achieved by means of external diastase enzymes injected into the host.

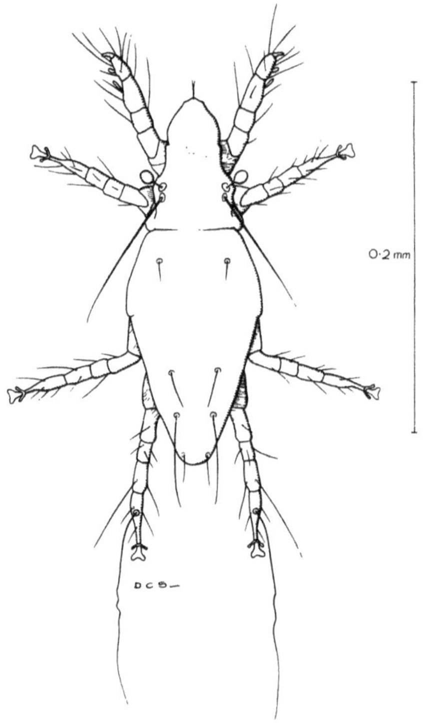

Fig. 18.1. *Pyemotes* species, adult female, dorsal view. Note the single claw on tarsus I and bifid claws with expanded pulvillus on tarsi II–IV. The pseudostigmatic organ can be seen between the bases of legs I and II. (From Swan 1934a, by courtesy of Prof. T. O. Browning, Waite Agricultural Research Institute, University of Adelaide, and by kind permission of the Editor of the *Journal of Agriculture and Industry of South Australia*)

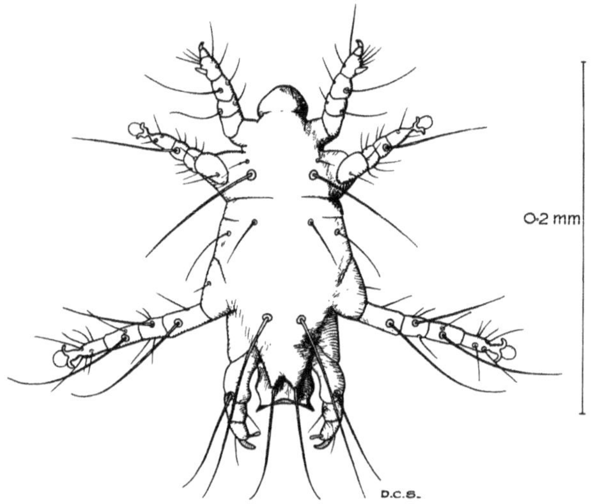

Fig. 18.2. *Pyemotes* species, adult male, dorsal view. Legs I–III are similar to those of the female (see Fig. 18.1). Leg IV has a short bent femur and the tarsus ends in a single stout claw. The male has no pseudostigmatic organ. (From Swan 1934a, by courtesy of Prof. T. O. Browning, Waite Agricultural Research Institute, University of Adelaide, and by kind permission of the Editor of the *Journal of Agriculture and Industry of South Australia*)

The liquefied body material is sucked into the mite through a modified tube made of the mouthparts (Voukassovitch and Dojmi 1937). During feeding the mite remains attached to the host, although in the early stages it may move to another site. As it feeds, the hysterosome swells until after 6 or 7 days—under the most favourable environmental conditions, including a temperature of 32°C (90°F)—it assumes a globular shape about 2 mm across (Fig. 18.3), the rest of the body appearing like an appendage of the gravid section. At this stage it is incapable of moving. Macroscopically the engorged females look like tiny vesicles on the surface of the host. Very occasionally they may cluster together in a mass appearing like a minute bunch of grapes. Inside the gravid female the developing mite hatches to a larva, then moults to a nymph and finally reaches the mature adult stage. This may take upwards of 6 days depending on environmental temperature. The mature adults emerge, the few males (less than 4% of the total) appearing first; they cluster around the genital opening, serving as midwives for the young females, which they at once fertilise (Voukassovitch and Dojmi 1937). The males remain on the mother and feed off its shrunken body, whilst the newly fertilised females either commence feeding on the host or may spend from a few hours to a few days migrating. The total number of young produced by an individual female varies between 300 under the best conditions and about 50 with a temperature below 20°C. The period of birth is also temperature dependent, varying from 2 to 40 days, and may even be halted altogether if the temperature is too low, possibly for the whole winter (Voukassovitch and Dojmi 1937). This form of diapause is biologically advantageous to the species in that it gives a longer period of birth to the young, some of which are born after the host has been able to renew itself, thus ensuring the young mites' food supply. In rare instances Voukassovitch and his colleague have observed that the young gravid females feed and multiply on the parent's body. Parthenogenetic reproduction sometimes occurs

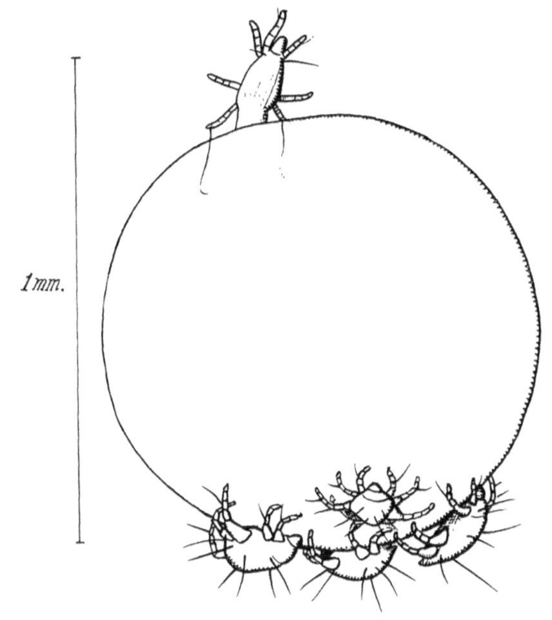

Fig. 18.3. *Pyemotes* species, gravid female, showing the enormously distended abdominal segment, with the rest of the mite appearing almost as an appendage. Four recently born males are clustered around the genital opening awaiting the birth of the females. (From Swan 1934a, by courtesy of Prof. T. O. Browning, Waite Agricultural Research Institute, University of Adelaide, and by kind permission of the Editor of the *Journal of Agriculture and Industry of South Australia*)

but all progeny are male (Newport 1853; Voukassovitch and Dojmi 1937). Unfed females can only survive for 24 h if the temperature is high and humidity low, but at lower temperatures the survival time is considerably longer (Swan 1934a). Lagrèze–Fossat and Montané were able to examine live mites up to 3 weeks after collecting them. If the mites happen to be born at a time when the host larva pupates or emerges as an adult, their source of food is removed. They then seek other sources and will attack man or other animals.

The digestive secretions of the various species of *Pyemotes* are more or less equally toxic to their insect hosts, but that of *P. tritici* is much more injurious to man than is that of *P. ventricosus* (Moser 1975). Jurukoff (1937) considered that the individual human reaction was uniform against the *Pyemotes*, but Voukassof and Dojmi (1937) maintained that there was great variety in response.

Control of *Pyemotes*

Since control of *Pyemotes* involves control of the host insects, the appropriate entomological advice should always be sought. As an example of the importance of knowledge of the host and its biology the following information from Webster (1908) and Webster and Reeves (1909) is worth studying.

The adult joint worm fly (*Harmolita tritici* Feld) deposits its eggs in the stem of the young growing wheat near the joints. The emergent larva feeds on the succulent stem cells, reaching maximum growth as the stem hardens. It overwinters in the hard stem either in stubble or in stored straw, emerging in adult form the following spring. It damages the wheat in a variety of ways, reducing the grain yield and rendering the straw useless for many purposes. The infested stubble or straw can introduce the pest into the next year's crop. Control measures include sowing early-ripening varieties and encouraging rapid growth with fertilisers, rotation of crops so that wheat is not grown on an infested area in successive years, burning of stubble in situ or raking it out and burning it, using infested straw as stable bedding and storing the sodden manure over the winter (which is fatal to the larvae) for spring use, never using such manure in the autumn of the year in which it was harvested and, finally, cutting the stubble as short as possible.

The wheat straw worm (*Harmolita* (*isosoma*) *grandis* Riley) produces two generations annually. The first, emerging in April, is wingless, with a travel capacity limited to about 3.5 m. Eggs are laid in emerging wheat seedlings just below the embryo head, which is eaten out by the developing larva. The adult of the second generation emerges in May, is winged and lays eggs in May and June in the stems of the most vigorously growing young wheat shoots left by the first generation. Whether the resulting larva remains in the stubble or is harvested with the grain depends on the growth stage reached when the eggs are laid. The effect is an overall reduction of grain yield (over 20%) of the wheat harvested. The parasite overwinters as a pupa in stubble or straw. The only effective measures are those of prevention of the breeding of the insect, which include crop rotation, clean early summer fallowing and the abandonment of spring culture. The burning of stubble and ploughing it in is ineffective, since the infested straw is damp and unaffected by these measures.

Management of Outbreaks

Treatment of Infested Persons

After removal from the source of infestation, with hospitalisation if necessary, the disease is self limiting. Symptomatic treatment preceded by a warm soapy bath is all that is required (Schamberg 1910)—a view that is in keeping with the original observation of Lagrèze-Fossat and Montané (1851) that a simple bath was effective. Topical application of simple antipruritics such as oily calamine lotion, crotamiton cream or weak corticosteroid/antibiotic creams together with oral antihistamines should be adequate to relieve itch. Oral antibiotics may be required for secondary infection and in rare instances of great severity a short course of oral corticosteroid therapy can be justified.

Prophylaxis for Workers

Lagrèze-Fossat and Montané (1851) suggested that smearing the skin all over with olive oil, in which the mites become helpless, would be effective in preventing lesions. The addition of miticidal substances such as sulphur or gamma-benzene hexachloride (in ointment) could improve this effect if used before work (Booth and Jones 1952). Hung-Chiung and Sung-Nien (1958) thought that sulphur-impregnated clothing, as suggested by Ewing (1921) as prophylaxis against chiggers, would be effective. It is probably better to change into such impregnated clothing at work when conditions indicate infestation and to change back again after work. This measure could be combined with protective ointments or oils.

Preventive Treatment Directed Against Host Insects

Measures in regard to such host insects have been discussed above. Appropriate action against other hosts should be taken after entomological advice. Disinfestation of grain not sufficiently damaged as to require destruction should be carried out using techniques designed to avoid rendering it toxic. Fumigation with methyl bromide might be suitable in some instances because it leaves no residue. Heat applied at 48.8°C for 1 hour was advised as adequate by Hung-Chiung and Sung-Nien (1958), who also recommend Swan's (1934b) technique of exposure to strong sunlight for several hours. This technique is particularly applicable to hay.

Disinfestation of Premises

Granaries, storehouses, shops, warehouses and ships' holds should be emptied and cleaned of all dust (which contains the majority of the mites in such premises). They should be fumigated with some substance which leaves behind a temporary residue that is toxic to insects and mites. Hung-Chiung and Sung-Nien (1958) advised 10% piperonyl butoxide and 1% pyretheum. Gamma-benzene hexachloride would also be effective, provided that the premises were adequately ventilated subsequently.

References

Ancona G (1923) Asma epidemico da *Pediculoides ventricosus.* Policlinico 30: 45–70

Aoki J, Hasegawa K (1966) On an epidemic of grain itch in barley storehouses in the central part of Japan and the mite concerned (in Japanese with English summary). Jpn J Sanit Zool 17: 29–36

Arnold HL, Haromoto FH (1962) Grain itch following fumigation for termites. Dermatol Trop 1: 37–39

Askins RA (1924) Dermatitis caused by *Pediculoides ventricosus.* Br Med J II: 950

*Booth BH, Jones RW (1952) Epidemiological and clinical study of grain itch. JAMA 150: 1575–1579

Davis JJ (1950) The 1950 epidemic of the straw itch mite. Proc Indiana Acad Sci 60: 183–184

Dorada FG, Vidal JMC (1946) Parasitismo cutaneo por el *Pediculoides ventricosus.* Rev Iber Parasitol 6: 293–308

Doucas CA (1942) Eine grosse Epidemie in Athens, hervorgerufen durch *Pediculoides ventricosus.* Dermatol Wochenschr 114: 46–49

Ewing HE (1921) Studies on the biology and control of chiggers. US Dept of Agriculture, Bureau of Entomology Bulletin No 986. US Govt Printing Office, Washington DC, pp 1–9

Fine RM, Scott HG (1963) Straw itch mite dermatitis caused by *Pyemotes ventricosus.* J Med Assoc Ga 52: 162–166

*Fine RM, Scott HG (1963) Straw itch mite dermatitis caused by *Pyemotes ventricosus*; comparative aspects. South Med J 58: 416–420

Flemming J (1884) Ueber eine geschlechtsreife Form als *Tarsonemus* beschreibenen Tiere. Z Gesamte Naturwiss Halle 57: 472. Cited by Schamberg (1910)

Glass FA (1948) Grain itch. A report of the first outbreak in the city of Baltimore. Ind Med 17: 95–96

Goldberger J, Schamberg JF (1909) Epidemic of an urticarioid dermatitis due to a small mite (*Pediculoides ventricosus*) in the straw of a mattress. Public Health Rep 24: 973–975

Gros H (1908) Sur un acarien parasite des teignes des céréales et cause accidentale d'éruption cutanée chez l'homme. Bull Soc Pathol Exot 1: 249–251

Grove EF (1926) Studies in specific hypersensitiveness. XXVI On asthma and dermatitis due to hypersensitivity to *Pediculoides ventricosus.* J Immunol 12: 263–271

Hewitt M, Barrow GI, Miller DC, Turk SM (1976) A case of *Pyemotes* dermatitis with a note on the role of these mites in skin diseases. Br J Dermatol 94: 423–430

Hickin NE (1969) The woodworm. Sci J 3: 64–70

Hone FS (1922) A series of cases closely resembling typhus fever. Med J Aust 1: 1–13

Hudelo, Dumet (1924) Dermatose par piqûres de *Pediculoides ventricosus* chez des ouvriers grainetiers. Bull Soc Fr Dermatol Syphiligr 31: 405–407

Hughes AM (1961) The mites of stored food. Tech Bull No 9 Ministry of Agriculture, Fisheries and Food. HMSO, London

*Hung-Chiung L, Sung-Nien T (1958) An outbreak of acarodermatitis urticarioides among workers in a department store. Chin Med J 76: 135–143

Jurukoff R (1937) Massenhafte Erkrankungen beim Menschen hervorgerufen durch *Pediculoides ventricosus*. Arch Schiffs Trop Hyg 41: 337–341

Katzenellenbogen I (1947) Acarodermatitis urticarioides. Arch Dermatol Syphilol 55: 621–629

Kennedy JD (1924) Acarodermatitis urticarioides (grain itch) in Turkey. J R Army Med Corps 43: 45–47

Kittredge HE (1933) Grain itch—report of two cases occurring in a small epidemic. Va Med Monthly 60: 357–360

Koller G (1882) Eine Getreide-Milbe als Krankheitserregerin. Pester Med Chir Presse 36: 127. Analysed in Biol Zentralbl (1884) 3: 127. Cited by Schamberg (1910)

Krczal H (1959) *Pyemotes boylei*, eine neue Pyemotid aus Hawaii. Zool Anzeiger (Berlin) 163: 148–152

*Lagrèze-Fossat A, Montané RJ (1851) Observation microscopique sur la mite du blé. Rec Agronom Soc Sci Agric Belles Lett Tarn-et-Garonne 32: 37–66

Larson AO (1920) A predaceous enemy of bean weevils. J Econ Entomol 13: 322–323

Llambias J, Lorenzo D (1920) Dermatose causée par un parasite du blé. CR Soc Biol (Paris) 83: 1528

Loir, Legangneux (1919) Maladie cutanée provoquée par un pédiculoide trouvé dans un changement d'orge arrivant au Havre. Bull Acad Med Paris 82: 308–310

Mandoul R, Lepigre AL, Jacqueman (1950) À propos d'une nouvelle manifestation en Algérie de la gale des céréales à *Pediculoides ventricosus* Newport. Alg Med 6: 433–436

Mariani G (1952) Due episodi d'infestasione da *Pediculoides ventricosus* nel Bresciano. Rev Ital Igiene 12: 76–79

Micks DW (1963) An outbreak of dermatitis due to the grain itch mite, *Pyemotes ventricosus* Newport. Tex Rep Biol Med 26: 221–226

*Moser JC (1975) Biosystematics of the straw itch mite with special reference to nomenclature and dermatology. Trans R Entomol Soc Lond 127: 185–191

*Newport G (1853) Further observations on the habits of *Monodontomerus*; with some account of a new acarus (*Heteropus ventricosus*), a parasite in the nests of *Anthophora retusa*. Trans Linnaean Soc Lond 21: 95–102

Nixon JA (1915) Cotton seed dermatitis and its cause, *Pediculoides ventricosus*. Bristol Med Chirurg J 33: 73–81

O'Connor FW (1920) An outbreak of itch due to a predaceous mite, occurring in England amongst men engaged in unloading cotton seed from Egypt. Trans R Soc Trop Med 13: 10–13

Oudemans AC (1937) Oven de Veelhard der sorten van Pediculoiden. Tijdschr Entomol 80: 4

Pantaleoni P (1920) Vasta epidemia di acariasi da grano in Romagna. *Policlinico* 27: 1275

Pascal (1900) Erytheme scarlatiniforme desquamitif generalisé d'origine parasitaire. Ann Dermatol Syphiligr (Paris) 1: 947–957

*Philippson L (1914) Attorna alla dermatosi pruriginosa prodotta dall' acaro delle fave secche comparsa in forma epidemica a Palermo. Rev Sanit Siciliana 2 (18): 5–7

Rawles LT (1909) Dermatitis *Ditropenotus aureoviridis*; synonym straw itch. J Indiana State Med Assoc 2: 337–340

Rogers GK (1943) Grain itch. JAMA 123: 887–889

Sampaio M (1951) Un caso curioso de bioleoja do *Ped. ventr.* Trab Soc Port Dermatol Venereol 9: 19–22

*Schamberg JF (1910) Grain itch. J Cutan Genitourin Dis Syphil 28: 67–89

Sergent E, Alary A (1916) Petite épidémie d'acariose en Algérie. Bull Soc Pathol Exot 9: 771–773

*Swan DC (1934a) The hay itch mite, *Pediculoides ventricosus* (Newport) (Acarina: Pediculoididae) in South Australia. J Agric Ind S Aust 37: 1289–1299

Swan DC (1934b) Dermatitis caused by a mite (*Pediculoides ventricosus*) and its occurrence in Australia. Med J Aust 2: 573–577

Thompson AGG (1925) Barley itch. Br Med J 1: 71

*Voukassovitch P, Dojmi L (1937) Contribution a l'étude biologique de *Pediculoides ventricosus*. CR Soc Biol (Paris) 126: 549–552

Webster FM (1908) The joint-worm (*Isosoma tritici* Fitch). US Dept of Agriculture Circular No 66, Dec 28. US Govt Printing Office, Washington DC, pp 1–7

Webster FM (1910) A predaceous mite proves noxious to men. US Dept of Agriculture, Bureau of Entomology Circular No 118, April. US Govt Printing Office, Washington DC, pp 1–24

Webster FM, Reeves GI (1909) The wheat straw worm. US Dept of Agriculture Circular No 106, Dec 28. US Govt Printing Office, Washington DC, pp 1–15

Willcocks FC (1914) The predaceous mite, *Pediculoides ventricosus*, Newport. Agric J Egypt 4: 31–51

Wills WK (1909) Barley itch. Br J Dermatol 21: 249–252

19 Infestation with Cheyletiellid Mites

Parasite infestation of domestic pets is becoming increasingly recognised as a source of human skin disease. Cheyletiellid mites are the commonest such parasites at present. They were first reported as attacking man by Lomholt (1918) in Copenhagen on the owners of infested cats. It has since been established that dogs, cats and rabbits are the principal hosts of the mites of the genus *Cheyletiella*, three of which are pathogenic to man. A knowledge of their morphology and their relationship to their natural hosts is valuable because accurate diagnosis and management of the human eruption is nearly always dependent on finding the parasite on the patients' pets.

Clinical Features

Patients usually present because of a severely itching, excoriated eruption, with a history of intermittent exacerbation. Other persons in the household may be affected. Occasionally a pet animal may be incriminated as the cause. The itch may be aggravated by warmth or be especially noticeable after contact with the offending animal (Fox and Reed 1978). In the absence of new lesions the itch subsides in a few days. The lesions often occur in the circumscribed areas and tend to be grouped three or four together (Davies 1938; Fig. 19.1), but discrete, isolated lesions may also occur (Davies 1938; Pirila and Muroma 1957; Fox and Reed 1978). Davies' patient showed red, acuminate, oedematous papules. Muller and Kirk (1976) stated that the lesions went through a progression of changes from papule to vesicle to pustule to crust with some central necrosis in the pustule (Fig. 19.2). Although vesicles are not always present, other workers have also noted necrotic changes (Walton 1970; Bagnall and Rook 1977; Cohen 1980; Fox and Reed 1978). The lesions are usually bright red but may be paler. (Fernstrom and Gentele 1960) and may persist as a firm, pale, waxy papule (Van Bronswijk, et al. 1972). In this respect it is interesting that in unsensitised individuals exposed experimentally to cheyletiellid mites Bjarke et al. (1973) observed that evanescent papules fading within a few hours appeared at first; however, with repeated exposures to bites, sensitisation occurred and the papu-

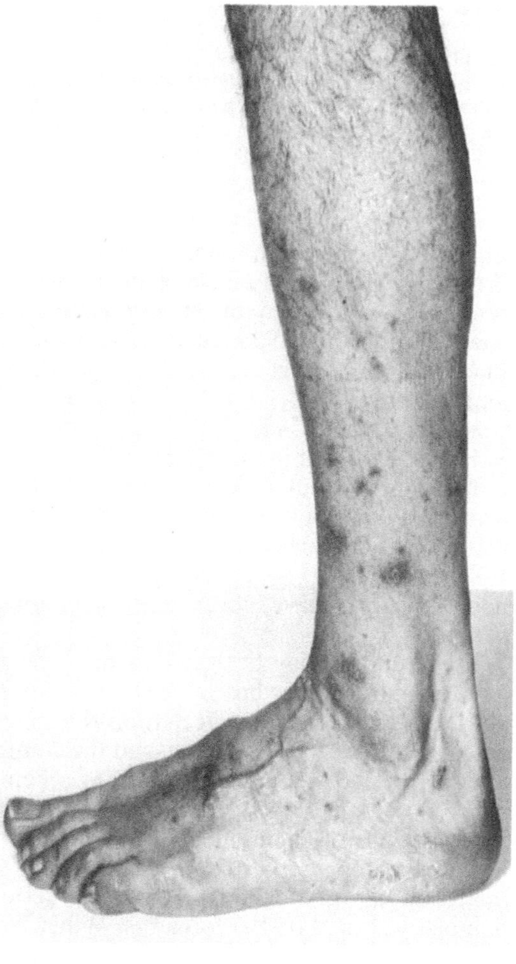

Fig. 19.1. Papulopustular eruption produced by *Cheyletiella yasguri*. (Courtesy of Prof. R. M. MacKie, University of Glasgow)

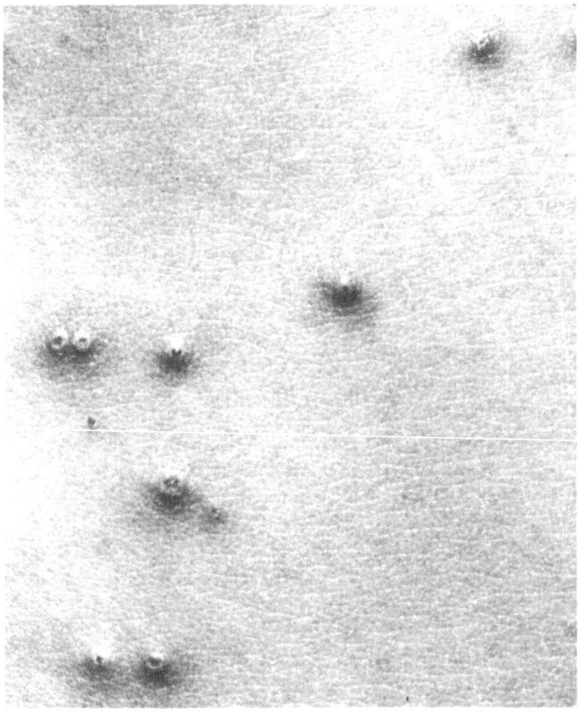

Fig. 19.2. *Cheyletiella* dermatitis. Crop of older vesiculopustular lesions on the lower anterior abdominal wall. Note the central vesicle, which tends to become necrotic. [From Bjarke et al. 1973, by kind permission of the author and the Editor of *Acta Dermato-venerealogica* (*Stockholm*)]

lar lesions then became more persistent. Lesions vary in size from 1 to 5 mm in diameter, which may be increased to 1 cm by an erythematous halo (Hart and Malone 1958; Bakkers and Fain 1972; Van Bronswijk et al. 1972). There is no visible central punctum (Bagnall and Rook 1977), although Cohen (1980) held that a tiny central eschar was present in all lesions. Thomsett (1968) stated that vesicular sensitisation could occur, whilst residual pigmentation was noted by Fernstrom and Gentele (1960) and by Bakkers and Fain (1972). All patients scratch, producing excoriations. Burrows have never been seen on these patients.

The eruption may be localised or widespread. Localisation depends on circumstances, for example Davies' patient was affected on the inner and anterior surfaces of the left arm and the contiguous area of the left side of the chest, these being the areas of contact with her cat when she carried it. Likewise, one of Thomsett's (1968) patients nursed her infested dog on her lap and developed lesions on the front of each thigh, on the anterior abdominal wall and on the forearms. Whilst Walton (1970) felt that exposed skin was most liable to attack, it is commonly the case that lesions quickly become widespread and involve upper and lower limbs and the trunk, especially around the waistline. Thomsett (1968) enumerated the frequency with which various regions were involved in 43 patients (see Table 19.1). Mougeot and Poirot (1975) recorded a patient with pruritus ani caused by *Cheyletiella* species.

Table 19.1. The site of lesions in 50 persons infested with *Cheyletiella* species. (Based on Thomsett 1968)

Site	No. of persons
Torso	2
Legs	2
Neck, arms and torso	4
Arms, torso and legs	5
Neck, arms, torso and legs	6
Arms	7
Arms and torso	24

Histopathology

Van Bronswijk et al. (1972) described acanthosis which progressed to spongiosis and vesicle formation with oedema of the subjacent upper dermis, accompanied by a chronic perivascular inflammatory infiltrate which included some eosinophils. Such a picture is non-specific and much less marked than that described in the dog by Schaffer et al. (1958), where many mites were found embedded in hyperkeratotic stratum corneum, the adjacent epidermis showing dyskeratosis, parakeratosis and vacuolation of malphighian cells, with the underlying dermis having a diffuse, intense pleomorphic cellular infiltrate containing mast cells, macrophages, neutrophils and a few eosinophils.

Diagnosis

The diagnosis depends upon

1. Suspicion of an ectoparasitic cause by virtue of the history and clinical appearance.
2. The intermittent nature of the eruption corresponding to periods of contact with a suspected source of infestation (Fernstrom and Gentele 1960; Brandrup et al. 1979).
3. The finding of the parasite on the suspected animal. This finding, combined with the disappearance of the lesions in the human *only* after appropriate treatment of the infested animal, provides proof of the diagnosis.

It is very unusual to find *Cheyletiella* on human patients, although it has been recorded (Fernstrom and Gentele 1960; Bakkers and Fain 1972). There are two possible useful techniques in this respect:

1. Examination of Sellotape strippings of the skin in the area of the bites as soon as possible after contact with the infested animal (Bagnall and Rook 1977 advise this for the animals).
2. Vigorous shaking of the victim's clothing inside a polythene bag (Hewitt et al. 1973) and examination of the collected dust microscopically. It is possible that mites could be found in this way, as both Thomsett (1968) and Walton (1970) stated that the mites could easily penetrate clothing.

Finding parasites on rabbits, cats or dogs may not always be easy. Obvious lesions should be gently scraped with a scalpel blade and the scales, crusts and other debris collected and examined on black filter paper by means of a dissecting microscope. Living and dead mites, which can easily be seen in this way, can be picked off and mounted in 30% potassium hydroxide or 80% lactic acid solutions and identified with ordinary microscope at 100 magnifications. Visualisation of the specific sensory organs on genu I will require 400 magnifications. In the absence of obvious lesions, the animal should be stood on a large sheet of paper or polythene and thoroughly groomed, the resultant dust being examined as for human clothing dust. Brushings or dust collected with a special vacuum collector (Sesay and Dobson 1972; Fig. 19.3) from the animal's bedding, the floor, carpets, upholstery and owner's bedding should be similarly examined. If abundant the excess gritty debris can be separated by the flotation technique recommended by Hewitt et al. (1973), leaving the mites in the supernatant.

The differential diagnosis is the same as for infestation with gamasid mites (see p. 305).

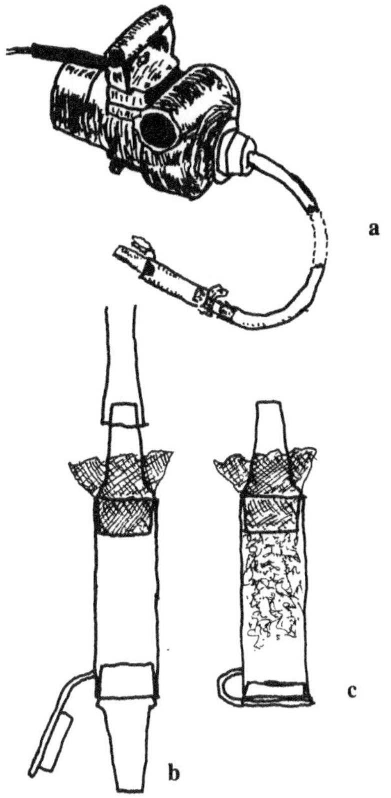

Fig. 19.3a-c. Apparatus for collecting dust samples for examination for mites. Originally designed for house dust samples but equally applicable to sample collection from dogs, cats, etc. for *Cheyletiella*. **a** Complete apparatus with suction and sampling units; **b** sampling unit as when taking samples; **c** sampling unit containing sample and sealed for storage. (After Sesay and Dobson 1972, by kind permission of Dr. R. M. Dobson and the Editor of *Acarologia*)

Morphology of *Cheyletiella*

Cheyletiella mites belong to the family Cheyletiellidae (Prostigmata). Like the related Cheyletidae they have short piercing chelicerae and stout pincer-like palpi tipped with strong tibial claws. In the Cheyletidae these serve the purpose of grasping prey, but in the Cheyletiellidae they are curved ventrally for grasping fur and feather (see Fig. 3.4a, p. 13). The elaborate comb-like setae on the palpal tarsi of Cheyletidae (see Fig. 3.4b) are replaced by simple setae in Cheyletiellidae. Most of the latter have claws on each tarsal pulvillus, but *Cheyletiella* is one of two genera in which these are replaced by a rayed or feathered structure (Fig. 19.4); Hirst 1917; Smiley 1970). For full details consult Smiley (1970).

Three species of *Cheyletiella*—*C. parasitovorax* (Megnin 1878), *C. yasguri* (Smiley 1965) and *C. blakei* (Smiley 1965)—are known to produce skin lesions in man and are differentiated from one another by the shape of the special sensory organ on the dorsal surface of genu I (Fig. 19.5). Foxx and Ewing (1969), on the basis of an average of 25 specimens at each stage, gave the dimensions of *C. yasguri* as follows: adult female 502 μm by 318 μm; male 349 μm by 223 μm; first nymph 267 μm by 208 μm; second nymph 416 μm by 293 μm; larva 229 μm by 180 μm. The other species have approximately the same dimensions and all are therefore rather small mites, about the size of *Sarcoptes scabiei* (Figs. 19.6, 19.7).

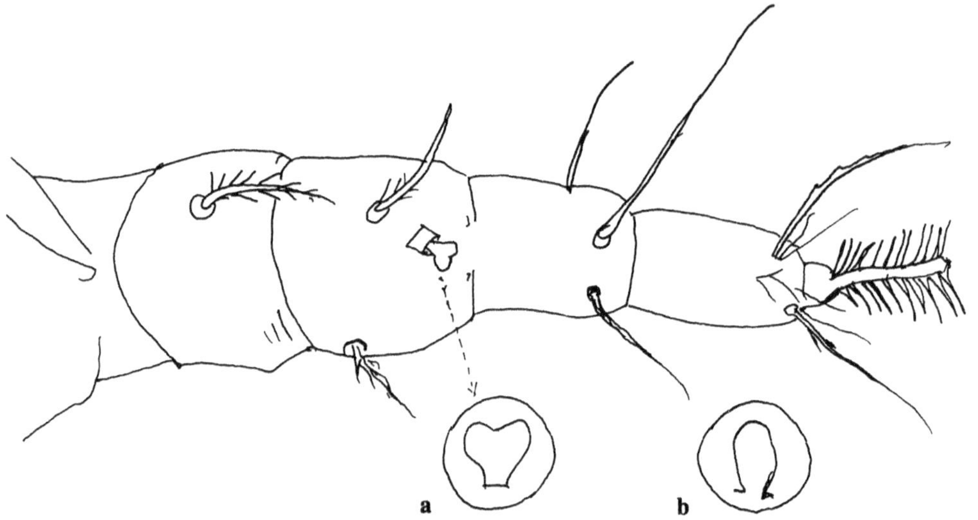

Fig. 19.4. *Cheyletiella yasguri*. Female leg I showing the sensory organ on the genu. **a** and **b** illustrate the difference between the sensory organs of *C. yasguri* and *C. parasitovorax*. Note also the rayed empodium on the pulvillus. [After Hewitt M and Turk SM (1974) *Cheyletiella* sp. in the personal environment. Br J Dermatol 90:679–683, by kind permission of Dr. M. Hewitt and the Editor of the *British Journal of Dermatology*]

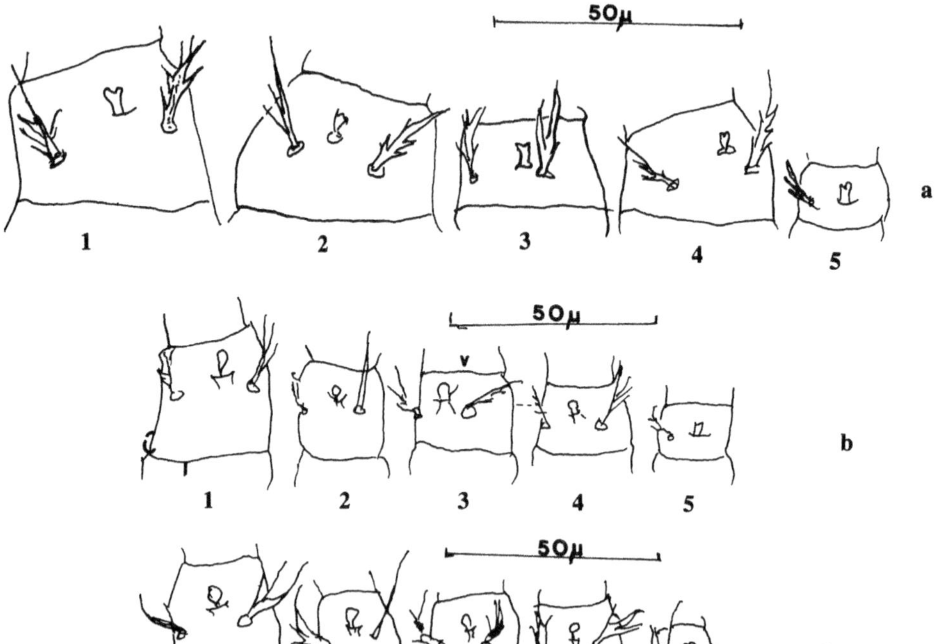

Fig. 19.5. Showing the special sensory organ on genu I in **a** *Cheyletiella yasguri*, **b** *C. blakei* and **c** *C. parasitovorax*, in the various stages of development. Van Bronswijk and De Kreek (1976) have pointed out that it is advisable to examine several adult specimens to be certain of the form of the sensory organ. Its shape in immature forms is an unreliable guide. [After Van Bronswijk JEMH and De Kreek EJ (1976) *Cheyletiella* (Acari: Cheyletiellidae) of dog, cat and domesticated rabbit; a review. J Med Entomol 13: 315–327, by kind permission of the authors and the Editor of the *Journal of Medical Entomology*]

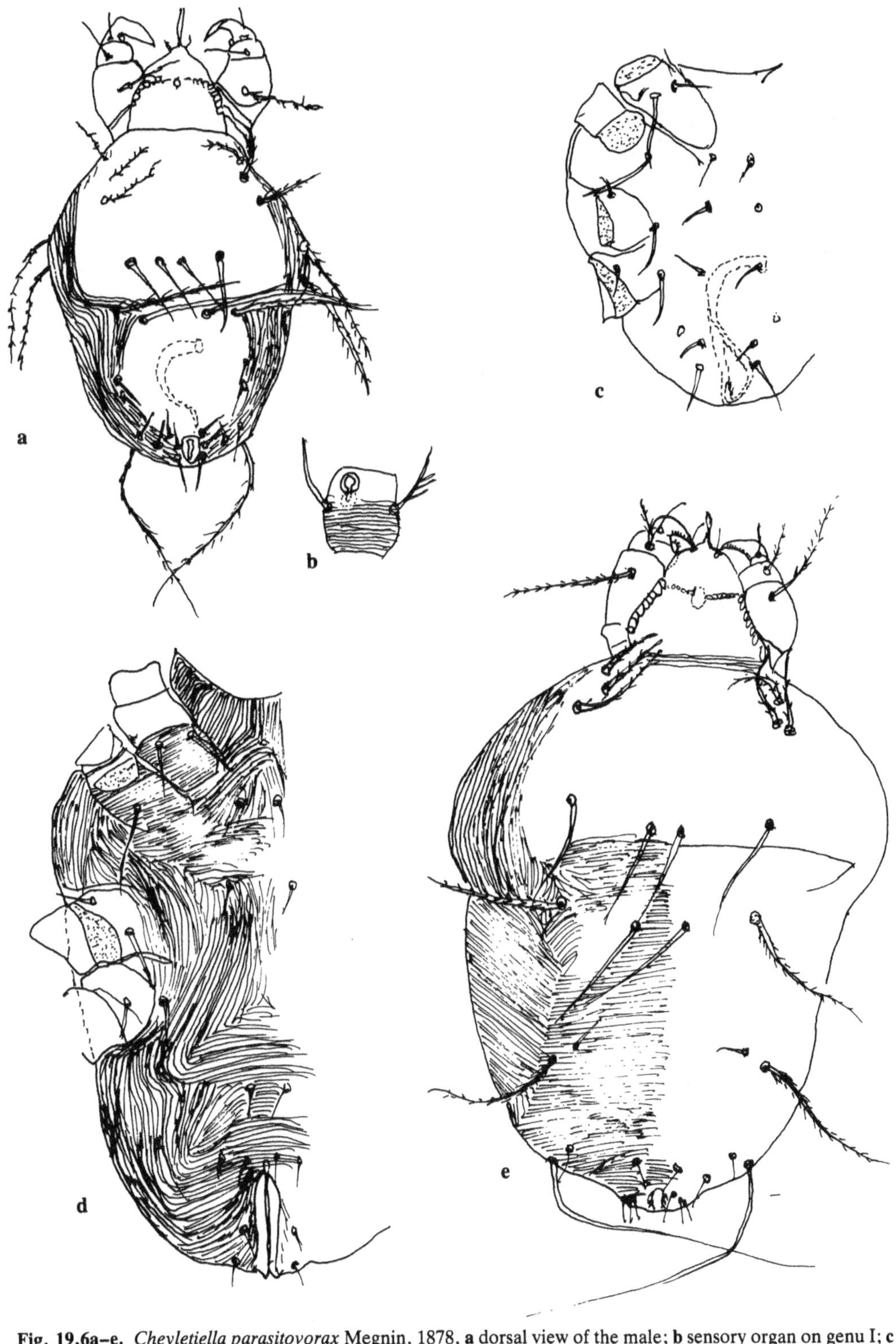

Fig. 19.6a–e. *Cheyletiella parasitovorax* Megnin, 1878, **a** dorsal view of the male; **b** sensory organ on genu I; **c** ventral view of male; **d** ventral view of female; **e** dorsal view of female. The distal portions of the limbs are omitted. Note the incurving claws of the pedipalps. (After Smiley 1970, by kind permission of the author and the Editor of the *Annals of the Entomological Society of America*)

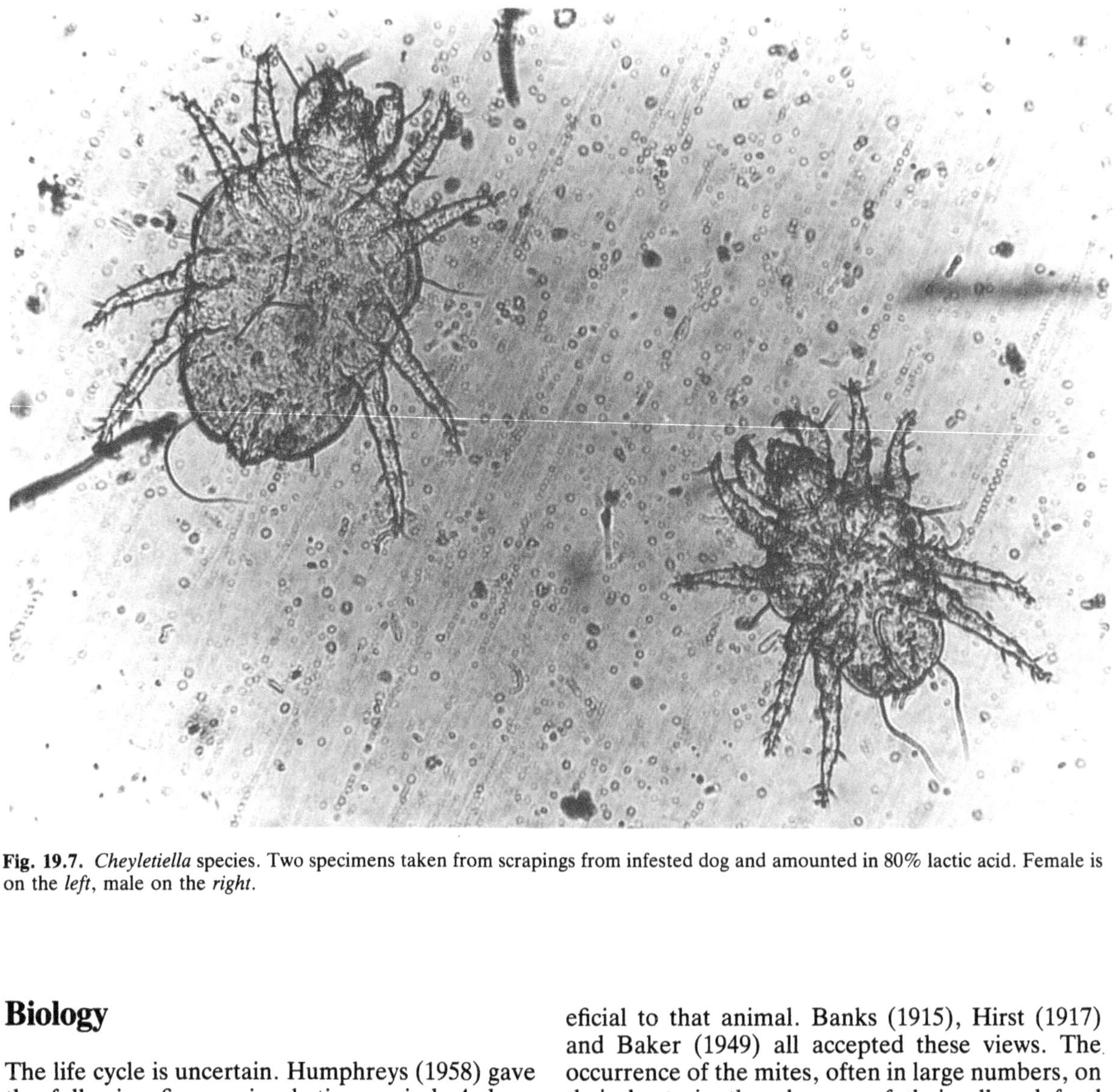

Fig. 19.7. *Cheyletiella* species. Two specimens taken from scrapings from infested dog and amounted in 80% lactic acid. Female is on the *left*, male on the *right*.

Biology

The life cycle is uncertain. Humphreys (1958) gave the following figures: incubation period, 4 days; larval stage, 7.5 days; first nymphal stage, 4.5 days; second nymphal stage, 5 days; adult stage, 13 days. These figures had no supporting evidence and remain unconfirmed. Foxx and Ewing (1969) were unable to rear these mites experimentally as the larva could survive for only 24 h and the adults for only 48 h away from their host animal. Under refrigerated conditions they found that adult females could survive for 10 days.

The role of *Cheyletiella* species on animals has been disputed (Megnin 1878). Kuscher (1940) and Cooper (1946) maintained that cheyletiellid mites were free-living predators feeding on various fur mites, whilst Rothschild (1969) has observed them feeding on rabbit fleas. Kuscher (1940) held that their preying on *Demodex* on the dog was beneficial to that animal. Banks (1915), Hirst (1917) and Baker (1949) all accepted these views. The occurrence of the mites, often in large numbers, on their hosts in the absence of their alleged food source was unexplained (Barr 1955). Foxx and Ewing (1969) could not induce *Cheyletiella* to attack fur mites but confirmed the observation of Mykytowycz (1957) that they feed on the host by engorging themselves with fluid from the latter's tissues. Along with Smiley's (1970) description of the palpal claws as being adapted for clasping hair, these findings support the opinion of Beesley (1963) and of Foxx and Ewing (1969) that *Cheyletiella* species pathogenic to man are obligatory parasites of their animal hosts.

Until Smiley's papers in 1965 and 1970 the pathogenic specimens were all thought to be *C. parasitovorax*. It is now accepted that most were in fact *C. yasguri*, with the proven exception of the cases recorded by Brockis (1971). This is also the present writer's experience. Gething and Walton (1972) considered that *C. parasitovorax* was parasitic on rabbits, *C. yasguri* on dogs and *C. blakei* on cats. They never found *C. yasguri* on rabbits and only on cats when there was also an infested dog on the premises.

Foxx and Ewing (1969) noted that the mites were usually found on the scapular area in rabbits and on the rump in dogs, and Cooper (1946) found they were most likely to be found between the scapulae in cats. Pillers (1925) noted that the whole length of the spinal region from scapulae to sacrum was involved in rabbits. The infestation of these three animals varied considerably. It was most intense and generalised in the younger animals. Foxx and Ewing (1969) observed that dogs between 2 and 8 weeks old suffered the most. Hundreds of mites could be removed after brushing off debris from the skin in this age group, whereas older dogs, whether associated with infested puppies or not, were usually only lightly infested, and only a few mites or eggs could be recovered as a rule. The reactions of the host to the mite varied. In many infested animals there were no obvious symptoms, the only evidence of the presence of mites being some slight scurfiness of the coat and perhaps a somewhat oily appearance. This might be accompanied by hyperaesthesia (Thomsett 1968). If the hair along the back was gently brushed "against the grain" with the hand, there was an acute scratch reaction on the part of the animal. In other instances there could be a much more severe reaction with circumscribed matting of the hair followed by some hair loss accompanied by erythema of the underlying skin. This could progress to acute weeping inflammation with total alopecia of the affected area, the whole becoming covered with a crust composed of a mixture of scales and dried serous exudate, teeming with mites.

Epidemiology

Cheyletiellid infestation involving man has a wide distribution. It has been recorded in many European countries as well as in the United States, Australia and New Zealand (Moxham et al. 1967; Taylor 1969; Dodd 1970; Rack 1971 and many others already mentioned).

It is closely associated with the handling of pet animals. Thomsett (1969) noted that its incidence was related to the way pets were kept. Infestation may arise in those who allow their pets to sleep in or on their beds (Olsen and Roth 1947; Hart and Malone 1958; Keh 1973). Children frequently carry their pets about and consequently the areas of contact are attacked (Davies 1938; Bjarke et al. 1973; Cohen 1980). Adults who sit with their pets on their lap easily become infested (Pirila and Muroma 1957; Thomsett 1968; Keh 1973). On the other hand, persons in an infested household who do not have such contact often escape attack. Persons of any age or either sex are liable to be affected. Ethnic limitations are probably closely related to the attitude of different races to pets. Apart from domestic infestation, the owners of boarding or breeding kennels are exposed to attack (Dodd 1970). Reed (1961) has noted that infestation in such kennels may be kept going by symptom-free adult dogs. Dogs which are exhibited at shows rarely have *Cheyletiella* mites on the skin or fur because of their repeated thorough grooming (Weitkamp 1964). Humphreys (1958) thought that his cases could have been infested by being exercised in an area where there were many rabbit victims from myxomatosis, for which *Cheyletiella* species are vectors (Mykytowykcz 1970).

Immunology

There is no specific information available concerning immunity in this condition. Children appear to react more severely than adults. Bagnall and Rook (1977) noted that the experimental lesions produced by Bjarke et al. (1973) were initially transitory and later more persistent. This change could represent a progression from an urticarial (immediate) response to a cellular (delayed) response.

With young dogs which are more prone to infestation the reaction may be very severe, whereas older animals show little or no evidence although harbouring large number of mites. This difference could represent immunity to attack.

Management

Human Patients

Topical application of simple antipruritic preparations such as oily calamine lotion or weak corticosteroid creams, either alone or in combination with antibacterial preparations (e.g. Vioform), is adequate. Oral antihistamines may help the itch. Simultaneous elimination of the source of the infestation is essential.

Animals

Acaricidal powders such as gamma-benzene hexachloride, pyrethrum, lime and sulphur (Walton 1970) or methylcarbamate (Fox and Hewes 1976) are usually successful. All infested animals should be treated simultaneously; if a large group of animals, such as the inmates of kennels, are involved, all should be treated irrespective of whether they are proved to have infestation or not (Walton 1970). Reed (1961) considered this to be important because the persistence of infestation in kennels was due to failure to treat infested animals which were symptom free and unsuspected. Yasgur (1968) advised removal of infested animals after treatment and thorough cleansing of the premises because he thought that persistence of infestation was due to mites surviving in a free-living state on the premises. This is as yet unsubstantiated and at variance with the opinion of Foxx and Ewing (1969) on the survival capacity of mites (see p. 332). Nevertheless, it is as well to disinfest premises and also pets' bedding etc., until stronger evidence is forthcoming. Preparations containing 0.5% chlordane or 4% malathion are suitable for this purpose. Yasgur has also suggested professional fumigation.

It seems to the present writer that failure to treat all animals on the premises is probably the reason for persistence of infestation, as Reed and Walton have said. It is also advisable to inspect all newcomers to kennels very carefully to exclude a new source of infestation.

References

Bagnall B, Rook A (1977) Arthropods and the skin. In: Rook A (ed) Recent advances in dermatology 4. Churchill, Edinburgh

Baker EW (1949) A review of mites of family Cheyletidae. Proc US Nat Museum 99: 267–320

Bakkers EJM, Fain A (1972) Dermatitis in man and in a dog caused by the mite *Cheyletiella yasguri* Smiley. Br J Dermatol 87: 245–247

Banks N (1915) The acarina or mites. US Dept of Agriculture, Bureau of Entomology Report No 108. US Govt Printing Office, Washington DC, pp 1–151

Barr AR (1955) A case of "mange" of the domestic rabbit due to *Cheyletiella parasitovorax* (Megnin). J Parasitol 41: 323

Beesley WN (1963) *Cheyletiella parasitovorax* (Acarina: Trombidioidae) as a parasitic mite in Britain. Parasitology 53: 651–652

*Bjarke T, Hellgren L, Orstadius K (1973) *Cheyletiella parasitovorax* dermatitis in man. Acta Derm Venereol (Stockh) 53: 217–224

Brandrup F, Andersen KE, Kristensen ST (1979) Infestation with the mite *Cheyletiella yasguri* Smiley in man and dog. Hautarzt 30: 497–500

Brockis DC (1971) Scurf in dogs. Vet Rec 89: 473

Cohen SR (1980) *Cheyletiella* dermatitis, a mite infestation of rabbit, cat, dog and man, Arch Dermatol 116: 435–437

Cooper KW (1946) The occurrence of the mite *Cheyletiella parasitovorax* (Megnin) in North America with notes on its synonymy and "parasitic" habit. 32: 480–482

Davies JHT (1938) Another acarine disease. Br J Dermatol 50: 243–244

Dodd K (1970) Skin lesions associated with *Cheyletiella yasguri* infestation. J Irish Med Assoc 63: 413–414

Fernstrom AJB, Gentele H (1960) Dermatitis caused by mites living on cats. Acta Paediatr Scand 49: 752–753

Fox JG, Hewes K (1976) *Cheyletiella* infestation in cats. J Am Vet Med Assoc 169: 332–333

Fox JG, Reed C (1978) *Cheyletiella* infestation of cats and their owners. Arch Dermatol 114: 1233–1234

*Foxx TS, Ewing SA (1969) Morphologic features, behaviour and life history of *Cheyletiella yasguri*. Am J Vet Res 30: 269–285

Gething MA, Walton GS (1972) Possible host specificity of *Cheyletiella* mites. Vet Rec 88: 512

Hart CB, Malone JC (1958) The occurrence of the rabbit fur mite *Cheyletiella parasitovorax* (Megnin 1878) on the dog. Vet Rec 70: 991–993

Hewitt M, Barrow GI, Miller DO, Turk F, Turk S (1973) Mites in the personal environment and their role in skin disorders. Br J Dermatol 89: 401–409

Hirst S (1917) On the occurrence of a pseudoparasitic mite (*Cheyletiella parasitovorax*, Megnin) on the domestic cat. Ann Mag Nat Hist 20: 132–133

Humphreys M (1958) *Cheyletiella parasitovorax* infestation of the dog. Vet Rec 70: 442

Keh B (1973) Dermatitis in man traced to dog infested with *Cheyletiella yasguri* Smiley (Acari: Cheyletiellidae) in California. Cal Vector Views 20: 77–79

Kuscher A (1940) Raumilben beim Hund (*Cheyletiella parasitovorax*). Wien Tierarzt Monatsschr 27: 10–16

Lomholt S (1918) To tilfaelde of dyrefuat hos mennesket (*Cheyletiella parasitovorax*). Hospitalstidende 61: 1098–1099

Megnin P (1878) Memoires sur les cheyletides parasites. J Anat Physiol (Paris) 14: 416–441

Mougeot G, Poirot JL (1975) Larves de *Cheyletiella* responsable d'un prurit anal tenace. Nouv Presse Med 4: 1509. Cited in Rev Appl Entomol (1976) 64: 2985

Moxham JW, Goldfinch TJ, Heath ACG (1967) *Cheyletiella parasitovorax* infestation of cats associated with skin lesions of man. NZ Vet J 16: 50–52

Muller GH, Kirk RW (1976) Small animal dermatology, 2nd edn. Saunders, Philadelphia, pp 375–380

Mykytowycz R (1957) Parasitic habit of the rabbit mite *Cheyletiella parasitovorax* (Megnin). CSIRO Wildlife Res 2: 164

Olsen SJ, Roth H (1947) On the mite *Cheyletiella parasitovorax* occurring on cats as a facultative parasite of man. J Parasitol 33: 444–445

Pillers AWN (1925) *Cheyletiella parasitovorax* Megnin, causing lesions in the domestic rabbit. Vet J 81: 96–97

Pirila V, Muroma A (1957) Dermatitis caused by mites (*Cheyletiella parasitovorax*) living on cats. Acta Derm Venereol (Stockh) 37: 376–381

Rack G (1971) *Cheyletiella yasguri* Smiley 1965 (Acarina: Cheyletiellidae) ein fakultative menschen pathogene Parasit des Hundes. Z Parasitenkr 36: 321–334

Reed CM (1961) Infestation of pups. J Am Vet Med Assoc 138: 306–307

Rothschild M (1969) *Cheyletiella parasitovorax* feeding upon the rabbit flea. Entomol Monthly Mag 105: 1262

Schaffer MH, Baker NF, Kennedy PC (1958) Parasitism by *Cheyletiella parasitovorax*, a case report on the infestation in a female dog and its litter. Cornell Vet 47: 440–447

Sesay HR, Dobson RM (1972) Studies on the mite fauna of house dust in Scotland with special reference to that of bedding. Acarologia 14: 384–392

Smiley RL (1965) Two new species of the genus *Cheyletiella* (Acarina: Cheyletidae). Proc Entomol Soc Washington 67: 75–79

*Smiley RL (1970) A review of the family Cheyletiellidae (Acarina) Ann Entomol Soc Am 63: 1056–1078

Taylor RM (1969) *Cheyletiella parasitovorax* infestation of a cat and associated skin lesions of man. Aust Vet J 45: 435

*Thomsett LR (1968) Mite infestations of man contracted from dogs and cats. Br Med J 3: 93–95

Van Bronswijk JEMH Jansen LH, Ophof AJ (1972) Invasion of a house by the dog parasite *Cheyletiella yasguri* (Smiley 1965), a mite causing prurigo in man. Dermatologica 145: 338–343

Walton GS (1970) *Cheyletiella* infestation of man and domestic animals. Vet Rec 87, Members Inf Suppl: 95–96

Weitkamp RA (1964) *Cheyletiella parasitovorax* parasitism in dog. J Am Vet Med Assoc 144: 597–599

Yasgur I (1968) *Cheyletiella dermatitis*. In: Kirk RW (ed) Current veterinary therapy, vol III. Saunders, Philadelphia, pp 266–267

20 House Dust Mites and Skin Disease in Humans

Mite Content of House Dust

Dust associated with mite-infested stored grain, food, copra etc. is so full of mites, shed exuvia and mite excretory products as to consist of little else. House dust throughout the world also contains a variety of mites, although never to the same extent. Cunnington (1967) listed 19 species in dust collected from the houses of asthmatics in the London area, whilst Hewitt et al. (1973) identified 38 different species in dust from houses, clothing and the persons of patients with various skin diseases. Others have supported these findings (Oshima 1964; Voorhorst 1967; Cunnington and Gregory 1968; Maunsell et al. 1968; Haarvøv and Alani 1970; Sesay and Dobson 1972; personal observations by the present writer). *Dermatophagoides pteronyssinus* (Fig. 20.1) and *D. farinae* (Fig. 20.2) were the dominant species, and others commonly found were *Euroglyphus maynei* (Fig. 20.3), *Goheria fusca* (Fig. 20.4), *Acarus siro* (see Fig. 3.2, p. 12), *Glycyphagus domesticus* (see Fig. 21.4, p. 349), *Tyrophagus putrescentiae* (see Fig. 21.1, p. 347) and predatory mites of the genus *Cheyletus* (Fig. 20.5). Some species were found only in tropical house dust (Fain et al. 1969; Hunponu-Wusu and Somorin 1978).

Asthma has been known for some time to be induced by *Pyemotes* mites (Ancona 1923; Grove 1926). Voorhorst et al. (1964) blamed *D. pteronyssinus* as the principal cause of asthma. They were supported by evidence correlating asthmatic activity with the numbers of mites in such dust under the influence of dampness, altitude and season (Varekamp et al. 1966; Voorhorst 1967; Spieksma et al. 1971), as well as the correspondence between the antigenic activity of extracts of house dust and of mites and the dependence of house dust antigenicity on the mite content of the dust concerned (Bachofen et al. 1967; Wraith 1967; Maunsell et al. 1968; El-Hefny and Frankland 1970; Voorhorst 1970).

MacKenzie (1923) and Mekie (1926) recorded finding several species of mites in urine, which were subsequently demonstrated to be contaminants—in MacKenzie's case on laboratory glassware. Hinman and Kampmeier (1934) found *Tyrophagus* (= *Tyroglyphus*) *longior* in the faeces of two patients with diarrhoea and cited instances of vulvovaginitis and scrotal cyst said to be due to mite infestation. Sasa (1950, 1951) attributed pathogenic significance to the presence of *Dermatophagoides* species in the sputum and urine of patients. Furusho et al. (1981) postulated that *D. pteronyssinus* was the cause of Kawasaki disease (acute febrile mucocutaneous lymph node syndrome) in 20 Japanese children, on the grounds of their presence in large numbers in house dust from the children's homes and the markedly increased IgG and IgE antibodies to these mites in the serum of their patients. An Editorial (1982) in the *Lancet* discusses further work on this subject, which would seem to implicate house dust mites as vectors for a possible rickettsial organism causing the disease.

Possible Pathogenic Role

These instances of disorders provoked by mites prompt the question "Do house dust mites evoke skin eruptions in man?" The only proven instance of this was in the woman patient reported by Hepple and McMillan (1973) with a recurrent generalised transient purpuric capillaritis 36–55 h after systemic absorption of house dust antigen. Her serum contained IgG and IgE antibodies to house dust mite. She showed exacerbations during bed making, when mites were found in the bedding, but not after the bedding had been made mite free. There is also the question whether the eczematous and urticarial reactions of atopy are mite induced. Eczema and asthma certainly occur in the same patients. Smith (1970) noted that 25% of childhood asthmatics had or had had eczema.

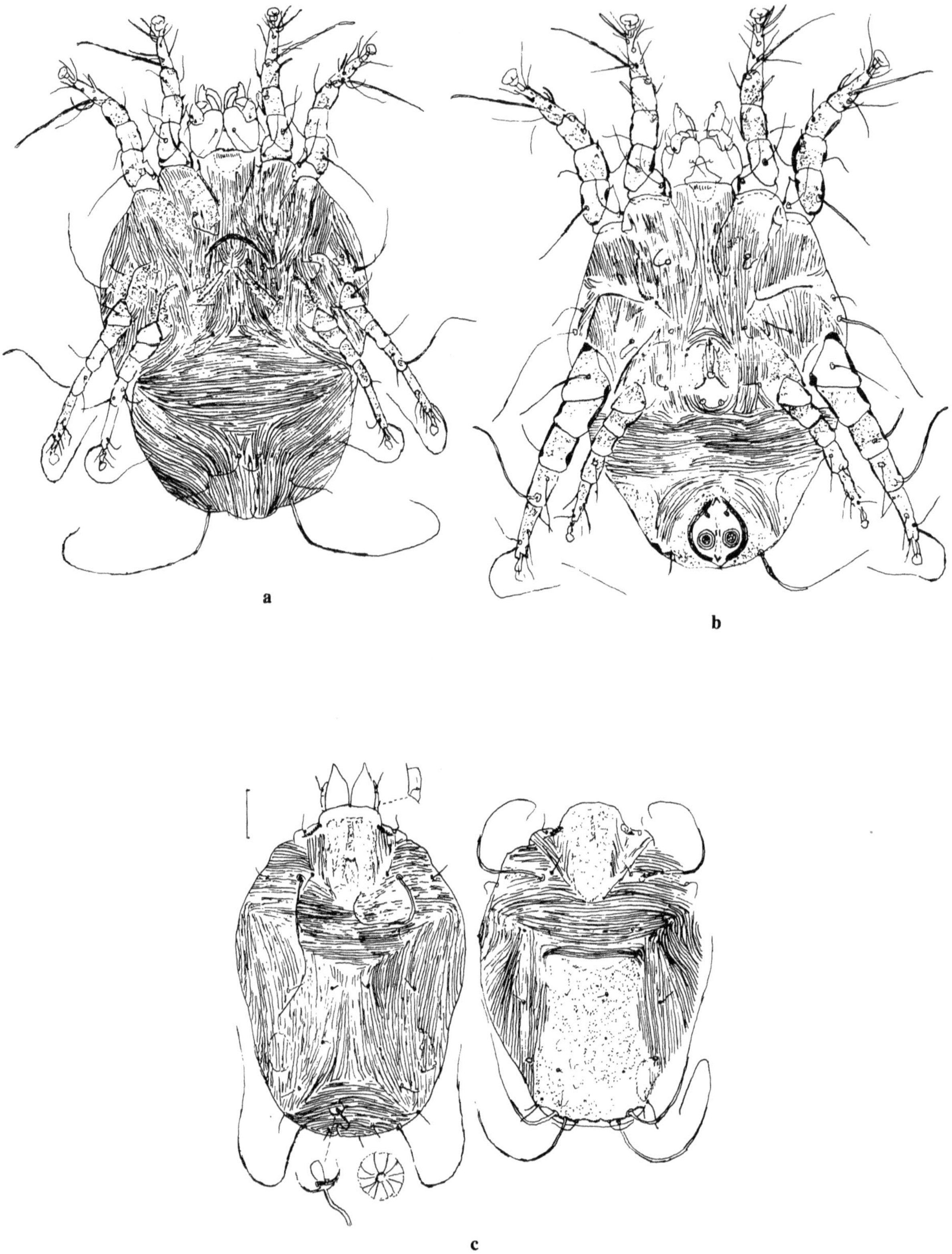

Fig. 20.1a–c. *Dermatophagoides pteronyssinus* (Trouessart). **a** ventral view of the female; **b** ventral view of the male; **c** dorsal view of female (*left*) and male (*right*). Note the enlarged view of the copulatory bursa of the female. The scale marking refers only to **c**. (After Fain 1966, by kind permission of the author and the Editor of *Acarologia*)

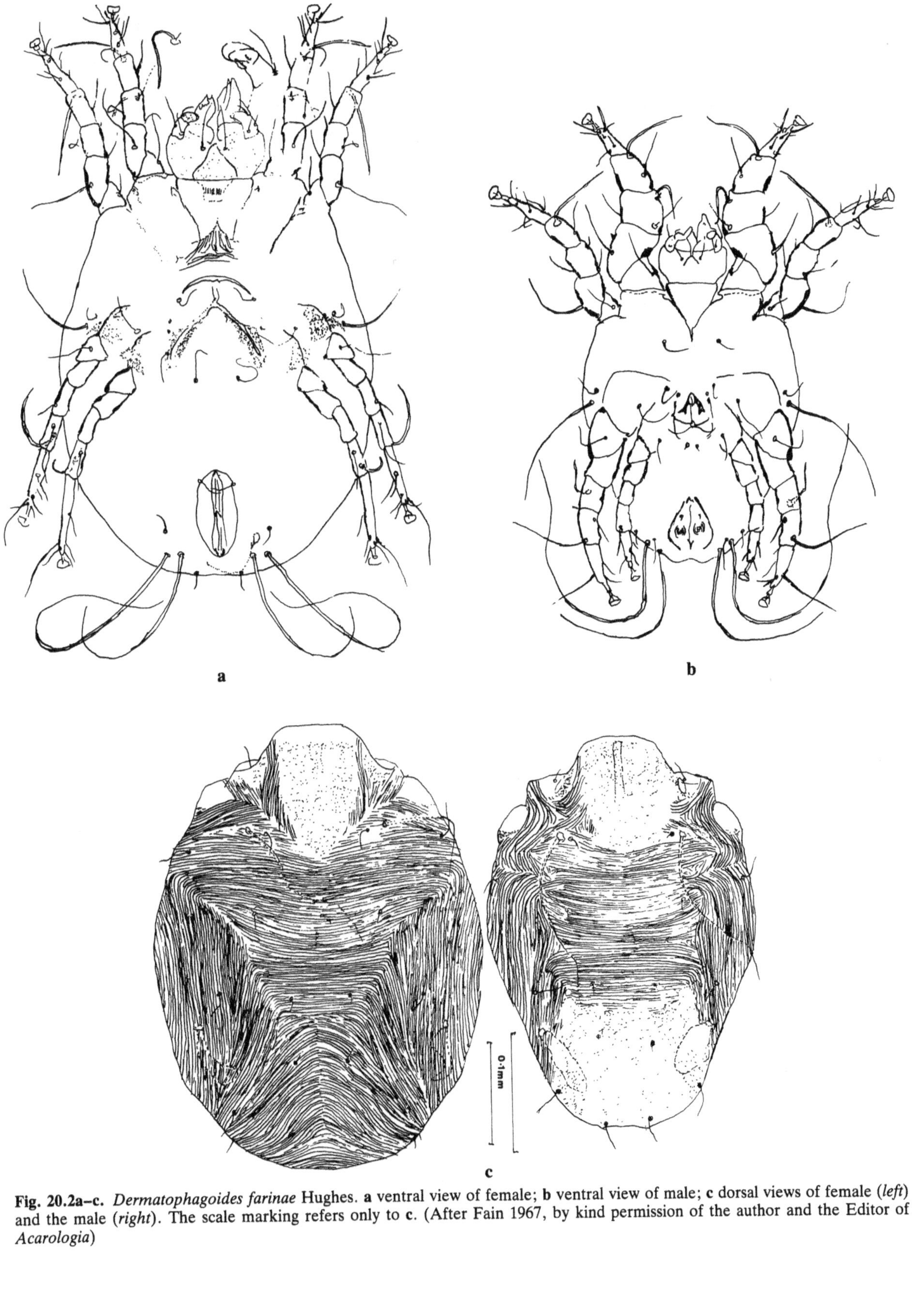

Fig. 20.2a–c. *Dermatophagoides farinae* Hughes. **a** ventral view of female; **b** ventral view of male; **c** dorsal views of female (*left*) and the male (*right*). The scale marking refers only to **c**. (After Fain 1967, by kind permission of the author and the Editor of *Acarologia*)

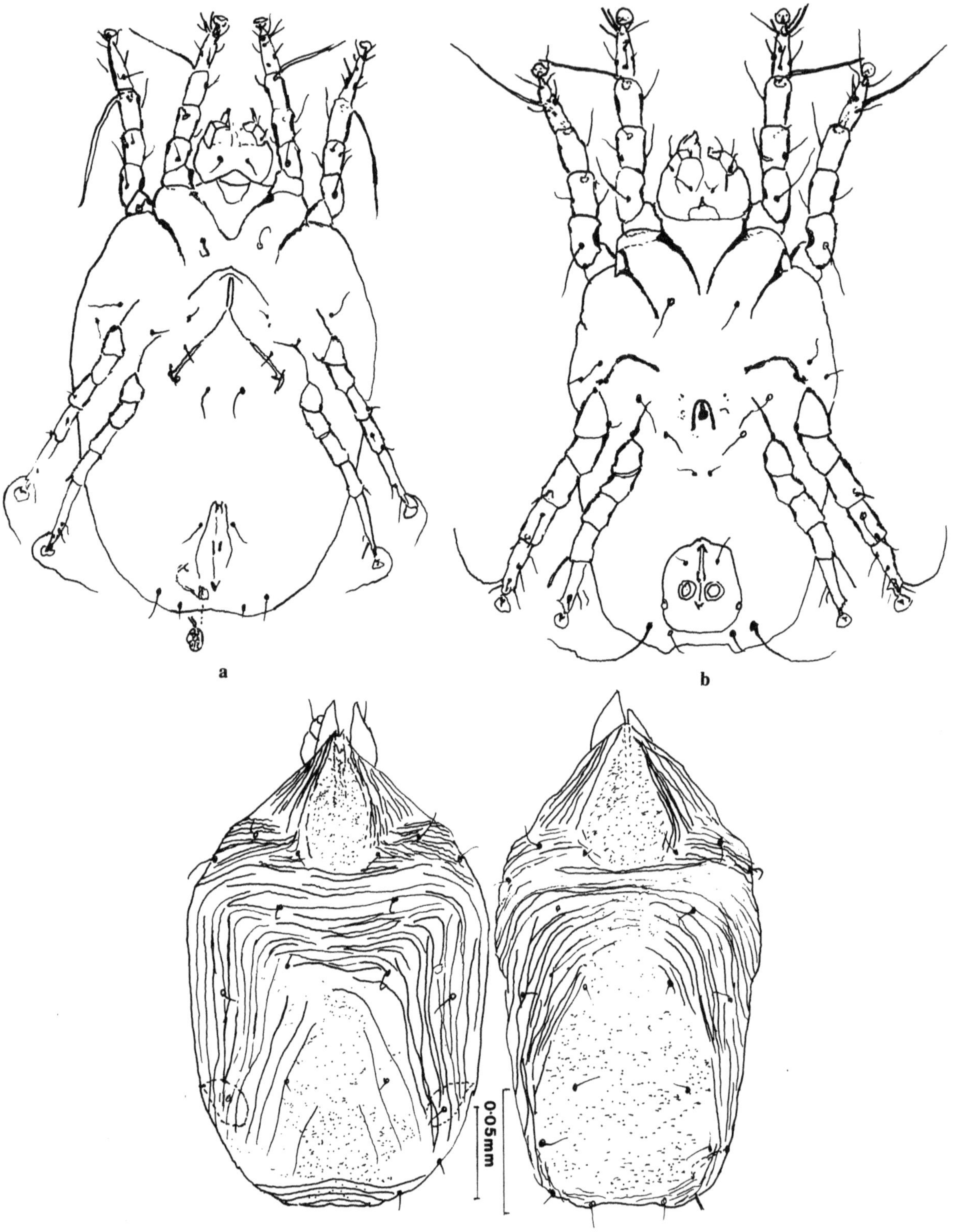

Fig. 20.3a–c. *Euroglyphus maynei* (Cooreman). **a** ventral view of female; **b** ventral view of male; **c** dorsal views of female (*left*) and male (*right*). Note the different patterns of the anal plate suckers in the males in Fig. 20.1, 20.2 and 20.3 The scale marking refers only to **c**. (After Fain 1965, by kind permission of the author and the Editor of *Revue Botanique et Zoologique d'Afrique*)

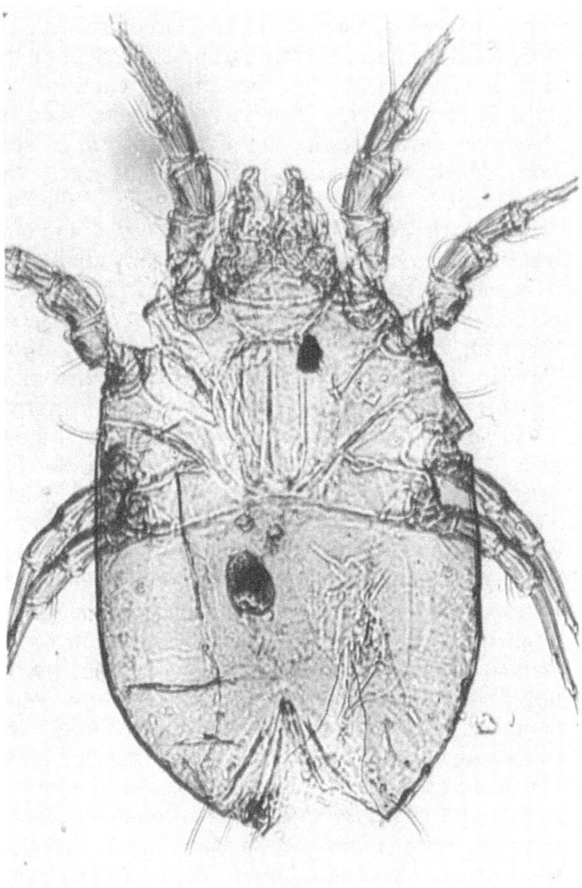

Fig. 20.4 *Goheria fusca* (Oudemans 1902). Photograph of a specimen found in mattress dust in Glasgow.

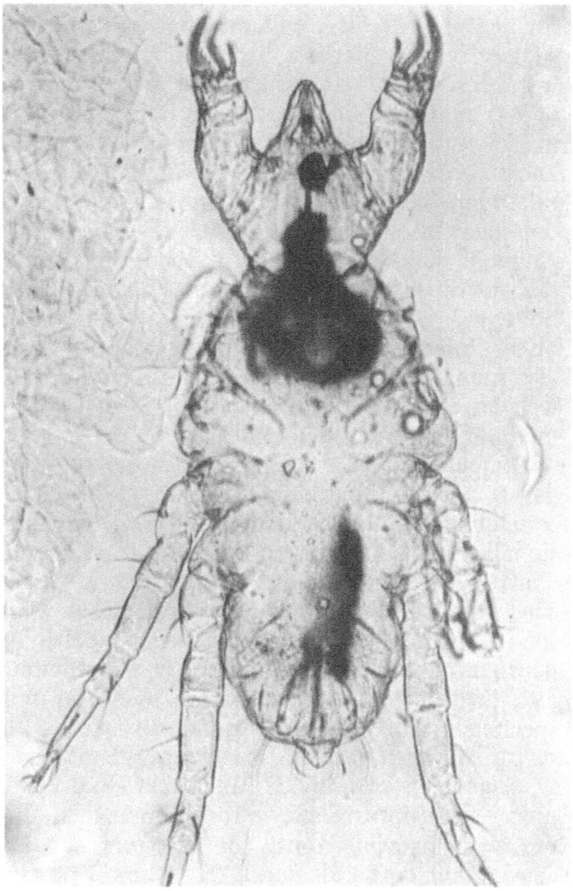

Fig. 20.5 *Cheyletus* species. Photograph of a specimen found in mattress dust in Glasgow.

Busvine (1977) considered that atopic eczema, which behaved very like asthma, could be due to the same cause. Hewitt and his colleagues (1973) made an examination for mites in house dust, clothing and skin scrapings from patients with a variety of skin diseases. The dominant and commoner species of the 38 they identified were similar to those enumerated above. The number from any individual or his clothing seldom exceeded one or two. Four patients, described in some detail, had positive patch test results to house dust, mites or mite extracts, but serum antibodies were not given. Change of environment in relation to mites benefited three patients, who showed exacerbation on re-exposure. The fourth patient with neurodermatitis cleared with topical steriod cum antibiotic therapy. Mites were found most often in this type of condition.

The present writer held a similar opinion but could not produce any positive evidence to support it. Many patients with atopic eczema had high serum IgE levels but no correlation between these levels or RAST results and eczematous activity could be obtained. RAST results were just as frequently positive for other antigens as for house dust mites. Clinically the evidence consisted of association with asthma and of the occasional patient who experienced very severe nocturnal exacerbations of eczema (as also happens among asthmatics). In at least two instances this was associated with a severe generalised itch and somewhat oedematous erythema suggestive of an acute allergic reaction and responding to treatment appropriate for the latter. Attempts to hyposensitise such patients did not give encouraging results.

Alexander (1972) showed that there was a high density of mites in house dust (over 1000/g of dust) in the dwellings of 34% of a group of children with papular urticaria. Positive results from intradermal tests against *Dermatophagoides* spp. extract were obtained in 10 of 34 patients (30%). All the controls gave negative results but were not matched for age and sex. This evidence was no more than suggestive that papular urticaria might in some instances be due to house dust mites. Oshima (1964) examined floor dust from different schools in Tokyo and found that *D. farinae* (*D. culinae*) and *D. scheremetewskyi* were the dominant species (although in 1967 he found *Euroglyphus maynei* dominant in one school). He felt that these mites could be held responsible for the skin eruption present on many of the children. In one school, however, where 78% of the girls suffered from bites, *Ornithonyssinus bacoti* and Pyemotidae were also found in several samples of dust. These could well have accounted for the skin lesions without incriminating any other mites.

The pathogenic role of *D. scheremetewskyi* Bogdanov 1864 is doubtful. Vitzthum (1929), cited by Dubinin et al. (1956), noted that it was occasionally found in human skin scales in scabietics. Traver (1951), a zoologist, claimed that it was the cause of a long-standing dermatosis from which she suffered and which had been labelled as neurodermatitis by more than one dermatologist. Over a number of years she found ten mite specimens on her skin, principally from the scalp. At least one of these was identified as *D. scheremetewskyi* by E. W. Baker. She attributed several bizarre effects to the mite, including burrowing subcutaneously on the forehead and causing her partial deafness. The clinical description of the eruption and its behaviour over the years was that of a classic neurodermatitis upon which was superimposed a delusion of cutaneous parasitosis (see Chap. 25). The activities attributed to the mites were incompatible with their morphology and known habits. Fisher et al. (1951) thought that the mites in Traver's case were much more likely to have been casual contaminants, a view supported by Fain (1967, 1969), who stated that *D. scheremetewskyi* was not a pathogen. He examined the mites which Traver had isolated from her skin and concluded that they were *D. pteronyssinus* or *D. farinae* and not *D. scheremetewskyi*. He blamed the dusty environment for the contamination and pointed out that *D. scheremetewskyi* was only reported as occurring in existing scaling dermatoses such as scabies or fungal infections, as in the case reported by Fisher et al. (1951). This also applied to the nine instances recorded by Dubinin and his colleagues (1956).

Consideration of Morphological and Biological Characteristics

It is important when postulating that a mite could be responsible for a particular skin disorder to consider the morphological and biological characteristics of the mite. Merely finding a few mites on the skin does not mean that they are the cause of any existing dermatosis. Known pathogens such as *Pyemotes*, *Cheyletiella* or *Ornithonyssinus* spp. bite, whilst the vast majority of dust mites are long-legged "nibblers" and "chewers". On the other hand, mites like *Sarcoptes scabiei* and *Demodex folliculorum* are morphologically adapted to living in the confines of burrows and hair follicles respectively. Free-living mites are not constructed for living in, let alone excavating, burrows. Being foragers and scavengers, however, they are quite capable of rummaging their way about amongst loose scales and crusts on the surface of human skin. They are also easily airborne and could thus readily contaminate skin, whether diseased or not. This would account for their presence on those occasions when they were recorded. The present writer has encountered this situation where the mites obviously had no pathogenic significance. It might be added that similar contamination of the skin in Japanese people is rendered easier by the habit of sleeping on mats laid on the floor, especially in view of the statement that mites are becoming more numerous in house dust in Japan (Furusho et al. 1981). If such mites contaminated the skin in very large numbers—as could occur, for example, with *Acarus siro* in granary dust, but only in grossly contaminated house dust with thousands of mites per gram—they might be harmless or could induce irritation and scratching because of the sensations resulting from their crawling or because of the inoculation of their bodies, dead or alive, or their excretory products into the skin by rubbing. Such inoculation might even induce sensitisation, and this is a possible explanation of the effect, if any, in atopics (i.e. atopic eczema). On the other hand, Van Bronswijk and Sinha (1971) failed to produce any skin reaction to live mites (*D. pteronyssinus*) placed on the skin for a period of 2 days. This problem requires further systematic investigation.

References

Alexander JO'D (1972) Mites and skin diseases. Clin Med 79: 14–19

Ancona G (1923) Asma epidemico da *Pediculoides ventricosus*. Policlinica 30: 45–70

Bachofen H, Scherrer M, Trautlein F and Wyss F (1967) Ist das Hausstaubasthma ein Milbenasthma? Dtsch Med Wochenschr 92: 1597–1602

Busvine JR (1977) Dermatoses due to arthropods other than scabies mites. In: Orkin M, Maibach HI, Parish HL, Schwartzman RM (eds) Scabies and pediculosis. Lippincott, Philadelphia, pp 132–138

*Cunnington AM (1967) The mite fauna of house dust. Acta Allergol (Kbh) 22: 415
Cunnington AM, Gregory PM (1968) Mites in bedroom air. Nature 217: 1271–1272
Dubinin VB, Guselnikova MI, Razatovsky IM (1956) Discovery of skin ticks (*Dermatophagoides scheremetewskyi* Bogdanov 1864) in some human skin diseases (in Russian). Bull Moscow Soc Exp Nat Sci (Dep Biol) 61: 43–53
Editorial (1982) The house dust mite and atopic dermatitis. Lancet II: 806–807
El-Hefny AM, Frankland AW (1970) House dust and mites as cause of inhalant allergic problems in the U.A.R. Excerpta Medica Int Congr Ser 211: 3–4
Fain A (1965) Les acariens nidicoles et détricoles de la famille Pyroglyphidae Cunliffe (Sarcoptiformes). Rev Bot Zool Afr 72: 257–288
Fain A (1966) Nouvellè description de *Dermatophagoides pteronyssinus* (Trouessart 1897). Importance de cet acarien en pathologie humaine (Psoroptidae: Sarcoptiformes). Acarologia 8: 320–327
Fain A (1967) Le genre *Dermatophagoides* Bogdanov 1864. Son importance dans les allergies respiratoires et cutanées chez l'homme (Psoroptidae: Sarcoptiformes). Acarologia 9: 179–225
Fain A (1969) Gale et dermatites produites par les acariens. Louvain Med 88: 755–764
Fain A, Cunnington AM, Spieksma FThM (1969) *Malayoglyphus intermedius* n.g., n.sp., a new mite from house dust in Singapore and Djakarta (Pyroglyphidar: Sarcoptiformes). Acarologia 11: 121–126
Fisher AA, Franks AG, Wolf M, Leider M (1951) Concurrent infestation with a rare mite and infection with a common dermatophyte. Arch Dermatol Syphilol 63: 336–342
Furusho K, Ohba T, Soeda T, Kimoto K, Okabe T, Hirota T (1981) Possible role for mite antigen in Kawasaki disease. Lancet II: 194–195
Grove EF (1926) Studies in specific hypersensitiveness. XXVI. On asthma and dermatitis due to hypersensitivity to *Pediculoides ventricosus*. J Immunol 12: 263–271
Haarvøv N, Alani M (1970) House dust mites (*Dermatophagoides pteronyssinus* (Trt), *D. farinae* Hughes, *Euroglyphus maynei* (Cooreman) Fain) in Denmark (Acarinae). Entomol Scand 1: 301–306
Hepple S, McMillan AL (1973) Purpuric dermatosis due to house dust mite (*Dermatophagoides* spp.) allergy: a case report. Clin Allergy 3: 23–31
*Hewitt M, Barrow GI, Miller DC, Turk F, Turk S (1973) Mites in the personal environment and their role in skin disorders. Br J Dermatol 89: 401–409
Hinman EH, Kampmeier RH (1934) Intestinal acariasis due to *Tyroglyphus longior* Gervais. Am J Trop Med 14: 355–362
Hunponu-Wasu OO, Somorin AO (1978) Epidemiological aspects of house dust allergy in Nigeria. J Dermatol (Tokyo) 5: 27–32
MacKenzie J (1923) Acari in specimens of urine. J R Army Med Corps 41: 157–158
Maunsell K, Wraith DG, Cunnington AM (1968) Mites and house dust allergy in bronchial asthma. Lancet I: 1267–1270
Mekie EC (1926) Parasitic infection of the urinary tract. Edinburgh Med J 33: 708–719
Oshima S (1964) Observations of floor mites collected in Yokohama. I. On the mites found in several schools in summer. Jpn J Sanit Zool 15: 233–244
Oshima S (1967) Studies on the genus *Dermatophagoides* (Psoroptidae: Acarina) as floor mites, with special reference to the medical importance. Jpn J Sanit Zool 18: 213–215
Sasa M (1950) Mites of the genus *Dermatophagoides* Bogdanoff 1864 found from cases of human acariasis. Jpn J Exp Med 20: 519–525
Sasa M (1951) Further notes on mites of the genus *Dermatophagoides* Bogdanoff found from human acariasis (Acarinae: Epidermoptidae). Jpn J Exp Med 21: 199–203
Sesay HR, Dobson RM (1972) Studies on the mite fauna of house dust in Scotland with special reference to that of bedding. Acarologia 14: 384–392
Smith JM (1970) Clinical findings in children with allergy to the house dust mite. Acta Allergol (Kbh) 25: 37–40
Spieksma FThM, Zuidema P, Leupen MJ (1971) High altitude and house dust mites. Br Med J I: 82–84
Traver JR (1951) Unusual scalp dermatitis in humans caused by the mite *Dermatophagoides* (Acarinae: Epidermoptidae). Proc Entomol Soc Washington 53: 1–25
Van Bronswijk JEMH, Sinha RN (1971) Pyroglyphid mites (Acari) and house dust allergy. J Allergy 47: 31–52
Varekamp H, Spieksma FThM, Leupen MJ, Lyklema AW (1966) House dust mites in their relation to dampness of houses and the allergen content of house dust. Proceedings of the 5th inter-asma congress, Utrecht, 1966, pp 256–268
Voorhorst R (1967) The house dust mite (*Dermatophagoides pteronyssinus*) and the allergen it produces, identity with the house dust allergen. Acta Allergol (Kbh) 22: 412–413
Voorhorst R (1970) Quantitative aspects of the problem of house dust atopy and house dust mites. Acta Allergol (Kbh) 25: 237–254
Voorhorst R, Spieksma-Boezeman MIA, Spieksma FThM (1964) Is a mite (*Dermatophagoides* sp.) the producer of the house dust allergen? Allergie Asthma 10: 329–334
Wraith DG (1967) Skin tests with extracts of mites. Acta Allergol (Kbh) 22: 414

21 Skin Eruptions Caused by Mites from Stored Food

Mites infesting food and other organic materials which are stored in bulk can cause serious economic loss and may from time to time cause reactions on the human skin. These eruptions, with various names such as "copra itch", "grocer's itch" and *Kramerkratze*, are probably commoner than the authenticated published reports would suggest. Outbreaks may be confined to one or two persons or appear in the form of small epidemics. They may occur in almost any part of the world, regardless of climate or the ethnic origin of the victims. The mites, mainly Acaridae, have been found on many substrates, a list of which was given by Browning (1942) and included groceries, seeds, bulbs, feathers, hay and many other items. The clinical features, although non-specific, suggest an arthropod origin to the experienced dermatologist. A single clinical description will suffice for the whole group.

Clinical Features

Itching, sometimes slight (Oppenheim and Taglicht 1925), sometimes almost intolerably severe (Pawlowsky and Stein 1929; Rokstad 1943) occurs in all patients. It may be accompanied by a pricking sensation (O'Donovan 1922; Thomas 1942). Whilst in some patients the onset may develop shortly after starting work (Castellani 1912–1913), in the majority it is generally about 24 h before such symptoms become evident. Sweating has been held to aggravate itch in some patients (Ditlevsen 1916; Fields et al. 1968).

Soon after itching is felt, and certainly within 48 h, an eruption appears on the skin. As a general rule the uncovered areas of face, neck, forearms and back of the hands are affected. Other regions such as the upper arms (Oppenheim and Taglicht 1925; Cleveland 1940), the shoulders (Rokstad 1943; Kilpio and Pirila 1952), legs (Castellani 1912–1913) and even the whole body (Castellani 1912–1913; Ditlevsen 1916) may be involved. Castellani's patients were never affected on the face, whereas it was always the first area to be attacked in Ditlevsen's patients. Both groups of patients worked with copra. In Castellani's group the copra was heavily infested with living mites, whereas Ditlevsen's patients handled copra which was heavily infested, but in which all the mites were dead, and worked in the enclosed dust-laden atmosphere of a ship's hold. Two patients of Kilpio and Pirila (1952) also showed widespread lesions. Cleveland's (1940) patients showed somewhat localised eruptions. In those who carried copra, the left side of the face and neck and the left arm were mostly affected, whilst in others who lifted infested cheeses from shelves the submental region was attacked, in addition to the same areas as in the copra porters. The patients reported by Anderson and Fishman (1948) carried large "wheels" of cheese in their arms and held them against the chest; both these areas became affected. Almost all the other workers who have been reported as showing skin lesions associated with handling stored food were either shovelling (O'Donovan 1922) or sorting and cleaning the infested material (Oppenheim and Taglicht 1925; Pawlowsky and Stein 1929; Pirila 1951; Pirila and Kilpio 1954; Fields et al. 1968).

The initial lesions may consist of erythema of the face with acute oedema of the eyelids (Ditlevsen 1916; Thomas 1942; Kilpio and Pirila 1952). This oedema may be very slight or, as Oppenheim and Taglicht (1925) observed, may involve most of the face. In other patients the first visible evidence is acute erythema, which may initially be confined to the face and hands and remain so, or may then spread over most or all of the body (Ditlevsen 1916), or which may be diffuse from the onset, when it is generally associated with a concomitant eczematous change (Oppenheim and Taglicht 1925; Thomas 1942; Rokstad 1943). A more common appearance than eczema is an eruption of small bright-red pinhead to pea-sized papules, which tend to be more marked on the face and forearms. They may be so numerous as to be confluent (Rokstad 1943). Sometimes some or all of them may look vesicular, although not actually so

(Oppenheim and Taglicht 1925), whilst others are truly vesicular. Such vesicles may rupture and become encrusted (Anderson and Fishman 1948), or may sometimes become pustular by secondary infection (Castellani 1912–1913; Cleveland 1940) or frankly eczematous and weeping (Oppenheim and Taglicht 1925). Sometimes the papular lesions are scanty and pale with a diffuse erythematous background (Ditlevsen 1916). Oppenheim and his colleague observed brownish-coloured nodules on one occasion.

These lesions will persist or continue to erupt as long as contact with the infested material is maintained. There is a distinct tendency towards eczematisation with such prolonged contact. When the patient ceases work or is moved away to another job the itch and skin lesions quickly subside. The time taken depends on the severity of the eruption and varies from a few days to just over a week. Even eczematised lesions will clear up in this manner (Ditlevsen 1916).

Castellani (1912–1913) and Ditlevsen (1916) both noted that some persons were not affected at all. Ditlevsen observed that the wife and children of one patient were also attacked when the man took a small quantity of copra home. The wife ate a little and developed redness inside the mouth and scaling on the lips.

Histopathology

Only very slight changes were found by Pawlowsky and Stein (1929). These included mild thickening of the stratum corneum and rete pegs with slight separation of epidermal cells. The dermal papillae were somewhat flattened and the collagen bundles a little separated. There was slight epidermal exocytosis but marked chronic perivascular infiltrate with minimally dilated and congested blood vessels with slight endothelial swelling.

Diagnosis

The diagnosis depends upon the clinical appearance and distribution of the eruption and upon the equally important history of occupation at the time of onset. The combination of what would appear to be an acute contact reaction on the face and hands with discrete lesions on the arms, neck and other exposed areas strongly suggests an arthropod cause. The finding of mites in the dust increases the certainty of this suggestion, and the occurrence of other cases amongst the patient's workmates confirms the diagnosis. The absence of familial cases (but note the exception of Ditlevsen's case) makes scabies seem unlikely, as does the absence of the clinical features of that disease. Other diseases caused by mites, such as *Pyemotes* infestation, will have to be excluded by identification of the mites in question, whilst acarine ectoparasites of birds and other animals are excluded by the history. The acute onset and distribution may suggest seborrhoeic eczema, but the equally rapid subsidence after removal from the source of irritation will soon exclude this diagnosis.

Table 21.1. Association of various species of mites reported to have occurred in foodstuffs, the handling of which has resulted in skin eruptions in man

Stored substance	Mites	References
Bacon	*Glycyphagus domesticus*	Czernecki and Kraus (1978)
Bulbs	*Rhizoglyphus hyacinthi*	Pawlowsky and Stein (1929)
Cheese	*Tyrophagus longior*, *Acarus siro*	Cleveland (1940); Thomas (1942); Anderson and Fishman (1948); Pirila (1951); Fields et al. (1968)
Copra	*T. longior*, *T. putrescentia*, *Caloglyphus krameri*	Castellani (1912–1913); Macleod (1915); Whitfield (1915); Ditlevsen (1916); Cleveland (1940); Laarman (1952)
Dates	*Carpoglyphus passularum*[a]	Oppenheim and Taglicht (1925)
Figs	*C. passularum*	O'Donovan (1922); Erhart (1925); Spitzer (1927); Rokstad (1943); Pirila (1951)
Plums	*C. passularum*	Oppenheim and Taglicht (1925); Spitzer (1927)
Prunes	*C. passularum*	Oppenheim and Taglicht (1925); Spitzer (1927); Pirila and Kilpio (1954)
Tobacco	*Carpoglyphus* species	Rokstad (1943)
Wheat pollards	*Suidasia nesbitti*	Kilpio and Pirila (1952)

[a] *Carpoglyphus passularum* is now called *C. lactis*.

Fig. 21.1a–d. *Tyrophagus putrescentiae* (Shrank 1781). (Synonym *T. castellani* Hirst 1912). **a** dorsal view of male; **b** anal region of male; **c** dorsal view of right leg I of male; **d** ventral view of female. (After Hughes 1961, by kind permission of the author and the Ministry of Agriculture, Fisheries and Food)

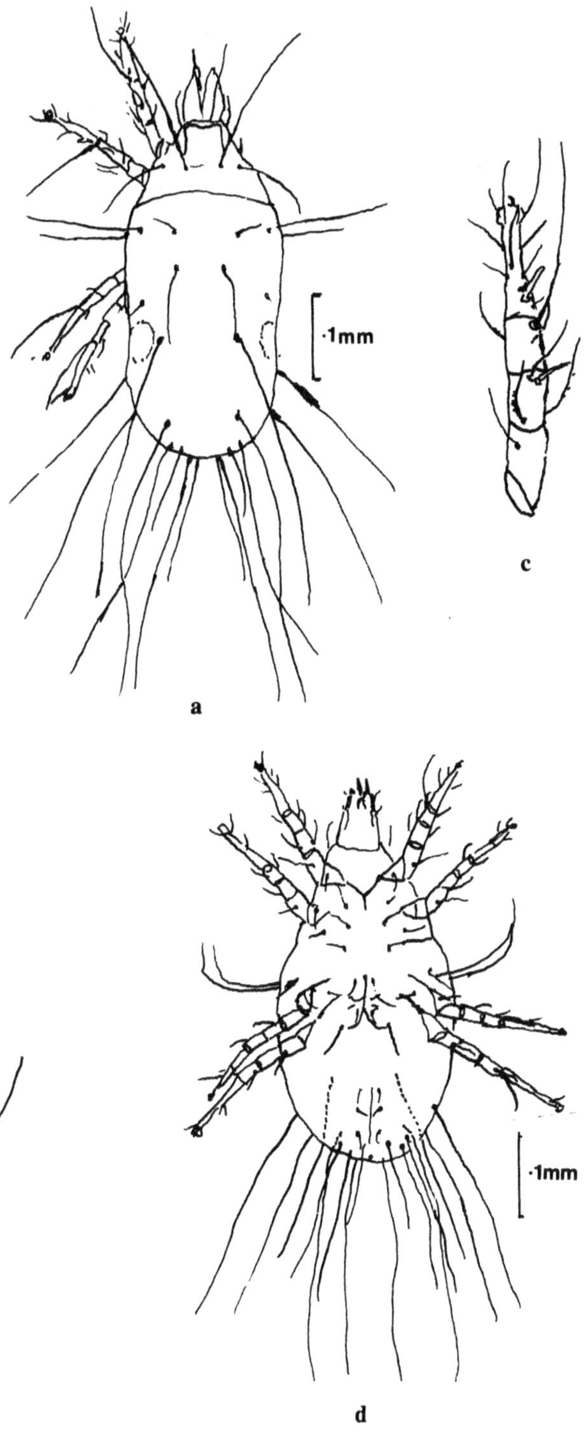

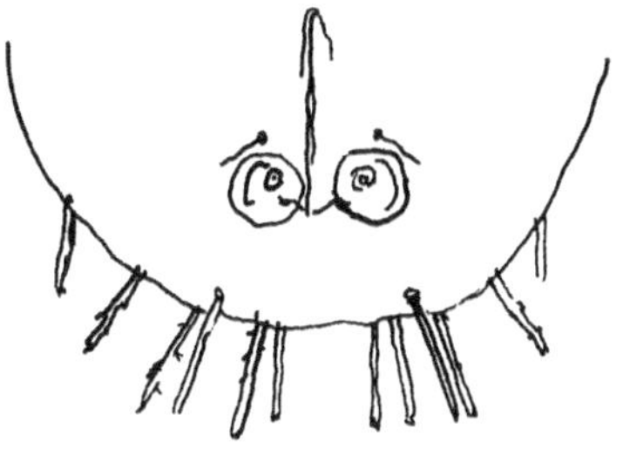

Mite Species Involved

Mites infesting stored food belong to the subfamilies Acaridae (the majority), Oribatei, Mesostigmata, Tarsonemini and Prostigmata (Hughes 1961). The number of species is very large, but only a few have been incriminated as causes of skin lesions in man. Table 21.1 lists some of these together with the foodstuffs (or other material) with which they have been associated. Figures 21.1–21.6, illustrate the salient features of most of

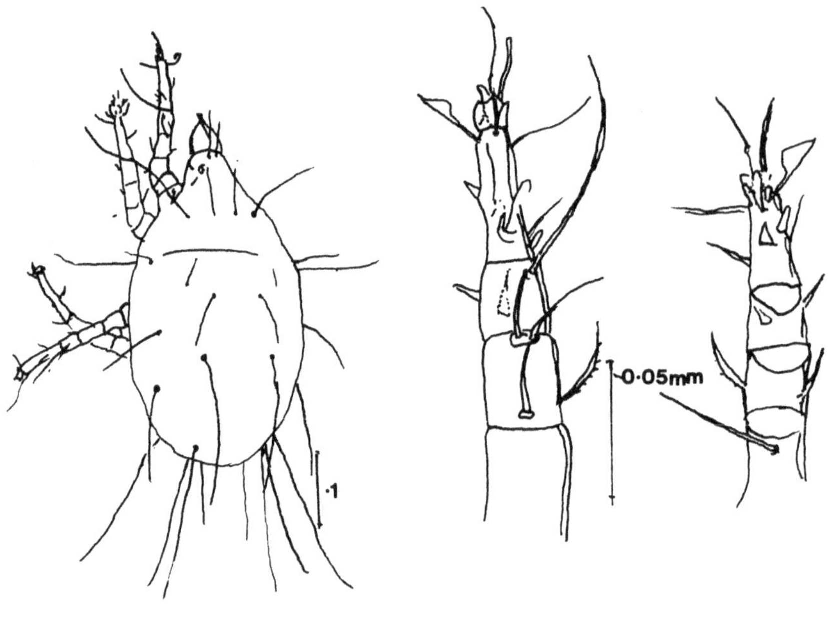

Fig. 21.2a, b. *Caloglyphus krameri* (Berlese 1881). (Synonym *Cosmoglyphus krameri* Oud. 1932). **a** dorsal view of male; **b** dorsal and ventral views of right leg I. (After Hughes 1961, by kind permission of the author and the Ministry of Agriculture, Fisheries and Food)

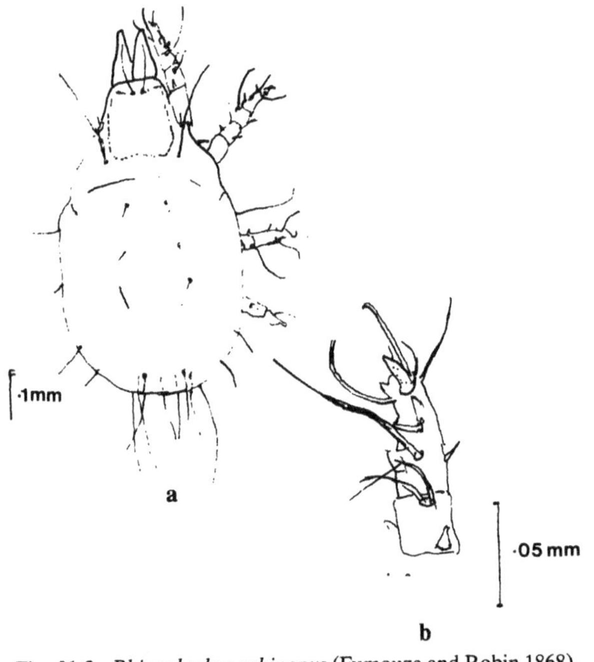

Fig. 21.3. *Rhizoglyphus echinopus* (Fumouze and Robin 1868). (Synonyms *Tyroglyphus hyacinthi* and probably *Rhizoglyphus hyacinthi*.) **a** Dorsal view of male; **b** details of right leg I of male. (After Hughes 1961, by kind permission of the author and the Ministry of Agriculture, Fisheries and Food)

these species (see also Fig. 3.2, p. 12, and Fig. 20.4, p. 341). The differences between some species are difficult to discover. In a book of the present size it is manifestly impracticable to elaborate on the minute details which require considerable experience to identify with accuracy. It should be stressed that advice from an expert acarologist is always desirable although not always immediately available. It is satisfying if one can accomplish this identification without help. In order to be able to make a start on identification until such time as confirmatory assistance is forthcoming, the interested reader is referred to the elementary outline of the features determining the various order, suborder, families etc. of mites set out in Chapter 3; with this and the help of Hughes' book, *The Mites of Stored Food*, success may be achieved. Identification of the species involved is valuable as it may confirm the suspected source of the trouble and facilitate the subsequent management.

Nesbitt (1945) has pointed out that Acaridae can be found in any climate from Arctic tundra to tropical rainforest. They flourish best between temperatures of 10°C and 20°C and at a relative humidity of 80%–85% (Solomon 1962). Some species prefer food with a low moisture content, such as grain and stored farinaceous products. Only the germs of grains are eaten (Nesbitt 1945; Solomon

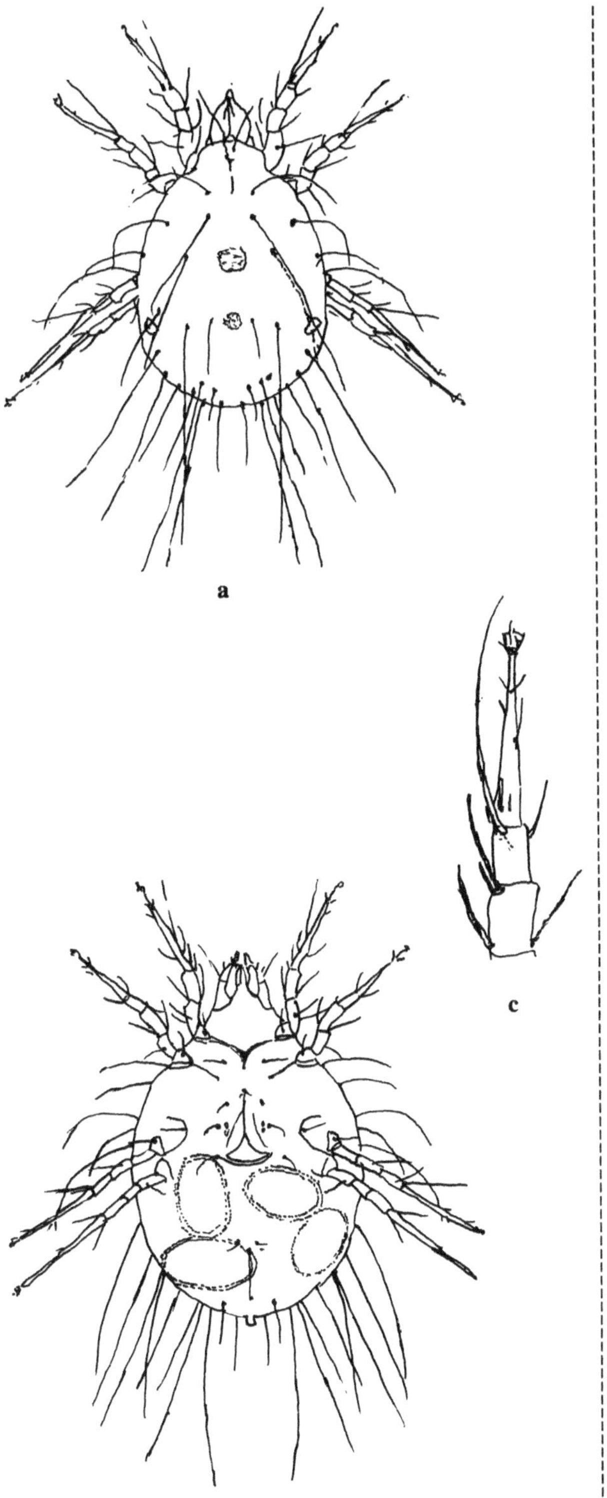

Fig. 21.4a–c. *Glycyphagus domesticus* (DeGeer). **a** dorsal view of male; **b** ventral view of female; **c** details of right leg I of male. (After Hughes 1961, by kind permission of the author and the Ministry of Agriculture, Fisheries and Food)

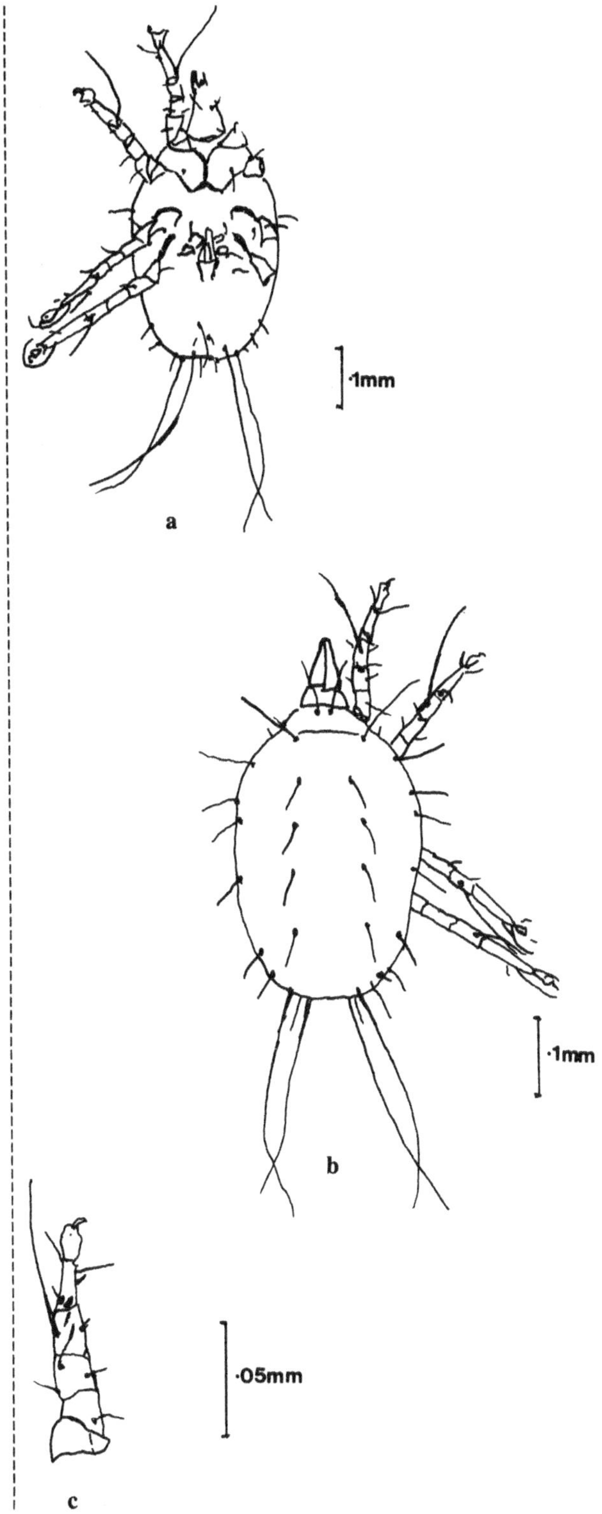

Fig. 21.5a–c. *Carpoglyphus lactis* (L. 1758). (Also referred to as *C. passularum* or *Acarus passularum*.) **a** ventral view of male; **b** dorsal view of female; **c** dorsal view of left leg I of male. (After Hughes 1961, by kind permission of the author and the Ministry of Agriculture, Fisheries and Food)

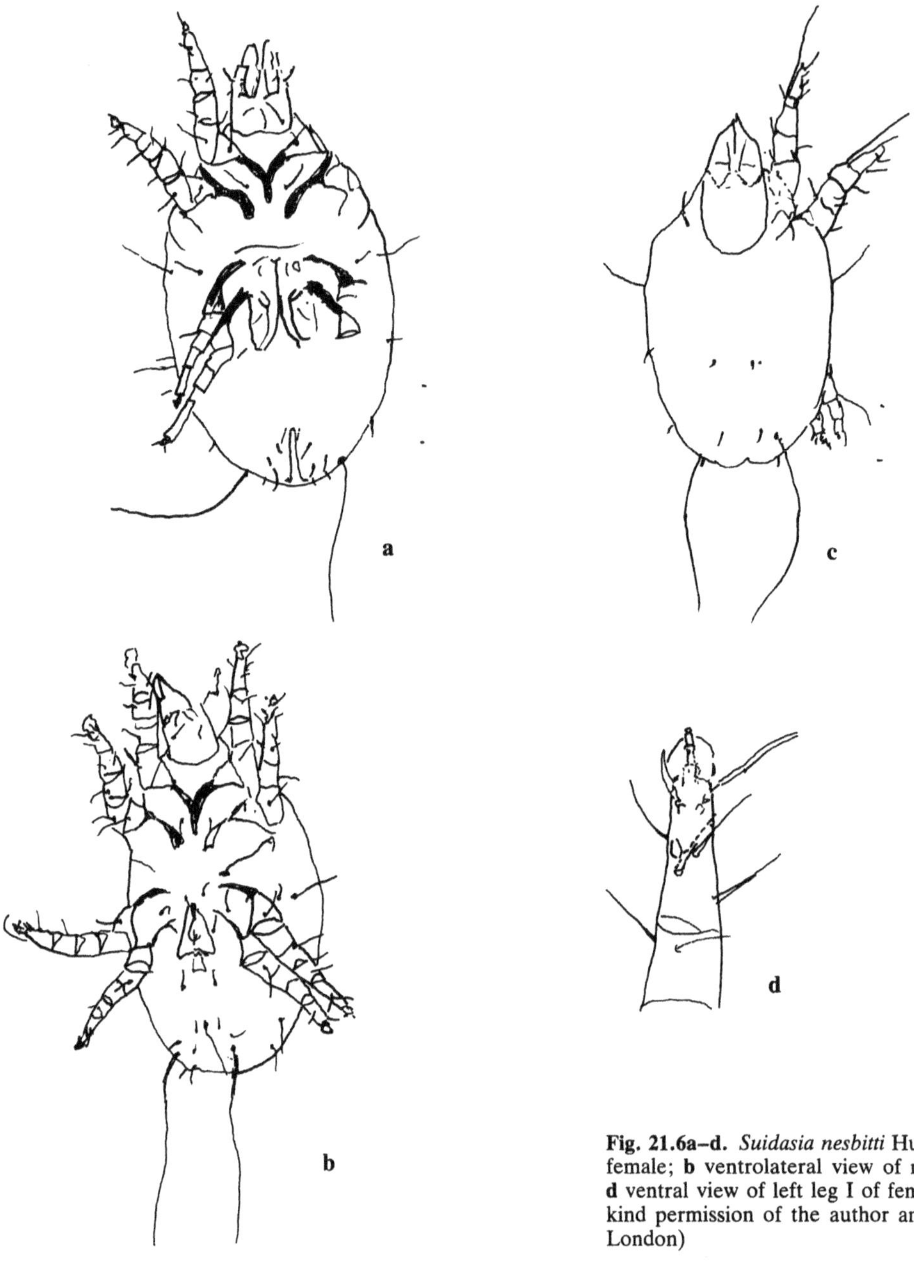

Fig. 21.6a–d. *Suidasia nesbitti* Hughes, 1948. **a** ventral view of female; **b** ventrolateral view of male; **c** dorsal view of male; **d** ventral view of left leg I of female. (After Hughes 1948, by kind permission of the author and The Zoological Society of London)

1962), but Solomon also pointed out that other parts are eaten if they are mouldy and he emphasised that in general these mites feed mainly on fungi. This is especially applicable to those mites which prefer food with a higher moisture content (Sinha 1964a). As far as grain is concerned, Pulpan and Verner (1965) observed that the mites proliferated in proportion to the moisture content of the grain, which was in turn dependent on the condition in which it was put into store and on the suitability of the storage premises. On foods like bacon the mites live exclusively on moulds.

Infested material may be handled in loose bulk, in bales or bags, or in prepared form such as cheeses, hams or sides of bacon. The method of handling, whether shovelling, sifting, sorting, carrying or simply moving, together with the prevailing atmospheric conditions (e.g. the dusty confines of a ship's hold or granary), determine the distribution and severity of the skin eruption.

All the infested material is coated with a fine, musty-smelling, brown, brownish-red or white dust up to several millimetres thick. It consists of myriads of living and dead mites, their excreta and food debris. Inspection of a small sample on a sheet of paper, using a hand lens, may reveal movement of the living mites.

As a result of patch tests and rubbing dead mites into the skin the consensus of opinion among researchers has been that the skin lesions were the result of primary irritation from some mite toxin and not allergy (Rokstad 1943; Pirila 1951; Fields et al. 1968). Thomas (1942) held that the effect was like that of a contact reaction. Oppenheim and Taglicht (1925) thought that the affected patients had a predisposition; however, as Laarman (1952) pointed out, there is perhaps a relationship between the number of mites and the severity of the reaction, which would explain why some people were unaffected (a similar view, attributed to Robertson, was cited by Zdarkova 1967). The contamination of their skin was relatively slight.

Pawlowsky and Stein (1929) achieved particularly interesting results. A reaction to dead mites was obtained only when the skin was mildly scarified, whereas if live mites were applied to the skin and confined to a defined area for 24 h rows of papules appeared at the periphery of the area similar to the arrangement of lesions in the same circumstances when *Pyemotes* mites were being tested (Goldberger and Schamberg 1909). Pawlowsky and his colleague observed faecal deposits from the mites on the skin in these tests after 48 h and thus inferred that the mites were behaving physiologically. Defaecation usually meant that the mites were hungry and probably fed by chewing epidermal scales, their chelicerae being well adapted for this purpose. This activity would produce papules as a result of the irritant digestive juices secreted from external predigestion. There would be no puncturing of the skin as with blood-sucking mites, no central punctum and no residual pigmentation for this reason (Laarman 1952). There is no evidence to support the suggestion of Fields et al. (1968) that the mites burrow into the scales. It would thus appear that these acarid mites can cause a skin reaction either by these toxic products (faecal or secretory) being rubbed into the skin and giving a contact effect, or by superficial feeding producing discrete papular lesions with no residuum. In very dusty atmospheres the contact type of reaction would be the more severe, whereas constant contact with less atmospheric dust would favour the papular type. Indeed, this distinction seems to exist.

Management of Patients

The skin eruption subsides in a few days if the patient is removed from the source of irritation. The application of oily calamine lotion is usually sufficient to relieve irritation, but in severe cases topical corticosteroid cum antibiotic preparations may be indicated.

Prevention can be largely achieved by the application of white soft paraffin to the exposed parts of the body before work, together with the wearing of protective gloves and long-sleeved overalls (Cleveland 1940; Anderson and Fishman 1948; Pirila 1951). It is especially important when working in enclosed dusty atmospheres to apply soft paraffin to the face. Fields et al. (1968) have observed that silicone protective lotions are useless. The wearing of goggles to protect the eyelids and conjunctivae might also be advisable. Thorough washing and changing clothes immediately after work is also necessary, preferably at the place of work.

Prevention and Management of Food Infestation

The technical problems involved vary with the materials concerned. Environmental conditions are of enormous importance. Where possible, temperature and relative humidity must be maintained to suit each individual foodstuff. The condition of the foodstuff when first stored or shipped should be as good as possible. The importance of this precaution was well exemplified in the outbreaks of copra itch in certain European ports in the report compiled by Ditlevsen (1916). He showed that those cargoes shipped in a good state from sources where the conditions were good seldom deteriorated and did not become infested, whereas those cargoes which were in poor condition at the time of shipment showed rapid deterioration with fungal growth and subsequent acarid invasion, which flourished in bad shipping facilities. The prevention of mite infestation in cheeses is easily achieved by a sound, intact coating of paraffin wax, which should be regularly inspected for breaks in continuity. Dried fruit should be clean and sound before being put into storage and maintained in a dry, cool atmosphere. Again regular inspection should be made for rotten specimens, the fruit being turned over and washed if necessary to avoid moulds developing. Grain should be sifted occasionally and regularly inspected. Good ventilation is essential in all warehouses.

Control of mite infestation has been achieved in Czechoslovakia (Pulpan and Verner 1965) and Canada (Sinha 1964a) by the deliberate use of *Cheyletus* species (*C. eruditus*)—an idea originally suggested by Ewing (1912). This is a purely predaceous mite, one of which per 100 kg of grain is sufficient to keep *Acarus siro* and other infesting acarids within acceptable limits, provided that environmental conditions are suitable (Pulpan and Verner 1965). In Canada the optimum effect is achieved in March and April (Sinha 1964b). In countries with less stable climates this technique is not very useful. Reliance must then be placed on fumigation with substances like methyl bromide (Solomon 1962).

References

Anderson NP, Fishman HP (1948) Cheese mite dermatitis in the United States. Arch Dermatol Syphilol 57: 227–234

Browning E (1942) Cited in Thomas (1942)

Castellani A (1912–1913) Note on copra itch. Proc R Soc Med (Sec Dermatol) 6: 28–29

Cleveland DEH (1940) Mite dermatitis. Arch Dermatol Syphilol 41: 831–832

Czernecki N, Kraus H (1978) Milbendermatitis durch *Tyrophagus dimidiatus*. Z Hautkr 53: 414–416 Extracted in Rev Appl Entomol (1979) (Ser B) 67: 324

*Ditlevsen C (1916) Acarodermatitis e copra. Arch Schiffs Trop Hyg 20: 503–511

Erhart F (1925) Uber eine akute Gewerbedermatitis. Arch Dermatol Syphilis 148: 516–518

Ewing HE (1912) The life history and habits of *Cheyletus seminivorus* Packard. J Econ Entomol 5: 412–420

Fields JP, Hoke AW, Cronce PC (1968) Cheese mite dermatitis. Arch Dermatol 98: 669–670

Goldberger J, Schamberg JF (1909) Epidemic of an urticarioid dermatitis due to a small mite (*Pediculoides ventricosus*) in the straw of a mattress. Public Health Rep 24: 973–975

Hughes AM (1948) A new tyroglyphid mite *Suidasai nesbitti* sp. n. Proc R Zool Soc Lond 118: 543–552

*Hughes AM (1961) The mites of stored food. Ministry of Agriculture, Fisheries and Food Technical Bulletin No 9. HMSO, London

Kilpio O, Pirila V (1952) A new tyroglyphid mite causing dermatitis. Acta Derm Venereol (Stockh) 32 (Suppl 29): 197–200

Laarman JJ (1952) Copra itch in the Netherlands. Doc Med Geogr Trop 4: 268–272

McLeod JMH (1915) Note on a case of acute dermatitis due to copra dust. Br J Dermatol 27: 118–119

Nesbitt HHJ (1945) A revision of the family acaridae (Tyroglyphidae), order Acari, based on comparative morphological studies. Can J Res 25: 139–185

O'Donovan WJ (1922) Discussion on occupational dermatitis. Br Med J 2: 499–504

*Oppenheim M, Taglicht H (1925) Über zwei Falle im Milbenkrankheiten bei Datterpackerinnen. Wien Med Wochenschr 75: 364–368

Pawlowsky EN, Stein AK (1929) Experimentelle Untersuchung über die Wirkung da eine eigenartige Dermatitis beim Menschen hervorgerufenden Milbe *Rhyzoglyphus hyacinthi* (Fam. Tyroglyphidae). Arch Dermatol Syphilis 158: 443–448

Pirila V (1951) On cheese and fig mite dermatitis. Acta Derm Venereol (Stockh) 31: 630–637

Pirila V, Kilpio O (1954) Occupational mite dermatitis; a further report from Finland. Acta Derm Venereol (Stockh) 34: 368–371

*Pulpan J, Verner PH (1965) Control of tyroglyphide mites in stored grain by the predatory mite *Cheyletus eruditus* (Schrank). Can J Res 43: 417–432

Rockstad I (1943) Endemic outbreaks of skin eruption caused by mites from food stuffs (figs) and tobacco. Acta Derm Venereol (Stockh) 24: 113–129

Sinha RN (1964a) Mites of stored grain in Western Canada. Ecology and methods of survey. Proc Entomol Soc Manitoba 20: 19–33

Sinha RN (1964b) Ecological relationships of stored product mites and seed-borne fungi. Proceedings of the first international congress of acarology, Acarologia 6: 372–389

Solomon ME (1962) Ecology of the flour mite *Acarus siro* L (= *Tyroglyphus farinae DeG*). Ann Appl Biol 50: 178–184

Spitzer E (1927) Dermatitis papulo-vesiculosa durch Beschaftigung mit milbigen Dorrpflaumen. Zentralbl Haut Geschlechtkr 22: 310–311

Thomas EWP (1942) Dermatitis due to *Tyroglyphus longior* Gerv. var Castellani, Hirst in cheese dust. Br J Dermatol 54: 313–319

Whitfield (1915) Acarus from a case of copra itch. Br J Dermatol 27: 125–126

Zdarkova E (1967) Stored food mites in Czechoslovakia. J Stored Food Products Res 3: 155–175

22 Infestation with Trombiculid Mite Larvae

Harvest mites are the larvae of trombiculid mites (see Table 22.1 for other common names). They have been a known cause of skin irritation, often very severe, for a long time and have a worldwide distribution. The first species to be identified, now called *Neotrombicula autumnalis*, was described in 1790 by Shaw. In 1834 it was recognised by Duges as the larval form of a mite (Toomey 1921). The adult stages are seldom seen, although a great deal of investigation about them has been done. Womersley and Heaslip (1943), in their comprehensive review of Far Eastern trombiculids, noted that only two of 15 species were fully documented in larval, nymphal and adult forms. Because of this they are classified on the basis of the morphology of the larvae (Finnegan 1945). Certain species in the Far East (*Leptotrombidium akamushi* and *L. deliense*) are known to be vectors of Japanese river fever (scrub typhus, rickettsial typhus, tsutsugamushi fever). The relationship between these mites and the typhus-like disease was first suggested by Palm (1878), an Edinburgh surgeon, who described cases he saw in Japan. However, trombiculids are just as well known because of the irritating skin eruption that follows their invasion of man's skin. Table 22.2 lists the species known to bite man. Included in this table are zoological synonyms, since the literature on the subject abounds with a large number of confusing names and it is difficult to ascertain which mite is meant.

Table 22.1. Common names used for trombiculid larvae in various part of the world. Collected from numerous papers and books in the reference list. Toomey (1921) gives a long list containing many not included here

Common name	Country
Harvest mite; harvest bug; red bug; berry bug	United Kingdom
Orange tawny	Ireland
Mower's mite	United Kingdom
Aoutat; *rouget*	France
Herbstgrasmilbe; *Erntemilbe*; *Grasmilbe*	Germany
Chigger; red bug	USA
Tlalzuatl	Mexico
Bicho colorado	Panama; Argentina
Coloradillo	Mexico; Panama; Honduras
Kedani; *akamushi*	Japan
Gonone	Celebes, Indonesia
Scrub itch; ti-tree itch	Australia
Mokka	New Guinea

Morphology of Trombiculids

The following description of the harvest mite *N. autumnalis* is based on that of Hirst (1915). It is the larva of an acarine mite some 150–300 μm long (Gordon and Lavoipierre 1962) with an unsegmented body, a gnathosome and three pairs of legs (Fig. 22.1). The body is oval with a transverse, slightly concave anterior margin. On the anterior half of the dorsal aspect is the sclerotised scutum, which is wider than it is long and also has a transverse anterior border but a slightly convex posterior edge. It has seven setae arranged as shown, those on the pseudostigmata being especially long. A pair of what appear to be eyes are situated on either side of the scutum. There are several rows of serrated setae arranged transversely. The number of setae in these rows varies slightly but generally seems to be used as one of several distinguishing anatomical features. Hirst did not regard them as very reliable identifying features, but Womersley and Heaslip (1943), Jenkins (1949) and Fuller (1952) all used them as characteristics which had different arrangements in different species. The palps (Fig. 22.1c, Fig. 22.2) are very distinctive because of the plumose setae, which are mainly on the ventral aspect. Some quite smooth setae occur on the lateral and dorsal aspects. There are six or seven feathered setae on the palpal tarsus, which ends in a marked three-pronged claw, the central prong being easily the most prominent. The legs are as shown in

Table 22.2. Species of trombidiform or prostigmatic mites, the larvae of which cause skin lesions in man. Generic placements according to Vercammen-Grandjean (1965, 1968). Synonymy after Wharton and Fuller (1952)

Species	Synonyms in literature	Distribution
Trombiculidae		
Neotrombicula autumnalis	*Leptus autumnalis*; *Microthrombidium autumnalis*; *Trombicula autumnalis*; *T. tlalzahuatl*[c]	Europe; United Kingdom
N. desaleri	*Trombicula desaleri*	
N. falrenholzi	*Microthrombidium falrenholzi*	
N. inoperatus	*Trombicula inoperatus*[a]	
Eutrombicula alfreddugesi	*E. tropica*; *Neotrombicula alfredduyesi*; *Trombidium cinnabarensis*; *T. irritans*; *Trombicula tlalzahuatl*[c]	USA; Central America; northern South America
E. batatas	*E. hominis*	South and east coasts of USA; Central America; northern South America
E. samboni		Central America
E. wichmanni	*Trombicula pseudoakamushi*; *T. minor*	Southeast Asia; Philippines; Australia; New Guinea
Blankartia acuscutellaris	*Trombicula acuscutellaris*	Sumatra; Selangor
Leptotrombidium akamushi	*Trombicula akamushi*[b]; *T. fletcheri*	Japan; New Guinea, Sumatra
L. deliensis	*Leeuwenhoekia deliensis*[b]	Malay; East Indies; New Guinea; Australia
Acariscus masoni	*Eutrombicula masoni*; *E. splendens*	South coast and southeast of USA
Doloisia brasiliensis	*Eutrombicula brasiliensis*	Brazil
Schoengastia katoni		
S. schuffneri		Sumatra; New Guinea
S. vandersandei		Dutch East Indies; New Guinea
Derrickiella coorongensis	*Schoengastia coorongensis*	Australia
Parascoschoengastia nunezi	*Euschoengastia nunezi*; *Neoschoengastia nunezi*	Mexico
Leeuwenhoekiidae		
Odontacarus australiensis	*Acomatacarus australiensis*	Australia
O. hirsti	*Leeuwenhoekia hirsti*	Far East; New Guinea; Australia
Trombidiidae		
Allothrombidium fuliginosum		France; Europe

[a] Doubtful species.
[b] Vectors of scrub typhus.
[c] Wharton and Fuller (1952) regard *T. tlalzahuatl* as a mixture of *N. autumnalis* and *E. alfreddugesi*.

Fig. 22.1a, the tarsi terminating in a pair of curved narrow claws and a claw-like empodium.

The features used for classification include the shape of the scutum, the characteristics and positioning of the seven setae of the scutum, the shape of the palps and their chaetotaxy, together with the arrangements of the rows of setae on the dorsal aspect of the body. Interested readers should consult special reference works, such as *A Manual of Parasitic Mites of Medical and Economic Importance* by Baker et al. (1956), which has a very useful bibliography.

Biology of Trombiculids

No two authors agree about the duration of the life cycle. This is partly because different species are discussed but principally because of the difficulty in following the full life history of an individual species. The stages through which trombiculid mites pass are egg, deutovum (mature embryo), larva, protonymph (nymphochrysalis), nymph, pre-adult (deutonymph; imagochrysalis) and adult. The total life cycle can be up to 1 year but is greatly

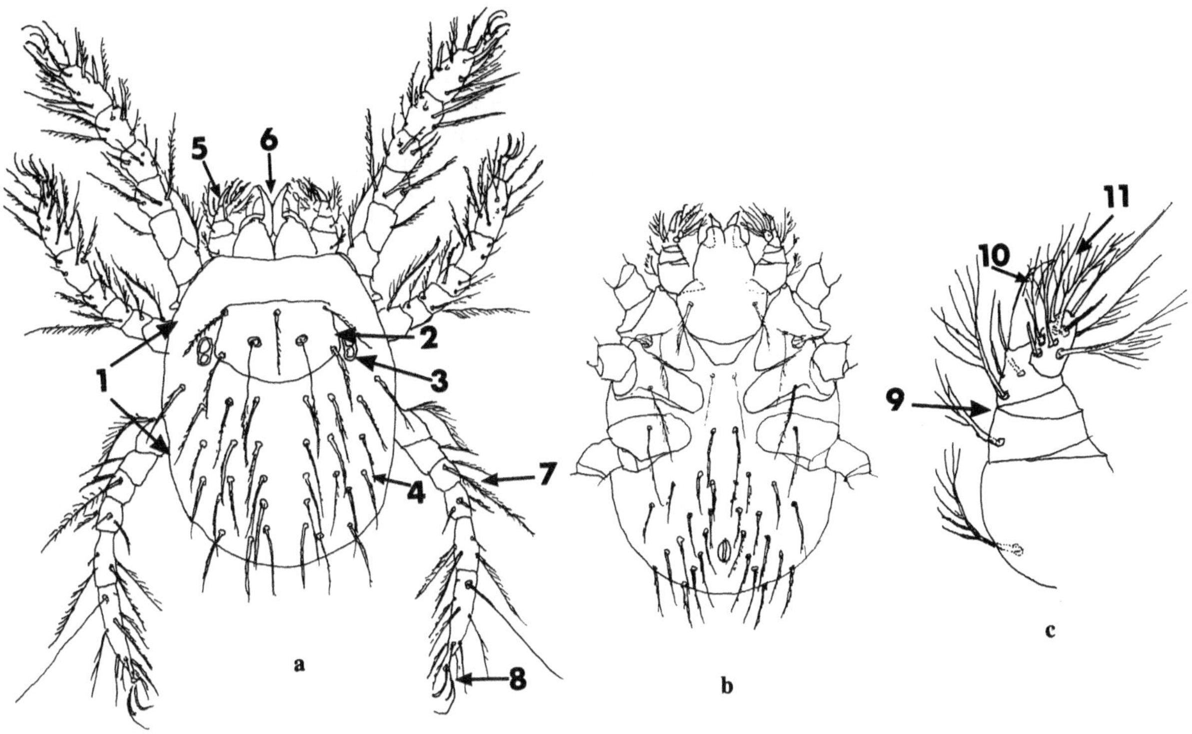

Fig. 22.1a–c. *Neotrombicula autumnalis*, Shaw. **a** Larva, dorsal view. Note seven setae on scutum. **b** Larva, ventral view. **c** Palp, ventral view. Note the plumed setae. *1*, body; *2*, scutum; *3*, pseudostigmata; *4*, transverse rows of body setae; *5*, palp; *6*, chelicerae; *7*, leg; *8*, claws and clawed empodium; *9*, palp with details of chaetotaxy; *10*, palpal claw; *11*, plumed tarsal setae (After Hirst 1915)

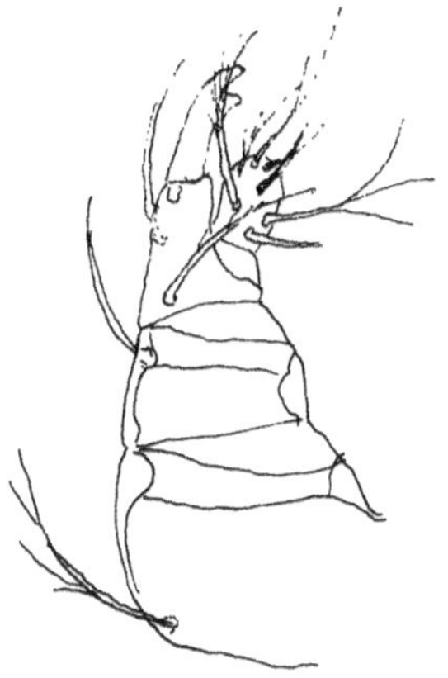

Fig. 22.2. Palp of *Eutrombicula wichmanni*, for comparison with Fig. 22.1c. (After Sambon 1927)

influenced by environmental temperature, relative humidity and availability of food sources. In tropical climates, where eggs are laid all the year round, there may be two generations or even more per annum, whereas in temperate zones reproductive activity is confined to the spring and summer (Gordon and Lavoipierre 1962). The spherical eggs, measuring about 150 μm in diameter, are deposited in clumps of up to 100 in soil (André 1937). According to Gordon and his colleague (1962), about 30–40 per month are laid, although Jenkins (1948) stated that in the laboratory the number was from 7 to 15 daily with some variation between species. The rate diminishes with fall in the temperature. Jenkins also observed an ovulation cycle of 14 days independent of any outside influence.

The eggs hatch after some 7–14 days, the period varying with the species. In some cases the latter half of the period is spent as a deutovum or embryo which lies dormant in a broken egg casing (Michener 1946). The larvae which emerge are very active and swarm over the surface of the soil and onto low vegetation such as grass and low-lying leaves. They tend to congregate on the edges of the leaves or tops of pebbles waiting for a passing host and are never more than a few centimetres from the ground (André 1938; Jenkins 1948). Ewing (1921) denied that the larvae ever left the ground, but Shelmire (1937) reported that he had deliberately induced infestation in people by making them sit on a moving vehicle and dangling their feet into low grass without touching the ground. Most workers are now agreed that the larvae do in fact climb onto low vegetation in the search for a vertebrate host. Some species, e.g. *Eutrombicula batatas*, prefer moist sunny areas with low leaf shade (Michener 1946), others such as *Acariscus masoni* like swampy, damp, deciduous areas, whilst *E. alfreddugesi* prefer wooded areas (Jenkins 1948). *N. autumnalis* has a preference for chalky soil, although this is not absolute. The larvae do not always find a host immediately and, according to Jenkins, can withstand starvation for up to 30 days. In an enclosed area such as a walled garden all the larvae tend to congregate on the sunny side beneath the shade of low leaves or grass. They are gregarious and in the evening collect in masses some 4–5 mm across to spend the night before dispersing again the next day (André 1937). The larvae of some species spend the cold months on a vertebrate host. Birds (D'Alberto 1875, cited by Musgrave 1943) and some reptiles (Chandler 1961) have been noted to have reddish or orange spots or tubercles on their skin, which on close examination have proved to be massed clumps of trombiculid larvae. This is a means of dispersing the species to find other hosts.

When a host is found the larvae transfer to it at once and seek out an area where the skin is soft, such as the ears, genitalia, axillae, mammae (Gordon and Lavoipierre 1962). These areas, together with those on man where there is constriction caused by clothing, are always the most heavily infested. Engorgement takes on average from 1 to 4 days but on some reptiles may require up to 48 days (Jenkins 1948). Whilst the larvae may overwinter on a host, such as in the ear of a rabbit (Keay 1934; Chandler 1961), they generally fall to the ground after feeding, creep into the surface soil and emerge after varying periods—1 month (André 1938), about 7 days (Herms 1950 Gordon and Lavoipierre 1962), 5–7 days (Michener 1946), 2 days (Jenkins 1948)—as an octopod nymph, which, after another week or so, becomes an adult. Nymphs and adults live amongst the surface soil feeding on insects, their eggs and general vegetable debris. However, they have been found at a depth of 1.8 m (6 ft) (Howard 1934, cited by André 1937). Richards (1950) said that in general the adults lived at a depth of about 1 m (3 ft), approaching the surface in warm weather but driven deeper by ground frost. The tendency of the adults to oviposit in the same area year after year prompted Gordon and Lavoipierre (1962) to regard them as habitat specific rather than host specific. The variety of animals which can serve as hosts would seem to support this viewpoint. Richards (1950) has also pointed out that whilst the adult population remains more or less constant, the larvae have a seasonal incidence, at least in temperate climates.

The animals which can act as hosts are very numerous. Jenkins (1948) listed 83 species, which include rodents and other small mammals, turtles, lizards, snakes and domestic animals, as well as man.

Clinical Features

The following account is based on that by Toomey (1921), except where stated. Many features described are common to all species. The moment of actual invasion is usually unnoticed. The larvae wander over the infested person's skin seeking a suitable feeding place. Hirst (1925) indicated that these were moist areas such as axillae, groins and cubital and popliteal fossae. Gordon and Lavoipierre (1962) regarded these areas as places of preference because the skin is thinner there, whereas Allington and Allington (1954) stated that trombiculids preferred covered areas for feeding, especially where the clothing was restricted. When the lesions first appear it is generally around the ankles, spreading to the dorsum and sides of the feet (Fig. 22.3). These latter areas are more commonly attacked in children. Lesions between the toes and over the toe joints are very frequent. However, the commonest area of attack on the feet is along the line of the top of the shoes, which agrees with a similar view expressed by MacLennan (1905), who also found lesions at the top of leggings and in the region of garters. Lesions are especially liable to occur in the popliteal fossae. The thighs are less commonly involved, but areas of predilection are the iliac crests, sacral region and around the waist, as well as in the groins and on the genitalia. Sometimes only the buttocks are affected. On the upper part of the body the thorax, upper back and upper abdominal wall are involved more often than the upper limbs; when the latter are affected the lesions occur commonly on the wrists, cubital fossae or axillae. A few lesions may appear on the collar line. Tropical species have a special preference for the prepuce, umbilicus and eyelids. In Mexico the species *Neoschongastia nunezi*, which is parasitic on poultry, attacks man on the scalp, neck, back, axillae and retroauricular folds (Nuñez-Andrade 1960).

Maude (1901), MacLennan (1905) and Chittenden (1915) agreed that those parts nearest to the ground suffered most, although Parkhurst (1937) pointed out that the upper trunk is so often in-

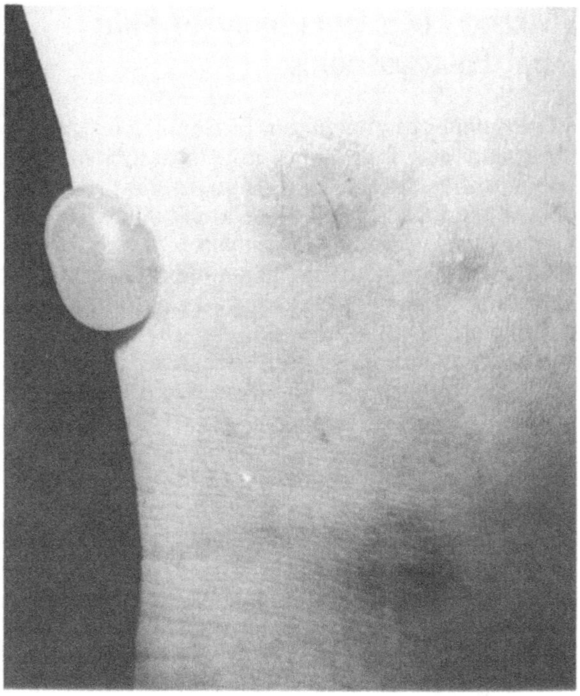

Fig. 22.3. Urticarial and bullous lesions around the ankle, thought to be caused by the bite of *Neotrombicula autumnalis*. Bullae are not uncommonly found around the ankle from this cause. Note also in the *centre* of the picture at the same level as the bulla a tiny papular lesion with an erythematous halo and at the *bottom* a similar lesion with a central haemorrhagic punctum.

volved that he suspected infestation from shoulder-high sources. Most other workers, however, consider this to be incorrect and that the upper trunk is involved because of the wandering propensities of the larvae or possibly because the subject has been lying on the ground. All are agreed that areas where the clothing causes constriction (e.g. under garters, the elastic in the legs and waistbands of undergarments, belts or brassières) are special targets for attack. In heavy infestation the whole body may be covered with lesions (D'Alberto 1875; Gunther 1938, both cited by Musgrave 1943).

Some 2–4 h after initial exposure the patient experiences a tingling sensation accompanied by pale anaemic macules about 2–3 mm in diameter. In the centre of some of these one or possibly two mites may be seen as minute red points. Over the next 10–16 h the macule increases in size and develops a central, red, dome-shaped papule (acuminate if at a hair follicle orifice). In those lesions described in Australia by Musgrave there were no symptoms for 6–12 h after exposure and then a papule 3–6 mm in diameter with a red areola appeared. When these papular lesions appear, itching begins, increasing rapidly in severity over the next 20–30 h. It has a smarting, burning character, is intermittent and unrelieved by scratching (Parkhurst 1937). It may progress further to an oedematous weal with a tiny central vesicle, the whole persisting for some 8–15 days before beginning to subside. These papular or urticarial lesions may become haemorrhagic with a dull purple hue, especially on the abdomen and lower limbs (Frazier 1969). The itch disappears as the papules involute, but if the latter are haemorrhagic the itch persists until the haemorrhagic element has cleared. Vesicles, when present, may subside, dry up and fall off as a scale but more usually they are scratched and replaced by a tiny crust. Very occasionally bullae may occur (Fig. 22.3). Maude (1901) recorded the appearances of tiny ulcers early on in the course of the disorder. Musgrave (1943) also noted these and observed that they tended to enlarge and take a long time to heal. Sambon (1927) cited Jackson [1908] as noting that the "legs below the knees were quickly reduced to a raw state because of the intense irritation" (and scratching). The shape and size of the lesions, especially the papules, depends rather on the site of the lesions than the species of mite (Gordon and Lavoipierre 1962). When the lesions heal they may leave residual pigmentation (MacLennan 1905; Frazier 1969). According to Toomey (1921), persistent nodules may also occur occasionally. He stated that pustules never appear; however, Pernet (1901) reported two instances, and in the eruption caused by *N. nunezi* in Mexico not only do pustules occur but some are umbilicated (Nuñez-Andrade 1960) and may be followed by scarring (Andrews and Domonkos 1971). When the genitalia are involved the oedematous phase may be very severe. In young uncircumcised boys this may cause painful paraphimosis (Frazier 1969).

Complications

The commonest complication is secondary infection, usually staphylococcal, from scratching, with lymphangitis and lymphadenopathy (Parkhurst 1937). Chittenden (1915) noted that occasionally erysipelas might supervene. Generalised urticaria has been reported (Maude 1901; Parkhurst 1937; Andrews and Domonkos 1971). Andrews and Domonkos also noted occasional widespread erythema.

Immunology

Very little has been written about the immunology of trombiculid infestation. As with other arthropods it appears that natives or long-term residents in endemic areas are relatively immune. Parkhurst (1937) remarked that some racial groups appear to be particularly resistant to the larval bite and cited the Papuans of New Guinea. On the other hand, Sambon (1927) was equally emphatic that, in addition to Australians in general, the Aboriginal inhabitants of that continent also suffered from bites. Ewing (1921) stated that no one had been clearly shown to be immune. Moreover, visitors to an endemic area are especially susceptible and may suffer severely.

The development of immunity to trombiculid larval bites is similar to that in relation to other arthropods, as described in Chapter 2. Those who are exposed in childhood probably initially suffer in the same manner as visitors but quickly develop an increasing tolerance. The general impression is thus given that the indigenous population is immune (Parkhurst 1937; Finnegan 1945; Chandler 1961). The itching felt seems to have two sources. Firstly the digestive enzymes in the mite's saliva causes a burning, smarting sensation, as do other arthropod salivary secretions and proteolytic enzymes. The more widespread itch is the result of acquired sensitivity to the antigenic material in those secretions. In fact, Parkhurst (1937) noted that antibodies to trombiculid saliva had been demonstrated by the Prausnitz–Kustner reaction.

Permanent residents in an infested area develop a high degree of tolerance to *continued* bites, and since these are probably regular throughout the season of larval abundance the immunity increases. After the larvae disappear no further biting occurs until the next year. After the new brood appears the first bites may provoke an itching reaction but act as an immunity booster dose so that no further reactions occur during the season (Chandler 1961). Visitors, however, are only attacked irregularly over short periods and develop no immunity. Therefore they continue to react unless they are regular visitors, in which case a partial immunity may develop. The occurrence of occasional outbreaks of urticaria is an indication of hypersensitivity. Parkhurst (1937) noted that in some areas with many chiggers no one seems to get bitten.

Method of Attachment to Skin and Histopathology

The manner of attachment of trombiculid larvae to the skin was for a long time a source of much debate. At first it was thought that the larva became attached rather like a tick and extended a long tongue through the puncture wound torn in the epidermis by the chelicerae (Trouessart 1899). However, Ewing (1921) showed clearly that it was firmly attached to the skin by the palpal claws forced downwards and backwards into the epidermis, whilst the chelicerae with their ventral barbs pierced the upper dermis only. Feng and Hoeppli (1933) studied experimental trombiculid bites and feeding on the skin of the gecko and also in the mosquito. They noted a homogeneous, eosinophilic, cell- and nuclear-free zone extending from the mouthparts inwards. This represented host tissue altered by mite salivary secretion. It was toughened by coagulation so as to remain rigid. Continuing mite secretion dissolved the centre forming a hollow tube. Ewing (1944) studied mite attachment on his own skin and noted similar changes. At no time was the formed tube part of the mite itself. Finnegan (1945) described the whole process succinctly. She stated that after attachment a histiolytic substance was secreted which broke down the tissues of the host. In the centre of this lysed tissue a clear canal appeared which gradually lengthened (up to 120 μm). It was straight or curved, looking like a hyaline tube which was continuous with the chelicerae, and could be separated from the surrounding tissues by dissection. Finnegan called it a "histiosiphon", which did not imply any affinity with any mouthpart (and it was the equivalent of Trouessart's "langue" and the "stylostome" of Jourdain 1899). It was soluble in concentrated alkali, which distinguished it from any chitinous structure. This description has not been bettered. The mite continues to secrete saliva with its contained digestive enzymes into the tube and sucks up liquid digest. Jones (1950) considered the secretion and sucking as alternating processes. The larva does not feed on blood. Ewing (1921) described the detachment of the larva as the result of wriggling backwards and forwards and sideways for several minutes.

The histological changes around and accompanying the formation of the histiosiphon have been described at various times by different writers and at different stages of the process. They are in fact a continuous series of changes, the severity of the response being dependent on the irritating quality of the saliva of the different species (Rook 1979).

The following description is based on Toomey's (1921) clinical stages.

1. The early stage of spastic ischaemia corresponds to the pale anaemic macules clinically. No histology of this stage has been published.
2. In the next stage of arteriolar vasodilation the papillary vessels are not engorged or dilated, those affected being the larger vessels of the mid-corium, around which there is a cuff of lymphocytes. The upper corium is oedematous, spreading from below upwards with some fibrin deposition but no cellular infiltrate. There is some early collagen degeneration, early lysis of lymphocytes and the appearance of an occasional polymorphonuclear cell.
3. The third or haemorrhagic stage is an accentuation of the second with the addition of capillary haemorrhage and some epidermal intracellular oedema. The haemorrhage quickly coagulates.
4. Epidermal oedema now appears with tiny subepidermal vesicles forming, the contents of which are sterile and consist of a few lymphocytes. The digestive damage by mite saliva in the corium is at its height at this stage.
5. This is the involutionary stage when the damaged tissues, cells and hyaline tube are gradually absorbed. Blood pigment appears amongst the dermal tissues. If the reaction has been especially severe there may be some fibrosis or even the formation of nodules.

There is often a tiny collar of hyperkeratosis around the puncture wound forming a support to the mouthparts of the mite (Parkhurst 1937). Rook (1979) has added that in very acute reactions (such as that mentioned by Jackson in Australia and cited by Sambon 1927) there would be epidermal changes of an eczematous nature with oedema and a neutrophil infiltrate in the corium giving rise later to a lymphocytic infiltrate and a granulomatous reaction.

Epidemiology

Harvest bugs attack both sexes indiscriminately but may appear to favour one or the other because of the extent or type of exposure. For example, women have been held to be more liable to attack because of the delicacy of their skin (Thresh 1906; Chittenden 1915), when in fact the reason is more likely to be the greater extent to which the skin around their ankles is exposed to infestation than that of men. Conversely, men are said to be more frequently bitten, but if this is the case it is because they are more likely to be exposed on account of their outdoor occupations (Armstrong 1901). With equal exposure, such as sitting or lying on infested grass at a picnic or beneath trees, especially ti-trees (tea-trees; Hirst 1929), the liability to be bitten applies equally to men and women. Clayton-Jones (1901) maintained that men wearing trousers were better protected than men wearing knee britches (see also under Management, p. 361).

Similar arguments apply to age as to sex. Children may be more easily bitten because they are more likely to go barefoot (Chittenden 1915) or wear sandals without socks (MacLennan 1905). They may develop extensive eruptions as a result of lying in grass (Clayton-Jones 1901).

There appears to be no ethnic difference in susceptibility, except in so far as persons of a certain racial group may be the indigenous population of an infested area, and it is then a question of acquired immunity.

In temperate climates the larvae usually appear in late summer and autumn (July to October in the northern hemisphere and December to April in the southern hemisphere). Farkaš (1977) noted their appearance in the Bratislava area of Czechoslovakia in May to June and again in September to October. Outbreaks in the United States occur at different times according to the climatic conditions and the species of trombiculids concerned (Jenkins 1948). In tropical climates man may be bitten at any time of the year because the environmental temperature is constantly favourable to proliferation of the mites.

Different species are involved in different areas (see Table 22.2). The epidemiology of scrub typhus is similar in this respect. The mites in these cases are abundant in the underbrush and debris of the floor of the rainforests, especially alongside water. Schüffner (1915) recorded that on an estate in Sumatra the workers were particularly liable to attack and to development of the fever. In most of Southeast Asia and New Guinea the chief sufferers were soldiers who developed scrub typhus or scrub itch. (It was said that the bites resulting from those species which vectored typhus did not itch; see below). A notable exception was in northern Burma where trombiculid bites, at least those resulting in scrub typhus, caused no lesions in World War II (Fuller 1947). Herms (1959) noted that scrub typhus, whilst endemic in Southeast Asia, occurred only at low altitudes in Formosa, although in India it was seen at heights of between 1980 m (6500 ft) and 2430 m (8000 ft). The coastal area of Queensland and the margins of the tropical rainforests there are also endemic areas of scrub typhus, where the trombiculid mites are said to be disseminated by lizard and bird hosts (Southcott 1947). Different species of mites, not vectors of typhus but causing a scrub itch, also occur in these and other Australian areas (Sambon 1927; Musgrave 1943; Derrick and Womersley 1954; Campbell and Domrow 1974). In general terms trombiculid larvae are few or absent in well-cultivated areas in these and other regions (Chittenden 1915). In both the United Kingdom and the United States they are said to be associated with gooseberry bushes and raspberry canes (Chittenden 1915; Ewing 1921), but whether this is correct is somewhat doubtful in view of their preference for low-lying vegetation. Perhaps red spider mites (Tetranychidae) were mistaken for trombiculids in these instances.

The severity of attacks in any of these areas depends on the number of mites involved, which in turn depends on host availability. In the tropical regions the hosts are mainly small rodents, which are abundant, although birds, reptiles and even amphibia can act as hosts. Audy (1951), in a study of the relationship between these mites and their hosts, noted that the longer the association, in evolutionary terms, between parasite and host the less likely the former was to harm the latter. Conversely, when the normal host and accidental host (man) are less closely related the more likely reactions are to arise in the accidental host. A marked reaction on the part of the host indicates that the parasite is exploring a new field. Audy then suggested that those larvae causing severe reactions (scrub itch) were normally parasitic on reptiles and birds, whereas the mites which act as vectors for scrub typhus are parasitic on mammals, which are much more closely related to man, and therefore an itching skin reaction is less likely.

Diagnosis

Diagnosis depends upon a number of factors. A history of exposure to harvest bugs and the finding and identification of one or more provide positive proof, but are not always forthcoming. The clinical picture of multiple itching lesions appearing suddenly should raise the suspicion of arthropod origin. The distribution, especially around the ankles as well as elsewhere, including beneath tight clothing, is of some importance, indicating that the arthropods in question probably come from close to the ground. Clinically the individual lesions cannot readily be distinguished from the bites of several other arthropods such as gamasid mites, *Pyemotes* or *Cheyletiella* species, but these have a somewhat different distribution on the body. Inquiry as to the possibility of exposure such as at picnics or working in known infested areas should help, as would knowledge of the existence of infestation in other persons in the same area. A biopsy in a doubtful case might show the characteristic histiosiphon. The differential diagnosis includes scabies, pediculosis corporis, other mite infestations mentioned above, bites or stings from flying insects (which seldom affect covered areas), bugs and fleas and also papular urticaria. Non-parasitic diseases which might be confused with harvest bug infestation include eczema, lichen planus, dermatitis herpetiformis and pruritus (e.g. caused by biliary cirrhosis or a drug), in which there is little to see except scratch marks. All of these conditions have their own specific features, which must be looked for and excluded. Other arthropods, when present, should be identified if possible.

Management

There are three aspects to management, namely *palliative*, to relieve itch and destroy larva on the skin; *preventive*, to deter larvae from biting; and *environmental*, to eradicate the mite from the infested area.

Itch can be relieved with simple antipruritics such as 1% phenol or menthol in oily calamine lotion. If severe, topical corticosteroids with an anti-infective agent such as chinoform or aureomycin can be used. Secondary infection, if it arises, may require appropriate systemic antibiotics. Pillsbury et al (1942), Ebeling (1975) and the United States Department of Agriculture (1976) all recommended a topical preparation containing benzocaine. This is to be deprecated since it offers little advantage and has the great disadvantage that topical benzocaine is a powerful sensitising agent. It is important, especially in those areas where scrub typhus is endemic, that exposed persons should have a warm soapy bath as soon as they return from an infested area to get rid of any larvae which remain on the skin. Almost all workers in the study of trombiculids have advised this.

The prevention of bites by various means is more important than the topical treatment of actual bites, especially if there is a risk of scrub typhus. This can be achieved by the application of insecticidal repellents to the skin and particularly to the clothing. Prior to World War II, by far the most useful substance in this respect was sulphur, although Toomey (1921) considered it to be useless. It can be applied as an ointment direct to the skin but is only partially effective unless it is applied in sufficient quantity for the grease to act as an additional deterrent barrier for the mites. In fact Armstrong (1901), Clayton-Jones (1901), Chittenden (1915) and Toomey himself (1921) all advocated simple Vaseline, probably for the same reason. However, when sulphur is applied to the clothing it has a more effective repellent action. Many workers, including Ewing (1921), advised that it should be dusted into the clothing, but later Ewing (1925) noted that it tended to collect in the folds and could thus cause dermatitis. He therefore recommended that it should be mixed in strong soap solution and the inner and outer garments should be soaked in this and allowed to dry. This solution he claimed, afforded 100% protection. Madden et al. (1944) confirmed that it was effective for some hours but regarded it as unreliable and also prone to cause dermatitis. They found the best repellents were MYL (an antilouse powder, see Chap. 5), dimethylphthallate (DMP) solution or 2% rotenone in pyrophyllite powder. Pillsbury and his colleagues (1942), however, said that rotenone caused scrotal dermatitis. Madden et al. finally concluded that DMP solution was the best and cheapest repellent, whilst Indalone spray was also very efficient but more expensive. Other substances which have given good protection are diethyltoluamide (DEET), ethylhexanediol (Rutgers 612), dibutylphthallate and dimethylcarbate (DMC) (Finnegan 1945; Chandler 1961; Gouck 1966; Ebeling 1975; United States Department of Agriculture 1976).

Additional protection can be afforded by clothing made of fine-weave cloth (Ewing 1944), the cuff and trouser bottoms of which should be close fitting. Boots (especially long boots) are preferable to shoes, and puttees give added protection. Ewing also advised that it was only necessary to impregnate socks, trouser bottoms, sleeve cuffs and shirt collars to prevent mites from gaining access to the body.

Mites should also be eradicated by "environmental manipulation" (Philip and Woodward 1946). Undergrowth should be cut down, grass kept short, paths in infested forests should be at least 1.2 m (4 ft) wide (Musgrave 1943), debris which has been cut out should be burnt and rodents and other small mammalian hosts in infested areas should be destroyed. Apart from keeping lawns mowed, Chittenden (1915) advised keeping sheep in pastures as the best method of keeping the mites within bounds.

Cultivation of infested ground is one of the best means of reducing the population of trombiculids. At one time Ewing recommended dusting such ground with sulphur (50 lb/acre). Nowadays more effective chemicals such as toxaphene or chlordane (2 lb/acre) or gamma-benzene hexachloride ($\frac{1}{2}$ lb/acre) or dieldrin are used (Gordon and Lavoipierre 1962; Chandler 1961; Ebeling 1975). Where work of this kind has to be done, Philip and Kohls (1948) recommended employing local labourers because they would be more likely to be resistant to bite reactions and would probably have acquired an immunity to scrub typhus.

Other measures which have been advised include proper garbage disposal in camp sites (Musgrave 1943), never sleeping directly on infested ground in such camps (Frazier 1969) and education of those who have to work in infested regions (Finnegan 1945).

References

Allington HV, Allington RR (1954) Insect bites. JAMA, 155: 240–247
André M (1937) Sur l'apparition brusque des aoutats ou rouget (larves de *Thrombicula autumnalis* Shaw) (acariens). Bull Museum Nat Hist Nat 2(Ser 9): 378–383
André M (1938) Quelques observations sur la larve du *Thrombicula autumnalis* Shaw a l'état de vie libre. Bull Soc Zool Fr 63: 45–47
Andrews GC, Domonkos A (1971) Diseases of the skin, 6th edn. Saunders, Philadelphia, pp 390–391
Armstrong EA (1901) Harvest bugs. Lancet II: 709
Audy JR (1951) Trombiculid mites and scrub itch. Aust J Sci 14: 94–96
*Baker EW, Evans TM, Gould DT, Hull WE, Keegan HL (1956) A manual of parasitic mites of medical or economic importance. National Pest Control Association Inc, New York
Campbell RW, Domrow R (1974) Rickettsioses in Australia; isolation of *Rickettsia tsutsugamushi* and *R. australia* from naturally infected arthropods. Trans R Soc Trop Med Hyg 68: 395–402
Chandler AC (1961) Introduction to parasitology with special reference to the parasites of man, 10th edn. Wiley, New York, pp 531–536
Chittenden FH (1915) Harvest mites or 'chiggers'. US Dept of Agriculture Farmers Bulletin No 671. US Govt Printing Office, Washington DC, pp 1–7
Clayton-Jones O (1901) Harvest bugs. Lancet II: 758
Derrick EH, Womersley H (1954) The scrub-itch mite of Southeast Queensland. Aust J Sci 16: 238–239
Ebeling W (1975) Urban entomology. University of California, Division of Agricultural Science, Los Angeles, Cal
*Ewing HE (1921) Studies on the biology and control of chiggers. US Dept of Agriculture Bureau of Entomology Bulletin No 986. US Govt Printing Office, Washington DC, pp 1–19
Ewing HE (1925) Sulphur impregnated clothing to protect against chiggers. J Econ Entomol 18: 827–829
Ewing HE (1944) The trombiculid mites (chigger mites) and their relation to disease. J Parasitol 30: 339–365
Farkaš J (1977) Problems of trombiculosis and its sporadic incidence (in Czech). Cesk Dermatol 52: 100–106
*Feng LL, Hoeppli R (1933) On some histological changes caused by mites. Chin Med J 47: 1191–1199
*Finnegan S (1945) Acari as agents transmitting typhus in India, Australia and the Far East. British Museum (Natural History)

Economic Series No 16. London, Trustees of the British Museum, pp 7–78
Frazier CA (1969) Insect allergy (allergic reaction to bites of insects and other arthropods). Warren H. Green, St. Louis
Fuller HS (1947) Infestation of man in Burma with trombiculid mites, with special reference to *Trombicula deliensis*. Am J Hyg 45: 363–371
Fuller HS (1952) The mite larvae of the family Trombiculidae in the Oudemans Collection: Taxonomy and medical importance. Zool Verhandelingen No 18. E.J. Bell, Leiden, pp 1–261
Gordon RM, Lavoipierre MMJ (1962) Entomology for students of medicine. Blackwell, Oxford, pp 267–272
Gouck HS (1966) Protection from ticks, fleas, chiggers and leeches. Arch Dermatol 93: 112–113
Herms WB (1950) Medical entomology, 4th edn. Macmillan Company, New York
Hirst S (1915) On the "harvest bug" (*Microtrombidium autumnalis*, Shaw). J Econ Entomol 10: 73–77
Hirst S (1925) On a harvest bug (*Leeuwenhoekia australiensis* sp. n.) attacking human beings at Sydney, New South Wales. Trans R Soc Trop Med Hyg 19: 150–152
Hirst S (1929) Note on the "Tea-tree itch mite" (*Trombicula hirsti*, Sambon. — *T. pseudo-akamushi*, Hato.) Annu Mag Nat Hist 3(Ser 10): 564–565
Jenkins DW (1948) Trombiculid mites affecting man. I. Bionomics with reference to epidemiology in the United States. Am J Hyg 48: 22–35
Jenkins DW (1949) Trombiculid mites affecting man. III. *Trombicula (Eutrombicula) splendens* Ewing in North America. J Parasitol 35: 201–204
Jones BM (1950) The penetration of the host tissue by the harvest mite *Trombicula autumnalis* Shaw. Parasitology 40: 247–260
Jourdain (1899) Le styloproct de l'uropode végétant et le stylostoma des larves de trombidon. Arch Parasitol 11: 28–33. Cited by Trouessart (1899)
Keay G (1937) The ecology of the harvest mite (*Trombicula autumnalis*) in the British Isles. J Anim Ecol 6: 23–35
MacLennan W (1905) The *Leptus autumnalis* and its skin lesions. Lancet II: 1765–1766
Madden AH, Lindqvist AW, Knipling EF (1944) Tests of repellents against chiggers. J Econ Entomol 37: 283–286
Maude A (1901) Harvest bugs. Lancet II: 562
Michener CD (1946) Observation on the habits and life history of a chigger mite, *Eutrombicula batatas* (Acarinae: Trombiculinae). Ann Entomol Soc Am 39: 101–118
Musgrave A (1943) Some arachnids and millipedes from New Guinea. Austr Museum Mag 8: 132–135
Nuñez-Andrade R (1960) Dermatozoonosis. Rev Med Mex 40: 449–467
Palm TA (1878) Some account of a disease called "shimamushi" or "island insect disease" by the natives of Japan; peculiar, it is believed, to that country and hitherto not described. Edinburgh Med J 24: 128–132
Parkhurst HJ (1937) Trombidiosis (infestation with chiggers). Arch Dermatol Syphilol 35: 1011–1036
Pernet G (1901) Harvest bugs. Lancet II: 616, 758
Philip CB, Kohls GM (1948) Mites and scrub typhus. Proceedings of the 4th international congress of tropical medicine and hygiene, May 1948, Washington DC. 2: 1656–1663
Philip CB, Woodward TE (1946) Tsutsugamushi disease (scrub- or mite-borne typhus) in the Philippine Islands during American re-occupation in 1944–1945. II Observations on trombiculid mites. J Parasitol 32: 502–515
Pillsbury DH, Sulzberger MB, Livingood CS (1942) Manual of dermatology. Saunders, Philadelphia, pp 329–340
Richards WS (1950) The distribution and biology of the harvest mite in Great Britain (Trombiculidae: Acarina) Parasitology 40: 118–126
Rook A (1979) Skin diseases caused by arthropods and other venomous or noxious animals, In: Rook A, Wilkinson DS, Ebeling FJG (eds) Textbook of dermatology, 3rd edn. Blackwell, Oxford, pp 911–954
Sambon LW (1927) The "scrub-itch mite" of North Queensland: a new species of Trombicula. Annu Mag Nat Hist 20(Ser 10): 157–161
Schüffner W (1915) Pseudotyphoid fever in Deli, Sumatra (a variety of Japanese kedani fever). Philippine J Sci (Biol) 10: 345–351
Shelmire B (1937) In discussion of Parkhurst (1937). Arch Dermatol Syphilol 35: 1011–1036
Southcott RV (1947) Observations on the epidemiology of tsutsugamushi disease in North Queensland. Med J Aust 2: 441–450
Thresh JC (1906) Erythema autumnale, harvest rash or prurigo du rouget. Lancet II: 1277
*Toomey N (1921) Trombidiasis (*Leptus autumnalis*). Urol Cutan Rev 25: 598–608
Touraine A (1947) Les traitements actuels des parasites animales de la peau. Baillière, Paris, pp 133–135
Trouessart EL (1899) Sur la pique de rouget. Arch Parasitol 11: 286–290
United States Department of Agriculture (1976) Home and Garden Bulletin No 137 Agricultural Research Service. US Govt Printing Office, Washington DC, pp 1-10
Vercammen-Grandjean P-H (1965) Revision of the genera *Eltonella* Audy 1956 and *Microtrombicula* Ewing 1950 with description of fifty new species and transferal of sub-genus *Chiroptella* to genus *Leptotrombidium* (Acarina: Trombiculidae). Acarologia 7(Suppl): 34–257
Vercammen-Grandjean P-H (1968) Chiggers of the Far East (Acarina: Trombiculiidae; and Leeuwenhoekiidae), vol 1. US Army Medical Research Development Command, Washington DC, p 138
Wharton GW, Fuller HS (1952) A manual of the chiggers. Mem Entomol Soc Washington 4: 1–185
Womersley H, Heaslip WG (1943) The Trombiculinae (Acarina) or itch mite of the Austro Malayan and oriental regions. Trans R Soc S Aust 67: 68–142

23 The Effects of Tick Bites

Ticks are the largest creatures of the class Acarina. They are very common, with many species and worldwide distribution. They are natural parasites of a great variety of animals, whether mammals, birds, reptiles or amphibians, but also cause numerous disorders in man. The form of reaction to their attachment to the skin may be as a foreign body effect, a local reaction to salivary secretion, a reaction to injected tick toxin, a generalised hypersensitivity reaction or even an animal's exsanguination through the sheer number of ticks involved. Hunter and Hooker (1901, cited by James and Harwood 1969) estimated that up to 200 lb of blood (about 100 litres) could be withdrawn by ticks from a large host animal in a single season. The greatest danger to man and animals, however, lies in the numerous infectious diseases which can be transmitted by ticks. Such diseases, caused by viruses, bacteria, spirochaetes, rickettsiae and protozoa, are listed in Table 23.1. Apart from listing the diseases it is not proposed to go any further into this aspect of tick bites, except where pertinent to the present subject. It is interesting that *Ixodes*-borne babeosis in animals was the first disease in which an arthropod was identified as a vector in 1893 (Ruebush et al. 1977).

Ticks attach to man for feeding purposes only, albeit out of biological necessity. In contrast, for example, to haematophagous flies, which bite, and then feed rapidly and very briefly, ticks remain attached to the human host for several days, feeding until so engorged with blood as to be several times their original size. They then detach themselves spontaneously, fall to the ground and continue their life cycle.

Morphology of Ticks

Ticks (Acarina: Parasitiformes; Metastigmata) are typical arachnids with an unsegmented body, a gnathosome (referred to as capitulum in the literature on ticks), consisting of the various mouthparts, and eight legs; the larvae have six legs (see Chap. 4). There are two groups of ticks, those which have a hard chitinous shield or scutum dorsally, the hard ticks or Ixodidae, and those without such a scutum, the soft ticks or Argasidae. The mouthparts of the Ixodidae project beyond the anterior end of the somewhat pear-shaped body and are visible viewed from above or below, whereas the body of the Argasidae completely conceals the mouthparts when viewed from above (see Fig. 23.6), and in this group the mouthparts can only be seen from the ventral aspect (see Fig. 23.7). The principal anatomical features of ixodid and argasid ticks are shown in Figs. 23.1 and 23.2 respectively. Note the position of the eyes, which are not always present, and the relative positions of the legs in the two families. In Ixodidae the shield completely covers the male, but in the female it is much smaller and only covers a small area posterior to the capitulum.

The mouthparts are shown in more detail in Figs. 23.3–23.5. A more intimate knowledge of their structure and function is necessary to understand the method of attachment to the host and why its premature removal before full engorgement, whilst essential for the host's well-being, should be carried out with great care so that portions of the capitulum should not break and be left behind in the skin. The gnathosome as a whole has a fused base which, viewed dorsally, varies in shape depending on the species (Arthur 1961). Its three distinct components, pedipalps, chelicerae and hypostome, are separated, except at the base. Laterally there is a pair of four-jointed pedipalps, the terminal segment of which is reduced in size and carries chemoreceptor sensillae. Medial to these on the dorsal surface are the two chelicerae, which, in addition to a bulbous base, have a straight, rigid, sclerotised shaft and a toothed terminal digit. Ventral to the chelicerae lies the hypostome, a stout single structure with backward-pointing teeth on its shaft. The gnathosome is longer in ixodid than in argasid ticks and in female

Table 23.1. Infectious diseases for which ticks act as vectors, with the principal ticks concerned. (Based on James and Harwood 1969)

Infectious disease	Tick vector	Remarks
Arboviruses		
1. Russian spring–summer encephalitis (RSSE)	*Ixodes persulcatus*	25–30% mortality
2. Central European tick-borne encephalitis	*Ixodes ricinus*	
3. Omsk haemorrhagic fever virus	*Dermacentor pictus*; *D. marginatus*; *Ixodes persulcatus*	0.5–3% mortality; rodents are reservoir hosts
4. Kyanasan Forest disease virus (Mysore, India)	*Haemaphysalis spinigera*; *H. turturis*	Virus also found in other spp., but not known whether they spread to man
5. Powassan virus (North America)	*Dermacentor andersoni*; *Ixodes spinipalpus*	*I. cookei and I. marxi* harbour virus, but not known whether they spread disease to man
Ungrouped viruses		
6. Colorado tick-fever virus (North America)	*Dermacentor andersoni*; *D. occidentalis*	Mostly children; virus also found in *Otobius lagophilus*; *D. parumpertus*; *Haemaphysalis leporispalustris*
7. Kemerovo virus (western Siberia)	*Ixodes persulcatus*	
8. Tribec virus (Czechoslovakia)	*Ixodes ricinus*	
9. Louping ill (United Kingdom)	*Ixodes ricinus*	Disease of sheep; can affect human contacts via ticks
10. Crimean haemorrhagic fever virus	*Hyalomma marginatum*	
11. Uzbekistan haemorrhagic fever virus (Central Asia)	*Hyalomma anatolicum*; *H. detritum*; *Rhipicephalus turanicus*	
12. Japanese encephalitis	*Ixodes*, *Haemaphysalis* and *Dermacentor* spp.	Less well established as tick-borne diseases, but the respective viruses have been found in the species of tick named
13. West Nile virus	*Argas reflexus hermanni*	
14. Equine encephalitis	*Hyalomma anatolicum*	
15. Lymphocytic choriomeningitis	*Amblyomma variegatum*; *Rhipicephalus sanguineus*	
Rickettsiae		
16. Rocky Mountain spotted fever	*Dermacentor andersoni*; *Haemaphysalis leporispalustris*	
17. Siberian tick typhus	Ixodid spp.	
18. Boutonneuse fever	*Rhipicephalus sanguineus* and spp. of *Haemaphysalis*; *Hyalomma*; *Amblyomma*; *Boophilus*; *Rhipicephalus*	Africa; Mediterranean coast; Southeast Asia. Almost any species of tick is or may be a vector
19. Epidemic typhus (louse-borne)		Can be tick transmitted in Ethiopia
20. Queensland tick typhus	*Ixodes holocyclus*	Clinically resembles rickettsialpox
21. Q fever		Worldwide; tick-borne in some areas, e.g. Queensland, Morocco, western Montana
22. Various veterinary Rickettsiae		May be important to man
Bacterial and spirochaetal		
23. Relapsing fever	*Ornithodorus* spp.	Reservoir in burrowing animals; mortality 2% (endemic) and up to 50% (epidemic)
24. Avian spirochaetosis	*Argas persicus*	Does not affect man
25. Tularaemia	*Dermacentor andersoni*; other ixodid ticks	Also direct infection without vector
Piroplasmosis		
26. Texan cattle fever	*Boophilus* spp.	Man unaffected
27. Equine piroplasmosis	Various spp. of various genera	Animal babeosis
28. Human babeosis	*Ixodes scapularis*; *I. dammini*	New England states; scattered areas in Europe
29. East Coast fevers	Several spp. of adults only	90% fatal to cattle; man unaffected
30. Bovine anaplasmosis	Several spp. of tick	Animals only, but worldwide; tabanids also vectors

than in male ixodids. The number and size of the teeth vary from species to species according to whether they are rapid or slow feeders. The latter, needing a longer period of attachment, have stronger and more numerous teeth.

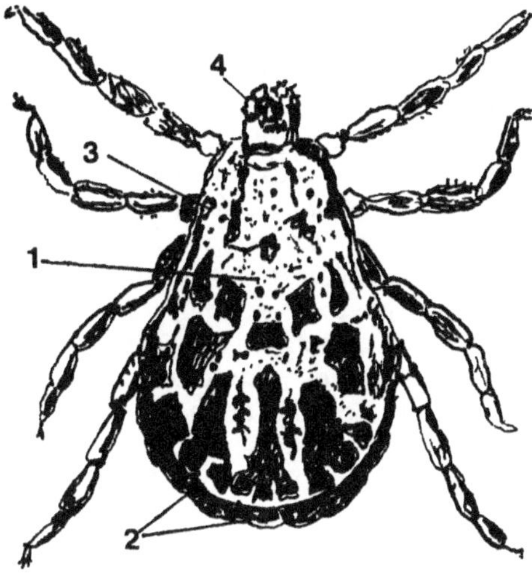

a

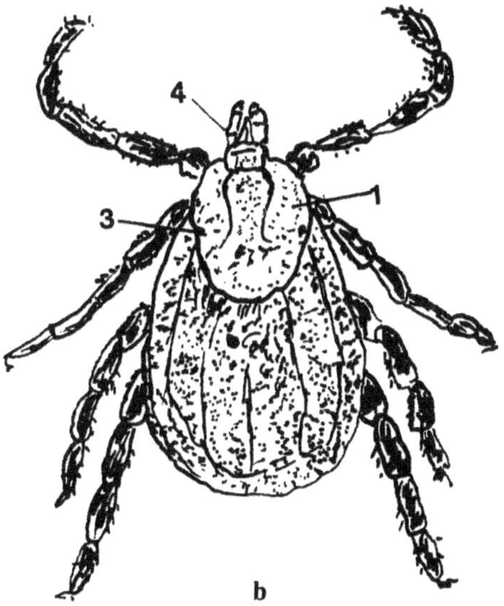

b

Fig. 23.1a, b. Ixodid tick (*Dermacentor venustus*) **a** dorsal view of male; **b** dorsal view of female. Note the scutum completely covers the male and has a characteristic pattern which varies from species to species. Female scutum is very much smaller. *1*, scutum; *2*, festoons on margins of male scutum; *3*, eye; *4*, mouthparts. [After Patton WS (1931) Insects, ticks, mites and venomous animals of medical and veterinary importance. Part II Public Health. H. R. Grubb, Croydon]

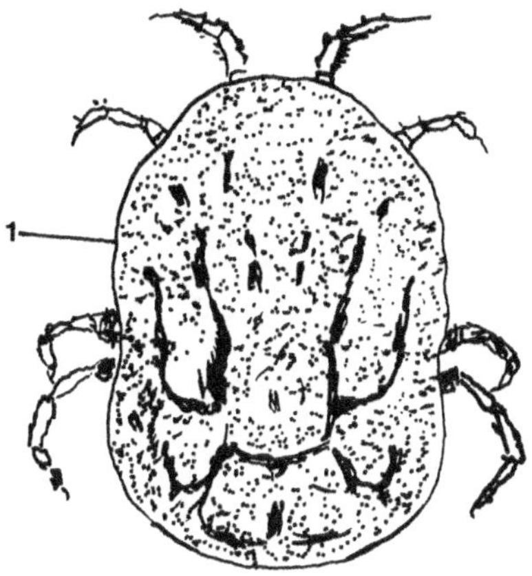

a

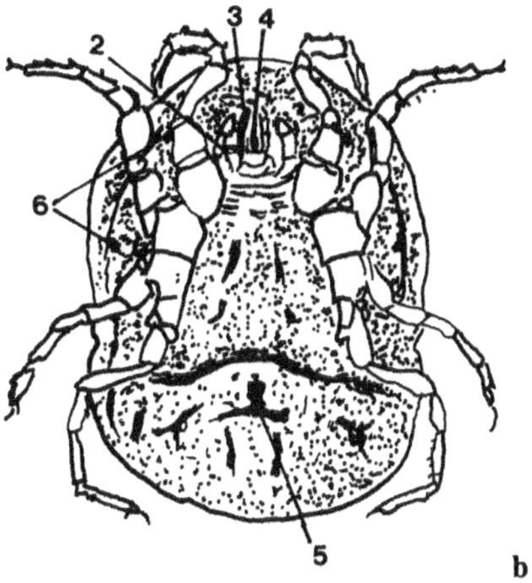

b

Fig. 23.2a, b. Argasid tick (*Ornithodorus savignyi*) **a** Dorsal view of female. Note the absence of a scutum and that the mouthparts are completely concealed. **b** Ventral view of female. *1*, soft body covering; *2*, pedipalps; *3*, chelicerae; *4*, hypostome; *5*, anal opening; *6*, eyes. [After Patton WS (1931) Insects, ticks, mites and venomous animals of medical and veterinary importance. Part II Public Health. H. R. Grubb, Croydon]

Attachment of Ticks to Host and Feeding Technique

When attaching itself to the host's skin the tick uses the rigid toothed chelicerae in a lateral tearing movement. This lacerates and cuts open the surface epidermis. At the same time salivary secretion may assist by softening tissues. This enables the toothed hypostome to be thrust into the opening, an operation which is assisted by the tick lifting itself at an angle by straightening its hindmost legs.

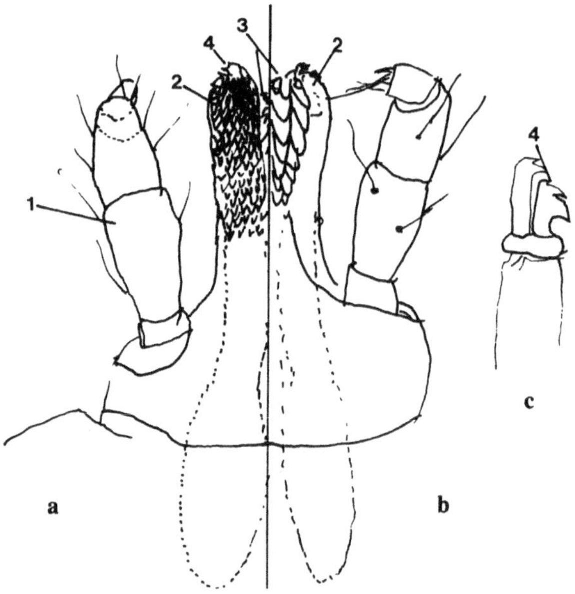

Fig. 23.3. Compound drawing of mouthparts of a tick (larva of *Amblyomma cajennense*), showing **a** dorsal view, **b** ventral view and **c** enlarged view of cheliceral teeth. *1*, pedipalp; *2*, chelicerae; *3*, toothed hypostome; *4*, teeth at tip of chelicera. [Modified from Patton WS (1931) Insects, ticks, mites and venomous animals of medical and veterinary importance. Part II Public Health. H. R. Grubb, Croydon]

As the tick penetrates deeper and becomes more fixed its body ultimately assumes a vertical stance. A cement-like substance is secreted intermittently in the saliva; this flows around the hypostome, setting hard in a laminated, interdigitating sheath which finally anchors the tick securely to the skin. Those ticks which are brief rapid feeders with shorter hypostomata, such as in the argasid group, are probably fixed in a somewhat similar manner, but most of the cement is near or on the surface, thus forming an adhesive union which is more easily separated.

When the tick is firmly attached there is haemorrhage around the tip of the hypostome as a result of the cytolytic and anticoagulant properties of the saliva. This liquid food source is rapidly sucked up via the hypostome into the hypopharynx and thence to the tick's gut. The feeding process continues whilst the tick slowly swells to many times its usual size. When it is completely engorged, which may take 6 or 7 days in ixodid ticks, its size may have increased a hundredfold or more. At this point it may remain attached to the host for an indeterminate period but usually it loosens its hold, wrenches its hypostome free and falls to the ground. [Fielding (1926), Arthur (1961) and Sheals (1973) are the source of much of this information.]

Biology and Habits of Ticks

Arthur's (1961) book contains a wealth of information on all aspects of tick biology. Ixodid ticks go through four stages, egg, larva, nymph and adult, a blood meal being required before any active stage can proceed to the next one. One, two or three different hosts may be necessary for these meals, depending on the species. There may be a considerable interval between the end of a meal and the development to the next stage, which makes the total life cycle vary greatly in length. For example, Nuttall et al. (1926) gave the duration of the cycle for *Amblyomma maculatum* (a host tick) as 110–359 days; for *A. americanum* it was 66–158 days. Some ticks appear to be parthenogenetic because the males have never been found on the host. Nuttall and his colleagues suggested that this could mean that the males were to be found in the habitat of the host rather than on the host itself and would require much further search.

The larvae of ixodid ticks find their host by chance. After emerging from the egg they climb to the top of grass stems or shrub twigs and await the passing of a suitable host. The presence of the latter is signalled chiefly by odour, but vibration, air current, interruption of incident light, warmth and moisture may all be stimulating factors (Arthur 1961). When the host brushes past, the tick (larva, nymph or adult) will cling to its coat or, in the case of man, to clothing.

Argasid ticks have a somewhat different life cycle. They may go through several moults of different nymph stages. There is little sexual dimorphism and they do not greatly increase in size as a result of feeding. Their principal hosts are birds, bats and man. They are commoner in warmer climates but do occur in colder regions, choosing a habitat (e.g. dwellings) which gives them protection: For example *Ornithodorus moubata* is found in native huts, especially in cracks in the walls or on the floor; *Argas vespertilionis* (Figs. 23.6, 23.7) lives in bat colonies, whilst *A. reflexus* inhabits pigeon coops or poultry houses. Both these genera are nocturnal, intermittent feeders, which find their hosts easily because they live in close proximity.

Most ticks can fast for long periods but do not live on the vegetable material which they inhabit (Newstead 1909). Large numbers of eggs are laid, in batches of up to 300, and the total in a life span may be as high as 7000, depending on species (Newstead 1909). The life may extend up to 15 or 16 years.

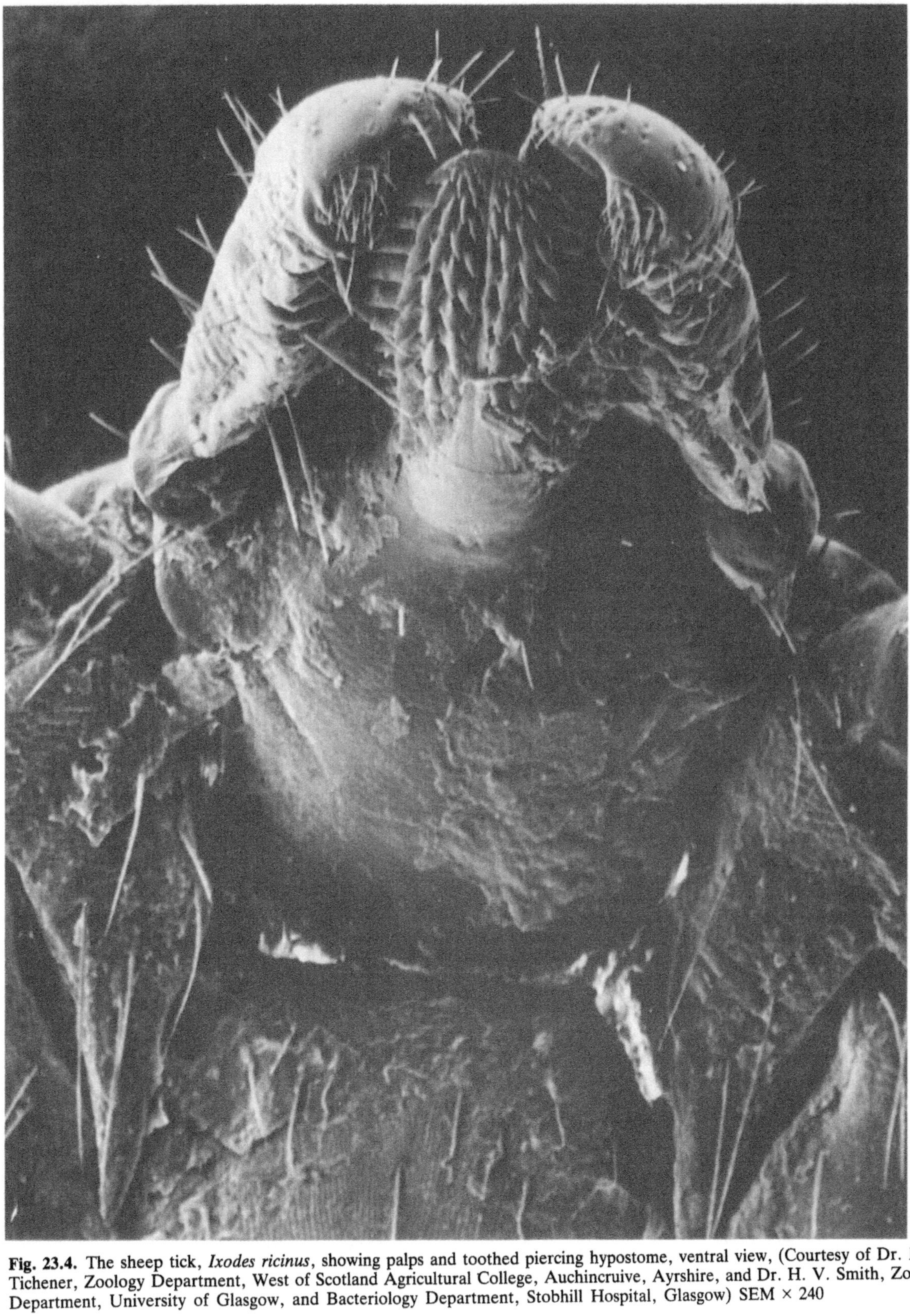

Fig. 23.4. The sheep tick, *Ixodes ricinus*, showing palps and toothed piercing hypostome, ventral view, (Courtesy of Dr. R. N. Tichener, Zoology Department, West of Scotland Agricultural College, Auchincruive, Ayrshire, and Dr. H. V. Smith, Zoology Department, University of Glasgow, and Bacteriology Department, Stobhill Hospital, Glasgow) SEM × 240

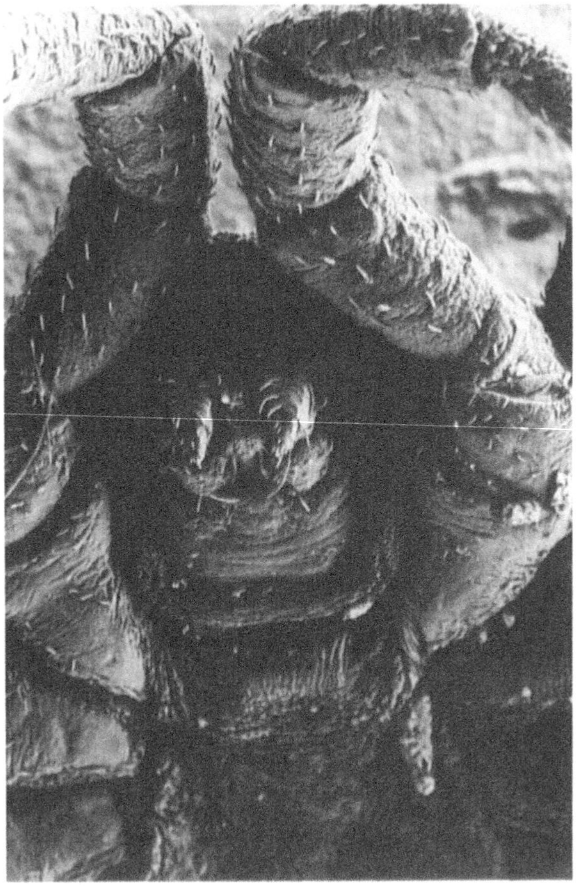

Fig. 23.5.

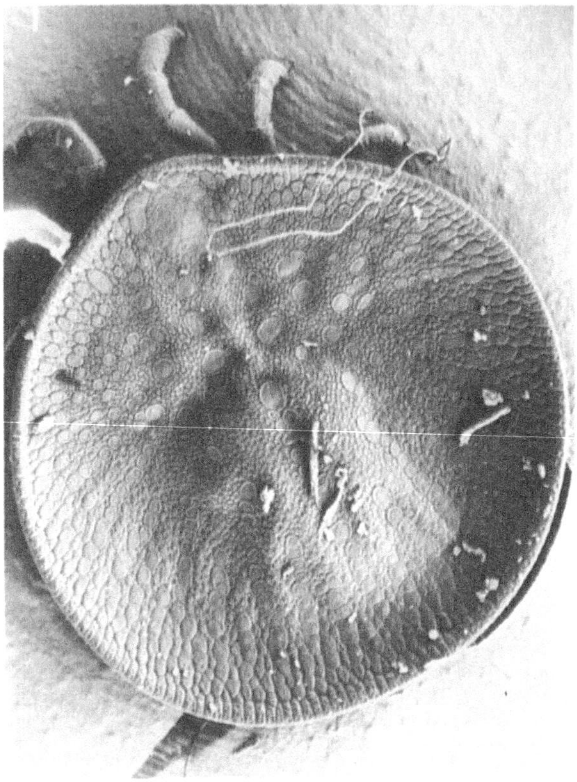

Fig. 23.6.

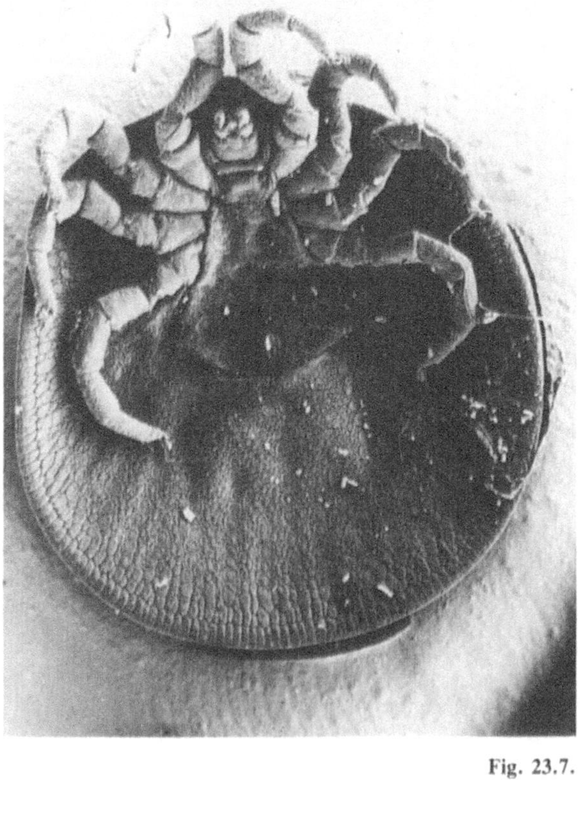

Fig. 23.7.

Fig. 23.5. *Argas vespertilionis*. Mouthparts seen from below. Note the paired central palps and the tip of the hypostome between them. (Courtesy of Dr. H. V. Smith, Zoology Department, University of Glasgow, and Bacteriology Department, Stobhill Hospital, Glasgow, and Dr. R. N. Titchener, Zoology Department, West of Scotland College of Agriculture, Auchincruive, Ayrshire) SEM × 80

Fig. 23.6. *Argas vespertilionis*, dorsal view. Note that the mouthparts are completely hidden. (Courtesy of Dr. H. V. Smith, Zoology Department, University of Glasgow, and Bacteriology Department, Stobhill Hospital, Glasgow, and Dr. R. N. Titchener, Zoology Department, West of Scotland College of Agriculture, Auchincruive, Ayrshire) SEM × 60

Fig. 23.7. *Argas vespertilionis*, ventral view, showing how the mouthparts are completely beneath the dorsal shield. (Courtesy of Dr. H. V. Smith, Zoology Department, University of Glasgow, and Bacteriology Department, Stobhill Hospital, Glasgow, and Dr. R. N. Titchener, Zoology Department, West of Scotland College of Agriculture, Auchincruive, Ayrshire) SEM × 60

The conditions of life vary from species to species. For example *Ixodes scapularis*, the cause (or causal agent) of Lyme disease, is dependent on the distribution of the hosts of its immature and adult forms, white-footed mice and white-tailed deer respectively (Wallis et al. 1978). Other species may live in arid regions on a variety of hosts. *Otobius megnini*, for instance, passes through its larval and nymphal to adult stages in the ear canals of these hosts, incidentally making this site attractive to myiasis-producing Diptera such as screwworm flies (Peacock 1958; Arthur 1961).

Man may be attacked in a variety of circumstances, picnicking in infested woods (*Dermacentor andersoni*), living in a heavily infested area (*D. variabilis*), having hosts infesting his house (e.g. bats with *Argas vespertilionis*), camping in infested caves (Condy et al. 1980) or in tents on infested ground (Hoogstraal and Gallagher 1982).

Ticks are of economic as well as medical importance. Apart from the physical damage they cause to animal hides, ticks, by virtue of their numbers, may interfere with milk, meat and egg production.

Tick Bite Reaction

Clinical Picture

Any part of the body may be bitten by ticks. The head and neck are common sites in children, whereas the trunk and distal parts of the legs seem to be the most frequently affected sites in adults. Grosshans et al. (1980) have noted that lesions very occasionally occur around the nipple area, which is a favourite site in animals. Some tick bites are painful, especially those inflicted by *Ornithodorus coriaceus*, whilst others evince little or no pain (see Table 23.2). The bites may also itch, sometimes at night only (Yesudian and Thambiah 1973), whilst in other cases the onset of itch may be delayed but may persist for months (Condy et al. 1980). The bite site itself may first be noticed by the patient because of the presence of the tick. In the first day or two it is about the size of a grain of rice (Maie and Ohsumi 1974; Sakai et al. 1976), its colour varying from a creamy white (Arthur 1947) to brown or greyish-brown (Patterson et al. 1979), depending on the species. As it becomes more firmly attached and begins to engorge with blood it assumes an erect posture, slowly enlarges and takes on a dark-purple colour. Its position and the cutaneous reaction around the embedded mouthparts cause the legs to be clustered together and protrude around the point of attachment like small black hairs (Maie et al. 1974; Sakai et al. 1976; Fig. 23.8). It is not uncommon for the tick to remain attached after it has become fully engorged (more than 7 days). If this occurs on the scalp it may pass unnoticed (as may happen in small girls with tick paralysis), but elsewhere, for example on the trunk, it may be mistaken for a warty tumour (Goldman 1963), especially if it can be felt but not seen by the patient.

Table 23.2. Species of tick, in classified order, which are known to have bitten man, with their approximate geographical distribution and important references (see footnotes and reference list)

Species	Geographical location	Remarks and references
IXODIDAE		
Ixodinae		
Ixodes actitarsus[1]	Japan	Maie and Ohsumi (1974); Sakai et al. (1976)
I. cookei	North America	
I. dammini	Eastern North America	Spielman et al. (1979)
I. eichhorni	New Guinea	[d]
I. granulatus	Malaysia	[d]
I. hexagonus[1]	USA; Canada; France; United Kingdom	[a,b,j]
I. holocyclus	Australia	Paralysis;[a,d,e,f,j,k]
I. lividus	Eurasia	
I. marxi	North America	[b]
I. monospinosus	Japan	Sakai et al. (1976)
I. nipponensis[1]	Japan	Sakai et al. (1976)
I. ovatus[1]	Japan	Sakai et al. (1976); Aoki et al. (1982)
I. pacificus	Western USA	[j]
I. persulcatus[1]	Eurasia; Far East, esp. Japan	Forest tick; Maie and Ohsumi (1974); Sakai et al. (1976)
I. petrus	Africa	
I. pilosus	South Africa	[a]Hamilton (1940)

Table 23.2. (*continued*)

Species	Geographical location	Remarks and references
IXODIDAE	Japan	Maie and Ohsumi (1974); Sakai et al. (1976)
I. ricinus[m]	Europe; Asia	Sheep tick; caster bean tick[a,b,e,f]
I. r. californicus	USA; Canada	[i]
I. rubicundicus	South Africa	Karoo paralysis tick; Erasmus (1952)
I. scapularis	Eastern North America	Steere et al. (1978); Wallis et al. (1978)
I. spinipalpis	North America	[e,f]
Amblyomminae		
Amblyomma americanum	North, Central and South America	Lone star tick; severe biter[e,f,h,i]
A. brasiliense	North, Central and South America	
A. cajennense	Central America; Caribbean; west coast of USA	Cayenne tick; silver tick; *mostacilla*; a severe pest[e,g,h,i]
A. hebraeum[l]	South Africa	Bont tick; Gear and Bevan (1936)[h]
A. integrum	India	Yesudian and Thambiah (1973)
A. maculatum	Southern USA	Gulf coast tick; pimento tick[e,f,g,h]
A. nuttalli	Mozambique	[b]
A. ovale (= *striatum*)	Northern Central and South America (Mexico to Argentina)	[h]
A. pomposum	Africa	[b]
A. testudinarium[l]	Japan	Toad tick; bites man; Sakai et al. (1976); Aoki et al. (1982)
A. variegatum	East and West Africa; West Indies	Bont tick[h]
Dermacentor albipictus	Northwestern USA	[f]
D. andersoni (= *venustus*)	North America	American wood tick[a,d,e,f,i,k]
D. auratus	Himalayan area	
D. marginatus	Russia	[f]
D. nuttalli	Asiatic Russia	[b]
D. hiveus	Russia	
D. occidentalis	West coast of USA	Western dog tick; Pacific tick[e,f,i]
D. parumpertus	Southwestern USA	Rabbit tick[e]
D. pictus	Russia; Eurasia	[f]
D. reticulatus	Palaearctic	[d]
D. silvarum	Palaearctic	[b]
D. variabilis	Eastern USA	American dog tick[a,e,f,i,k]
Haemaphysalis bispinosa[l]	Australia; Japan	Maie et al. (1974); Sakai et al. (1976)[d]
H. chordeilis	USA; Canada	[b]
H. cinnabarina	Northwest America	[k]
H. concinna	Eastern Siberia	[b]
H. detritum	North Africa; Russia	
H. japonica	Japan	
H. leachi leachi	South Africa	Yellow dog tick; Gear (1939)[d]
H. leporis palustris	North America	Rabbit tick[f,i]
H. papuana	India; New Guinea	[b,d]
H. punctata	Eurasian Russia; Mediterranean	[a]
H. spinigera	India; Australia	[d]
H. sulcata		
H. turturus	India	[b]
Rhipicephalinae		
Rhipicephalus appendiculata	Central and South Africa	Brown tick; Gear and Bevan (1936)
R. bursa	Eurasia; Russia	[b,d]
R. evertsi	Africa	Red tick[b,d]
R. cuspidalis	Portuguese Guinea	[b]
R. parvus	Africa	[b]
R. rossicus	Russia	[b]
R. sanguineus	Texas; Europe; Asia; Africa; Australia	Brown dog tick[d,e,g,i]
R. schulzi	Russia; Eurasia	[b]
R. simus	South Africa	[f,j]
R. turanicus	Eurasia	[f]
Hyalomma aegypticum	Tropical	Megaw (1934)[d]
H. anatolicum (= *excavatum*)	Central Asia	[f]
H. asiaticum		
H. detritum	Russia; North Africa	[b,f]
H. dromedarii	Eastern Russia	[b]
H. marginatum	Crimea	[f]

Table 23.2. *(continued)*

Species	Geographical location	Remarks and references
IXODIDAE	Japan	Maie and Ohsumi (1974); Sakai et al. (1976)
H. rufipes	South Africa	[b]
H. savignyi	Russia	[b]
H. transiens (= *truncatum*)	South Africa; Russia	Male tick bites; Erasmus (1952)[f,j]
H. tunicator	Western USA	
Boophilus annulatus	Yugoslavia	[a,b]
B. decoloratus	South Africa	Bene tick; Gear and Bevan (1936)[b]
Margaropus annulatus	North America; neotropical	North American cattle tick; larva the worst pest[e,h]
M. a. australis	Australia; Japan; South Africa	Australian cattle tick; lowland tick[e,g]
M. a. decoloratus		[e]
Aponomma exornatum	Portuguese Guinea	[b]
ARGASIDAE		
Argas arboreus	Egypt	
A. brumpti[m]	Egypt; Southern Africa	Negatively heliotropic; Condy et al. (1980)[h]
A. minanensis	Iran	[b]
A. persicus	Cosmopolitan	Fowl tick; nocturnal[d,g,h,k]
A. reflexus[m]	Egypt	Pigeon tick; nocturnal[b,h]
A. vespertilionis	Widespread	Bat tick; Titchener (1983 personal commun.)[d]
Otobius megnini	South Africa	Peacock (1958)[b]
O. lagophilus	Canada; USA	[e,j]
Ornithodorus brumpti[m]		[j]
O. coriaceus	Mediterranean; tropical neotropical; Central Asia	Maie et al. (1974)[b,g,i]
O. dugesi		[b]
O. erraticus	Egypt	[b]
O. foleyi		Severe bites[b]
O. gurneyi	Australia	Paralysis; blindness; coma[b]
O. hermsi	USA	[b,i]
O. lahorensis	Central Asia	Peacock (1958)[b]
O. moubata[m]	Africa; Iberian peninsula	In native huts[d,h,j]
O. (= *Alectorobius*) *muesbecki*	Persian Gulf area	Arabian tick; Hoogstraal and Gallagher (1982)
O. neneensis		[b]
O. nicollei	Neotropical	
O. parimentosus		Severe bite[b]
O. parkeri	USA	[b]
O. rostratus	Neotropical	Ecchymotic bites[b]
O. rudis	Neotropical	[b]
O. savignyi	Africa	Native huts[d,h]
O. talaje	Australia; South and Central America	Nocturnal; bite itches[d,h]
O. tartahorskyi	Russia; Iran	[b]
O. tholozani	Central Asia	Ecchymotic bites[b,h]
O. turicata[l]	USA and Mexico	[b,h]
O. verrucosus	Russia	[b]

The superscript letters in column three indicate the following references: [a] Abbott (1943); [b] Arthur (1961); [c] Ebeling (1975); [d] Fielding (1926); [e] Hooker et al. (1912); [f] James and Harwood (1969); [g] Newstead (1909); [h] Nuttall et al. (1926); [i] Parker et al. (1937); [j] Gregson (1973); [k] Murnaghan and O'Rourke (1978).

[l] Ticks whose bite is usually painless.

[m] Painful biters.

Local Effects

The local lesion caused by ticks is initially a slightly red papule, which quickly develops inflammatory swelling and an erythematous halo, having a diameter of up to 4 cm (Fig. 23.9). It may be very tender (Bancroft 1884) or sometimes develops paraesthesia or surrounding numbness (Goffinet and Laterre (1978). If the reaction is very acute, blistering may appear (Nuttall et al. 1926; Yesudian and Thambiah 1973; Hoogstraal and Gallagher 1982; Fig. 23.10), and these cases itch severely. The erythematous halo may become ecchymotic (Nuttall et al. 1926). After a few days the cellular

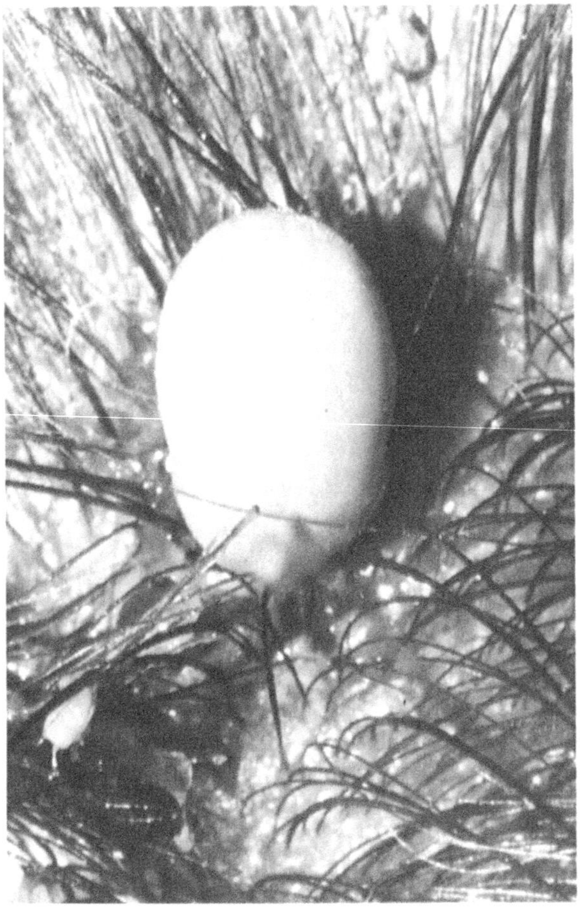

Fig. 23.8. Showing a tick (unidentified) attached to the scalp of a small girl. The white egg-shaped structure is the distended abdomen. At the bottom the front legs can just be discerned as dark thick "hairs". (Courtesy of Dr. W. S. Douglas and Dr. A. M. M. Strong, Monklands District Hospital, Airdrie, Lanarkshire)

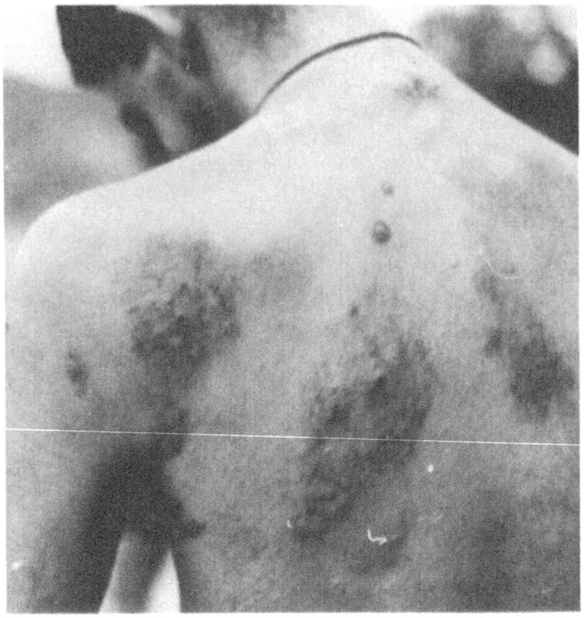

Fig. 23.9. Tick bites showing nodular lesions with tiny central blood crusts and large "halo" area of bruising around each. (From Condy et al. 1980, by kind permission of Dr. Condy and the Editor of the *Central African Journal of Medicine*)

reaction to the tick makes the lesions more nodular and the immediately surrounding halo may become indurated. Some of the nodules may persist and if they are multiple can closely resemble prurigo (Yesudian and Thambiah 1973). Nuttall and his colleagues also observed that many lesions could become surmounted by tiny blood crusts, such as are often seen with insect bites, especially those which are excoriated by the patient. Wakkerman and van Rijn (1965) described an eruption like papular urticaria caused by larvae of an unidentified *Ixodes* tick amongst bilberry pickers.

The inflammation may sometimes give rise to central necrosis and perhaps the formation of a small ulcer. Larger lesions of this type which give rise to abscesses or cellulitis are generally the result of secondary bacterial infection (Nuttall et al.

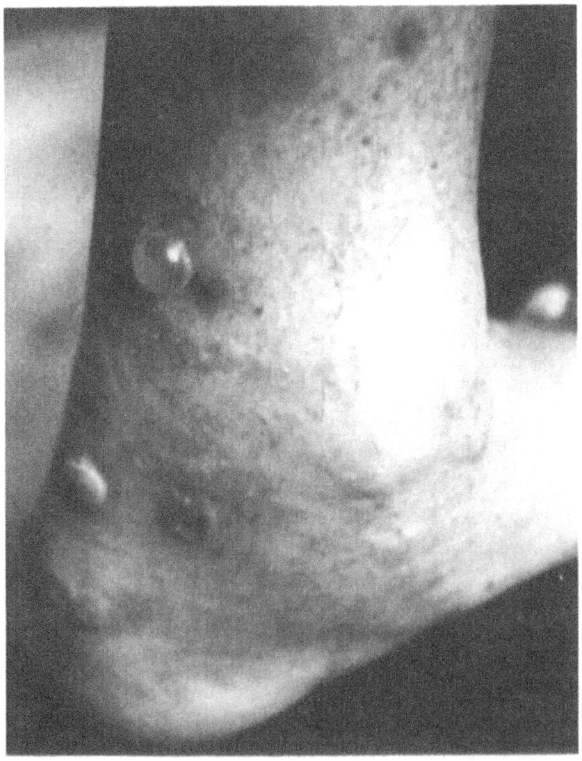

Fig. 23.10. Bullous eruption from tick bites. (From Hoogstraal and Gallagher 1982, by kind permission of the authors and the Editor of the *Lancet*)

1926). Very localised central necrosis without such infection causes a small central scar. Other complications arising from bites by *Ixodes ricinus* include local gangrene, erysipelatoid swelling, generalised erythema, generalised urticaria or psoriasiform eruption (Nuttall et al. 1926).

Healing of a tick bite takes at least 2–3 weeks but may take much longer. Itching nodules may persist for months, as many authors have testified. In some patients these itching nodules may recur for months (Goldman 1963; Condy et al. 1980) or even annually (McCaffrey 1916). Eczematous flare-up occurred in Shasky's (1972) patient when treatment was stopped.

Systemic Effects

Systemic symptoms were recorded in some patients by Nuttall and his team (1926). These included nausea, vomiting, diarrhoea, pulse irregularities and dyspnoea. Parker et al. (1937) noted fever with successive bites, subsiding each time when the tick was removed. Such symptoms may be confused with the more distant toxic reactions to certain tick bites. For example Arthur (1961) described listlessness, restlessness, troubled sleep followed by muscular weakness, gastrointestinal irritation and drooping of the eyelids, all of which disappeared within 24 h of removal of the tick. These symptoms are not unlike those of some instances of tick paralysis. On the other hand, the appearance of a lesion purplish-red in colour with central black particles—the broken-off remnants of tick mouthparts—described by Aoki et al. (1982) was not unlike the 2-cm diameter red papule with painless central black necrotic eschar described by Gear and Bevan (1936) which accompanied the symptoms of mild fever, headache, photophobia, delirium, hallucinations and generalised pain of tick typhus. These symptoms do not disappear with removal of the tick and are also associated with regional lymphadenitis, not generally seen with tick bites except when there is secondary infection.

Histology

It is difficult to describe the precise histology of a tick bite reaction in man, since the reported findings often contain no reference to the temporal relationship between the initial attachment of the tick and the biopsy. However, some help can be obtained from Trager's (1939) experimental work on immunity to tick bites in guinea pigs. He noted that a 4-day-old bite (with fully engorged tick larva still attached) in a non-immune (first infestation) guinea pig showed absence of epithelium at the point of attachment of the tick, a mass of pink staining material (? fibrin) around the embedded mouthparts, a small haemorrhagic area (the feeding pool) at the base of the lesion, but no dermal cellular reaction or epidermal thickening in the host tissue. On the other hand, in an "immune" animal (i.e. one previously infested) the "fibrin" mass was surrounded by a large inflammatory reaction consisting of a solid mass of neutrophils and "polyblasts" (immature neutrophils) and a few eosinophils. This infiltrate varied in intensity with different host biopsy specimens. The epidermis was thickened at the edges and growing down into the cellular infiltrate (i.e. showed pseudoepitheliomatous hyperplasia). The whole of the area was oedematous. There was no pool of red cells and the larva was unable fully to engorge because by the fourth day it was effectively walled off from its food source. Trager noted that this reaction was often visible clinically as a white blister.

At the actual point of penetration there is epidermal and dermal liquefaction necrosis extending as deep as the tip of the tick hypostome (Patterson et al. 1979). The hypostome itself is surrounded by a homogeneous secretion, probably tick saliva (resembling the so-called fibrin described by Trager), which shows indentation interdigitating with the hypostomal teeth, thus anchoring the tick firmly to the skin. The tissue reaction occurs around the necrotic area. The epidermis in the immediate vicinity of the puncture shows a parakeratotic surface "crust", spongiosis and in places vesiculation, the vesicles being filled with neutrophils and a few erythrocytes. There is some associated acanthosis (Yesudian and Thambiah 1973). Heyl (1982) noted pyknosis of the epidermal keratinocytes close to the tick puncture. Pseudoepitheliomatous hyperplasia occurs in many lesions (Marshall 1967; Shasky 1972).

There is pronounced vascular dilatation of the upper dermal blood vessels and sometimes also in the deeper ones. Erasmus (1952) noted endothelial swelling close to the "bite shaft". There is a dense perivascular cellular infiltrate which varies greatly in its content, with neutrophils and lymphocytes as a rule. Eosinophils may be present (Heyl 1982) or absent (Erasmus 1952). Histiocytes seem to be late arrivals, as are plasma cells. Fibroblasts have also been recorded. The cellular content would seem to be age dependent, although information on this point is scarce and vague. For example, in a 2-month-old nodule Goldman (1963) noted only lymphocytes, plasma cells and histiocytes. Patterson and his colleagues (1979) observed all the cells mentioned here in a lesion of unspecified age, whilst Yesudian and Thambiah (1973) recorded only a lymphocytic reaction in their cases. The infiltrate may also be periappendicular (Goldman 1963; Scrimenti 1970; Aoki et al. 1982) and may extend to the deeper dermis and subcutaneous tissues. This is probably applicable to those ticks with long mouthparts which penetrate deeply. In other instances the deep dermis and subcutaneous fat is not involved (Yesudian and Thambiah 1973). Marshall (1967) noted that the histological picture could be confused with Hodgkin's disease or other lymphoma, and, where pseudoepitheliomatous hyperplasia was prominent, tick bites have been mistaken for squamous carcinoma.

In many cases where the tick has been removed no remaining mouthparts can be found, but they are sometimes seen if the tick has been carelessly removed. It may be that the granuloma formation reported by some workers is related to retained parts, although Shasky (1972) recorded foreign body giant cells with a cellular reaction and proliferating blood vessels as a "typical tick-bite granuloma", even though no mouthparts were seen. Patterson et al. (1979) and Yesudian and Thambiah (1973) noted specifically that no granuloma was present.

Heyl (1982) emphasised in his cases of tick bite alopecia that, apart from the reaction in the immediate vicinity of the puncture, there was no cellular reaction 1.3 cm (half an inch) away.

Immunology

As with many other arthopods, persons with the longest exposure to tick bites are more resistant than newcomers. This is almost certainly because repeated exposure induces immune reactions. This was demonstrated experimentally in guinea pigs by Trager (1939), who showed that, on guinea pigs bitten for the first time, ticks engorged fully, but if such feeding was repeated several times the ticks ultimately failed to engorge and fell off after only a short feeding period. If several ticks were fed in a very localised area on a sensitised host a blister quickly formed below the ticks and caused them to detach. These experiments suggested that the host's tissues were reacting in a manner which prevented or discouraged the ticks from feeding. Histologically in these circumstances a cellular reaction developed which had the pleomorphic picture of a foreign body granulomatous reaction without the foreign body. Trager construed this as being an immunological reaction, which was also the view of Bagnall and Rook (1977). Gregson (1973) regarded the lymphocytic cells in this infiltrate as being the immunologically important element.

Trager (1939) had also implied the presence of circulating antibodies by successfully transferring passive immunity to tick bites to unexposed guinea pigs with serum from resistant animals. He considered that these antibodies stimulated and intensified the cellular reaction to the bite, the effect of which was to wall off the tick from its food supply.

Gregson (1973) also observed that an Arthus reaction follows tick bites in cattle. This has an irritating effect which induces increased grooming, thus leading to the earlier removal of the ticks. The antigenic stimulus for these immune reactions would appear to be proteins and/or haptens in the tick saliva. Much further research is needed both in regard to the nature of the antigen and also to the immune status of the lymphocytic infiltrate.

Tick Bite Alopecia

Ross and Friede (1955) described patchy alopecia occurring a week or two after tick bites on the occipital region of the scalp in two children. The lesions were somewhat ovate and about 1.3 cm (half an inch) long. There was neither erythema nor scaling and, except where the tick had been attached, no scarring. There was a history of tick bite, and in fact one engorged tick was still attached to the vertex of the scalp in one of the children. When the tick was removed it left an area about 6 mm (quarter of an inch) in diameter which was inflamed and slightly scaly. Marshall (1967) recorded a similar instance with an area of baldness resembling alopecia areata, 3–4 cm in diameter, a week following a tick bite on that area, whilst Heyl (1982) reported two similar cases both in children. In each case the hair loss began 1 week after removal of the tick and in each there was a small central scar at the bite site. The patch of alopecia in the younger of these two children showed several exclamation mark hairs typical of alopecia areata. Regrowth in each child began within 2 weeks and was complete in 2 months in one and almost complete in 1 month in the other.

Histologically Heyl's cases showed a dense perivascular infiltrate of neutrophils, lymphocytes, histiocytes and eosinophils in the immediate vicinity of the tick attachment site, with marked tissue necrosis involving both the connective tissue and one hair follicle. At a distance from the bite site but within the area of alopecia there was no necrosis, but the hair follicles were of telogen type with crumpled hair shafts.

The cause of the central hair loss is obviously the result of tissue necrosis; that in the surrounding area, however, appears to be of toxic origin. Heyle (1982) suggested it could be the combined effect of tick saliva and neutrophil lysomes, since there was no evidence of inflammatory or immunological reaction. It seems unlikely to the present writer that the effects of the lysosomes would occur at a considerable distance from the actual bite site. The toxin is more likely to have come from the tick saliva, and Heyl further suggested it might depend on the depth of penetration of the ticks with long hypostome. The suggestion of a toxin as the cause brings to mind the epilatory toxic effect of therapeutic doses of thallium acetate in the long-abandoned treatment of scalp ringworm. The hairs in such cases were put into the telogen phase by the poison. The delay in onset of alopecia after a tick bite is only to be expected, since hair fall is not immediate after the telogen phase sets in. A delay of 1–2 weeks would be expected, as occurred with thallium.

Tick Paralysis

The condition called "tick paralysis" has been known in Australia since 1824 (Abbott 1943). The first human case was described by Bancroft (1884), and the condition has since been recorded from a number of countries, particularly in the Canadian province of British Colombia (see Epidemiology p. 376).

Clinical Features

The clinical features of tick paralysis were comprehensively reviewed by Abbott (1943), from whose paper the following account has been compiled (unless otherwise stated). The appearances of the actual bite are no different from that in cases without paralysis. The paralysis is an acute ascending lower motor neurone paralysis of the Landry type. It usually starts with weakness of the lower limbs, progressing in a matter of hours to falling down and noticeable incoordination, which is principally due to muscle weakness, although rarely there may also be true ataxia. Phillips and Murphy (1950) considered ataxia appeared before muscle weakness. This is followed by inability to stand and then inability to sit up, with progressive weakness of the upper limbs, starting at the periphery. Finally cranial nerve weakness with dysarthria and dysphagia leads to bulbar paralysis, respiratory failure and death. Localised paralysis may sometimes occur (Hamilton 1940) when the tick is attached to certain areas such as the external auditory meatus—facial paralysis (Crossle 1932); behind the ear—photophobia (Abbott 1943) or blurring of vision (Bancroft 1884); or on the side of the forehead—frontalis and orbicularis oculi paralysis). Pain or numbness may sometimes precede the onset of paralysis (Erasmus 1952; Gregson 1973). In children restlessness and irritability, malaise and sometimes anorexia or vomiting are not uncommon presenting features. Most patients are afebrile. Examination reveals a progressive, complete, flaccid paralysis, the superficial and tendon reflexes disappearing from below upwards as the paralysis develops. The pupils are dilated and non-reactive to both light and accommodation. A morbilliform rash has been recorded (Taylor 1966).

If the tick is found and removed all the symptoms usually disappear very rapidly and in the reverse order from their appearance. Sometimes, however, recovery may be slower and rarely may take several weeks. Any residual permanent paralysis is exceedingly rare. Nevertheless, should the paralysis have progressed to involve the bulbar region and given rise to respiratory difficulty, the result may still be fatal even after the removal of the tick. In Australia, where the offending tick is *Ixodes holocyclus*, the symptoms may progress for up to 2 days after tick removal before recovery sets in, and here also fatalities occur. The majority of the patients are small children (see Epidemiology below).

The diagnosis of paralysis caused by a tick depends on finding the tick, on the condition occurring in an infested region and on the awareness of the physician of the disease. In this respect a careful history is important, and the views and information obtained from parents of paralysed children should always be listened to carefully (Taylor 1966). Occasionally the tick is only discovered after death (McCormack 1921), which makes it all the more important always to examine the patients with this type of paralysis very meticulously for the presence of ticks, paying special attention to the orifices and the scalp. This possibility should always be remembered when an unusual paralysis occurs in an uninfested region. The patient may have travelled a long distance (by aeroplane or train) before the paralysis starts. Differentiation from poliomyelitis is very important. Costa (1952) summarised the differences, and these have been set out in Table 23.3. Peacock (1958) has recorded one instance of tick paralysis in which the laboratory findings also suggested the possibility of poliomyelitis.

Epidemiology

Tick paralysis occurs in definite localities, in which it is associated with individual species of tick (see Table 23.4). A curious but unexplained fact is that the same tick may have a wide distribution but only cause paralysis in limited regions. For example *Dermacentor andersoni* causes paralysis much more frequently in northern Idaho than in the southern part of that state, whereas it serves as a vector for Rocky Mountain spotted fever in the same areas, but with a reverse incidence. *D. variabilis* likewise only causes paralysis in the southeastern United States but not in Canada, where it is just as common (Murnaghan and O'Rourke 1978). There is a seasonal incidence for tick paralysis, corresponding to the breeding season of the relevant tick species. This may enable it to be distinguished from poliomyelitis, which is a disease of summer and autumn. In some areas tick paralysis only appears in the spring (May to June in British Columbia), but in other areas the breeding season may overlap that of poliomyelitis (June to July for *D. variabilis* in the eastern United States; Gregson 1973).

This disease is more prevalent in children and most fatalities occur in children. Murnaghan and O'Rourke (1978) noted that in 139 of 166 cases in

Table 23.3. Essential clinical differences between tick paralysis and paralytic poliomyelitis

Feature	Tick paralysis	Poliomyelitis
Tick bite	Yes	No
Recovery after tick removal	Yes	No
Fever	No	Yes
Headache	Seldom	Severe
Muscle spasm	No	Yes
Neck and back stiffness	No	Yes
Preceding incoordination	Yes	No
Type of paralysis	Ascending; symmetrical	Regional
Reflexes	Absent very early	Absent
Sensory symptoms	Minor	Minor
CSF	Normal	Raised cell count; slightly raised protein
Accompanying encephalitis	No	Sometimes
Seasonal incidence[a]	Yes	Yes
Subsequent disability	No	Yes (50%)

[a] These do not always coincide.

Table 23.4. Geographical distribution of tick paralysis related to principal causal ticks. (Based on Abbott 1943)

Geographical location	Principal causal ticks
British Columbia; Northwestern United States	*Dermacentor andersoni*
Eastern United States	*Dermacentor variabilis*
East and west coasts of Australia	*Ixodes holocyclus*
South Africa	*Ixodes pilosus*[a]; *Hyalomma transiens*; *Otobius megnini*
Europe and Mediterranean:	
France	*Ixodes hexagonus*
Germany	*Rhipicephalus sanguineus*
Yugoslavia	Spp. of *Hyalomma, Boophilus* or *Rhipicephalus*
Crete	*Ixodes ricinus*; *Haemaphysalis punctata*

[a] Said by Arthur (1961) not to be a cause of paralysis.

British Columbia and the northwestern United States the patients were under 16 and the mortality was 12%. In the southeastern United States two of 40 patients died, one being adult, and the lower death rate was attributed to earlier removal of the tick. Of 21 cases in Australia 18 were children, and ten fatalities were recorded. Girls were more often affected in North America in *D. andersoni*-induced paralysis, but elsewhere there did not seem to be any sex difference in the children attacked. On the other hand, there was a preponderance of men (four or five for every woman) amongst affected adults because of their outdoor occupation.

Schmidt et al. (1969) noted that in 70% of 305 cases the tick was attached to the head or neck; the fatality rate was higher, but not significantly so, in this group.

Cause of the Paralysis

Woltman (1943) suggested that the symptoms resembled those of coniine poisoning. Rose and Gregson (1956) showed that there was a conduction block at the myoneural junction, suggesting a curare-like effect. Murnaghan (1955, cited by Gregson 1973) concluded that this caused failure of acetycholine liberation at the myoneural junction. Cherington and Snyder (1968) were essentially in agreement. However, Murnaghan and O'Rourke (1978) pointed out that whilst this held for most tick paralysis cases, those caused by *Ixodes holocyclus* were probably due to a disturbance of central nervous system transmission. No evidence has been adduced to incriminate a viral source for the toxin, which is still considered to be directly secreted by the tick. Paralysis with some ticks appears only to be associated with fast feeding (Gregson 1937; Mail and Gregson 1938), most of the toxin being produced on the fifth or sixth day at the end of engorgement. Rapid feeding in these ticks occurs in the breeding season (Gregson 1937); the toxin production is often said to be related to the presence of fertile eggs in the tick (cited by Abbott 1943). This is not universally applicable, because Erasmus (1952) recorded paralysis following the bite of a male tick, *Hyalomma transiens*. Nymphal ticks may be rare causes of paralysis (Gregson 1973), whilst in the case of the argasid tick *Otobius megnini* only nymphs cause paralysis since the adults are non-feeders (Peacock 1958).

Immunology

The immunology of tick paralysis is the same as for ticks in general—an immunity to tick bites developing in adults prevents the ticks from feeding to engorgement. This probably explains why the paralysis is much commoner in children on whom the tick engorges fully. Antibodies to the paralysis toxin can be developed for *I. holocyclus* in dogs, but not for *D. andersoni*, which suggested to Murnaghan and O'Rourke (1978) that the former toxin was probably a protein but the latter was not.

Histopathological changes in the brain nervous tissue are minimal. Murnaghan and O'Rourke (1978) stated that this fact indicated a biochemical rather than a structural change. Vascular engorgement with diffuse dense plasma cell infiltrate in brain tissue was found at post mortem in one case by Ferguson (1924).

Treatment

Recovery usually quickly follows removal of the tick. Persons who have visited tick-infested areas where paralysis is known to occur should have their bodies and clothing carefully inspected for ticks on return. Ticks do not always attach immediately and may thus easily be picked off before attachment. For established paralysis supportive therapy including assisted respiration and other measures of intensive care may be necessary until the process of spontaneous recovery begins. The use of dog anti-paralysis serum developed in Australia has not become established because of urticaria and other side-effects (Abbott 1943).

Erythema Chronicum Migrans and Lyme Disease

Erythema chronicum migrans (ECM), an expanding annular erythema, has been known for a long time as a complication of some tick bites (Afzelius 1910). Hellerstrom (1930) reported it occurring simultaneously with a tick-borne viral meningoencephalitis. Putkonen et al. (1962) recorded 31 cases of ECM in Helsinki between 1952 and 1960. They also encountered 29 cases of meningoencephalitis, but not in association with ECM. They noted that only six instances of both diseases in the same patient had been mentioned in the literature. Steere et al. (1977a, b) described an outbreak of ECM followed by meningoencephalitis, cardiac or arthritic symptoms, which has been named "Lyme disease" after the district in Connecticut, USA where it occurred.

Clinically ECM appears from 4 to 20 days after a tick bite, and in Lyme disease a variety of

Table 23.5. Time relationship between the tick bite and the various symptoms of Lyme disease. (Schrock 1982)[a]

Feature	ECM	Neurological	Cardiac	Arthritic
Time of onset after tick bite:				
Usual	2 weeks	4 weeks	5 weeks	6 weeks
Range	4–20 days	2–11 weeks	3–21 weeks	2.6–24 weeks
Duration of symptoms:				
Usual	10 days	3 weeks	1 week	8 days
Range	3 days to $1\frac{1}{2}$ years	2–32 weeks	3 days to 6 weeks	1–90 days
Recurrent episodes	Yes	Yes	No	Yes but not always

[a] By kind permission of the author and the Editor of the *American Journal of Medicine*.

combinations of symptoms could occur thereafter, sometimes ECM being absent. Schrock (1982) has outlined the chronological order in which they may appear (Table 23.5) and the alternative combinations in the syndrome (Table 23.6). ECM starts as a red macule or papule with a central punctum representing the point of attachment of the tick (Naverson and Gardner 1978). It extends peripherally in ring form and may encircle half the body (Scrimenti 1970). The margin may be oedematous, the centre clearing partially or completely, without scaling or crusting. There may be more than one lesion, but in uncomplicated cases there are no other symptoms, neither lymphangitis nor lymphadenitis, and the general health is good.

With Lyme disease, however, whether it starts with ECM or not, associated symptoms may occur ranging from nil to malaise, fatigue, chills, fever, headache, stiff neck, backache, myalgia, nausea, vomiting and sore throat (Steere et al. 1978). In a review of 314 cases Steere et al. (1983b) tabulated a long list of early signs and symptoms in Lyme disease, which are shown in Table 23.7. After varying periods (see Table 23.5) mono- or oligoarthritis or migratory polyarthritis occur, sometimes with characteristic recurrent episodes of pain and swelling. Meningoencephalitis with cranial nerve neuropathies or sensory root symptoms may follow, or occasionally disorders of myocardial conduction, but these two groups never occurred together. It is interesting to note the relevant data in 11 patients with European lymphocytic meningoradiculitis (Bannwarth's syndrome) reported by Ryberg et al. (1983), which are shown in Table 23.8.

Table 23.6. Variations in presentation of Lyme disease. (Schrock 1982)[a]

Clinical features	Incidence
ECM + arthritis	53%
Arthritis alone	24%
ECM alone	14%
ECM, neurologic and arthritis	4%
ECM and neurologic	3%
Neurologic and arthritis	1%
Neurologic alone	1%

[a] By kind permission of the author and the Editor of the *American Journal of Medicine*.

Histopathology

Histopathological changes in the skin show the usual reaction to the tick bite in the centre of the ECM lesion with, at the periphery, dermal changes only, consisting of a "leucocyte" infiltrate around the skin appendages with slight surrounding oedema (Scrimenti 1970). Stewart et al. (1983) noted a perivascular lymphocytic infiltrate in their patient's lesion; this finding was confirmed by Berger and his colleagues (1983), who added that the lymphocytes were often accompanied by plasma cells or eosinophils, or both. The eosinophils were seen chiefly in biopsies from the centre of lesions, whilst plasma cells were present in biopsies from the periphery of lesions.

Cause

Careful epidemiological studies in the Lyme area of Connecticut by Steere et al. (1978) and by Wallis et al. (1978) of the distribution of cases and of tick species indicated that *Ixodes scapularis* was the probable agent in the United States; however, *I. dammini* has also been incriminated (Schrock 1982). In Europe ECM and meningoencephalitis have long been associated with the closely related *I. ricinus* (Putkonen et al. 1962; Von Thöne 1968).

Table 23.7. Early signs and symptoms of Lyme disease found amongst 314 patients reviewed. (Steere et al. 1983b)[a]

Signs	% Pos.	Symptoms	% Pos.
1. ECM	100	1. Malaise, fatigue, lethargy	80
2. Multiple lesions of ECM	48	2. Headache	64
3. Regional lymphadenopathy	41	3. Fevers and chills	59
4. Generalised lymphadenopathy	20	4. Stiff neck	48
5. Pain in neck flexion	17	5. Arthralgias	48
6. Malar rash	13	6. Myalgias	43
7. Erythematous throat	12	7. Backache	26
8. Conjunctivitis	11	8. Anorexia	23
9. Frank arthritis	6	9. Sore throat	17
10. Splenomegaly	6	10. Nausea	17
11. Hepatomegaly	5	11. Dysaesthesia	11
12. Muscle tenderness	4	12. Vomiting	10
13. R. upper quadrant tenderness		13. Abdominal pain	8
in the abdomen	8	14. Photophobia	6
14. Periorbital oedema	3	15. Hand stiffness	5
15. Evanescent skin lesions	3	16. Dizziness	5
16. Abdominal tenderness	2	17. Cough	5
17. Testicular swelling	1	18. Chest pains	4
		19. Ear pain	4
		20. Diarrhoea	2

[a] By kind permission of the authors and the Editor of the *Annals of Internal Medicine*.

Table 23.8. Clinical and laboratory features found in 11 patients with European meningoradiculitis. The IgG index was of antibodies to Lyme disease spirochaete (LDS). (Ryberg et al. 1983)[b]

Feature	Number affected
1. General symptoms	6
2. Headache	8
3. Other regional pain	11
4. Slight neck stiffness	1
5. Mild fever	2
6. Mild sensory disturbance	9
7. Cranial nerve palsy	10
a) Facial nerve, unilateral	3
b) Facial nerve, bilateral	7
c) Other cranial nerve upset	4
8. Other paralysis	2
9. History of tick or insect bite	4
10. ECM	3
11. Elevated CSF protein	10
12. CSF pleocytosis	11
13. Plasma cells in CSF	8[a]
14. Elevated CSF IgG index	8[a]
15. CSF oligoclonal pattern	8[a]

[a] Only nine patients were examined for these features.

[b] By kind permission of the authors and the Editor of the *Lancet*.

Stewart et al. (1983) recorded the first case of Lyme disease in Australia, in the Hunter valley of New South Wales, although they were unable to identify the arthropod responsible.

Degos et al. (1962) claimed to have shown by agglutination tests that ECM was due to a rickettsial organism, but they were unable to isolate any microbial agent for ECM. Of course, viruses have been isolated as causal agents for the different meningoencephalitic disorders of Europe, the USSR and the United States. The beneficial effect of penicillin and tetracycline suggests that an infective agent transmissable by ticks is the cause, and Schrock (1982) thought the later symptoms could be immunologically mediated, a view supported by the demonstration of circulating complexes and cryoglobulins.

More recent positive support for the infective theory has been the finding of spirochaetes in *I. dammini* and *I. ricinus*, associated respectively with Lyme disease and ECM. Moreover, experimental rabbits developed lesions of ECM 4 weeks after the infected ticks had fed on them (Burgdorfer and Kierans 1983). Ackerman (1983) demonstrated antibodies to *Borrelia duttoni* (a spirochaete) in six patients with ECM and eight patients with tick-borne meningopolyneuritis by indirect immunofluorescene. Barbour et al. (1983) demonstrated antibodies to the spirochaete isolated from *I. dammini* (IDS) in patients with Lyme disease but not in controls. Berger et al. (1983) demonstrated spirochaetes in the periphery of lesions of ECM in association with plasma cells, whilst Waldo and Sidhu (1983) showed that the spirochaetes present were morphologically akin to IDS, having a *Treponema*-like configuration. Benach et al. (1983) found spirochaetes in the blood of two patients with Lyme disease. Burgdorfer et al. (1982) showed that the IDS fluoresced in the serum from patients with Lyme disease, indicating the presence of specific antibodies in such serum.

The evidence presented is overwhelmingly in favour of ECM and Lyme disease being a tick-borne spirochaetosis. Its elucidation was initiated by the persistently expressed suspicions of the mother of one of the original Lyme patients (Harris 1983).

Epidemiology

Lyme disease has a seasonal incidence, with its onset from May to November but mostly in June and July. Children are rather more commonly affected than adults, 39 of the original 51 patients studied by Steer and his colleagues being children. Over 500 cases have now been encountered in the northeastern United States extending as far west as Minnesota (Schrock 1982). Burgdorfer et al. (1983a) concluded that Lyme disease is probably much more widespread in the United States than hitherto suspected. The causal ticks belong to the *I. ricinus* group. In the United States *I. scapularis* and *I. dammini* have been incriminated (Editorial 1979; Schrock 1982). They are frequently overlooked because of their small size. Von Thöne (1968) has pointed out that many of the bites are given by nymphal forms, which cause a stronger reaction than the adults. He has suggested that some persons with ECM of unknown origin may have been bitten by an *I. ricinus* nymph, because these creatures only remain on the host a relatively short time (up to 24 h) and may easily be missed.

Diagnosis

In an epidemic area diagnosis is not difficult with ECM and other symptoms, but in the absence of skin lesions may not be easy. A history of tick bite is helpful. The arthritis in children is reminiscent of juvenile rheumatoid arthritis but of shorter duration. This time factor also applies to the other manifestations (Steere et al. 1978). Laboratory tests for confirmation of the diagnosis include histopathology to show the pathological changes and, with appropriate staining, to demonstrate spirochaetes, and immunological examination for circulating immune complexes, raised IgG and IgM and also antibodies to IDS.

Treatment

ECM responds to either penicillin or tetracycline (Putkonen et al. 1962; Scrimenti 1970; Naverson and Gardner 1978; Schrock 1982). According to Schrock, antibiotic therapy reduced the subsequent incidence of arthritis. Steere et al. (1983a) concluded that for adults oral tetracycline (250 mg q.i.d.) or phenoxymethylpenicillin (500 mg q.i.d.) given for 10 or preferably 20 days was the best regimen. For children they recommended phenoxymethylpenicillin (50 mg/kg to a total of 1–2 g daily) for similar periods. For those children sensitive to penicillin, erythromycin (20 mg/kg) was advised. Relapses may occur with inadequate dosage or length of treatment. It is interesting to note that as long ago as 1948 Lennhoff claimed to have found spirochaetes in the lesions of ECM, but these findings were discounted because of similar claims made in respect of psoriasis and pityriasis rosea. The use of penicillin and tetracycline were originally based on Lennhoff's findings.

General Treatment of Tick Bites

Removal of attached ticks must be done with care. Under no circumstances should forcible removal of any kind be attempted. This will only result in breaking off mouthparts and leaving them in situ to cause irritation and reactionary foreign body granulomata. Blocking tick respiration by covering with soft paraffin (or liquid paraffin in sites such as the external auditory meatus) is very effective but requires up to 2 or 3 h or more before the tick releases itself. More rapid results may be achieved by applying chloroform or ether to the attached tick or even warming it by a match flame. A rapid and certain method is by excision or punch biopsy under local anaesthesia.

Persistent nodules left after the tick has fallen can be treated by the topical application of potent corticosteroids such as flurandrenalone (Goldman 1963), but these are not always effective. Yesudian and Thambiah (1973) found intralesional injection of triamcinolone acetonide at a dose of 1 mg to be very effective. Trice (1953) recommended electrodessication for such nodules. However, most bites heal quickly after the tick has left or been removed.

Prevention of Tick Bites

Prevention of bites by repellents is only partially effective. Hoogstraal and Gallagher (1982) obtained no protection from clothing impregnated with dimethylphthallate but reported that oil-based dimethylphthallate applied to the skin helped and that the frequent use of a spray containing pyrethrum (Pif Paf) was fairly effective.

Control of Ticks

Control of ticks is difficult. Domestic animals should be dipped in an appropriate anti-tick solution at intervals, if practicable. Crop rotation may be helpful but only feasible in some locations (Newstead 1909). Burning pasture land with lime may also help but requires the removal of all livestock for some weeks to allow eggs to hatch before applying the lime. Wild animals will re-infest this land in time. Poultry, which enjoy eating ticks, are useful in controlling the tick numbers in smallholdings.

References

*Abbott KH (1943) Tick paralysis; a review. Proc Mayo Clin 18: 39–45, 59–64

Ackermann R (1983) Erythema chronicum migrans und durch Zecken übertragene Meningopolyneuritis (Garin–Bujadoux–Bannwath); Borrelien-Infektionen? Dtsch Med Wochenschr 108: 577–580

Afzelius A (1910) Verhandlungen der dermatologischen Gesellschaft zer Stockholm 16 December 1909. Arch Dermatol Syphilis 101: 404–407

Aoki K, Mori M, Kamata H, Suzuki H (1982) Tick bites; a study using scanning electron microscopy. J Dermatol 9: 79–84

Arthur DR (1947) Observations on *Ixodes hexagonus* Leach 1815 (Acarina: Ixodidae). Entomol Monthly Mag 83: 69–76

*Arthur DR (1961) Ticks and disease. Pergamon, Oxford

Bagnall B, Rook A (1977) Arthropods and the skin. In: Rook A (ed) Recent advances in dermatology 4. Churchill, Edinburgh, pp 59–90

Bancroft J (1884) Queensland ticks and tick blindness. Aust Med Gaz 4: 37–38

Barbour AG, Burgdorfer W, Grunwaldt E, Steere AC (1983) Antibodies of patients with Lyme disease to components of the *Ixodes dammini* spirochaete. J Clin Invest 72: 504–515

Benach BW, Bosler EM, Hanrahan JP et al. (1983) Spirochaetes isolated from the blood of two patients with Lyme disease. N Engl J Med 308: 740–742

Berger BW, Clemmensen OJ, Ackerman AB (1983) Lyme disease is a spirochaetosis. Am J Dermatopathol 5: 111–124

Burgdorfer W, Keirans JE (1983) Ticks and Lyme disease in the United States. Ann Intern Med 99: 121

Burgdorfer W, Barbour AG, Hayes SF, Benach JL, Grunwaldt E, Davis JP (1982) Lyme disease—a tick-borne spirochaetosis? Science 216: 1317–1319

Burgdorfer W, Barbour AG, Hayes SF, Peter O, Aeschlimann A (1983) Erythema chronicum migrans—a tick-borne spirochaetosis. Acta Trop (Basel) 40: 79–83

Cherington M, Snyder RD (1968) Tick paralysis: neurophysiologic studies. N Engl J Med 278: 95–97

Condy JR, Norval RAI, Blackburn NK, Clemence P (1980) The effects of the bites of *Argas brumpti* (Acarina: Argasidae) on humans. Cent Afr J Med 26: 212–213

Costa JA (1952) Tick paralysis on the Atlantic seaboard. Am J Dis Child 83: 336–342

Crossle FC (1932) Facial paralysis following tick-bite. Med J Aust 2: 764

Degos R, Touraine R, Arouette J (1962) L'erythema chronicum migrans. Discussion d'une origine rickettsienne. Ann Dermatol Syphiligr (Paris) 89: 247–260

Ebeling W (1975) Urban entomology. University of California, Division of Agricultural Science, Los Angeles, Cal

Editorial (1979) New tick troubles in the U.S.A. Lancet II: 450

Erasmus LD (1952) Regional tick paralysis. Sensory and motor changes caused by a male tick, genus *Hyalomma*. S Afr Med J 26: 985–987

Ferguson EW (1924) Deaths from tick paralysis in human beings. Med J Aust 2: 346–348

*Fielding JW (1926) Australasian ticks. Service Publication (Tropical Division) No 9. Commonwealth of Australia, Department of Health, Melbourne, pp 1–114

Gear J (1939) Complications of tick bite fever. A survey of fifty cases. S Afr Med J 13: 35–36

Gear JHS, Bevan C (1936) An outbreak of tick bite fever. S Afr Med J 10: 485–488

Goffinet AM, Laterre C (1978) Méningoradiculite par piqûre de tique. Acta Neurol Belg 78: 217–222

Goldman L (1963) Tick bite granuloma; failure of prevention of lesion by excision of tick bite area. Am J Trop Med Hyg 12: 246–248

*Gregson JD (1937) Studies on the rate of tick feeding in relation to disease. Proc Entomol Soc Br Columbia 33: 15–21

*Gregson JD (1973) Tick paralysis: an appraisal of natural and experimental data. Canadian Department of Agriculture Monograph No 9. Ottawa, Acland, pp 5–109

Grosshans E, Meyer M, Capesius C, Stoeckel E (1980) Les infiltrations lymphocytaires aréolo-mammelonnaires. Le lymphocytome cutane benin de l'aréole mammaire. Ann Dermatol Venereol 107: 153–161

*Hamilton DG (1940) Tick paralysis: a dangerous disease in children. Med J Aust 1: 759–765

Harris ED (1983) Lyme disease. Success for academia and the community. N Engl J Med 308: 773–775

Hellerstrom S (1930) Erythema chronicum migrans Afzelii. Acta Derm Venereol (Stockh) 11: 315–321

*Heyl T (1982) Tick bite alopecia. Clin Exp Dermatol 7: 537–542

Hoogstraal H, Gallagher MD (1982) Blisters, pruritus and fever after bites by the Arabian tick *Ornithodorus* (*Alectorobius*) *muesebecki*. Lancet II: 288–289

*Hooker WA, Bishopp FC, Wood HP (1912) The life history and bionomics of some North American ticks. US Department of Agriculture Bureau of Entomology Bulletin No 106. US Govt Printing Office, Washington DC, pp 1–239

*James MT, Harwood RF (1969) Herms's medical entomology, 6th edn. Macmillan, London, pp 320–361

Lenhoff C (1948) Spirochaetes in aetiologically obscure disease. Acta Derm Venereol (Stockh) 28: 295–324. Cited by Waldo and Sidhu (1983)

McCaffrey D (1916) The effect of tick bites on man. J Parasitol 2: 193–194

McCormack PD (1921) Paralysis in children due to the bite of wood ticks. JAMA 77: 260–263

Maie O, Ohsumi T (1974) A case of tick bite. J Dermatol 1: 29–31

Mail GA, Gregson JD (1938) Tick paralysis in British Columbia. Can Med Assoc J 39: 532–537

Marshall J (1967) Ticks and the human skin. Dermatologica 135: 60–65

Megaw J (1934) Typhus fevers in the tropics. Br Med J II: 244–246

*Murnaghan MF, O'Rourke FJ (1978) Tick paralysis. In: Bettini S (ed) Arthropod venoms. Springer, Berlin Heidelberg New York, pp 419–464 (Handbook of experimental pharmacology, vol 48)

Naverson DN, Gardner LW (1978) Erythema chronicum migrans in America. Arch Dermatol 114: 253–254

Newstead R (1909) Reports of the twenty-first expedition of the Liverpool School of Tropical Medicine; Jamaica 1908–1909. Section I. Medical and economic entomology. Ann Trop Med Parasitol 3: 421–469

*Nuttall GHF, Warburton C, Cooper WF, Robinson EE (1926) Ticks—a monograph of the Ixodidae. Cambridge University Press, Cambridge.

Parker PR, Philip CB, Davis GE, Conley RA (1937) Ticks of the United States in relation to disease in man. J Econ Entomol 30: 51–69

Patterson JW, Fitzwater JE, Connell J (1979) Localised tick bite reaction. Cutis 24: 168–172

Peacock PB (1958) Tick bite paralysis or poliomyelitis. S Afr Med J 32: 201–202

Phillips P, Murphy MA (1950) Tick paralysis. Can Med Assoc J 63: 38–39

Putkonen T, Mustakallio KK, Salminen A (1962) Erythema chronicum migrans with meningitis: a rare coincidence of two tick-borne diseases. Dermatologica 125: 184–188

Rose I, Gregson JD (1956) Evidence of a neuromuscular block in tick paralysis. Nature 178: 95–96

Ross MS, Friede H (1955) Alopecia due to tick bite. Arch Dermatol 71: 524–525

Ruebush TK, Cassaday P, Marsh HJ, Lisker SO, Voorhees DB, Mahoney EB, Healy GR (1977) Human babeosis on Nantucket Island. Ann Intern Med 86: 6–9

*Ryberg B, Nilsson B, Burgdorfer W, Barbour AG (1983) Antibodies to Lyme disease spirochaete in European lymphocytic meningoradiculitis (Bannwarth's Syndrome). Lancet II: 519

Sakai S, Noguchi M, Sufuni S, Fukushi G, Yamaguchi T, Takada N (1976) Five cases of tick bite. J Dermatol 3: 121–125

Schmidt N, Bowmer EJ, Gregson JD (1969) Tick paralysis in British Columbia. Can Med Assoc J 100: 417–421

Schrock CG (1982) Lyme disease: additional evidence of widespread distribution. Recognition of a tick-borne dermatitis-encephalitis-arthritis syndrome in an area of known *Ixodes* tick distribution. Am J Med 72: 700–702

Scrimenti RJ (1970) Erythema chronica migrans. Arch Dermatol 102: 104–105

Shasky DR (1972) Tick bite granuloma with auto-eczematisation. Arch Dermatol 106: 916

*Sheals JG (1973) Arachnida (scorpions, spiders, ticks, etc.) In: Smith KGV (ed) Insects and other arthropods of medical importance. Trustees of the British Museum (Natural History), London, pp 432–451

Spielman A, Clifford CM, Piesman J, Corwin MD (1979) Human babeosis on Nantucket Islands, U.S.A.: Description of the vector, *Ixodes* (*Ixodes*) *dammini* n.sp. J Med Entomol 15: 218–234

Steere AC, Malawista SE, Hardin JA, Ruddy S, Askenase PW, Andiman WA (1977a) Erythema chronicum migrans and Lyme arthritis. The enlarging clinical spectrum. Ann Intern Med 86: 685–698

*Steere AC, Malawista SE, Snydman DR, Shope RE, Andiman WA, Ross MR, Steele FM (1977b) Lyme arthritis. An epidemic of oligoarthritis in children and adults in their Connecticut communities. Arthr Rheum 20: 7–17

*Steere AC, Broderick TP, Malawista SE (1978) Erythema chronicum migrans and Lyme arthritis: epidemiologic evidence for a tick vector. Am J Epidemiol 108: 312–321

*Steere AC, Hutchinson GJ, Rahn DW, Sigal LH, Craft JE, DeSanna ET, Malawista SE (1983a) Treatment of the early manifestations of Lyme disease. Ann of Intern Med 99: 22–26

*Steere AC, Baartenhagen NH, Craft JE, Hutchinson GJ, Newman JG, Rahn DW, Sigal LH, Spieler RN, Steim KS, Malawista SE (1983b) The early clinical manifestations of Lyme disease. Ann Intern Med 99: 76–82

Stewart A, Glass J, Patel A, Watt G, Cripps A, Clancy R (1983) Lyme arthritis in the Hunter valley. Med J Aust 1: 139

Taylor CW (1966) Tick paralysis. Can Med Assoc J 95: 125

*Trager W (1939) Acquired immunity to ticks. J Parasitol 25: 57–81

Trice ER (1953) Conization treatment of insect bite granuloma. Arch Dermatol Syphilol 68: 586–588

Von Thöne AW (1968) *Ixodes ricinus* und Erythema chronicum migrans (Afzelius). Dermatologica 136: 57–60

Wakkerman CThB, van Rijn JFA (1965) Strophulus arthropodicus verursacht durch Ixodidan. Hautarzt 16: 37–38

Waldo ED, Sidhu GS (1983) The spirochaete in erythema chronicum migrans. Demonstration by light and electron microscopy. Am J Dermatopathol 5: 125–127

Wallis RL, Brown SE, Kloter KO, Main AJ (1978) Erythema chronicum migrans and Lyme arthritis; field study of ticks. Am J Epidemiol 108: 322–327

Woltman HW (1943) In discussion of Abbot (1943) Proc Mayo Clin 18: 39–45, 59–64

Yesudian P, Thambiah AS (1973) Persistent papules after tick bites. Dermatologica 147: 214–218

24 Centipede Bites and Millipede Burns

Centipede Bites

Centipedes (Chilopoda) are common, the giant species particularly so in the tropics and subtropics (Remington 1950). In some parts of the world they are regarded with fear as dangerous creatures. The majority of writers consider that they do not endanger life, although Remington felt that they were potentially dangerous. They can cause severe injury in some localities, and Pineda (1923) recorded a fatality in a 7-year-old boy in the Philippines. They do not inflict damage with their mouthparts or by stinging but through sharpened claws on their modified first pair of legs with which they grip their prey (for they are predaceous). The hardened claws on these legs have each a slit-like opening on the dorsal curvature through which is discharged venom from the poison gland situated in the basal segment of these modified legs. The poison is thus injected at the time the claw perforates the skin of the human victim, usually at night.

Clinical Features

The clinical features of centipede bites vary with species and locality. Baerg (1924, 1925) described the bite as sharp and needle-like; the effect lasted only 15–30 min with bites from *Scolopendra sumichrasti* and *Theatops spinicaudus*, whereas with *S. polymorpha* it persisted for 3 h with localised sweating and a sensation like an embedded splinter. Andrews and Domonkos (1971) described the puncture wound as haemorrhagic. *S. heros* is the species most frequently mentioned. According to Baerg, it caused immediate pain with some swelling and local tenderness persisting for over 3 h. Bayley-DeCastro (1921), on the other hand, dealt with many patients bitten by this species in the Andaman Islands, in the Bay of Bengal. The effects were uniformly severe. There was an immediate feeling of heat and tingling, quickly followed by severe pain, which lasted for several hours. At the bite site two haemorrhagic points appeared, which within 24 h had enlarged and progressed to localised necrosis. Intense inflammatory oedema extending to deeper tissues developed, along with pronounced lymphangitis and regional lymphadenopathy. The necrosis spread as deep as the subcutaneous fascia, often reaching considerably beyond the immediate bite site, and then sloughed off. Subsequently healing was usually rapid but occasionally extended over several weeks or even months, and scarring resulted. In the more severe instances there was pyrexia tachycardia, tachypnoea, anxiety, headache and even rarely a stuporose condition.

Bayley-DeCastro (1921) pointed out that the same species had relatively insignificant effects in India and Burma. Reactions in Malaya were fairly severe, but only transient in New Guinea (Ariff 1956; Keegan 1963). Cloudsley-Thompson (1958) and Ebeling (1975) both noted sharp pain with associated swelling around the bites in their patients. Remington (1950) described an epidemic of centipede bites in soldiers in the Philippines in World War II. He himself was bitten in the axilla; the almost unbearable pain subsided in about an hour to be followed by severe axillary swelling next day, and mild pain and tenderness persisted for 3 weeks. In Texas, Micks (1960) collected eight examples of centipede bite, six with severe pain and swelling and two with marked but unspecified systemic symptoms. Severe itch sometimes occurs (Andrews and Domonkos 1971).

Treatment

There is no specific treatment for centipede bites. As a first aid measure, rubbing potassium permanganate crystals into a small incision over the bite within an hour is said to lessen damage (Bayley-DeCastro 1921). Simultaneous disinfection is advisable. The injection of local anaesthetic (2% procaine or equivalent) into the bite site is the single most useful measure (Remington 1950). Analgesics such as pethidine or even morphia are recommended (Ariff 1956; Southcott 1978). The latter authors also advise antitetanus measures. Established inflammatory lesions require appropriate antibiotics. Ariff (1956) claimed that a 24-h course of corticosteroids would initiate involution of lesions, and Micks (1960) found these compounds necessary to control systemic symptoms. For necrotic lesions, rest in bed, preferably in hospital, is required.

Morphology of Centipedes

Sheals and Rice (1973) gave the following description of centipedes:

> Centipedes are elongated, many-legged, tracheate arthropods with a distinct head and a dorso-ventrally flattened body. The head has a single pair of antennae and three pairs of trophic appendages, one of mandibles and two of maxillae. The trunk cannot be differentiated into regions. There is one pair of legs to each segment, of which there are from 15 to over 100. The first pair of trunk appendages, the maxillipedes or toxognaths, are provided with powerful claws, at the tips of which are the orifices of ducts leading from large venom glands.

Fig. 24.1 shows the poison claws on the modified first pair of legs.

There are five orders of centipedes (see Table 24.1), although most authorities group Craterostigmamorpha with Lithobiomorpha. Other details of the various species are also shown in Table 24.1, including the few instances where species other than scolopendromorphs have attacked man.

The giant scolopendromorphs cause the great majority of skin lesions in man. They can be up to 30 cm long, are often of spectacular colour (green, blue and yellow) and are nocturnal. Some species feed not only on insects but also on small mice and birds (Keegan 1963). According to Cloudsley-Thompson (1958), even the largest specimens do not bite unless molested, but Keegan (1963) maintained that they would bite instantly if touched. They dislike light and prefer to live in humid situations such as beneath stones, leaves, bark or logs. In India they are said to be found beneath roof mats. They will at times enter houses or tents and bite the occupants (Remington 1950).

The nature of the venom, which is clear is some species and opalescent in others, is uncertain. Cornwall (1915–1916) was of the opinion that it was composed principally of digestive enzymes. Bayley-Decastro (1921) was able to reproduce exactly the changes which occurred after centipede bites in man by injecting venom into rabbits.

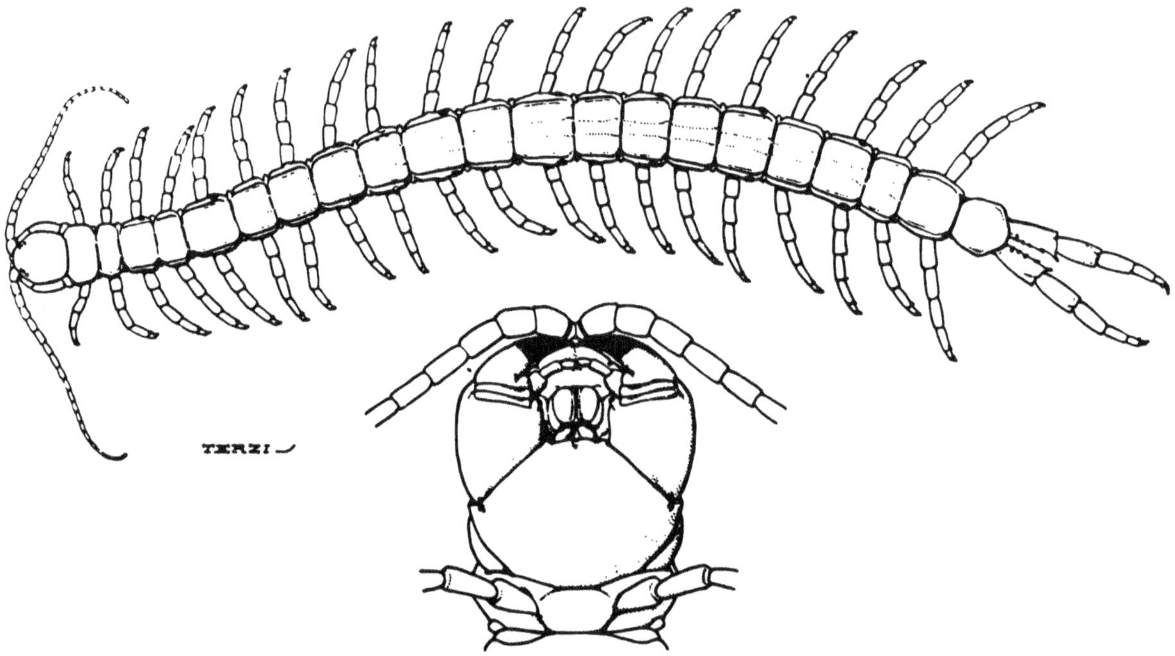

Fig. 24.1. Giant centipede, *Scolopendra morsitans*. The anterior view of the head shows the modified pair of legs with posion claws. The tips of the claws (shown as black in the drawing) are inserted by lateral pressure. (Courtesy of the Director of The Wellcome Museum of Medical Science, Dr. A. J. Duggan)

Table 24.1. Different orders of centipedes with relevant details. (Compiled from various sources, but principally Cloudsley-Thompson 1958)

Order	Legs (pairs)	Antennal segments	Eyes	Remarks
Geophilomorpha	31–177	14	O	Very agile; do not bite man
Lithobiomorpha	15	20–50	O	Most species unable to penetrate human skin. *Lithobius forficatus* causes needle-like prick but no lesion
Craterostigmamorpha	15		O	Contains one genus, *Craterostigmus*; Australian; usually put in Lithobiomorpha
Scutigeromorpha	15	Very long	C P	So-called house centipedes. Widespread; originally outdoor spp. but can live and multiply indoors. Very agile; sheds legs when gripped. Six larval and four adolescent stages. *Scutigerus forceps* can give very painful bite
Scolopendromorpha	23	17–30	O	Beautifully coloured according to locality. Giant species widespread throughout the tropics and subtropics. Spread by modern commercial transport. Severe bites caused by *Scolopendra* spp.

O, ocelli; C, compound; P, protruding.

Prevention of Centipede Attacks

In areas where centipedes are common, the doors and windows of houses should be effectively screened to prevent their entry. Mosquito nets on beds, especially in camps, are a further safeguard, as is the careful handling of clothing which has been left on the ground overnight. In houses to which centipedes have already gained access the use of insecticides is advised, e.g. 2% chlordane, 1% lindane or 2%–4% malathion, with appropriate precautions (Keegan 1963).

Millipede Burns

Millipedes are generally regarded as harmless. Halstead and Ryckman (1949) noted that no mention of them was made in several well-known textbooks of medical entomology. However, they can cause injury to man when acting defensively. Those few reports which have been published indicate that the occurrences are not quite so uncommon as had been thought and that the effects can be very severe. Very young children and "ignorant scientists who disregard local advice" are the most likely victims (Radford 1975b). Others are usually affected when asleep on the ground (Radford 1975a).

Clinical Effects

Millipede lesions are the result of contamination by a toxic liquid which emanates from the millipede's body. The areas liable to be involved are exposed skin surfaces and the eyes. On the skin a marked prickling and burning sensation is felt almost immediately, and the lesion is like a corrosive burn (Radford 1975b). The skin becomes yellowish-brown in colour, turning to a dark mahogany brown over the next 24 h. This discolouration generally masks any underlying inflammatory erythema. Within 24 h after contamination the surface becomes blistered, the blisters being maximal where the noxious fluid was most concentrated (Loomis 1936). If the contamination is very slight there may be no blisters. With prolonged contact before first aid is applied—as happened to Burtt (1938) when he kept a large live millipede in his hip pocket for an hour—the whole area of contact may be badly burned and blistered. Blisters may burst leaving a raw, eroded surface, which usually heals within 2 weeks without a scar (Fig. 24.2), because the burn is superficial and the raw area is an erosion and not an ulcer. In children healing usually occurs in this manner. In adults the blisters may not rupture, being less pronounced, but they dry up and desquamate after 6 or 7 days. Scarring will only occur if secondary infection supervenes and involves deeper structures. Discolouration may persist for months. In dark-skinned persons persistent hypopigmentation is a common sequel (Radford 1975b; see Fig. 24.2). Burtt's (1938) lesion was visible 14 months after it was sustained, possibly because of deeper involvement and scarring. If eyelids and cheeks are involved, as is to be expected if the eyes are attacked, there is noticeable oedema for several days.

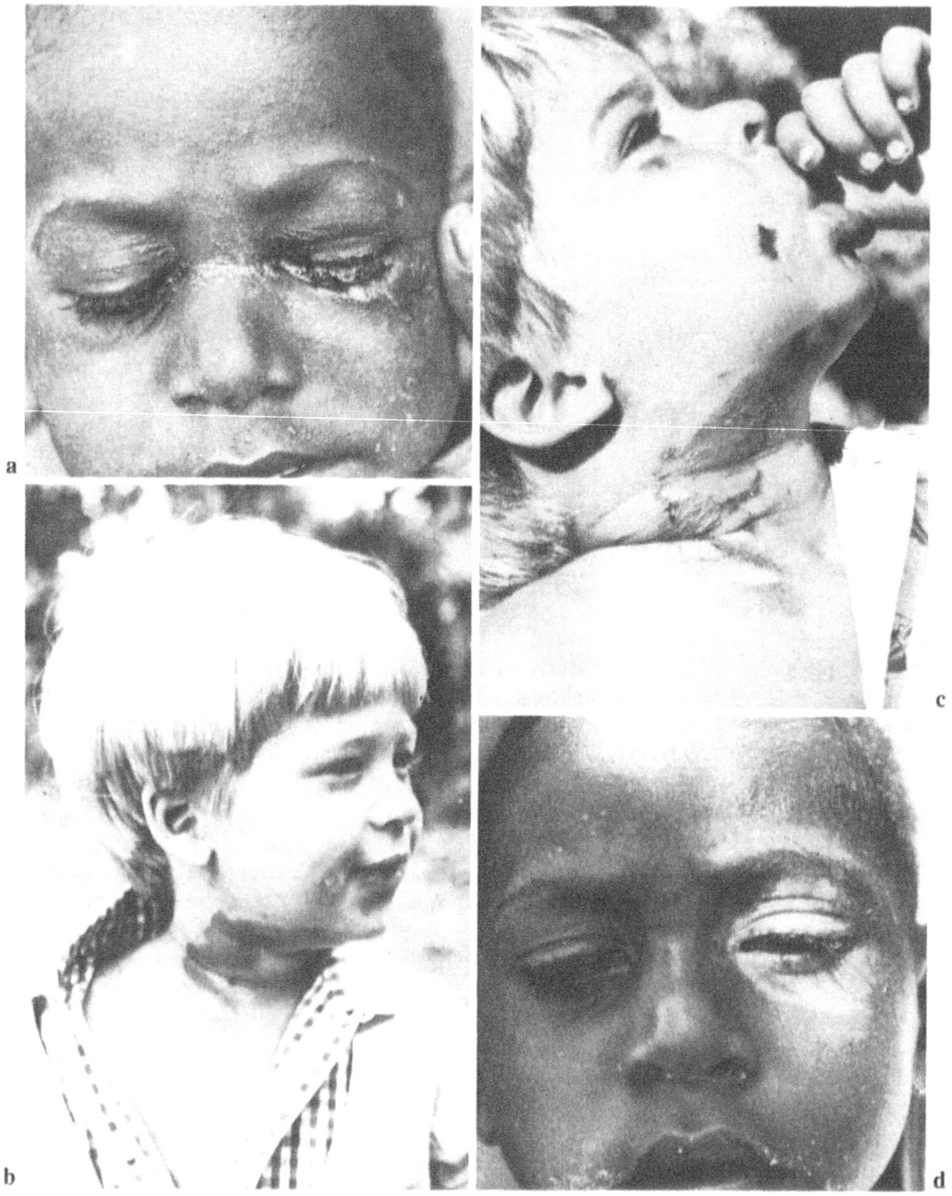

Fig. 24.2a–d. Millipede burns. **a** eye lesion in Papuan child; **b** neck and perioral lesions; **c** raw, weeping surface following lifting of blisters; **d** hypopigmented periorbital skin after healing (cf. **a**). (From Radford 1975b, by kind permission of the author and the Editor of *Tropical and Geographical Medicine*)

The most prominent feature of eye involvement is the instantaneous and exceedingly severe pain, which may persist continously for 2–3 days. It is of an intense burning and smarting character, as if the eye had been touched with a red-hot needle (Loomis 1936). Both Loomis and Radford noted that the pain was in no way diminished by repeated eye lavage. The pain is accompanied by copious lacrimation, chemosis, conjunctival injection and swelling of the tarsal conjunctiva (Haneveld 1958). Uncontrollable blepharospasm is also present. Corneal ulceration may occur but is not invariable. There is a recurrent periorbital swelling for about 3 days. In Loomis's case this involved the eyelids and the malar area of the cheek, which were also contaminated. A whitish conjunctival discharge may be noticeable. Although the eye symptoms are very severe, they appear to settle down after a few days without sequelae as a rule.

Serious Consequences

Natives in Papua New Guinea were insistent that millipedes could cause blindness, and McNamara (cited by Musgrave 1943), who disbelieved, had the proof forcibly demonstrated when his dog sustained a millipede burn of one eye and was blind in that eye in a week. The same result has also been reported in chickens in Haiti (Loomis 1936), and it seems quite possible that it could happen to very young children who play on the ground. Burns in the mouth, acquired by a young child as the result of putting a millipede in its mouth, have been recorded (Radford 1975a). Haneveld (1958) suffered pain on closing his eyes for weeks after his attack.

Diagnosis

The diagnosis is usually obvious. The occurrence of the lesion in a region known to be inhabited by millipedes of the species which can produce burns should alert suspicion. The diagnostic features are as follows: (1) in the case of eye involvement, the dramatically sudden onset of very severe pain in one eye with the accompanying symptoms described above; and (2) in the case of skin involvement only, the lesion is single, there is skin pigmentation, burning and later blistering. There is also a foul smell from the liquid at first.

Treatment

If skin only is affected the damaged part should be washed as soon as possible with copious amounts of water. Ether or alcohol, if available, are better solvents of the contaminating liquid. Blistering can be treated by painting the lesion with 1% gentian violet or 1% acriflavine solution and leaving it uncovered. If erosions are present they can be quite adequately managed by a simple dressing of calico cloth dipped in liquid paraffin or some mild astringent soak such as 1% aluminium acetate solution. Antibiotics are required if secondary infection is suspected.

Eye involvement requires immediate copious lavage with water to minimise the risk of further damage. Even a 5-min delay could have serious consequences (Haneveld 1958). This lavage can be repeated for a day or two. Local anaesthetic ointments can be used, but local instillation of 1% to 5% cocaine solution, as advised by Haneveld (1958), is better. The ointments carry a risk of sensitisation if they came into contact with damaged skin. Sulphonamide or antibiotic drops are also advisable (neomycin carries a risk of sensitisation). Atropine drops are essential, if corneal ulceration is present, to avoid adhesion of the iris. The eye should be covered, and periorbital oedema should be reduced by cold compresses.

Morphology of Millipedes

Millipedes or Diplopoda are elongate, tracheate arthropods with a distinct head and trunk composed of large numbers of apparent segments, each of which, with the exception of the first four, bears two pairs of legs. They have a single pair of antennae on the head, and a head plate or gnathochilarium is formed by a pair of mandibles and a pair of maxillae (Sheals and Rice 1973). There are two sub-classes, the Selapognaths and the Chilognaths. The former are inconspicuous, soft-bodied harmless creatures. The latter are hard-bodied arthropods whose burnished, often brightly coloured, chitinous exoskeleton is reinforced with calcareous material (Burtt 1947). Most millipedes are Chilognaths, and all the species causing injury to men belong to the family Juliaformia. The genera concerned and the geographical location from which they have been reported are shown in Table 24.2. Some of the larger tropical species can reach a length of 30 cm (Figs. 24.3, 24.4). During their life cycle they may pass through from 2 to 7 instars between egg and adult, each instar adding several new segments.

Millipedes are nocturnal vegetarians, with a preference for soft, decomposed plant matter. Since they are moisture dependent and dislike light, their natural habitat is in shaded, humid spots such as under stones and amongst dead leaves and bark (Cloudsley-Thompson 1958; Haneveld 1958). When disturbed they coil into a tight spiral (Fig. 24.5) and when approached they discharge a foul-smelling defensive liquid, which resembles, according to species and secretion, chlorine, bromine, iodine, bitter almonds, urine, faeces, garlic etc. (Radford 1975b). The fluid is formed in repugnatorial glands, one on each side of each segment, and is discharged through a pore which is normally closed by a chitinous rod. When the millipede is about to discharge the fluid the plug is withdrawn by muscular action and the liquid is expelled by pressure from surrounding tissues (Burtt 1947). In the larger millipedes this pressure is sufficient for a fine jet, invisible to the naked eye, to be propelled for a distance of up to 84 cm (Loomis 1936).

Table 24.2. Species of millipedes which have been recorded as causing injuries to man. (Based on Radford 1975b)

Species	Where recorded	References
Rhinocrichus lethifer	Haiti	Loomis (1936)
Rhinocrichus latespagor	Haiti	Loomis (1936)
Polyconoceras attems	Papua New Guinea	Jolivet (1970)
Spirostreptus genus	Indonesia	Kopstein (1932); Haneveld (1958)
Julus genus	Indonesia	Kopstein (1932)
Spirobolus genus	Tanzania	Burtt (1938)
Orthoporus genus	Mexico	Halstead and Ryckman (1949)

Several of these millipedes have also been recorded from Panama, Nigeria, India, Australia and Malaysia

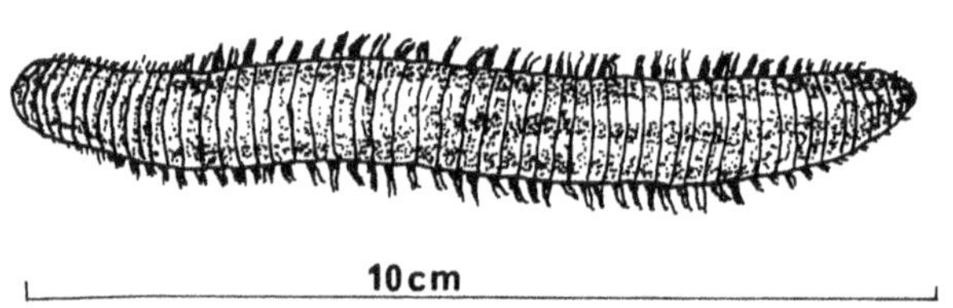

Fig. 24.3. A large tropical millipede, *Rhinocricus lethifer*, natural size. [From Sheals and Rice 1973, by kind permission of the authors and the publishers, the Trustees of the British Museum (Natural History)]

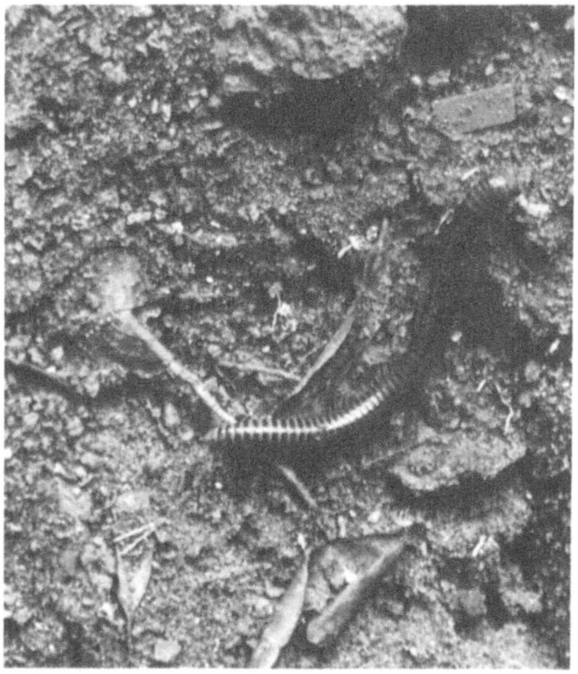

Fig. 24.4. Unidentified millipede from Thailand. Estimated length 25 cm. (Courtesy of Dr. A. Lyell, Glasgow)

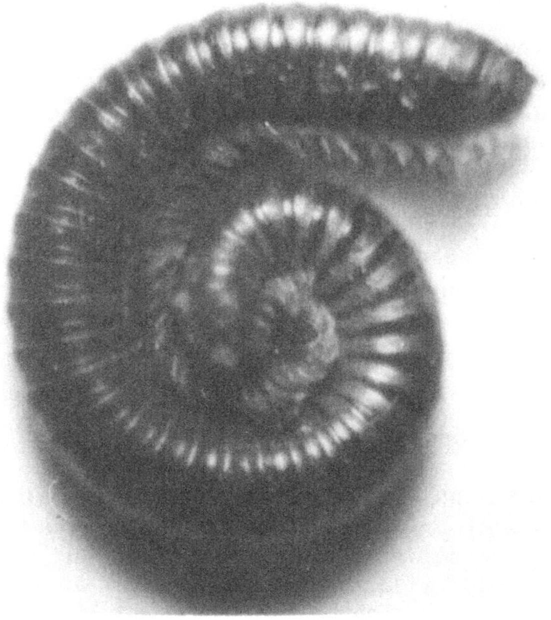

Fig. 24.5. Harmless millipede (about 2.5 cm long), found in the present writer's garden, showing the tight coil position millipedes adopt when disturbed.

The secretion may consist of *p*-benzoquinone or other quinones for *Julida, Spirobolida* and *Spirostreptida*, *p*-cresol for a single species of *Chordeumida* and benzaldehyde and/or hydrocyanic acid for some polydesmids. These are all defensive secretions (Meinwald et al. 1966). The discharge of cyanide is achieved by the admixture of two precursors from different chambers at the exact moment of discharge (Jolivet 1970).

References

Andrews GC, Domonkos A (1971) Centipede bites. In: Diseases of the skin, 6th edn. Saunders, Philadelphia, pp 376–377

Ariff AW (1956) Cortisone for centipede bites. Br Med J I: 986

Baerg WJ (1924) The effect of the venom of some supposedly poisonous arthropods. Ann Entomol Soc Am 17: 343–352

Baerg WJ (1925) The effect of the venom of some supposedly poisonous arthropods of the Canal Zone. Ann Entomol Soc Am 18: 471–478

*Bayley-DeCastro A (1921) The poison of the Scolopendridae being a special reference to the Andaman species. Indian Med Gaz 50: 207–209

Burtt E (1938) Irritant exudation from a millipede. Nature 142: 796

Burtt E (1947) Exudate from millipedes with particular reference to its injurious effects. Trop Dis Bull 44: 7–12

*Cloudsley-Thompson JL (1958) Spiders, scorpions, centipedes and mites. Pergamon, London

Cornwall JW (1915–1916) Some centipedes and their venom. Indian J Med Res 3: 541–557

Ebeling W (1975) Urban entomology. University of California, Division of Agricultural Science, Los Angeles Cal, pp 345–346

Halstead BW, Ryckman R (1949) Injurious effects from contacts with millipedes. Med Arts Sci 3: 16–18

Haneveld GT (1958) Eye lesions caused by the exudate of tropical millipedes. Trop Geogr Med 10: 165–167

*Jolivet P (1970) À propos de l' extrème toxicite d'une espèce geante de Myriapode Diplopode de la Nouvelle Guinée australienne appartenant au genre *Polyconoceras attems* (Rhinocrididae). Entomologiste 26: 30–40, 47–54

Keegan HL (1963) Centipedes and millipedes as pests in tropical aras. In: Keegan HL, MacFarlane WV (eds) Venomous and poisonous animals and noxious plants of the Pacific region, Pergamon, Oxford, pp 161–163

Kopstein F (1932) Die Gifttiere Javas und ihre Bedeutung für den Menschen. Med Volksgezondh Ned Indië 21: 222–256

*Loomis HF (1936) The millipedes of Hispaniola with description of a new family, new genera and new species. Bull Museum Comp Zool Harvard 80: 1–191

Meinwald YC, Meinwald J, Eisner T (1966) 1,2-Diallyl-4(3H)-quinazolinones in the defensive secretion of a millipede (*Glomeris marginata*). Science 154: 390–391

Micks DW (1960) Insects and other arthropods of medical importance in Texas. Tex Rep Biol Med 18: 624–635

Musgrave A (1943) Some arachnids and millipedes from New Guinea. Aust Museum Mag 8: 132–135

Pineda EV (1923) A fatal case of centipede bite. J Philippine Islands Med Assoc 3: 59–61

Radford AJ (1975a) Giant millipede burns in Papua New Guinea. Papua New Guinea Med J 18: 138–141

*Radford AJ (1975b) Millipede burns in man. Trop Geogr Med 27: 279–287

Remington CL (1950) The bite and habits of a giant centipede (*Scolopendra subprincipes*) in the Philippines. Am J Trop Med 30: 435–455

Sheals JG, Rice AL (1973) Diplopoda (millipedes). In: Smith KGV (ed) Insects and other arthropods of medical importance. Trustees of The British Museum (Natural History), London, pp 473–478

Southcott RV (1978) Australian harmful arachnids and their allies. Southcott, Mitcham, Adelaide, pp 32–33

25 Delusion of Cutaneous Parasitosis

Most dermatologists and some physicians, general practitioners, psychiatrists and entomologists have encountered patients who are convinced that their skin is infested with animal parasites in the absence of any evidence to support their belief. Delusion of parasitosis is a distressing complaint but one which should not be overlooked in the present context. Patients suffering from it require full examination and careful management. Whilst it is uncommon, it is not nearly as rare as the number of reported instances would seem to indicate (Evans and Merskey 1972; Bishopp 1980; Munro 1980). W. G. Waldron, an entomologist, who had personally seen over 100 cases in a period of 5 years, stated that every entomologist who had contact with the public was aware of this problem—often by referral from a dermatologist or a family physician (Schrut and Waldron 1963).

Clinical Features

The patient is usually a woman aged over 50, but the age and sex incidence of this condition depend to some extent on the patient's constitutional background. Munro (1980) said that the sex incidence was equal, but Skott (1978) noted that women predominated to the extent of three to one. Most of the patients under 40 are men, unless the condition affects members of the same family group, when younger women may also be involved. Women over 70 are not uncommonly affected.

The condition commences with itching, usually in a fairly localised area such as the scalp or exposed parts of the skin before ultimately becoming widespread (Obermayer 1961). The itching, which persists night and day, may be accompanied or even replaced by sensations of crawling, creeping, stinging, biting or burning (McNamara 1928; Wilson and Miller 1946). More than half of Skott's (1978) patients had no skin lesions at all; however, other patients react by scratching or rubbing, which produces changes in the skin varying from trivial marks to widespread excoriations. These may have the bizarre character and distribution of dermatitis artefacta (Evans and Merskey 1972). Over a long period the scratching, which develops into digging or picking at the skin, may result in quite severe mutilation (McAndrews et al. 1956) and may seriously interfere with sleep.

Very soon after the onset of the irritation the patient begins to imagine that it is caused by infestation by some sort of insect. Occasionally the idea of parasites comes to the patient like a flash of inspiration (A. Lyell 1982, personal communication). This belief or conviction, which increases with time, assumes a quite disproportionate importance in the mind of the patient, whose behaviour becomes governed by the reaction to the idea of parasites (Tullett 1965). Initially the patient scratches or rubs the skin to relieve the itch, but these activities are soon transformed into digging or picking to remove the "parasites". Some patients, however, do not indulge in this activity (A. Lyell 1982, personal communication). The fingernails may be assisted by pins, needles, hairpins, knife or scissors points (Obermayer 1961). Tiny pieces of skin are removed, together with fragments of scale, crust, hair or the debris of fluff, feathers or dust which may collect on the clothing and skin. They are all carefully stored in small pieces of paper, matchboxes or similar receptacles, and these pathetic objects are then produced for inspection as "evidence" of the "parasites" present. The material is claimed to consist of dead insects and much information is given about it (see below). The presentation of such "evidence", together with the intensity of the patient's belief is almost pathognomonic of the disorder.

Further questioning may reveal other steps which have been taken to get rid of the "parasites". Compulsive washing and scrubbing of the skin, often several times daily, is sometimes observed (Munro 1978a). Similarly energetic cleaning and disinfecting of the whole house and all the furniture is regularly performed, more often than would ordinarily be deemed necessary and no matter how inconvenient to the patient or her family. The obsession may drive the patient to change the furniture more than once (Evans and Merskey 1972) or even to change residence, not once but several times (Schrut and Waldron 1963; Evans and Merskey 1972), only for the "parasites" to establish themselves quickly in the new abode. Because these patients believe themselves to be infested they naturally regard themselves as a source of contagion to others (Perrin 1896) and take preventive measures accordingly. They may stop work, isolate themselves at home or even move away from the family (Perrin 1896; Schrut and Waldron 1963); they may impose similar precautions on their families. Not infrequently they are so convinced of their infestation and its contagion as to persuade one or more members of the household that they too are infested. Such induced beliefs are constantly reinforced by the instigator and may become as firmly held by the recipient, the so-called folie-à-deux.

Medical consultation, which is sought not so much to relieve the itch as to get rid of the "parasites", quickly reveals another facet of the condition. If, after examination, the doctor expresses doubt as to the presence of any insects or states categorically that there are none, he will arouse instant resentment in the patient. "Evidence" is produced to prove that he is wrong. As Evans and Merskey (1972) reported, "The dermatologist's assertion that the material was mere flotsam was met with a heated indignation. They [the patients] felt that doctors treated their complaints in a most unreasonable and unsympathetic manner".

The "parasites" and their alleged habits are described in detail. A feature of such descriptions is that they conform to the patient's idea of what parasites should look like and how they should behave (McNamara 1928). This, incidentally, also applies to the symptoms—they are what the patient feels they ought to be. Sometimes the insects are "new to science"' (Wilson and Miller 1946), and on rare occasions more than one kind of insect is said to be present (Vacek 1982). Their colour, shape, size, situation on the patient and source in the house may all be given. Some of the descriptions are quite fantastic. One patient of Schrut and Waldron (1963) demonstrated the jumping ability of the "parasites" when the fragments of "evidence" were pushed along a plastic strip with a steel knife. The static electricity generated caused jumping movement. Another patient confided to her doctor during her last illness that she had 227 "parasites" (which she called "capricornes") in her ear and under the skin of her left malar region (Fauré et al. 1957).

An important point made by Schrut and Waldron (1963) was that the illness lasts for 2–3 months or longer, whereas actual arthropod infestation seldom does this. This distinction is probably true, with the exception of scabies and pediculosis, which are usually easily excluded by the patient's doctor.

All the patient's remarks about the "parasites" are argued with apparent logic from the original, rigidly held false belief. It has been remarked by all observers that the majority of these patients appear to be of average intelligence, coherent and able to exercise good judgement in other matters. According to A. Lyell (1982, personal communication) the patient is desperate to maintain his/her sanity. Therefore, what the dermatologist says, in effect, when he tells the patient that there are no parasites, is "You are mad"—an opinion which is confirmed for the patient when the next statement is to the effect that referral to a psychiatrist is desirable. This is really tantamount to saying that the patient knows that what he believes is not true.

R. M. Herrington (1982, personal communication) puts it in another way. He suggests that the patient is stimulated by a need to explain a symptom; once it has been explained, there is an end to abnormal thoughts as no other delusory ideas are necessary. Subsequent behaviour arises from the original delusion, which is firmly held. This firm belief is what makes the patients so plausible. (Patients with senile dementia must obviously be excluded from this generalisation.) Should the doctor whom they have consulted continue to disbelieve them, they will seek other advice; indeed it is characteristic that many doctors are consulted. The patient of McAndrews et al. (1956) consulted no fewer than 104 doctors and one veterinary surgeon in a period of 6 months. Many patients are loquacious about their complaint, especially when the delusion is shared with other members of the family, in which case the dominant partner can scarcely be prevailed upon to stop talking about it. Sometimes, however, taciturnity is the outstanding feature (Perrin 1896).

Unless there is evidence of organic brain damage as the result of a cerebral vascular incident or atherosclerosis, the patients are generally in good physical health. Spontaneous remission is uncommon and, according to Bers and Conrad (1954), has not been observed. Perrin (1896) appeared to hold the same opinion, but one of his own patients seemed to recover spontaneously, although she could hardly stop herself discussing the episode subsequently. One of Wilson's (1952) patients recovered completely and quickly after unwanted tenants, allegedly the source of the "infestation", left. This seems to have been a delusion with an ulterior motive and probably not genuine. The three patients described by Wolff (1957) lost their delusion after admission to hospital. Another patient, a nurse, lost her delusion after the relief of severe tension (A. Lyell 1982, personal communication). Thus not all delusions are permanent. Fear of infestation is not a feature of these cases. McAndrews and his colleagues (1956) have defined a delusion as a fixed and organised belief or judgement contrary to demonstrable fact. A delusion of cutaneous parasitosis implies an unfounded belief that the sufferer is infested by arthropod parasites. Acarophobia, a term sometimes mistakenly used to mean delusion of parasitosis, describes a *fear* of infestation with mites (usually *Sarcoptes*) and does not include other arthropods (Evans and Merskey 1972). Patients with a delusion lack insight, whereas those who suffer from a phobia realise their fears are groundless but require constant reassurance to that effect. The only real fear of those suffering from a delusion of cutaneous parasitosis is that they will infest others. They *know* that they themselves are already infested.

Background to Delusions of Cutaneous Parasitosis

There are four aspects to the background to delusions of cutaneous parasitosis. In addition to social factors there are the underlying mental state of the patient, the previous relationship to parasitic infestation and the precipitating factors.

Social Factors

According to Munro (1980), patients with delusions tend to come from the lower socioeconomic group, but not all workers agree with this (Reilly 1977). Alcohol and drug abuse are a feature in about half the men affected, and younger women with drug addiction could also be at risk in respect of delusions.

Marital difficulties seem to play an important part. Unmarried men or those with broken marriages are much more often affected than are those with stable family life (Munro 1980). Munro has also noted that in married women patients with delusions of parasitosis the reproductive rate is below average. A. Lyell (1982, personal communication) has remarked on the number of instances of marital difficulty, infidelity, separation, divorce etc. which has preceded the onset of delusion. Social isolation is also an important factor.

Psychiatric Factors

There has been considerable debate and not a little difference of opinion about the mental state of the patient with this condition. However, this has been somewhat clarified by recent papers by Munro (1977, 1978a, c, 1980) and by Reilly (1977; Reilly and Beard 1976) Some workers hold that the delusion is related to paranoid disorders (Munro 1978c) or that there is a pronounced paranoid tendency (Halprin 1966). Munro (1978a) felt that a suspicious, paranoid attitude was typical. There was a strong relationship to schizophrenia in some (Bebbington 1976). Faure and his colleagues (1957) considered it to be part of a global psychosis, exactly the opposite to the view taken by Ekbom (1938). Both Baumer (1951) and Krafchuk (1956) thought that it was a genuine psychosis, but others (Ladée 1966; Hopkinson 1970; Skurczynski 1971; Gould and Gragg 1976) held that there was no uniform aetiology, some patients being paranoid and others having organic brain damage as the result of atrophy or vascular damage. Goltz and Derbes (1977) grouped patients with delusion of parasitosis into five categories:

1. Post-infestation
2. Associated with organic brain damage or drug-induced toxic states—including amphetamines (Alapin 1977; Munro 1980)
3. Schizophrenia
4. Associated with depression
5. Idiopathic

Munro (1980) emphasised that one group hitherto regarded by psychiatrists as rare was in fact not at all uncommon. This was the group of patients included in the disorder called "monosymptomatic hypochondriacal psychosis" (MHP). He defined this as a condition in which the patient had a single hypochondriacal delusion (not necessarily of cutaneous parasitosis) extending over a considerable period, not secondary to any other illness and in which the personality remained well preserved. Reilly (1977) noted that this did not imply the absence of symptoms of psychiatric disability but merely that such symptoms, if present, were not part of the primary psychotic illness but represented a reaction to it. Munro (1980) recognised two groups of patients: firstly, young men, many of whom had a history of drug or alcohol abuse, and, secondly, older women. (The diagnostic features of this state as given by Munro are listed under Diagnosis, p. 396). Such patients, however, are not the only ones who may suffer from delusion of cutaneous parasitosis. The grouping proposed by Goltz and Derbes (1977) could perhaps be modified to read as follows:

1. MHP, including drug-induced psychosis
2. Post-infestational
3. Associated with organic brain disease
4. Schizophrenia
5. Associated with depression

The sensation of creeping on the skin (formication) may be a feature of group 2. Group 1 corresponds to what Perrin (1896) regarded as secondary "parasitophobia", the other four groups equating with his primary "parasitophobia". The obvious difficulty in deciding to which group in any classification a particular patient belongs was aptly summed up by the writer of an Editorial (1977) in the *British Medical Journal* who said that the psychiatric state was difficult to assess (an opinion shared by Tullett 1965). However, one fact does seem certain—the majority of the patients recorded prior to 1875 were either depressed in association with involutionary processes or had brain damage brought on by vascular accident or degeneration-producing senile dementia.

Consideration of Vitamin Deficiency

In addition to the psychiatric background mention must be made of certain rare instances where the cause was shown to be vitamin deficiency. Pellagra was noted to be the responsible agent by Myerson (1924), by Aleshire (1954) and by Obermayer (1961). Incidentally, one of Aleshire's patients was taking amphetamine at the time of onset of her delusion (see p. 397). Pope (1970) recorded a rare instance of a patient whose symptoms of delusion of parasitosis were associated with pernicious anaemia and disappeared within a week of the administration of vitamin B_{12} (cyanocobalamin).

Previous Association with Parasitic Infestation

Because of the extent of the skin as a body organ (it is the largest in the body), it is not surprising that, as Klauder (1936) observed, it becomes the object of concern in both health and sickness more than any other organ. Moreover, Giacardy (1923) stated that amongst the "maladies imaginaires" those which arouse the fear of dermatosis are assuredly the most numerous. Trivial skin lesions and the mildest itch, he claimed could be increased by the stress of such influences as heat, sweating, bathing etc. They could also be stimulated by suggestion. The idea of a skin disease is not difficult to imagine under such conditions, especially if the patient has an unstable background.

Previous association with parasitic infestation is thus an important factor in determining the nature of the delusion. Such association may be direct, in that the patient may have suffered in the past (often the immediate past) an infestation (e.g. scabies or lice)—as suggested by Perry (1876) in his patient with delusion of pediculosis, which ultimately cleared spontaneously. There may have been a parasitic infestation in the family or amongst the neighbours, or the patient may have been involved with an animal with cutaneous parasitosis. There may have only been rumours circulating about the risks of parasitic infestation, such as were cited by Wilhelmi (1935) as being rife in Germany in members of the armed forces after World War I and exacerbated by sensational propaganda in the popular press. Schrut and Waldron (1963) stated that "in practically all instances investigated there had been an original and very real arthropod infestation noted to precede and probably trigger the parasitic delusion". Whilst it is perhaps going too far to insist that this applies to all patients, it is undoubtedly important.

Myerson (1924) pointed out that delusion of cutaneous parasitosis is founded on the nature of the paraesthesiae. He wrote that

> ... man seeks constantly to understand his sensation, seeking constantly that mental resting place which is an explanation. Skin sensations are primordially related to insects and a persistent sensation can easily be conceived as bringing out an idea of bugs. For untold centuries parasites have lived in the skin, hair and [skin] appendages of man, and it is only recently, and in a relatively small part of the human population, that parasites have been expelled from their habitat on the surface of the human being.

Added to this primeval instinct are the patient's mistaken ideas of what parasites can do and what constitutes a rash. Giacardy (1923) pointed out that even "goose flesh" can be mistaken for a rash and the most trivial acneiform spots can be magnified into parasite-induced lesions. This is particularly liable to occur in those persons with obsessional personalities and with high standards of cleanliness, who are particularly prone to develop monosymptomatic hypochondriacal delusions (Sargant 1964, cited by Tullett 1965). In fact, it can well be said that whilst no man "by taking thought can add an cubit to his stature", persons suffering from a delusion of cutaneous parasitosis can add very substantially to the meaning of trivial scratch marks and occasional minute follicular pustules or papules, about which the average individual would not think twice. Wilson (1952) has also suggested that some instances of delusional parasitosis may originate in an unconscious desire to end the sharing of their dwellings with an unwelcome visitor or tenant.

Precipitating Factors

It is not always possible to pinpoint an incident which could be said to precipitate the onset of the itch and delusion. Such incidents have, however, been recorded far too often to be mere coincidental findings. Delusion has been reported following immediately after a sudden family bereavement, usually of spouse or parent (Dewhurst and Todd 1956; Fauré et al. 1957; Evans and Merskey 1972); following flooding in the patient's home (Fauré et al. 1957); after a cruel practical joke involving the supposed ingestion of maggots (Perrin 1896); after injury (Ekbom 1938; Pope 1970); after contact with persons alleged to have had parasitic infestation, whether proven or imaginary (Perrin 1896; Giacardy 1923; Wilson and Miller 1946); after association with parasitised animals (McNamara 1928; McAndrews et al. 1956); after it had been suggested by a third party, without foundation, that the patient was infested (Perrin 1896; Wilson and Miller 1946); and for no apparent reason abruptly after the appearance of vitiliginous plaques in two quite unconnected cases (Myerson 1954). All these factors amount to what could be termed personal or family disasters of one kind or another, contact with real or imaginary infestation being regarded as a personal disaster by the obsessively cleanly person.

Shared Delusion of Cutaneous Parasitosis

"Folie à deux" is a neat phrase coined by Lasegue and Falret in 1877 (Dewhurst and Todd 1956) to denote a delusion shared by two persons. Since more than two people can be involved, Evans and Merskey (1972) preferred "Folie partagée". "Shared delusion" is equally meaningful. Baillarger [1860], cited by Greenberg (1954), originally defined the condition as "two or more members of the same family suffering from monomania, the characteristic delusional state being identical . . . the outbreak not being simultaneous but one anteceding the other by several months". The induced person is genuinely deluded, although the induction of false beliefs is associated with a varying degree of commitment on the part of the induced person (Evans and Merskey 1972). For example, in the two instances of folie à deux cited by Greenberg (1954) one of the secondary victims only shared the belief in question from awe of his marital partner and the other from filial devotion, although basically psychotic himself. Another patient said subsequently that he only expressed belief for the sake of domestic harmony. Dewhurst and Todd (1956) stressed the importance of the nature of the delusion and its value to the person induced, in determining the strength of his conviction. They also pointed out that the stability of the delusion might be partly dependent on the degree of suggestibility of the induced person.

The moving spirit in the majority of the cases of shared delusion of cutaneous parasitosis is the mother of the family. Wolff (1957) emphasised that in his example of three persons showing such a delusion there was a hierarchical element. The wife was the first to develop the delusion. She then persuaded her husband to accept it and he in his turn assisted his wife to convert his brother to the same belief. When all three were admitted to hospital for treatment the combined effect of some degree of separation from one another and the loss of family segregation from others brought about a remission in all three. The wife subsequently relapsed 3 years later but failed to induce the other two to accept the delusion again. This example also emphasises the importance of social isolation in the development of delusions.

The clinical features of shared delusion of cutaneous parasitosis are similar to those of one person deluded with added factors. In the instance recorded by Giacardy (1923) a man, his wife and daughter mistakenly believed they were suffering from scabies alleged to have been contracted from a neighbour's Spanish maidservant. Although the husband sought treatment first, the condition had actually started with his wife. Numerous measures to get rid of the "parasites" had already been taken when the husband and wife were interviewed together. The husband had a few banal spots on his arms about which he spoke but made little fuss. His wife, who did most ot the talking, embroidered the facts, commented on them and developed them. The couple's communication was clearly stamped with the force of her personality. As Giacardy observed, "the fire of her conviction, the abundance of her energy had created in her entourage an atmosphere of itching. They were on the look-out for the slightest pimple and the most inoffensive acne was subjected to the most energetic treatment. A woman of fertile imagination, she had imposed scabies on her daughter, husband and neighbour." This description emphasises that the dominant role is played by the person who first has the delusion, that it is usually the mother of a household and that all the members have to undergo the treatment she dictates.

Diagnosis

Although the diagnosis of delusion of cutaneous parasitosis may be obvious, it should be made by a dermatologist; the exclusion of true parasitosis is sometimes difficult and the dermatologist has the necessary expertise. It can only be done by a thorough examination of the patient and the patient's clothing, if indicated. Microscopic examination of specimens should also be made; if a mite is found it should be identified, because the chance of an occasional house dust mite being found does not imply a diagnosis of parasitosis. The present writer has seen an instance of folie à deux in which the patients brought with them specimens mounted on a slide and one or two house dust mites were found. Only when these are present in very large numbers and then only in special circumstances can they be regarded as pathogenic. The patient reported by Traver (1951) further emphasises this point (see Chap. 20). The diagnosis of delusion of cutaneous parasitosis should not be entertained until pathogenic parasites as well as any other cause of unexplained generalised itching (Ayres 1953) have been excluded. Additional points of diagnosis are the characteristics outlined by Munro (1980), many of which apply to patients with delusion of parasitosis but not necessarily belonging to his group of MHP:

1. Patient's insistence on a physical aetiology
2. The same unvaried stereotyped story
3. Great imagination about points of therapy
4. Persistence in seeking medical opinion
5. Demand for his/her diagnosis to be confirmed
6. Anger and disdain if diagnosis of parasitosis doubted
7. Suggestion of psychiatric basis met with vituperation
8. Psychiatrists are told the patient has been sent to them under false pretences
9. Corroboration of the patient's story by accompanying relatives
10. Cooperation grudging or absent
11. Persistence of the delusion long after symptoms have been successfully suppressed

Add to these items the presentation of "evidence", and, when two or more members of the family are affected, the garrulity of the instigator of the delusion and the onset at intervals in the case of folie à deux. On the other hand, it must also be stressed that a diagnosis of scabies in two or more members of the same family should not be made until a mite or burrow has been positively identified. This is particularly important in the present context (Giacardy 1923). Accuracy of the diagnosis is very important with regard to treatment (Reilly 1977; Munro 1980). Bishopp's (1980) suggestion that the presence of a psychiatrist at an outpatient visit would be very valuable in this respect is a good one, provided that he or she is presented to the patient as a medical colleague and not as a psychiatrist.

Management

The general management of patients with delusion of cutaneous parasitosis has been well summarised by Gould and Gragg (1976), whose views are the basis of what follows. Be certain of the diagnosis but do not exaggerate the attempt to find parasites. Take the patient seriously and listen to what he or she has to say, noting unusual facets. Inquire how the disorder has affected the patient's life; try to gain the patient's confidence and distract him or her from the obsessional belief. Be on the look-out for signs that the patient is likely to accept *any* help, not necessarily technical. Talk to such patients as long as necessary in order to indicate to them that they are not sources of contagion. If necessary, enlist the help of a psychiatrist but do not refer to the latter as such directly. Patients with paranoid tendencies are resentful of suggestions that they should see a psychiatrist and are likely to become uncooperative. Offer relief for the irritation but not thereby implying that this should be antiparasitic.

McFarland (1953) found that a placebo gave relief for about 2 weeks, whilst Ayres (1953) thought that patience allied with firmness was often successful treatment for patients with delusion of recent origin. Hamann and Avnstrop (1982) were of the opinion that a dermatologist should supervise the treatment of these patients because their delusion was monosymptomatic with dermatological manifestations.

If the delusion is toxic in origin or due to some vitamin deficiency the correction of the cause is usually sufficient to result in the disappearance of the symptoms in time, often rapidly.

The use of specific psychiatric measures such as ECT (Baumer 1951; Bers and Conrad 1954) have helped some patients in the past and may still do so occasionally if indicated for underlying reasons of psychiatric abnormality. Antidepressant drugs have helped some patients. Hopkinson (1970) obtained good results in three depressed patients using imipramine. Roberts and Roberts (1977) found Parstelin very effective and claimed that the monoamine oxidase (MOA) inhibitor contained in it was responsible. However, Reilly (1977) was of the opinion that the benefit was due to trifluoperazine, which is also an ingredient. This compound drug does not seem particularly suitable for most patients with this delusion, who are elderly, because the MOA inhibitor element is contraindicated in cardiovascular disorders, which may be the background pathology.

In 1971 Skurczynski reported good results with neuroleptic drugs, stating that they controlled tthe symptoms. He used thioridazine (Melleril), metotenazate (Frenolon) and perazine (Taxilan) in combination. Riding and Munro (1975), confirmed by Reilly (1975), Reilly et al. (1978), Munro (1977, 1978a, b, c, 1980) and by Hamann and Avnstrop (1982), the latter using a double blind cross-over clinical trial, reported most encouraging improvement in many patients given pimozide, which is also a neuroleptic drug. Bishopp (1983) considered that only those cases of MSH with a psychotic background would benefit from pimozide, but Duke (1983) also found that simple neurotic excoriations might be greatly improved by it. It is thus apparently extremely valuable in treating patients with MHP, of which delusion of cutaneous parasitosis is a good example. In his 1980 series Munro achieved excellent results in 19 of 26 patients and improvement in the other seven. The drug is given daily, preferably in a single oral dose in the morning. The dosage is from 2 to 12 mg daily (Reilly 1977), depending on the individual response of each patient. Favourable response occurs within the first week of treatment, and as the delusion diminishes or disappears so the dose may be reduced to a smaller maintenance level. The latter is necessary, since the drug only suppresses the symptoms, but does so completely in many cases. On the other hand, withdrawal of the drug results in an equally dramatic relapse. The present writer's patients with folie à deux responded quickly and completely to pimozide. Toxic side-effects are seldom encountered at low dosage levels but may occur at doses over 8 mg daily. They include initial drowsiness and later a pleasurable sense of alertness, episodes of depression (Hamann and Avnstrop 1982), tension symptoms, postural hypotension occasionally, extrapyramidal dysfunction (parkinsonism) and indigestion (Reilly 1977; Munro 1980). Duke (1983) added a number of other behavioural reactions, such as restlessness, inattention, aggressiveness etc.; dystonic reactions (e.g. torticollis, tardive dyskinesis); autonomic reactions, including dry mouth, visual disturbances and incontinence; changes in blood pressure and ECG; menstrual disorders; allergic reaction and blood dyscrasias. Reilly said that parkinsonian symptoms could easily be combated by anticholinergic drugs such as orphenadrine 50 mg three times daily. A warning note should be sounded, however, since a very severe case of parkinsonism and another with severe oculogyric crises both occurred after small doses of pimozide. Both recovered when the drug was withdrawn and suitable counter measures were adopted (R. M. Herrington 1982, personal communication).

It would appear (Munro 1980) that the symptoms of MHP are possibly induced by dopamine hyperfunction, a state which, for example, can be induced by dexamphetamine. Dopamine transmission to the brain can be prevented by several neuroleptic drugs through selective receptor blockade. This may explain their antipsychotic action and the relapse when they are withdrawn. Butyrophenones (e.g. haloperidol) and especially diphenylbutyl-piperidine (pimozide) are highly specific dopamine blockers. Both drugs completely inhibit certain behavioural abnormalities induced by amphetamine. This explanation could also account for the beneficial effects of pimozide in MHP.

The prognosis is excellent for those delusions caused by toxic states or vitamin deficiency. With the advent of pimozide prognosis is also good for those patients with MHP manifested by delusion of cutaneous parasitosis. It is less favourable for those patients with a schizophrenic or depressive background, according to many authors (McAndrews et al. 1956; Obermayer 1961; Halprin 1966; Bebbington 1976; Reilly and Beard 1976; Editorial 1977), and much poorer when marked paranoia is present (McAndrews et al. 1956; Obermayer 1961). Nevertheless, pimozide has also greatly improved the outlook in many of these patients.

References

Alapin B (1977) In discussion of Reilly (1977) Br J Dermatol 98: 457–459

Aleshire I (1954) Delusion of parasitosis. JAMA 155: 15–17

Ayres S Jr (1953) In discussion of McFarland (1953) Arch Dermatol Syphilol 67: 278–283

Baumer L (1951) Die Behandlung des Juckreizes in besondere beim 'Dermatozoenwahn' mit Elektroschock. Hautarzt 2: 131–132

Bebbington PE (1976) Monosymptomatic hypochondriasis, abnormal illness behaviour and suicide. Br Psychiatry 128: 175–178

Bers N, Conrad K (1954) Die chronische taktile Halluzinose. Fortschr Neurol Psychiatr 22: 254–270

Bishopp ER (1980) Monosymptomatic hypochondriasis. Psychosomatics 21: 731–749

Bishopp ER (1983) Monosymptomatic hypochondriacal syndromes in dermatology. J Am Acad Dermatol 9: 152–158

Dewhurst K, Todd J (1956) The psychosis of association—folie à deux. J Nerv Ment Dis 124: 451–459

Duke EE (1983) Clinical experience with pimozide; emphasis on its use in post-herpetic neuralgia. J Am Acad Dermatol 8: 845–850

Ekbom KA (1938) Praeseniler Dermatozoenwahn. Acta Psychiatr Neurol 13: 227–259

Editorial (1977) Delusions of parasitosis. Br Med J I: 790–791

Evans P, Merskey H (1972) Shared beliefs of dermal parasitosis; folie partagée. Br J Med Psychol 45: 19–26

Fauré H, Berchtold R, Ebtinger R (1957) Sur les parasitoses délirantes. Evol Psychiatr (Paris) 1: 357–375

Giacardy P (1923) Un cas d'acarophobie familiale. J Med Bordeaux 53: 479–480

Goltz RW, Derbes V (1977) Delusion of parasitosis. In: Orkin M, Maibach HI, Parish LC, Schwartzman RM (eds) Scabies and Pediculosis. Lippincott, Philadelphia, pp 51–57

*Gould WM, Gragg TM (1976) Delusion of parasitosis. Arch Dermatol 112: 1745–1748

Greenberg HP (1954) Folie à deux. Guy's Hosp Rep 103: 381–392

Halprin K (1966) The art of self-mutilation. II. Delusions of parasitosis. JAMA 198: 1207

Hamann K, Avnstrop C (1982) Delusion of infestation treated by pimozide: a double blind cross-over clinical study. Acta Derm Venereol (Stockh) 62: 55–58

Hopkinson G (1970) Delusions of parasitosis. Acta Psychiatr Scand 46: 111–119

Klauder JV (1936) Psychogenic aspects of skin disease. J Nerv Ment Dis 84: 249–273

Krafchuk JD (1956) In discussion of McAndrews et al. (1956) J La State Med Assoc 108: 279–286

Ladée GA (1966) Delusion of parasitosis or of dermatozoiasis. In: Hypochondriacal syndromes. Elsevier, Amsterdam, pp 306–323

McAndrews J, Jung R, Derbes V (1956) Delusion of dermal parasitosis (acarophobia) manifested by folie à deux. J La State Med Assoc 108: 279–286

McFarland AR (1953) Mechanical trauma. Arch Dermatol Syphilol 67: 278–283

MacNamara ED (1928) A note on cutaneous and visual hallucinations in the chronic hallucinatory psychoses. Lancet I: 807

Munro A (1977) Delusion of parasitosis. Br Med J I: 1219

Munro A (1978a) Monosymptomatic hypochondriacal psychoses, a diagnostic entity which may respond to pimozide. Can Psychiatr Assoc J 23: 497–500

Munro A (1978b) Two cases of delusion of worm infestation. Am J Psychiatry 135: 234–235

Munro A (1978c) Monosymptomatic hypochondriacal psychosis manifesting as delusions of parasitosis. Arch Dermatol 114: 940–943

Munro A (1980) Monosymptomatic hypochondriacal psychosis. Br J Hosp Med 24: 34–38

Myerson A (1924) Two cases of acarophobia. Boston Med Surg J 184: 635–638

Obermayer ME (1961) Dynamics and management of self-induced eruptions. Cal Med 94: 61–65

Perrin L (1896) Des nevrodermies parasitophobies. Ann Dermatol Syphiligr (Paris) 7: 129–138

Perry JE (1876) Pediculophobia. Med Surg Registrar 34: 267–268

Pope FM (1970) Parasitophobia as the presenting symptom of vitamin B_{12} deficiency. Practitioner 204: 421–422

*Reilly TM (1975) Pimozide in monosymptomatic psychosis. Lancet I: 1385–1386

Reilly TM (1977) Monosymptomatic hypochondriacal psychosis; presentation and treatment. Proc R Soc Med 70: 39–43

Reilly TM, Beard AW (1976) Monosymptomatic hypochondriasis. Br J Psychiatry 129: 191–192

Reilly TM, Jopling WH, Beard AE (1978) Successful treatment with pimozide of delusional parasitosis. Br J Dermatol 98: 457–459

*Riding J, Munro A (1975) Pimozide in the treatment of monosymptomatic hypochondriacal psychosis. Acta Psychiatr Scand 52: 23–30

Roberts J, Roberts R (1977) Delusions of parasitosis. Br Med J I: 1219

Schrut AH, Waldron WG (1963) Psychiatric and entomological aspects of delusionary parasitosis. JAMA 186: 213–214

*Skott A (1978) Delusions of infestation: Reports from the Psychiatric Research Centre, No 13, St. Jorgens Hospital, University of Göteborg, Sweden

Skurczynski Z (1971) W sprawie tzw. obledu pasozytniiczego. Psychiatr Pol 5: 655–660

Traver JR (1951) Unusual scalp dermatitis in human caused by the mite *Dermatophagoides* (Acarina: Epidermoptidae) Proc Entomol Soc Washington 53: 1–25

Tullett GL (1965) Delusions of parasitosis. Br J Dermatol 77: 448–455

Vacek J (1982) Syndrom Bludove parasitozy (akarophobie) Cesk Dermatol 57: 94–102

Wilhelmi J (1935) Ungezieferwahn. Dtsch Med Wochensch 9: 351–352

Wilson JW (1952) Delusion of parasitosis (acarophobia). Further observations in clinical practice. Arch Dermatol Syphilol 66: 577–585

Wilson JW, Miller HE (1946) Delusion of parasitosis (acarophobia) Arch Dermatol Syphilol 54: 39–56

Wolff S (1957) Folie à trois; a clinical study. J Ment Sci 103: 355–363

26 Insecticides and Other Methods of Controlling Arthropods

Man may need to control, destroy or repel arthropods because of the damage they do to his food, livestock and other material, because they are vectors of many infectious diseases or because of the direct annoyance or harm they themselves cause to him. For the solitary annoying fly, bug, beetle, wasp etc., the natural reaction is to swat it or otherwise physically destroy it. However, this may be too late and, if the arthropods concerned are present in large numbers, futile. Other means may therefore have to be used. These include physical measures such as heat or cold; chemical poisoning (insecticides); dehydration; or biological interference with the arthropods' development in some way or another, by chemical repellents, by trapping by attractants, whether sexual or food, by destruction of their habitat, by preventing their ingress into dwellings etc. Each of these methods has been used, some extensively and universally, others specifically to eradicate a particular creature. Some have been described in detail elsewhere (e.g. the eradication of screwworms in Chap. 8). Many are only in the experimental or developmental stages and have not yet been fully utilised. It is beyond the scope of this book to discuss all of these in detail. Many are matters of agricultural, horticultural or veterinary use, especially where vectors or crop pests are concerned. However, insecticides and repellents are of great interest here, not only because they get rid of arthropods, but also because of their side-effects on man, whether as a patient or a person attending a patient or engaged in their manufacture and testing. Even so, only those substances used directly on man or his clothing or dwelling will be considered in some detail.

Insecticides

Insecticides are chemicals which cause the death of arthropods either by being absorbed through their integuments (contact poisons) or because they are ingested by the arthropod, fatally damaging some vital system such as the central nervous, circulatory or respiratory systems. They act in a variety of ways and are classified either according to their chemical action and origin or according to their physiological effect. Table 26.1 shows the generally accepted grouping of the different classes of insecticides.

Organochlorines

DDT (which stands for dichloro-diphenyl-trichloroethane) was discovered in Switzerland in 1939 but was not put into common use until towards the end of World War II. Its first great success was in destroying lice and bringing an epidemic of typhus in Naples to an end. (Burton 1945). It is simple and relatively cheap (Busvine 1980). It acts on the peripheral nervous system of insects, spiders and ticks, but mites in general are not affected by it, and its effects on scorpions are unsatisfactory (Ridgway et al. 1962). Its action appears to be that of an axon poison (Guthrie and Tindall 1968). Tremors develop, followed by uncoordinated movements. The insects then become paralysed, fall on their backs and die of dessication. DDT became very widespread in its use but has largely been superseded by newer and more effective insecticides because of the rapidly increasing number of insects which have become resistant to it.

Following the decline of DDT other organochlorines came to the fore and the most useful of these was lindane (HCH; γBHC). The action and effects of this compound have been fully discussed in Chap. 15. The other well-known substances in this group such as chlordane, dieldrin and aldrin (all 5-membered ring compounds), and toxaphene

Table 26.1. Grouping of the various chemicals and other methods used to destroy arthropods.[a] The systemic insecticides ingested by the host are not normally prescribed for this purpose but have been observed to have the effect attributed to them

General grouping	Specific examples	Notes
A. *Stomach poisons*		
1. Inorganic	Salts of mercury; arsenic; fluorides	Used horticulturally as insoluble salts. Mercury compounds in pediculosis. Now largely abandoned
2. Organic		
a) Poison bait	Organophosphorus compounds e.g. dichlorvos.	Normaly used as contact poisons
b) Mothproofing	Eulans; Mitin	Incorporated into wool to repel moth larvae
c) Systemic	Phenylbutazone; Tanderil; co-trimoxazole	All ingested by host. Blood-sucking arthropods poisoned. Obligatory parasites unable to become established (e.g. lice)
	Phenothiazine	Inhibits neuromuscular transmission and cytochrome oxidase activity
	Methotrexate	Kills *Demodex* in situ and temporarily inhibits *Sarcoptes*
	Coumaphos; dimethoate, etc.	Veterinary use for protection of cattle against warble fly larvae
B. *Contact poisons*		
1. Vegetable origin	Nicotine	Synapse poison
	Pyrethrum	Very rapid acting; an axon poison. Can cause contact dermatitis. Unreliable at low concentrations
	Rotenone (from derris)	Affects respiratory tissue
		All the so-called botanical insecticides are non-persistent and so less toxic for man
2. Miscellaneous synthetics	Thiocyanates; Lethane	Much used in 1940s against head lice
3. Synthetic pyrethroids	Allethrin Resmethrin (furan cyclic group) Permethrin (chlorinated) Decamethrin (brominated plus a cyanide group)	Chrysanthemic acid ester, as potent as pyrethrum; the others are placed in ascending order of potency. All are axon poisons and cytochrome oxidase inhibitors. Potentiated by piperonyl butoxide or sulphoxide. Very effective; low vertebrate toxicity.
4. Organochlorines	DDT and analogues	Axon poison. Many resistant species now. Abandoned mostly for ecological reasons
	Gamma-hexachlorocyclo-hexane (lindane; γBHC)	Synaptic poisons; lindane is the chlorine analogue of mucoinositol
	Chlorinated camphor (toxaphene)	
	Chlorinated cyclodienes (aldrin; chlordane; dieldrin etc.)	Water insoluble. Resistance to all the organochlorines has developed in many countries
5. Anticholinesterases		
a) Organophosphorus compounds	Parathion; malathion	Blocks action of cholinesterase by combining with it. Relatively low mammalian toxicity for malathion in the concentrations used
b) Carbamates	Physostigmine; carbaryl	Synaptic poison by competing with acetylcholine for fixation by the esterase. Some carbamates are synergised by Dimetilan
C. *Synergists*		
1. Containing a methylene dioxyphenol group	Piperonyl butoxide; sulphoxide	These inhibit microsomal mixed function oxidase systems, which are responsible for degradation toxins. This inhibition interferes with detoxifying of other insecticides, notably pyrethrins and carbamates, and greatly potentiates their effect
2. Containing a *N*-alkyl group	SKF 525A; WARF anti-resistant	
3. Containing *O*-2-propynyl group	NIA 16824	
D. *Contact poisons* (mites and ticks)		
1. DDT		Ineffective
2. Some DDT-related compounds	All contain 2-*p*-chlorobenzene groups	Effective
3. Organochlorines	Lindane	Effective against scabies but apparently banned for many other purposes.? Because of resistance

Table 26.1. *(continued)*

General grouping	Specific examples	Notes
4. Empirical	Benzyl benzoate; sulphur; dimethylthianthrene; tetraethylthiuram monosulphide; crotamiton	All are effective in scabies
E. *Juvenile Hormones* (and analogues)		Interfere with moulting and metamorphosis
F. *Fumigants*		
1. Gaseous	HCN; methyl bromide; ethylformate; dichlorvos	Some require expert application, others are comparatively safe. Dichlorvos is normally a contact poison and is persistent
2. *Vapours*	Mothballs (camphor)	Only in closed containers
G. *Chemosterilisants*		
1. Antimetabolites	Methotrexate	Interfere with normal egg and spermatozoa formation
2. Alkylating agents		
H. *Dehydrating agents*		
1. Finely divided hard gritty dust		These damage the surface cuticle causing water loss
2. Silica aerogels		These adsorb protective surface lipids leading to profound water loss
I. *Repellents*		
1. Against flying insects	Volatile repellents; contain citronella oil	Insects avoid these. They may cause contact dermatitis. Effective for a few hours
	Synthetics such as DMP or DEET	Especially active against mosquitoes and non-biting flies
2. Against crawling insects	Pyrethrins; thiocyanates; benzyl benzoate	Against ticks, fleas, cockroaches; non-persistent. Thiocyanates unsuitable for man. Some mites are repelled
J. *Attractants*		
1. Pheromones	Sex attractants; aggregation pheromones; trail makers	Specific for each species. Not all are effective
2. Exogenous	Food source	Attract certain insects (e.g. fruit flies and wasps by decaying fruit)
3. Odour	Trichlorethylene	Attracts seaweed flies

[a] The information has been collated from various sources mentioned in the preceding chapters and classified with help from Busvine (1980), Ebeling (1975) and Guthrie and Tindall (1968)

(a chlorinated pine oil) have high insecticidal properties but are also very toxic for mammals and are not used directly on man or his clothing. Aldrin and dieldrin are classified as Group I toxins (the most toxic group) and chlordane as Group II (Ebeling 1975).

Organophosphorus Compounds

Malathion

Malathion is one of the best organophosphorus insecticides. It acts by virtue of its anticholinesterase properties and, compared with many of the others in the same group has a low mammalian toxicity. Cole et al. (1958) showed that as a powder 1% malathion was more effective and 0.5% less effective than synergised pyrethrum powder against body lice. It appeared to be safe, and this was confirmed by Hayes et al. (1960), who could only detect a very slight change in human blood cholinesterase activity after several weeks' contact with 10% powder in clothing. Since it is never used at a concentration of above 1% powder and only in very infrequent applications, it has been deemed safe. Its absorption, if any, can be assessed by measuring the urinary output of its metabolites. Clinical trials as a lousicide (it is equally effective against many other arthropods) in areas where DDT and γBHC were becoming less than 100% effective, showed malathion to be more effective than either (Shawarby et al. 1963; Maunder 1971b). Its value was repeatedly confirmed in the laboratory by Cole et al. (1967), whilst the development of resistance seemed not to have occurred (Cole et al. 1969), although in their tests the number of generations tested was only 44. Some arthropods may take a good deal longer than this to develop resistance (but see below regarding resistance in general). Maunder (1971b), in fact, pointed out that in some areas of Africa some resistance to malathion was already beginning to appear and he estimated its useful life as an insecticide as between 10 and 20 years from that time. So far it is still very effective, probably because it is being used more intelligently as regards the development of resistance than were previous insecticides. Martinez et al. (1975) showed that used as a preventive against the bug *Triatoma infestans* in Argentina by spraying onto the walls of brick and adobe houses malathion was very efficient and did not cause any toxic effects in either the operatives or the residents, nor did it discolour the fabric of buildings or furniture or have any unpleasant smell.

In clinical use the great advantages of malathion are (1) it is 100% effective against mobile stages of arthropods; (2) it has an ovicidal effect resulting from its persistent residual action for up to 3 weeks (which prevents embryos from emerging from the eggs); (3) it has a residual effect in treatment of head lice which prevents re-infestation for up to 6 weeks because of its persistence on hair; (4) it does not interfere with treatment of secondary infection; (5) modern presentations have removed its unpleasant smell of mercaptan; and (6) it has been shown to be effective as a cream shampoo with 5-min application (Preston and Fry 1971), although on general principles this is too short a period to achieve any residual effect. As an 0.5% alcoholic solution (Prioderm) it is 100% adulticide and 95% ovicidal. If used at either double this concentration or for two applications of 0.5%, which is a theoretical overkill, it greatly reduces the likelihood of the emergence of resistant strains. Taplin et al. (1982), stressing this particular point, have indicated that education of medical, nursing, public health and pesticidal workers is very important if malathion and other insecticides which are effective at present are to be used worldwide in such a way as to avoid the development of resistance. Maunder (1981) has pointed out that its paralysing effects on embryos have produced some very curious anomalies in the appearances of the eggs of head lice (nits), which may lead to mistaken reports of ineffectiveness or resistance.

Dichlorvos

Dichlorvos, another organophosphorus compound, is a slow-acting stomach poison usually employed to give off an insecticidal vapour. It is thus used on sinks or baths to kill cockroaches, in closed containers holding louse-infested clothing (usually only small amounts of clothing, because of the difficulties of penetration; Grothaus and Cole 1973) or as a component of flea collars for dogs and cats.

Carbamates

Carbamates are salts or esters of carbamic acid (NH_2COOH). The only naturally occurring compound in this group is physostigmine, which is found in the seeds of the calabar bean, *Physostigma venenosum*. Carbamates are parasympathetico-mimetics with an anticholinesterase effect (Guthrie and Tindall 1968). This effect is said to be achieved by competing with acetylcholine for attachment to cholinesterase radicals (Busvine 1980). Although this mechanism differs from that of malathion, the effect on arthropods is the same, that of a synaptic poison inducing paralysis. There are similar effects on mammals, but some carbamates (e.g. 3-isopropylphenyl-*N*-methylcarbamate) are much more toxic than others such as carbaryl (Vandekar 1965). The latter is regarded as clinically safe, although when it is used as an agricultural spray operatives must take care not to get splashed (Vandekar 1965). Carbaryl is used clinically in man as an alcoholic lotion for killing head lice, and its effects on the latter have been fully described by Maunder (1981; see also Chap. 5). Lice resistant to carbaryl can be killed by synergised carbaryl (Clark and Cole 1967), but this is said to be uneconomical for general use (Cole 1973). A related compound, propoxur, is used as a contact insecticide spray for dwellings and crops.

Synergists

Synergists are substances which enhance the activity of insecticides but are themselves not necessarily insecticidal. They act in a variety of ways. They may, by oxidation, inhibit detoxifying microsomal enzymes, e.g. sulphoxide or piperonyl butoxide (Guthrie and Tindall 1968). They may chemically alter insecticides in the arthropod tissues to a more potent form or compete with the insecticide for uptake by inhibiting enzymes (Busvine 1980). They are used principally with pyrethroids and carbamates. See Busvine (1980) for fuller details.

Insecticide Resistance

Resistance to insecticides received little attention in the literature prior to the advent of DDT in the early 1940s. The instant and universal success of this insecticide resulted in its use on a vast scale worldwide. As early as 1947 it became apparent that some of the arthropods against which it was being used were becoming resistant to it. This was first noticed on some species of flies and mosquitoes, and in 1952 Hurlbutt and colleagues reported that it had failed to control an epidemic of body lice in Korea. They demonstrated that this was because the lice were mostly resistant to DDT, Kitaoka (1952) confirmed a similar event in Japan. In those localities where resistant lice occurred different insecticides had to be used. Resistance was not confined to DDT, however. Wright and Pal (1965) observed that there was a marked increase in the number of reports of resistance to organochlorines in general compared with a previous survey by Wright and Brown (1957). An ever-increasing number of arthropods are developing insecticide resistance. According to Busvine (1980), the number is now well over 300, of which one-third are of medical importance. Some species (e.g. *Phlebotomus*, *Glossina*) have not yet developed insecticide resistance.

Resistance to a particular chemical varies from species to species; some are susceptible, others tolerant. Conversely, a particular species may be susceptible to one insecticide but resistant to another. In general terms resistance to a particular insecticide extends to chemically related compounds. Shalaby (1971) suggested that the development of resistance depended on one or more prior exposures to the insecticide in question. This seemed to explain why lice in some areas were susceptible to lindane but in other areas the same species was resistant. Experimentally, by measuring the insecticide concentration necessary to cause a 50% mortality in a given time (LC 50), Clark and Cole (1964) showed that marked resistance to lindane developed quickly (8000-fold in 73 generations), whilst that to carbaryl was much slower and that to malathion even slower.

This resistance does not develop in an individual, as suggested by Gordon and Lavoipierre (1962), but is a genetic trait, according to Busvine (1980). Arthropods which possess it escape death on exposure, while the rest are killed by one or more exposures. In an outbreak of louse infestation this results in the death of susceptible lice and the survival of the few resistors. These are enabled to proliferate so that eventually the proportion of resistant lice in the general louse population rises rapidly. Thus colonies acquire resistance but individuals inherit it.

What causes resistance? Busvine (1980) indicated that it was due to the enhanced detoxification systems of the resistant arthropods. For example, the insecticide may be altered to a less toxic derivative by enzymatic action such as the transformation of DDT to DDE—a metabolite of DDT; 1,1-dichloro-2-2-bis (*p*-chlorophenyl) ethylene—or by attacking the carboxyl radical of malathion; or the microsomal oxidase detoxifying systems may be more active. It would seem that this latter action is likely, since Clark and Cole (1967) also showed that carbaryl-resistant lice were killed by synergised carbaryl and synergists are known to act by inhibiting microsomal oxidase systems. When resistance develops, some other form of insecticide will be required (as with the synergist and carbaryl) or an entirely different method of arthropod destruction will have to be used. Maunder (1971a) showed that lice were at that time resistant to both DDT and the lindane/dieldrin group of organochlorines but were fully susceptible to organophosphorus compounds such as malathion, carbaryl or propoxur.

Pyrethroids and Pyrethrum

Powdered pyrethrum flowers have long been used as an insecticide. The lethal properties are due to a toxic substance contained in a small oily fraction. The effect is very rapid and this is probably due to the low water–oil partition coefficient (Busvine 1980), which allows the athropod cuticle to be penetrated easily and quickly. The accumulated toxin then attacks the central nervous system and also inhibits cytochrome oxidase (Guthrie and Tindall 1968). One of the advantages of pyrethrum extract is its low mammalian toxicity. At weak concentrations, however, it is unreliable as an insecticide. Synthetic substitutes have been produced. The early ones were of similar potency to the natural extract, but later synthetics such as resmethrin, permethrin (chlorinated) and decamethrin (which contains a CN group and is brominated) are increasingly more effective (Busvine 1980) They are all potentiated by synergists.

Synthetic Juvenile Hormones

The normal maturation stages of an insect are controllable by at least two groups of hormones. Ecdyson controls metamorphosis, and juvenile hormone seems to exercise overall control of this process and the laying down of yolk in eggs (Chapman 1971). Synthetic substitutes have been produced which can be used to interfere with these processes. Ecdyson substitutes are steroidal in type and expensive (Busvine 1980). Synthetic juvenile hormones have been shown to inhibit moulting, fatally trapping the emerging insect (lice in this case) in its own moult (Vinson 1973). Where given in excess to adult females it inhibits the hatching of eggs (Cole and van Natta 1973), but it must be given continuously to louse colonies because within a day or two of a single application normal egg laying is resumed (Vinson 1973). These techniques, whilst most interesting and promising, are still really in the experimental stages.

Sorptive Dusts

Sorptive dusts have been known as a means of protecting stored grain for about 2000 years and have been intensively studied since the 1940s (Busvine 1980). According to Tarshis and Blinstrub (1963), sorptive dusts are dusts of very hard nature and very fine particle size which act either by abrasion of the chitinous arthropod cuticle, breaking its continuity, or by adsorption of the protective waterproof lipid of the epicuticle. In either case the result is a rapid and fatal water loss. An industrial silica aerogel Dri-Dri 67 has been shown to be effective against 40 species of arthropod. Its effectiveness can be accelerated by the addition of 2% Dibrom and 0.5% pyrethrum, which increases its action against fleas and cockroaches. In a clinical trial it killed pubic lice and their eggs on 10 students, two of whom found it very dry but tolerable for the 2 h necessary. Its action on infected premises has been shown to last for up to 3 years. It seems unlikely that resistance will develop as its effect is purely physical. It deserves thorough clinical trial.

Fumigants

There are many substances which in gaseous or vapour form are lethal to arthropods. Most, but not all, are also dangerous to man and domestic animals, and some such as prussic acid (HCN) or phosphine require special handling by trained operatives. Many are only available for large-scale use in disinfesting buildings or ships or for agricultural or horticultural purposes. A few are available on a personal level for disinfestation of clothing or use in houses. All require strict adherence to written instructions to avoid accidents and achieve optimal results.

Hot air at a controlled temperature above 60°C is probably the cheapest and most effective method of disinfesting clothing. On a small scale a hair dryer inside a polythene bag can be successful, but probably easier to use and more efficient is a tumble dryer, as recommended by Maunder (1983). A heat period of 15–30 min is usually adequate. Steam sterilisation is now obsolete because of the rather formidable equipment required.

Methyl bromide is a very effective fumigant, which is odourless, non-inflammable and does not damage or stain clothing. Portable kits are available in the form of 20 ml ampoules. One of these, together with the person's infested clothes, are placed together in a polythene bag, which is then sealed, and the ampoule is broken. This method can be used by untrained persons (Grothaus and Cole 1973). Ethyl formate can be used in a similar manner but has the disadvantage of being inflammable. Both of these chemicals are used chiefly against body lice.

Dichlorvos is applied on impregnated resin strips against lice. In the laboratory it is effective through 40 layers of cloth, but in practice is less efficient for disinfesting clothes. It is most likely to be successful with very small quantities of clothes. It is relatively safe (Grothaus and Cole 1973) and can also be used on similar strips placed in strategic spots against cockroaches.

Biological Means

Control of arthropods by biological means is really beyond the scope of this book, although reference could be made to the eradication of screwworm flies (Chap. 8, pp. 93–94) and the use of predators against mites attacking stored grain (Chap. 21, pp. 351–352). Male flies can be removed from circulation by baiting traps with either female pheromones or ultrasonic emission of sound synchronous with the wing beats of female flies. Destruction of nesting and breeding places are very important, but responsibility lies in the province of public health authorities and entomological services. Interested readers should consult Ebeling (1975) or Busvine (1980) and the WHO paper "Equipment for vector control" (1974).

Repellents

Intensive study of repellents was stimulated by World War II and the huge casualties directly or indirectly caused by arthropods (Sherman 1966). Much work then and since has been carried out by research entomologists of the United States Department of Agriculture at Orlando, Florida, and elsewhere in other centres throughout the world. Up to the time of the war citronella was the only useful repellent. However, investigations have since produced a host of chemicals with repellent properties. One of the earliest was MYL antilouse powder which contained

0.2% pyrethrins (as 20% pyrethrum concentrate) 2.0% 2-4-dinitroamide (an ovicide) 2.0% *N*-isobutyl undecyclenamide (a synergist) 0.25% phenol (antioxidant)	in pyrophyllite powder

This was not a true repellent but inhibited the establishment of lice on the body by killing mobile and egg stages (Knipling and Dove 1944). Further tests for materials which would protect the users by their application to the skin included three substances which have proved to be very effective. They are dimethylphthallate (DMP), 2-ethyl-1, 3-hexanediol (Rutgers 612) and the butyl ester of 3,4-dihydro-2-2-dimethyl-4-oxo-1, 2H-pyran-6-carboxylic acid (Indalone). Travis et al. (1946) confirmed the effectiveness of these materials, noting also that they were all powerful paint solvents and could cause mucosal irritation. They gave protection against various species of mosquito and *Stomoxys calcitrans* of from 2 to 6 h in laboratory tests. A combination of 60% DMP with 20% each of Rutgers and Indalone, referred to as 6-2-2-, was better than any of the individual ingredients. These workers also observed that different materials gave different protection times (PT) for the same species and that the same material could give different PT for different species. This has been confirmed by all subsequent workers. Their tests also showed that the insects were repelled on some occasions but fed through the repellent on others. Smith and Burnett (1949) and Travis et al. (1949) furnished huge lists of materials tested using DMP or Indalone as the substance for comparison. Only a very few came up to their standard.

Goldman (1949), reviewing the subject, concluded that the PT depended not only on the chemical itself but on the vehicle used, the area to which it was applied and the time at which it was used. He noted that any discomfort was usually due to the vehicle, the best of which was a cream. Application was most effective if it coincided with the period of the arthropod's greatest activity, especially with flying insects. He insisted that adherence to careful instructions as to use was most important to achieve the best results. Travis (1950) noted that the PT was inversely proportional to the rate of biting, which was itself dependent on the number of insects involved.

A further factor in the effectiveness of repellents was the individual being protected. Sweating reduced PT, as did insensitive perspiration (Rietscher and Spencer 1975), whilst hairy persons seemed to be more resistant even if shaved for experimental purposes. As far as sweating was concerned, its effect was probably on the loss of repellent by rubbing, evaporation or absorption (Smith 1966). Kasman et al. (1953) had indicated that the greatest loss was by absorption through the skin.

King (1951) added dimethylcarbate (DMC) and 2-phenoxyacetone to the list of useful repellents, whilst Travis and Smith (1951) noted that variants of 6-2-2- of equal effectiveness included the substitution of DMC or of 2-propyl-*N*-*N*-diethyl succinamate for Rutgers 612 in the formula. In 1955 Gilbert et al. introduced a potent new repellent *N*, *N*-diethyl-*m*-toluamide, known for short as DEET. This has remained one of the best of all repellents and was noted by Bar-Zeev and Ben-Tamar (1968) to be excellent in combination with Indalone and 2-propyl-*N*-*N*-diethyl succinamate in preventing insects from ovipositing in places where it had been applied.

The method of application of repellents involves the use of dusting powder (considered by Knipling and Dove 1944 to be the least effective vehicle), lotions or sprays, both usually in an alcoholic base—all of which are applied directly to the skin. Lotions have proved the most effective vehicle.

Impregnation of clothing is also a valuable method and probably the best single means of deterring arthropods. For trombiculid larvae impregnated socks, trouser bottoms, sleeve cuffs and collars are the important barriers to invasion and attack (Goldman 1949). Two properties of repellents are essential when used for impregnation. Firstly, they must have a long "shelf life" (i.e. they will remain active for long periods when treated clothing is stored). Secondly, they should be effective for reasonable periods of up to 1 week whilst the clothes are being worn (Smith 1966), and, furthermore, should be able to withstand rinsing in water without being removed. Gilbert (1957) demonstrated these properties in DEET, which has a shelf life of 26 days and withstands at least two rinsings. A good repellent should not deteriorate on the skin. One of the effects of some repellents is to reduce skin CO_2 release. CO_2 attracts mosquitoes (Smith 1966). Smith also noted that relatively large amounts of some repellents were required, but the amount varied with the chemical (e.g. 0.05 mg/cm^2 for DEET and 1.0 mg/cm^2 for

DMP). The best protection is afforded by wearing impregnated clothing and applying repellent to the skin. The most appropriate chemicals to use vary with the geographical area and the species to which exposure is likely. Table 26.2 indicates some of the choices.

Table 26.2. Some of the choices among repellents for impregnating clothing, in order of effectiveness (King 1951)

Arthropod group	Most appropriate repellents
A. Mosquitoes	1. Methyl, *N*, *N*-diisopropyladipamate[a]
	2. 2-Butyl-2-ethyl-1-3-propanediol[a]
	3. *N*-Butyl-1,2,3,6-tetrahydrophthalimide
	4. Indalone
	5. Undecylenic acid
	6. 2,4-Nonanedial
	7. α-Butoxyl-*N*-cyclohexylacetamide
	8. DMP[b]
	9. Rutgers 612b
B. Ticks	A4, 7 and 5
	1. *N*-Butylacetamide
	2. Hexylmandelate
	3. *N*-*N*-Dibutylacetoacetamide
	4. *N*-Propylacetamide
C. Fleas	A5
	B1, 4 and 2
	1. Benzyl benzoate
D. Trombiculid larvae	A8
	C1
	1. Diphenyl carbamate
	2. Benzil
	3. *p*-Tolyl benzoate[c]
	4. Dibutylphthallate[c]

[a] Shelf life of up to 149 days and active for 56 h of wear.
[b] Shelf life of up to 27 days and active for 16 h of wear.
[c] A combination of these two can withstand up to four launderings.

Sherman (1966) discussed the requirements for a systemic insecticide repellent (SIR). These were that it should be

1. Effective against a wide variety of species
2. Orally administered
3. Long acting, i.e. from 12 to 24 h
4. Of low toxicity
5. Possessed of long shelf life

An SIR fulfilling these criteria has yet to be produced. The stomach poisons indicated in Table 26.1 have some of these properties. Of those likely to affect man phenylbutazone (butazolidine) was shown by Cole and van Natta (1964) and by Shawarby et al. (1964) and a related compound, Tanderil, by Cole and van Natta (1967) to be lethal to lice feeding on rabbits which had been dosed with these drugs at levels of 20 mg/kg and 10 mg/kg respectively. Shawarby and his colleagues found butazolidine was partially effective clinically but required repeat treatment for complete success.

Co-trimoxazole (containing 80 mg trimethoprim and 400 mg sulphamethoxazole) was found, accidentally, to kill head lice when given orally to patients with pediculosis capitis. The individual ingredients were ineffective. Successfully treated patients developed intense itch of the scalp and neck and the lice left the scalp and died. There was no evidence of recurrence 15 days later (Shashindra et al. 1978).

Photosensitivity was induced in operatives spraying fruit trees with phenothiazine, presumably through absorption, since topical application caused no such effect (Deeds et al. 1940). It is known to induce photosensitivity in psychiatric patients and is probably unsuitable for use as an SIR in man. The effects of methotrexate on *Sarcoptes* and *Demodex* are discussed in Chaps. 15 and 16 respectively.

Toxic Effects of Insecticides

The toxic effects of insecticides on man, with special reference to the effects on man's skin, are of relevance to the subject of this book. Those who use insecticides, whether as repellents or for therapeutic purposes, and more especially those who apply them for pest destruction on crops or to disinfest farm buildings, as well as those who are engaged in their manufacture, are all exposed to possible risks from contact on the skin or by inhaling their toxic products. The hazards of scabiecides, including γBHC, have been described in Chap. 15.

Contact dermatitis with sensitisation can occur with any of the substances used. A few examples will suffice. Sulzberger and Weinberg (1930) reported an instance in a woman hotel worker who was repeatedly exposed to an insect powder containing pyrethrum. Patch tests and subsequent challenge both produced positive results. Mirakhmedou and Kasimov (1972) have recorded 112 cases amongst cotton workers of skin reactions to either DDT or γBHC; 38/49 gave positive patch test results to DDT and 47/63 to γBHC. The workers were contaminated either directly by crop spraying or indirectly through handling contaminated cotton. The eruptions were mostly acute but a few were chronic (up to 5 years). The occurrence was seasonal and confined to exposed skin surfaces. Normal skin was affected, but the reaction was aggravated by abrasion, fissuring, scratching and sweating.

Draize et al. (1944) had previously shown that solutions of DDT were liable to cause dermatitis with sensitisation, whereas this was less likely with the powder form. They pointed out that it could be absorbed through the skin; in animals the effects of such absorption included anorexia, weight loss, hyperexcitability and tremors, proceeding to clonic convulsions. Unlimited use of DDT solution was not therefore without risk. Moreover, when such organochlorines were used as sprays they could be inhaled and were then even more likely to cause systemic reactions.

Compounds such as malathion and parathion are also toxic, especially the latter. Dikshith and Datta (1972) noted that occupational poisoning by inhalation amongst manufacturers, dispensers and sprayers of parathion was common. Bhargava et al. (1977) reported an instance of an erythema multiforme-like eruption following contact with methyl parathion for destroying bedbugs. This was confirmed by a recurrence on re-exposure to this material as a snuff. The present writer has seen an exfoliative dermatitis in a window cleaner, which was confirmed as being caused by contact with 10% malathion dust used as a spray to kill clover mites in land adjoining a housing estate. He was employed to clean the layer of dust which had settled on the windows of the houses during the spraying.

Cronce and Alden (1968) reported four cases of dermatitis in pet owners from contact with "flea collars" impregnated with Vapona (dichlorvos). The reaction was confined to the forearms, cubital fossae and sides of the neck. All four gave positive patch test results to Vapona. Best and Murray (1962) recorded detectable absorption of carbaryl in the blood of workers engaged in the production, handling and shipping of this insecticide, but no symptoms resulted.

Rabinovitch (1966) and Lamberg and Mulrennan (1969) recorded contact dermatitis and a bullous dermatitis respectively from the use of DEET. Rabinovitch also noted some conjunctivitis and aggravation of acne in two of his cases. The bullous eruption recorded by Lamberg and Mulrennan was followed by skin necrosis and occurred only in the cubital fossae. An identical lesion was produced experimentally by the application of DEET.

From these few examples it can be seen that insecticides need careful handling and should always be kept away from children. The effects of swallowing them would be very similar to their effects on arthropods and quite likely to be fatal.

References

Bar-Zeev M, Ben-Tamar D (1968) The effectiveness of repellents on cloth as determined by oviposition of *Aedes aegypti* L. Mosquito News 28: 396–403

Best EM, Murray BL (1962) Observations on workers exposed to Sevin insecticide; a preliminary report. J Occup Med 4: 507–517

Bhargava RK, Singh V, Soni V (1977) Erythema multiforme resulting from insecticide spray. Arch Dermatol 113: 686–687

* Busvine JR (1980) Insects and hygiene, 3rd edn. Chapman and Hall, London

Buxton PA (1945) The use of the new insecticide DDT in relation to the problem of tropical medicine. Trans R Soc Trop Med Hyg 38: 367–400

Chapman RF (1971) The insects; structure and function, 2nd edn. The English Universities Press, London

Clark PH, Cole MM (1964) Laboratory studies on resistance of the body louse to insecticides. J Econ Entomol 57: 205–210

Clark PH, Cole MM (1967) Resistance of body lice to carbaryl. J Econ Entomol 60: 398–400

Cole MM (1973) Synergistic compounds. In: Proceedings of an international symposium on the control of lice and louse-borne diseases. PAHO/WHO scientific publ No 263. Pan American Health Organisation, Washington DC, pp 1–195

Cole MM, van Natta DL (1964) Tests with systemic insecticides in rabbits as toxicants for body lice. J Econ Entomol 57: 67–70

Cole MM, van Natta DL (1967) Further tests with systemic insecticides in rabbits as toxicants for body lice and new test for yellow fever mosquitoes. J Econ Entomol 60: 955–959

Cole MM, van Natta DL (1973) Synthetic juvenile hormones. In: Proceedings of an international symposium on control of lice and louse-borne diseases. PAHO/WHO scientific publ No 263. Pan American Health Organisation, Washington DC, pp 246–247

Cole MM, Clark PH, Weidman DC (1958) Sleeve tests with malathion powders against DDT resistant body lice. J Econ Entomol 51: 741–742

Cole MM, White SA, McWilliams JG (1967) Louse powders tested by a new method of sleeve tests. J Econ Entomol 60: 546–548

Cole MM, Clark PH, Weidman DC (1969) Failure of laboratory colonies of body lice to develop resistance to malathion. J Econ Entomol 62: 568–570

Cronce PC, Alden HS (1968) Flea-collar dermatitis. JAMA 206: 1563–1564

Deeds F, Wilson RH, Thomas JO (1940) Photosensitisation by phenothiazine. JAMA 114: 2095–2097

Dikshith TSS, Datta KK (1972) Effect of parathion on the skin of guinea pigs. Experientia 28: 169–171

Draize JH, Nelson AA, Calvery MO (1944) The percutaneous absorption of DDT (2,2–bis (*p*-chlorophenyl) 1,1,1-trichloroethane) in laboratory animals. J Pharmacol Exp Med 82: 159–166

*Ebeling (1975) Urban entomology. University of California, Division of Agricultural Science, Los Angeles, Cal

Gilbert IH (1957) Evaluation of repellents against mosquitoes and deer flies in Oregon. J Econ Entomol 50: 46–48

Gilbert IH, Gouck HK, Smith CN (1955) New mosquito repellents. J Econ Entomol 48: 741–743

Goldman L (1949) Use of repellents in clinical dermatology: general principles. Arch Dermatol Syphilol 60: 777–780

Gordon RM, Lavoipierre MMJ (1962) Entomology for students of medicine. Blackwell, Oxford

Grothaus RH, Cole MM (1973) Use of fumigants for control of body lice. In: Proceedings of an international symposium on control of lice and louse-borne diseases. PAHO/WHO scientific publ No 263. Pan American Health Organisation, Washington DC, pp 192–195

*Guthrie DH, Tindall AR (1968) The biology of the cockroach. Edward Arnold, London, pp 386–399

Hayes WJ, Mattson AM, Short JG, Witter RF (1960) Safety of malathion dusting powder for louse control. Bull WHO 22: 503–514

Hurlbutt HS, Altman RM, Nibley C (1952) DDT resistance in Korean body lice. Science 115: 11–12

Kasman S, Roadhouse LAO, Wright GF (1953) Studies in testing insect repellents. Mosquito News 13: 116–123

King WV (1951) Repellents and insecticides available for use against insects of medical importance. J Econ Entomol 44: 338–343

Kitaoka M (1952) DDT resistant louse in Tokyo. Jpn J Med Sci Biol 5: 75–88

Knipling EF, Dove WE (1944) Recent investigation of insecticides and repellents for the armed forces. J Econ Entomol 37: 477–480

Lamberg SI, Mulrennan JA (1969) Bullous reaction to diethyl toluamide (DEET). Arch Dermatol 100: 582–586

Martinez A, Cichero JA, Alania IR, Gonzalez FF (1975) Control of *Triatoma infestans* with malathion concentrates. J Med Entomol 11: 653–657

Maunder JW (1971a) Resistance to organochlorine insecticides in head lice, and trials using alternative compounds. Med Officer 125: 27–29

Maunder JW (1971b) Use of malathion in the treatment of lousy children. Community Med 126: 145–147

*Maunder JW (1981) Novel phenomena arising from the use of acetylcholinesterase inhibiting insecticides against human lice. Community Med 3: 31–37

Maunder JW (1983) Pediculosis corporis: an updating of attitudes. Environ Health 19: 130–131

Mirakhmedou UM, Karimov AM (1972) The effect of pesticides on the skin of agricultural workers (in Russian). Vestn Dermatol Venereol 46: 50–52

Preston S, Fry L (1977) Malathion lotion and shampoo. R Soc Health J 97: 291

Rabinovitch MV (1966) The effect of diethyl toluamide on the skin and eye mucous membranes in man (in Russian). Zh Mikrobiol Epidemiol Immunobiol 43: 109–112

Ridgway RL, McGregor T, Flanigan JF (1962) The effect of residual deposits of insecticides on the scorpion *Centruroides vittatus*. J Econ Entomol 55: 1012–1013

Rietscher RL, Spencer TS (1975) Correlation between mosquito repellent protection time and insensible water loss from the skin. J Invest Dermatol 65: 385–387

Shalaby AM (1971) Susceptibility of *Pediculus humanus capitis* and *Pediculus humanus corporis* to chlorinated hydrocarbons insecticides in Libya. Z Angew Entomol 69: 227–233

Shashindran CH, Ghandhi IS, Krishnasamy S, Ghosh MN (1978) Oral therapy of pediculosis capitis with cotrimoxazole. Br J Dermatol 98: 699–700

Shawarby AA, El-Refal AR, El-Hawary MFS, El-Essawi M (1963) Field and laboratory studies on the use of malathion for control of body lice in Egypt. Bull WHO 28: 111–120

Shawarby AA, Mahdi AH, Sadek S, Mahmoud W (1964) Laboratory and field trials of phenylbutazone as a systemic lousicide in man. J Egypt Public Health Assoc 39: 97–106

Sherman JL (1966) Development of a systemic insect repellent. JAMA 196: 166–168

Smith CN (1966) Personal protection from blood-sucking arthropods. JAMA 196: 146–149

Smith CN, Burnett D (1949) Effectiveness of repellents applied to clothing for protection against salt-marsh mosquitoes. J Econ Entomol 42: 439–444

Sulzberger MB, Weinberg CB (1930) Dermatitis due to insect powder. JAMA 95: 111–112

Taplin D, Castillero RM, Spiegel J, Mercer S, Rivera AA, Schachner L (1982) Malathion treatment of *Pediculus humanus* var *capitis* infestations. JAMA 247: 3103–3105

Tarshis B, Blinstrub R (1963) Preliminary studies in the use of sorptive dusts for the control of the human lice *Phthirus pubis* and *Pediculus humanus capitis* DeGeer. Am J Trop Med Hyg 12: 91–95

Travis BV (1950) Known factors causing variation in results of insect repellents. Mosquito News 10: 126–132

Travis BV, Morton FA, Cochran JH (1946) Insect repellents used as skin treatments by the armed forces. J Econ Entomol 39: 627–630

Travis BV, Morton FA, Jones HA, Robinson JH (1949) The more effective mosquito repellent tests at the Orlando, Fla., Laboratory 1942–47. J Econ Entomol 42: 686–694

Vandekar M (1965) Observations on the toxicity of carbaryl, folothion and 3-isopropylphenyl-*N*-methylcarbamate in a village-scale trial in Southern Nigeria. Bull WHO 33: 107–115

Vinson JN (1973) IID. Experimental louse control methods. In: Proceedings of an international symposium on control of lice and louse-borne diseases. PAHO/WHO scientific publ No 263. Pan American Health Organisation, Washington DC, pp 238–241

WHO (1974) Equipment for vector control. World Health Organisation, Geneva

*Wright JW, Brown AWA (1957) Survey of possible insecticide resistance in body lice. Bull WHO 16: 9–31

*Wright JW, Pal R (1965) Second survey of insecticide resistance in body lice 1958–1963. Bull WHO 33: 485–501

Taxonomic Index

This contains only the zoological names of species, genera, families etc. The page numbers refer to their morphology, biology, incidence etc. Those numbers printed in normal type refer to information in the text, those in bold type to tables and those in italic to illustrations.

Bacteria, rickettsiae and other organisms and plants are contained in the General Index.

General Index

Most of the information about the morphology, biology and incidence as causes of skin lesions of the arthropods mentioned in this book will be found in the Taxonomic Index. The General Index contains clinical, immunological, histopathological and other details about the reactions induced in man, and information about insecticides etc. Zoological names and the occasional botanical name are printed in italic. Page numbers printed in normal type refer to information in the text, those in bold type to tables and those in italic to illustrations.

GPSR Compliance

The European Union's (EU) General Product Safety Regulation (GPSR) is a set of rules that requires consumer products to be safe and our obligations to ensure this.

If you have any concerns about our products, you can contact us on ProductSafety@springernature.com

In case Publisher is established outside the EU, the EU authorized representative is:

Springer Nature Customer Service Center GmbH
Europaplatz 3
69115 Heidelberg, Germany

Batch number: 10838521

Printed by Printforce, the Netherlands